A PRACTICAL GUIDE FOR VETERINARIANS, VETERINARY STAFF, AND BREEDERS

CANINE
Reproduction and Neonatology

Marthina L. Greer, DVM, JD

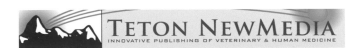

TETON NEWMEDIA
INNOVATIVE PUBLISHING OF VETERINARY & HUMAN MEDICINE

Executive Editor: Carroll C. Cann
Design and Production: www.fiftysixforty.com

Teton NewMedia
P.O. Box 4833
Jackson, WY 83001
1-888-770-3165
tetonnm.com

ISBN# 1-59161-041-9

Printed in the United States

Print Number 5 4 3 2 1

Library of Congress Cataloging-in-Publication Data on file

Preface

Breeder clients cannot be stereotyped and classified any more than the rest of your client base. The majority of our breeder clients are seeking a high level of care, both for fertility work and for emergency care. This is the client base for which this book is written.

In today's medical climate of "evidence-based medicine", there are still fields in veterinary care that cannot rely on this process. Although there are protocols where published and researched information can be applied, many decisions in the scope of the topics in this book are based on common sense, intuition and experience.

Many breeder clients are very well-informed and have a great deal of experience. They are often demanding and frequently require after-hours care for timed breedings, whelpings, as well as pediatric and prenatal care. We look at working with these clients as a joy and a challenge. We hope you find this book to be valuable when you need a readily retrievable, practical resource.

For the veterinarian without a great deal of experience in breeding and whelping dogs, working with breeders can be a great learning experience. For veterinarians with more experience, we find the most effective way to work with these clients is to listen carefully to their opinions, guide them to a compromise with the science on your side, and never doubt their gut instincts.

Dedication

I would like to dedicate this book to my family, staff, and clients.

To my parents, Dave and Nancy Greer, who taught me I could do anything in life I wanted to. And for putting me up and putting up with me during the warm Phoenix winters so I could get away from practice and school to concentrate on writing.

To my husband, Dan Griffiths and kids Katy and Karl, for picking up the slack.

To my fabulous staff, for always being there when we needed them. To Trish and Dr. Zella for pushing me hard enough to make this happen.

To my terrific clients, who taught me all you see represented in this book. To Ch. Jane Marple and her grand-dogs who taught me humility and boundaries.

To Carroll Cann, for his patience.

Table of Contents

Chapter 9: Infertility and Reproductive Problems in the Valuable Bitch

Chapter 10: Infertility and Reproductive Problems in the Valuable Stud Dog

Chapter 11: Special Breedings

References

Appendices

Index

CHAPTER 1
Working with Breeders

What is "Normal" reproduction?

As we have always been taught, you must know "normal" to know "abnormal". So how do we define "normal"?

As veterinarians, we seldom experience "normal" reproduction. This is because many breeders are very skilled in handling breeding timing, the actual breeding, the pregnancy and the whelping and require little veterinary intervention. However, according to current AKC records, 60% of all breedings are now handled by some form of artificial insemination and veterinarians are more likely to be involved. We will have more and more to offer these technically skilled clients as more sophisticated techniques become available, which now include shipping fresh and frozen semen necessitating veterinary assistance in insemination, and as clients come to expect more advanced care.

Veterinarians may think of "normal" as the breeder who owns both the stud dog and bitch or uses a stud dog near her home. In this scenario, the breeder makes his or her own arrangements for breeding including the timing based on behavior of the stud dog and bitch. They handle the breeding either by natural breeding by copulation or doing an artificial insemination themselves. They either assume their breeding has been successful or diagnose the pregnancy themselves based on palpation. They manage the bitch throughout her pregnancy. The whelping takes place uneventfully at their home or kennel and the breeder assesses that the bitch has completed whelping based on their own palpation or on another assumption. They handle the puppies through their neonatal period. All either goes off without a hitch or the breeder is willing to accept the situation and does not ask for veterinary intervention. Many breeders will seek out more advanced veterinary services if we are available to provide them.

Who are the breeders?

There are many different varieties of breeders, just as there are many different types of pet-owning clients. They can be categorized, but this is done at the risk of failing to recognize overlap between categories and of stereotyping. Nevertheless, it is helpful to know that there are differences.

Breeders involved in competitive events

These are breeders who are in some form of competition and thus breed with specific guidelines of the "perfect dog" in mind when selecting breeding stock. This may include dogs who compete in conformation (appearance, based on a breed standard), agility, flyball, tracking, herding, coursing, field and hunting dogs, earth dogs, bear and raccoon hunting, to name some representative categories. They tend to travel long distances to attend these events and may have professional trainers or hire handlers for competitive events.

These dogs are bred for a specific performance purpose following pedigree analysis by the breeder and they have been screened for genetic diseases.

Most of these breeders have several dogs, 2 to 20, of the same or related breeds (usually 1 or 2 breeds) and have devoted themselves to either maintaining or improving their breed for many years, sometimes a lifetime. These dogs tend to live in the home of the breeder or in a small well-maintained kennel built to the breeder's specifications.

Many breeders will produce one to several litters a year. They sell directly to the end consumer, your dog-owning client. They will have interviews with prospective puppy buyers and have a waiting list of potential homes. They rarely run ads to sell pups. These breeders are likely to keep one or more puppies from each litter to continue their performance involvement and breeding with young stock. The breeder will often keep the puppies until at least 8 weeks of age for socialization and determination of the pup they want to keep. Placement is based on which puppy is best suited for which family. In some cases, they may "run on several puppies", in other words, keep several littermates until they are adolescent when they are better able to tell which puppy they want to keep for performance and breeding.

To keep their numbers manageable, some breeders will place breeding age dogs in family homes and have them return briefly for breeding. Some prefer to place adult dogs in single dog homes after they are finished competing, breeding, and spaying or neutering.

This type of breeder is frequently a member of one or more dog breed clubs. They may belong to a local kennel club and also one or more breed specific clubs with restricted memberships. They often participate in breed specific "rescue", where if a dog of their breed is relinquished to a humane society or shelter, they will actively attempt to provide a foster home until they can re-home the dog.

Many of these breeders will sell dogs with health guarantees and on some type of contract with the buyer. Often, the contract will state that the pup is to be returned to the breeder if the family who has made the purchase cannot keep the dog – this minimizes the likelihood that their pups will end up in shelters and in rescue organizations. Many will sell the puppies with a "limited" AKC registration, meaning if these pups are used for breeding, their offspring cannot be registered with AKC. These pups are usually sold after being evaluated by a veterinarian. Some pups are wormed and vaccinated by the breeder and some by the attending veterinarian, but they tend to have supporting veterinary paperwork and a well-thought out vaccine and worming schedule.

Pet breeders

These breeders tend to breed for the pet dog market, but not for competition. They often own one or two dogs of their specific breed. These tend to live in the home or in a small kennel in the garage.

Some have a litter to expose their children to the wonders of birth. Many have only one or two litters total. Others breed their dogs because they purchased it as a puppy and want to "make some of the money back" that they spent on the purchase. Some breed because they have friends, family and co-workers who said they want one "just like her". Some breed to try to recreate the dog they have now.

Pet breeders are less likely to do health screening tests and research pedigrees when choosing a mate for the dog. They will often purchase a second dog of the opposite sex for breeding to their first dog. They frequently keep one of the pups as a replacement for the older dog. Some intentionally breed two different breeds together.

Commercial breeders

"Puppy mills" is a common but not necessarily accurate term used for commercial breeders. They tend to raise many puppies (in the double to quadruple digits), many different breeds (over five), and often raise mixed breed dogs (designer dogs – which changes with the public's preferences). They may have signs posted where they can change the listing of the breeds available and may run newspaper and internet ads listing all of the breeds available or run multiple ads by breed.

Some commercial breeders house the dogs in groups, in barns or other buildings converted for this purpose. As a result, the parentage may be difficult to ascertain. Some commercial breeders have facilities far superior to that of breeders who are involved in competitive events. If they sell directly to the consumer, the buyer, may not be invited to the premises (the breeder may meet the buyer off site – "we live way out in the country and it is so hard to find us") or you may not be allowed to see the dogs and the dog's parents where they are housed. Some sell directly to the public through another breeder-friend as a broker, but this is the only group of breeders who sell puppies through pet stores. Buyers often find them on the internet.

Commercial breeders often have USDA and/or state certification and are routinely inspected by USDA, the state, and/or AKC. The paperwork that accompanies the puppies may include USDA health papers since the puppies frequently cross state lines. There may not be any other veterinary records. Puppies are often sold and transported under 7 weeks of age. Vaccines tend to be given from a very early age (under 6 weeks), given frequently, and administered by the breeder. The vaccines used may be brands you do not use in your practice; worming protocols include drugs such as Ivermectin® and coccidiostats from a very early age (2 weeks) on. The pups often originate from Midwestern states in the U.S. or from outside the U.S. (Mexico and islands off the coast of the U.S.)

The buyers (who are your well-meaning clients) are often convinced that they are not buying from a commercial breeder, or make the purchase out of pity for the puppy. The commercial breeder will rarely sell the pups on a limited registration or with a contract with the buyer.

Why work with breeders?
The breeder client of all types can be a boon to your client base. Not only will they build your practice by being clients, but also by referring fellow dog-breeders and new puppy buyers to you. Some veterinarians begin to work with breeders when they are breeders themselves.

How to work with breeders
The "Competition breeder client"
The competitive breeder client is usually well-educated, challenging, and demanding. They know their lines of dogs, are well connected in the breed, and have many resources. They are very aware of the genetic screening tests available, often outpacing the veterinarian as this field is changing very rapidly. They have been breeding dogs for many years and usually have with great skills in breeding, whelping, and neonatal care.

The inexperienced veterinarian may find this group intimidating at first exposure. Unfortunately, the "breeder client" is not always well received in many veterinary clinics in the U.S. Veterinarians who seek to assist breeders find that when handled correctly, these clients are hungry to learn more, appreciate the services available, and can teach us as much as we teach them. Although the breeder may initiate the veterinary visit with a seemingly strong opinion, when countered with respect and a well-thought out scientific approach to the situation, they will frequently be convinced to treat as the veterinarian proposes or a medically appropriate compromise may be made.

If the veterinarian is willing to offer breeding services and develop a mutual exchange of information with the breeder client, a truly wonderful working relationship can evolve.

The breeder client will sometimes request a "breeder" discount. This may or may not be appropriate and each veterinary hospital must have its own policy. The hospital may choose to discount some, but not all services. For instance, you may discount vaccinations, but not reproductive services only sought out by breeders. The breeder client often brings in multiple puppies or adult dogs at one visit, making more efficient use of the veterinarian's time. They can also serve as a wonderful source of referrals when their puppies are placed in homes in your community. For a practice seeking a source of new clients, this can work out very well.

Additionally, the opportunity to aid breeders can be immensely rewarding. There are few procedures that bring greater joy in veterinary practice than a cooperative effort with a client that results in the birth of a healthy litter of puppies that you had a hand in producing.

The "Pet puppy breeder"
These clients can be less challenging regarding the services requested and the hours that they

expect you to be available. They ask less difficult questions and do not generally go to the same extremes as the competition breeder. They usually use a local dog and ask for less intervention on timing, prenatal care, and other services. They appreciate the assistance.

The "Commercial breeder"

These clients often use the veterinarian for USDA certificates and "herd management" issues but not individual pet care. These pets are at the greatest risk of diseases such as parasites and brucellosis as they move in and out of their kennels and those of others who transact business in the same way often overlooking the importance of testing and quarantining to prevent diseases.

What skills does a veterinarian need to develop to provide basic reproductive care?

1. Semen collection including sperm counts, motility, and morphology.
2. Artificial insemination – vaginal and surgical insemination.
3. Ovulation timing and breeding management.
4. Pregnancy diagnosis with ultrasound and radiographs, including estimations of litter size and due dates.
5. C-sections – surgical technique, dystocia management, and puppy resuscitation.
6. Prenatal and postpartum management of the bitch.
7. Neonatal and pediatric care.
8. Infertility evaluation and treatment for males and females.
9. Treatment options for pyometras, uterine disease, prostate disease, accidental breedings, and mammary disease.
10. Good client education tools, including handouts.

Caseload – Emergency care, weekends

Breedings and whelpings happen 365 days a year, holiday or weekend. Babies come when they are ready and bitches need to be bred when they have ovulated. If you choose to work with breeders and are willing to make yourself available to them on weekends, nights, and holidays, they will deeply appreciate your efforts. Of course, you should charge appropriately for these services and explain this to them if necessary.

As valuable as emergency clinic services are, they are usually not suited to assisting the breeder client with semen collection for shipment and weekend artificial breedings. They are often very busy with critically ill and injured patients and are neither staffed nor equipped to provide breeding services.

C-sections can frequently be handled very well by general practitioners, but in some situations are better handled at emergency and referral practices.

If the general practitioner has the veterinary and support staff and equipment to perform a successful C-section, this can be a wonderful service to offer to your breeder clients. Of course, this requires that you make proceeding to surgery a priority in the practice, whether during a routine day or after hours.

If the practice does not have sufficient staff to have a ratio of one support staff for every two anticipated puppies or does not have anesthesia and equipment for C-sections and the associated complications, it may be best to refer to an emergency clinic.

Whether in general, referral or emergency practice, we must remember our caesarian patient is not one patient but a group of patients. When faced with a bitch with a dystocia or premature labor, we must keep in mind that a delay in assessment and treatment or surgery is risking many patients.

Therefore to adequately provide services to these patients, they must be seen as patients who are in a life-threatening situation even if the bitch has the appearance of being stable. The staff must be empowered to make decisions on who can be rescheduled in general practice. Triage in emergency practices may require putting the pregnant bitch higher on the treatment list than the condition of the bitch alone would indicate if the pups are to be saved.

Your role in education, referrals and alternatives to conventional treatments

Remind your breeder clients that there are many procedures you offer as a licensed professional that they are not legally permitted to perform themselves. These vary from state to state and may include, but are not limited to administering rabies vaccinations and performing surgical procedures, such as ear crops and taildocks. Each state has its own veterinary practice act, which should be consulted if there is any question.

Help your clients cultivate the 8 skills they should have to become better breeders

You may ask why you should contribute to this aspect of assisting your breeder clients. Good question. Some will not require your assistance as they are skilled already. Some will not want your input. But most will need assistance at least with the veterinary aspects of which pup to sell, which to keep and which to breed. A complete physical examination of the patients and good written explanations of the exam findings and any abnormalities will be of great assistance to the breeder. We want our breeders to rely on us as the experts for their examinations and treatment planning. Use the skills and knowledge you have, and limit your services to what you know.

The following are skills you can help clients develop but are not skills you yourself will likely have or need to have first-hand knowledge of.

1. Know the breed standard

Each breeder should strive to know what their breed club has written as its "breed standard" – their ideal dog.

Illustrated standard

Many breed clubs not only have written descriptions but have included photographs and drawings of their standard. These can be found on-line or in published form from the breed clubs.

Mentor

Nearly every successful breeder has had someone take them under their wing early in their dog competition career. If you have the resources, assist fledging clients in hooking up with others in their breed or related breeds who would be interested in mentoring them.

Dog events

Locating and attending events is a great way to see many great specimens of their breed and network with others. Most areas also have all-breed clubs and single breed clubs that can be joined.

Internet

Many breed clubs have an on-line list or lists prospective breeders can join for advice and networking.

2. Breed knowledge
Know which lines "click"
This information is often found only as an oral tradition, discussed when breeders get together. It is better to find out from another's experience than to try the experiment again and again.

Identify and prioritize
Identify and prioritize the top 4 genetic problems in the breed: researching the breed on-line, through breed clubs, and in print can illuminate the most common disorders of a breed. As this can change from time to time, the breeder should continue to research their breed.

Focus on crippling, life-altering or fatal diseases first
These are the diseases that are the most damaging to the breed.

Avoid including genetic problems in the lines
Observation by the breeder, physical examination by the veterinarian, blood tests, radiographs, DNA testing and many other techniques exist or will exist in the near future to aid in selection.

3. Develop a method to select dams and sires

4. Pedigree analysis
Review the traditional AKC pedigree, the stick dog pedigree by Carmen Battaglia and the inheritance pedigree.

5. Develop a retrievable record keeping system
Complete paper or software records, photos and videos for each dog are essential.

6. Learn to evaluate litters
Sixty percent of dogs shown are not owned by the breeder, supporting the fact that many breeders sell the "wrong" dog, the one they should have kept.

7. Follow up all puppies at 6 months
Puppy parties (see chapter 2), videos and radiographs are all useful techniques. By doing this, the breeder can monitor the product of their breeding program.

8. Learn to manage, feed and condition a competition dog
Only 35% of a dog's presentation and appearance is genetic, 65% is management, nutrition, and training – aspects that the owner can control.

When to refer
Many conditions of the reproductive tract can be handled effectively by the general practitioner. However, there are some treatments that maintain fertility, such as medical therapy for pyometras, semen freezing, and alternatives to neutering for stud dogs with prostate or testicular disorders that are treatment options for the valuable breeding dog that are not first line treatments for pet dogs.

Some diagnostics and treatments, as well as complex breedings, are better handled by veterinarians who frequently deal with breeders and are skilled in these procedures or by board-certified Theriogenologists. In these cases, referrals to this group of veterinarians should be offered to the clients.

Screening for genetic selection

Dogs have been subjected to genetic selection ever since humans domesticated the dog. This is not new; this is how humans developed breeds intended for specific purposes over many centuries. However, here we are referring to a more sophisticated form of genetic selection.

Selection based on phenotype

This type of screening has been used for many years. There are two broad categories. First are general findings on physical examination of the dog. Second are specific disease-based screening tests developed by veterinary specialists to provide breeders with a standardized approach that can be used in evaluating their offspring and breeding stock.

General findings on physical examination

This is where the veterinarian or breeder classifies the dog's structure as normal, abnormal, or some gradation in between on physical characteristics found by examination (See Chapter 2).

Specific disease-based Screening Tests

These tests use the physical appearance of the dog to detect abnormalities. Perhaps the best known test in this category is the use of radiographs to screen for hip dysplasia utilizing OFA for analysis.

These specific evaluations are standardized and allow dogs to be certified in different categories so that the findings can be included in databases. These screenings are based on physical examination, radiographic and laboratory findings.

Selection based on genotype

There are four types of DNA tests: parentage tests, mutation-based tests, linked-marker tests and tests to identify the breeds but not the individual parents who contributed genetics to an individual dog. This type of genetic screening is the most rapidly evolving. Completion of the canine genome in 2004 and research at both commercial and non-commercial facilities is expanding the number of DNA tests exponentially. It is not likely that any veterinarian will be able to stay current with all of the available tests. Dog breed clubs will, however, have recommendations of the tests available for screening. Careful research into each test is needed to be certain that the test was evaluated for the breed in question before making a recommendation. DNA markers for one breed do not necessarily serve as the DNA marker for another breed. For our use in selecting potential breeding dogs, mutation-based tests and linked-marker tests provide diagnostic insights (See Chapter 2).

With all of these genetic findings available, the breeder may look to you for input on how to interpret the data and put it to use in their breeding program. Our clients trust us to aid them in limiting or eliminating genetic diseases in their breeding stock, while at the same time maintaining the diversity of their purebred dogs. Here is a great challenge for us as veterinarians: there is no genetically perfect dog; they all have at least one genotypic or phenotypic defect. And with the number of tests looming in our future, very few dogs will be candidates to be tested for every disorder for which a test exists. Our goal as consultants to our breeder clients is to assist them in making the best genetic decisions they can.

Veterinarians ARE the animal experts, the professionals our clients and the public put their faith in.

CHAPTER 2
Genetic Selection and Screening

Selecting breeding stock

As a veterinarian entrusted to aid a breeder, it is helpful to understand in general how breeders can be assisted as well as how individual breeders can use your expertise. You may be involved in selecting dogs to include, and more importantly, to exclude from a breeder's breeding stock. Most veterinary schools spend little time on teaching genetic counseling. Even if it was taught, the field has changed so rapidly, it is probable what was taught is now out of date.

To be most effective in this role, you will need to avoid the temptation to systematically eliminate every dog with a defect from the gene pool. This approach will quickly alienate the breeder who has come to you for assistance. The goal is not to say what the breeder wants to hear, but to aid them in selecting dogs to include in their breeding program to perpetuate the positive traits and eliminate the undesirable traits.

There are several flaws in systematically eliminating all dogs with a defect. First, our purebred dogs have been described as "endangered species" by Dr. Anne Traas. Pure-bred dogs cannot be interbred and still be considered pure-bred. If we keep dog breeds from intermingling (that is the purpose of the closed breed registries), each breed currently has all of the genetic material it will ever have. Genes cannot be gained by breeding, only eliminated. If we eliminate every dog with a defect, we will have few or no purebred dogs left in most breeds. Some breeds, such as the Otterhound, have less than 900 dogs world-wide; here there is already a dangerously small gene pool.

There is no perfect individual dog. By maintaining more dogs in the line, we maintain genetic diversity in the breed. We must not make the mistake of eliminating dogs with obvious but minor genetic defects (such as umbilical hernias and distichia) and inadvertently continue to breed dogs with more serious hidden defects (such as temperament concerns). So we must support and assist breeders in determining carefully how to select breeding dogs, not recommend the elimination of every dog with a defect.

Second, some individual dogs carry specific traits that are too valuable to the breed to be eliminated. A top-winning or high performing dog is often too highly valued, both emotionally and genetically, to be tossed out of a breeding program. Even if this top-winning dog carries or is affected by a genetic defect, it is not automatically "bad" genetically. These carrier or affected dogs are probably preserving essential genes. Remember, the defective gene was not created by the breeder, but by a genetic mutation. It then becomes magnified by "genetic bottlenecking" (repopulating a breed from a limited number of individuals) or "founder's effect", also known as popular sire syndrome (the disproportionate use of one individual in a breed, usually a male dog.). Most breeders have too much invested in a line of dogs just to start over. Neither the breeder nor the individual dog is to blame for the genetic defect. Random DNA mutations are the cause of genetic diseases.

One approach to classifying genetic disorders is to rank them in order of severity, arbitrarily numbered as below.

Group 1 disorders are genetic defects that are minor in their impact on the dog's health and owner's need for ongoing care. These are disorders such as umbilical hernias – these may require surgical repair (see AKC guidelines) but after correction, do not leave any lasting impact on the dog's health. These disorders are frequently the easiest of the three groups to detect, and are most often detected on the youngest dogs. It is too easy to mistakenly toss these dogs out of the gene pool; consider the option of leaving these affected dogs intact, allow them to grow up and later compare them with other dogs of their breed. The affected dog may turn out to have the least serious defect and the most valuable desirable traits, making them a valuable addition to their breed.

Group 2 disorders are genetic defects that are non-life threatening but have an ongoing impact on the dog's health and owner's need for ongoing care. Thyroid disease and, allergies are disorders that falls into this category – this requires lifetime medication and an ongoing expense but if well-managed, does not alter the dog's lifestyle or longevity.

Group 3 disorders are genetic defects that are life-changing disorders. These include seizures caused by epilepsy, genetic orthopedic disorders such as hip dysplasia, and temperament issues. Not only do these disorders require lifetime management, but they impact the dog's health, alter the lifestyle of the dog and owner, and often shorten the dog's life expectancy.

Using this type of classification is helpful to the client and veterinarian when determining if the individual dog should be included or excluded from the breeding stock.

Counseling the breeder/client

The best approach to adopt when providing genetic counseling for a breeder is to assist them in developing goals. Most breeders share the common goals of producing healthy dogs with longevity while either maintaining or improving their breed type. Within the same breed, breeders have their own opinions of what their breed should look like (breed type, conformation) and how they should perform (temperament and abilities). Once general goals are defined, more specific goals can be identified. The breeder should be encouraged to focus on correcting weaknesses in their pedigrees. The breeder can be aided in determining their personal thresholds for traits. Some traits are all or none, i.e. the dog must be free from a trait, i.e. cataracts, and other traits are on a continuum, i.e. hip scores. If the criteria the breeder establishes are too stringent, no or few dogs will be eligible to be bred, but if they are too lenient, improvement in their goals will be slow. A balance of all traits must be achieved; if only one trait is sought, too many other important qualities and traits may be eliminated from the line.

We can provide a valuable service to the breeder-client by helping them identify their goals. Diseases that most veterinarians and breeders identify for elimination from the breeding pool are those that cause death, are life-changing, or significant discomfort; or that have no available or affordable treatment options. Many geneticists suspect that a number of the diseases seen today have a genetic basis that has not yet been identified. In the future there will probably be DNA tests for diseases that at this time are not known to be genetic.

Some breeders forget when they breed a litter that most of the pups will end up as "pet" puppies, not show dogs. It is important that the pet puppies, those sold to families to become a beloved family member, must be of sound health and temperament. They must not knowingly produce pet dogs who will be difficult or dangerous to live with and/or that will be costly or impossible to provide with medical care.

On the rare occasion that a genetic defect is caused by a recent mutation which may only affect a small number of individuals, the breeder is well-advised to be severe in eliminating these individuals from their breeding program to avoid dispersing the new mutation into the whole gene pool. However, if a small-population breed (there are at least 44 recognized by AKC), has a wide-spread defective gene, breeders must systematically breed carriers to normals and gradually replace carrier breeding stock with normal-testing offspring. "Defective genes were not created by breeders. They are due to mutations, bottlenecking and founders effects in the development of breeds." (Bell, Jerold: "The Proper Use of Genetic Tests in Making Breeding Decisions." ESSFTA. Seattle, 28 Feb. 1998.)

As the number of genetic screening tests increase, breeders will have to determine which tests are appropriate for their individual situation. It will soon become cost-prohibitive to run all available tests on all breeding stock, unless these tests are "bundled". However, certain individuals within the breed, such as frequently used sires, should be screened more intensively. An owner of a frequently used stud dog should first screen the dog for the most common and serious diseases in their breed, and then continue to screen for as many disorders as possible. Another consideration is to bank the frequently used stud dog's DNA to use for testing later as more DNA tests become available. DNA can be banked as blood (whole or dried on an FTA card) or as frozen semen. This is important whether the dog is retired or deceased and no longer siring pups or if the dog's semen is banked and he continues to sire pups long after his reproductive life is over.

It is generally the bitch owner who researches pedigrees and seeks out males for compatibility and desirability. The most common categories of traits sought are conformation (meaning appearance and structure), health, performance and temperament. Usually, all four are desired and must be balanced.

Pedigree analysis is an important aspect of stud dog selection. Pedigree depth is vertical when the generations of dogs listed in the pedigree are evaluated. Pedigree breadth is horizontal when the siblings of the bitch and sire are evaluated. Both analyses are important. Websites such as the OFA and CHIC websites are valuable resources in researching some of the test results breeders will want to analyze. Other sources are breeder and club websites, breed publications, and direct communication with other experienced fanciers of the breed.

There are many ways to sort through strengths and weaknesses of individual dogs when selecting an appropriate mate. Stud dog selection is based on many criteria.

The most frequently identified reasons breeders select a stud dog are:
1. Convenience – knowledge of and proximity to a stud dog.
2. Cost – the expense of the stud fee and semen shipment/insemination costs
3. Pedigree – the desirability of the ancestors
4. Offspring produced – the success of previous offspring
(Battaglia, Carmen: "Breeding Better Dogs Seminar." Greater Racine Kennel Club. Racine, Wisconsin. 19 Feb. 2005.)

One technique is described by Carmen Battaglia, in his "Breeding Better Dogs" book. This technique uses "Stick Dog" figures and a symbols pedigree to help the breeder visualize the strengths and weaknesses of an individual dog's traits. Using this method, the breeder can more easily select dogs for their breeding program with physical traits they want to incorporate into their line. This technique emphasizes only physical appearance, and does not incorporate important traits related to health.

George Padgett D.V.M., geneticist and professor of pathology at Michigan State University, was a strong supporter of breeders sharing information among themselves. He emphasized the importance of revealing not only the good qualities of a dog to the owner of a potential mate to that dog, but also the inferior qualities emphasizing traits related to health. There is little question that revealing genetic information to others in your breed is necessary to prevent breeding two dogs together that share an undesirable trait (doubling up on that trait). Unfortunately, the world of dog breeders is fiercely competitive and some breeders fear this honesty will give their dog an undeserved poor reputation and drive potential mates or buyers away from their line of dogs. It is important we as veterinarians support the honest reporting of disorders by both reporting it to the owner of the bitch or stud dog and supporting them in sharing the information with others. However, as professionals, we must only report this to the owner(s) of the dogs and not share the information directly or indirectly with members of the dog-owning public who are not privileged to have access to this information.

Traits such as temperament are subjective. Researching for phenotypic and genotypic tests is time-intensive. Breed clubs often have resources on their websites. The CHIC website (http://www.caninehealthinfo.org) lists many but not all AKC breeds and is a good place to begin. This research should be left for the breeder to initiate, allowing the veterinarian to become involved in discussing frequency, severity of the disease and delivery of the testing services.

If the breeder has questions or a severe problems that are beyond the scope of the primary care veterinarian, a consultation with a geneticist should be recommended.

Hybrid dogs

There is a current trend in breeding and puppy sales of producing hybrid or "designer dogs." This is nothing more than intentionally producing mixed-breed dogs. There is an apparent misconception that by mixing breeds, the outcome will produce healthier puppies. Unfortunately, most of the dog owners participating in this process are not screening their sires and dams for genetic disorders. Hybrid vigor is not automatic; mixing 2 or more breeds together arbitrarily will not automatically sort out the "bad" genes and leave in only the good genes. If this were the case, practicing veterinarians would see only purebred dogs – the mixed breed dogs would be in perfect health and never need veterinary care. Of course, we all know that this is not the case.

Breeding "designer dogs" will produce dogs of unpredictable temperament, random size, and unpredictable health problems. Randomly mixing genetics from one breed of dog with another is likely to lead to more health and temperament problems than it solves since these dogs are usually not screened to prevent passing along known inherited diseases.

DNA and the canine genome

In 2004, the collaborative effort of many researchers culminated in discovering the canine genome. At the time of publishing, approximately 50 of the more than 360 known canine genetic diseases had DNA tests available. However this number is likely to increase exponentially. This increase will make it difficult and cost-prohibitive to have every individual screened for every disorder. However, by understanding the inheritance of disorders, veterinarians and breeders may identify key foundation dogs in the pedigrees and be able test only a limited number of dogs. When foundation dogs are available and can be identified as clear of a disorder, offspring may not need to be tested.

Researching the genetics of individual breeds

In the United States, breed clubs generally make recommendations but rarely mandate testing for specific traits or diseases. Recommendations may be based on the frequency and/or the severity of the disease. For instance, hip dysplasia affects 30 % or more of large breed dogs, so the frequency and severity of the condition drives the desire to screen for the disease. Other disorders, such as epilepsy, may be less frequently seen but it is a highly undesirable trait in a genetic line, due to both the emotional and financial cost of controlling the disease. For these reasons epilepsy too is an example of a disorder breeders strive to breed out of their lines.

The CHIC website (http://www.caninehealthinfo.org/), breed specific parent club websites, and website for institutions and companies offering DNA testing are excellent and up-to-date resources of tests suggested and currently available.

CHIC is co-sponsored by the OFA and the AKC Canine Health Foundation. CHIC works with parent clubs to identify health screening protocols appropriate for individual breeds and serves as their fee-based database. Dogs that are tested in accordance with the parent club established requirements, that have their results registered and made available in the public domain are issued CHIC numbers. CHIC's purpose is to encourage uniform health testing and sharing of all results, normal and abnormal, so that more informed breeding decisions can be made in an overall effort to reduce the incidence of genetic disease and improve canine health.

Selection based on phenotype

Phenotypic screening has been used for many years while genotypic testing, the gold standard for screening for genetic defects, is relatively new. However, most identified defects do not have a DNA test available. Until DNA genotype tests are available for more disorders and traits, we will continue to use phenotype testing.

There are two broad categories of phenotypic testing. First are the general findings on physical examination of the dog. Second are specific screening tests developed by veterinary specialists to provide breeders with a standardized approach they can use in evaluating their offspring and breeding stock. Perhaps the best known phenotype testing is the use of radiographs to screen for hip dysplasia utilizing OFA for analysis.

Physical evaluation for phenotypic abnormalities
General findings on physical examination
You do this every time you examine a litter of puppies or an adult dog that the owner is considering using for breeding, but you may not have thought of it this way before. This is a very economical method for breeders to screen for physical abnormalities. You and the breeder will both be doing phenotypic analysis, but you will be looking for different traits than the breeder will. You will be looking for undesirable traits such as a heart murmur, and they will be looking for traits such as the shape of the eye or the tailset. Both are important in selecting breeding stock.

The veterinary examination of adult or young dogs includes:
1. Evaluation of vital signs. Normal pups by 6 weeks and older should have a normal body temperature of 101.0° to 102.5°, heart rates of 100 to 250 beats per minute and a respiratory rate of 30 to 50 breaths per minute. Mucus membrane color may be slightly paler than in the adult as many pups have a normal physiological anemia.
2. Evaluation of the dentition. This includes the size and shape of the jaw, alignment of the incisor and canine teeth, and evaluation of the interdigitation of the premolars. It is believed the upper and lower jaws can be influenced by different genes and therefore grow at different rates. Alignment may change up to 8 months of age and older. In many breeds, having complete dentition is also a factor.
3. Evaluation of the oral cavity. The pup should be evaluated for a complete hard and soft palate and normal swallowing reflexes. Evaluation for elongation of the soft palate nearly always must be done with general anesthesia and is not part of a typical comprehensive physical examination. The size of the trachea is a valuable evaluation for the brachycephalic breeds, but as it requires a lateral thoracic radiograph for evaluation, this is also not part of a routine physical examination.
4. Evaluation of the nares includes the size of the nostril opening. No breed standards have specific requirement for this, but appearance of the dog can be influenced by this. As a matter of function, nostrils that are stenotic can impair the dog's respiratory capabilities.
5. Evaluation of the eyes. A complete examination for ERC or CERF requires the services of a board-certified veterinary ophthalmologist. However, some abnormalities are detectable by simple visual examination with good lighting and magnification. These include distichia, persistent pupillary membranes, dermoids, entropion and ectropion, epiphora, everted nictitans, and microophthalmia. Pups should be observed during the evaluation to assure that they have normal vision. Eye size and shape may be important to the breeder but is not usually clinically significant.
6. Evaluation of the ears. The ears should be evaluated for the presence of a complete pinna and ear canal on both sides of the head. Ear size, shape, and position are important to the breeder but few ear abnormalities are clinically significant. Hearing tests are addressed by BAER testing, described below.
7. Evaluation of the limbs. Pups should be observed on the floor to be certain that they have normal locomotion. With a few breed specific exceptions, the pups should not have deviation of the forelimbs – the front toes should point forwards. Some breeders are reluctant to allow

their pups to be placed on the floor at the veterinary clinic, so this is a challenge you may need to overcome to allow for complete evaluation. Limbs should be palpated for symmetry and swellings. The feet should be evaluated to be certain that all toes and footpads are present. Older pups can be evaluated with palpation for normal elbows and shoulders. You may be asked to check pups hips for an Ortolani sign. Patellar location and laxity can be assessed in even the very young puppy.

8. Evaluation of the thorax. The lungs should be clear on auscultation and the heart should be normal. Careful auscultation of the heart is essential. Both sides of the thorax should be evaluated, with the stethoscope placed over each valve. This can be difficult to achieve with a wiggly puppy and a room full of active littermates. It can be helpful to hold the pup in your lap or you may even leave the room with the pup so the pup and you are less distracted. Offering the pup baby food to lick can keep them more still during auscultation. The new electronic stethoscopes make detecting subtle murmurs much less challenging.

   An undetected heart murmur can lead to difficulties for you and the breeder if the pup is found to have a murmur by the new owner's veterinarian. Be very thorough in your auscultation. Any murmur, even grade 1 murmurs, must be reported to the breeder as they may intensify as the pup ages.

   Some murmurs are innocent murmurs and may disappear by 12 weeks of age. Some murmurs are so loud they are suspect from the first visit. If a pup is found to have a murmur, it is recommended the pup be held for subsequent evaluation or sold with full disclosure. If the murmur has not resolved by 12 weeks of age, the pup is smaller than its littermates, or if the pup seems to be exercise intolerant, a prompt referral to a veterinary cardiologist is recommended for a full cardiac evaluation.

9. Evaluation of the abdomen. The abdomen should be soft on abdominal palpation with no masses or intestinal abnormalities noted. Ropey intestines or pot-bellied appearance are a frequent finding in pups who have not been adequately treated with anthelminthics. The ventral abdominal wall should be evaluated for both umbilical and inguinal hernias. It may be useful to place gentle pressure on the mid-abdomen to detect small hernias. Small reducible hernias may resolve spontaneously but should be noted regardless as these are inherited and both the breeder and prospective puppy owner should be made aware of their presence.

10. Evaluation of the rectum. It is possible but unlikely that a young pup can have an incomplete GI tract and no rectum. If feces are found on the rectal thermometer, a complete GI tract can be assumed.

11. Evaluation of external genitalia.

    a. Male puppies should have their penis and testes evaluated. Both testes should be present in the scrotum by 3 weeks of age. If there is family history of penile defects, such as phimosis, penile frenulum or hypospadia, or there are abnormalities noted with urination, the penis should be exteriorized for visual examination. If the bladder is distended, the pup should be observed for urination because some very young male pups may develop urinary calculi and obstructive diseases.

    b. Female puppies should be carefully evaluated for location and size of the vulva and os clitoris as well as for vaginal discharge. The vulva is frequently small or more ventrally located than in the adult. If the os clitoris is enlarged or prominent, the possibility of an intersex pup should be considered. Many female pups have mild to moderate vaginal discharge associated with mild puppy vaginitis. This is not serious and may not require treatment unless the pup has clinical signs of urinary tract disease or discomfort.

12. Evaluation of the tail. The tail may be complete or shortened either by surgical docking or a genetic shortening. Clinically significant defects in the tail include kinks and skin folds. In most cases, the tail length and position is not of clinical significance.

Temperament and performance traits

Temperament qualities and desired performance traits vary with each individual breed and the preferences of each breeder. This is a subjective evaluation; there are no rules and no database. Current understanding of ethology suggests that temperament is a highly inherited trait. These decisions are generally made by the breeder and their network of fellow dog breeders. In some situations, veterinary participation and referral to a behaviorist with these skills may be beneficial to the breeder.

Longevity

Many traits, both physical and behavioral, play a role in achieving this goal. There is no one test or way to select for this.

Specific disease-based screening examinations and their respective databases

This type of evaluation uses the physical findings (phenotype) of the dog to detect abnormalities in its genetic make-up. Although DNA tests for specific diseases are the preferred method of screening for genetic diseases, in the absence of DNA tests, phenotypic evaluations are the only alternative. Applying results from the sire and dam, along with information on other close relatives such as siblings, half-siblings, aunts and uncles allows breeders to apply greater selective pressure to produce normal offspring and avoid affected offspring.

These specific tests are standardized evaluations. This permits breeders to compare dogs to an ideal standard and to one another. In some cases, the results are released only to the breeder, but in others, the results are included in databases. These screenings include findings based on physical examination, radiographs and laboratory testing. General information and websites will be included here to introduce each current category to the practicing veterinarian. Prior to a client visit requesting these screenings, it would be beneficial to visit the website and familiarize yourself with the tests requested.

Most of these tests are evaluations a general veterinary practitioner can offer as a service to their clients. Several evaluations, however, require specialized training and/or equipment and will require a referral to specialists. Many experienced breeders have already developed a network of preferred specialists and expect to visit several veterinarians to complete their screening prior to the sale of puppies or placing an individual dog in their breeding program.

Phenotypic screening
CERF (Canine Eye Registration Foundation) exams and ECR (Eye Certification Registry)

This is a complete ophthalmic examination, which must be completed by a board-certified veterinary ophthalmologist (a member of the ACVO). Upon completion of the examination, a form is prepared indicating normal and abnormal findings. A dog with normal findings or some limited abnormalities will be registered with ECR or CERF upon submission of the form and the appropriate fee. Breeding advice will be offered based on guidelines established for that particular breed by the Genetics Committee of the ACVO for dogs with abnormalities noted on examination.

There is great variation in the type of eye disorders and age of onset in different dog breeds. Therefore, there is great value in repeating the opthalmic examinations periodically throughout the life of any dog in a breeder's line that have offspring in an active breeding program. This certification is good for 12 months at a time so the dog must be reexamined and recertified to maintain its' registration with ECR or CERF. Patients can be as young as 6 weeks of age for their first evaluation and there is no upper age limit. Some breeders will have ophthalmic examinations completed prior to selling puppies as pets. As of January 1, 2001, patients are required to have permanent identification in the form of a microchip, DNA profile, or tattoo to be registered with ECR or CERF. Both will certify the eyes of normal hybrid dogs.

ECR and CERF exams are done on a regular schedule at most veterinary ophthalmologist's offices. They are also frequently held in conjunction with other canine performance events at the performance locations. Many breeders find it more convenient to attend an eye clinic.

ECR and CERF also maintains a data base based on dog breeds. This information will be used in generating research reports, but the individual dog's identities will become confidential and will never be released. CERF also has a publication called "OCULAR DISORDERS PRESUMED TO BE INHERITED IN DOGS." The 5th Edition, 2007 version is available on CD and is a valuable resource when assisting breeders in decisions about breeding programs. Additional information on CERF can be found at www.vmdb.org/history.html. Information about ECR can be found at www.offa.org.

OFA cardiac database

The purpose of the OFA cardiac database is to identify dogs which are phenotypically normal prior to inclusion in a breeding program. For the purposes of the database, a phenotypically normal dog is defined as either one without a cardiac murmur or one with an innocent heart murmur that is found to be otherwise normal by virtue of an echocardiographic examination which includes Doppler echocardiography. If a murmur is detected on evaluation, referral for echocardiography should be recommended both for the health of the patient and the information gathered for the breeding program. Murmurs are graded 1 through 6. These and other descriptive terms for murmurs may be found on the OFA cardiac website at www.offa.org/cardiacgrade.html.

Cardiac auscultation is the primary screening method for initial identification of Congenital Heart Disease (CHD) and the initial classification of dogs. This evaluation is completed by cardiac auscultation at rest and may include additional auscultation after exertion to detect murmurs. Complete instruction on how this examination should be performed is available on the OFA website. It may be performed by Board- Certified Cardiologists (preferred) (suffix on OFA number of C), internists or other Specialists (suffix S) or by General Practitioners (suffix P). In addition, Echocardiograms and/or Holter monitoring may be recommended for some breeds. (See following sections on testing for arrhythmias and echocardiographic exam.)

There are many forms of congenital heart disease in dogs which are caused by malformations of the heart or great vessels. The lesions characterizing congenital heart defects are present at birth and may develop more fully during perinatal and growth periods. Many congenital heart defects are thought to be genetically transmitted from parents to offspring; however, the exact modes of inheritance have not been precisely determined for all cardiovascular malformations. At this time, inherited developmental cardiac diseases like subaortic stenosis and cardiomyopathies are difficult to monitor since there is no clear cut distinction between normal and abnormal. The OFA states it plans to modify the congenital cardiac database when a proven diagnostic modality and normal parameters by breed are established. However at this time, the OFA cardiac database should not be considered as a screening tool for SAS or cardiomyopathies. Current information regarding the OFA cardiac database can be located at: http://www.offa.org/cardiacinfo.html.

OFA patellas

Patellar luxation can occur either in a medial or lateral position and may be either bilateral or unilateral. This disorder occurs in many breeds. Dogs can show symptoms as early as 8 weeks of age. In some cases, the affected dog has abnormal limb carriage from the time they begin to bear weight at 3 weeks of age. Frequently, the dogs have a knock-kneed (genu valgum) stance and the foot can be seen to twist laterally as weight is placed on the limb. In many cases, the dog presents acutely lame, often painful and non-weight-bearing on the first episode. The patella is usually reducible, and laxity of the medial collateral ligament may be palpable. The medial tissues of the stifle joint are often thickened.

Patellar luxation is diagnosed by palpation of the position of the patella with mild manipulation performed by any qualified veterinarian. Radiographic studies are not included in this evaluation. Evaluation of the patellar position can be done as early as 8 weeks of age. The patient should not be sedated and must be at least 12 months of age to be included in the database. Re-evaluation later in life is encouraged as some luxations become evident as the patient ages. The patella is classified as either being in a normal position, or if it is luxated, is categorized by grade. To receive OFA patellar certification, the patient is examined, the appropriate form is completed including the veterinarian's findings, signed by the veterinarian, and submitted to OFA with the associated fee. OFA encourages submission of all evaluations, normal or abnormal but does not charge a fee for abnormal patellar evaluations.

A method of classifying the degree of luxation and bony deformity is useful for diagnosis, and can be applied to either medial or lateral luxations by reversing the medial-lateral directional references. The position of the patella can easily be palpated starting at the tibial tubercle and working proximal along the patellar ligament to the patella.

Grade 1 patellar luxation
Manually the patella easily luxates at full extension of the stifle joint, but returns to the trochlea when released. No crepitation is apparent. The medial, or very occasionally, lateral deviation of the tibial crest (with lateral luxation of the patella) is only minimal, and there is very slight rotation of the tibia. Flexion and extension of the stifle is in a straight line with no abduction of the hock.

Grade 2 patellar luxation
There is frequent patellar luxation, which, in some cases, can become permanent. The limb is sometimes carried, although weight bearing routinely occurs with the stifle remaining slightly flexed. Especially under anesthesia it is often possible to reduce the luxation by manually turning the tibia laterally, but the patella reluxates with ease when manual tension of the joint is released. As much as 30 degrees of medial tibial torsion and a slight medial deviation of the tibial crest may exist. When the patella is resting medially the hock is slightly abducted. If the condition is bilateral, more weight is shifted onto the forelimbs.

Many dogs with this grade live with the condition reasonably well for many years, but the constant luxation of the patella over the medial trochlear ridge of the trochlea causes erosion of the articulating surface of the patella and also the proximal area of the medial lip. This results in crepitation becoming apparent when the patella is luxated manually.

Grade 3 patellar luxation
The patella is permanently luxated with torsion of the tibia and deviation of the tibial crest of between 30 degrees and 50 degrees from the cranial/caudal plane. Although the luxation is not intermittent, many animals use the limb with the stifle held in a semi flexed position. The trochlea is very shallow or even flattened.

Grade 4 patellar luxation
The tibia is medially twisted and the tibial crest may show further deviation medially with the result that it lies 50 degrees to 90 degrees from the cranial/caudal plane. The patella is permanently luxated. The patella lies just above the medial condyle and a space can be palpated between the

patellar ligament and the distal end of the femur. The trochlea is absent or even convex. The limb is carried, or the animal moves in a crouched position, with the limb flexed.

Patellar luxations fall into several categories. The first 3 are either known to be or suspected to be inherited. Medial luxations occur in toy, miniature, and large breeds. These patients have anatomic deformities that cause luxation. Lateral luxation occurs in toy and miniature breeds. These patients usually present in middle age. Lateral luxation occurs in large and giant breeds. These dogs usually present at 5 to 6 months of age, are usually affected bilaterally, and may have associated hip dysplasia. Luxation resulting from trauma occurs in various breeds, and is of no importance to the certification process. Unless there is deviation of the tibial crest, it may be difficult to differentiate traumatic from congenital patellar luxation. (See www.offa.org)

Testing for arrhythmias

Use of a 24 hour ECG using a Holter monitor is currently the preferred evaluation when testing a dog for arrhythmias. The Holter allows the monitoring over a period of approximately 100,000 heart beats, increasing the opportunity of detecting intermittent arrhythmias. Dogs which show runs of PVC's are at increased risk for syncope or sudden death. It is presumed there is an inherited component to this disease and in some breeds, screening for PVC's is recommended prior to breeding (Figure 2-1).

There are services that provide the equipment and interpretation of the results by a Board-certified Cardiologist. In general, breed clubs have already made these arrangements.

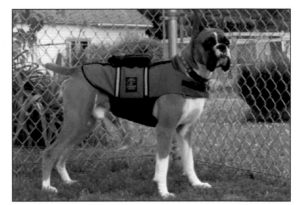

Figure 2-1.
Holter monitor for cardiac arrhythmias.

Screening for deafness

Congenital deafness in dogs (or other animals) can be acquired or inherited. Inherited deafness can be caused by a gene defect that is autosomal dominant, recessive, or may involve multiple genes. Congenital deafness has been recognized in approximately 80 dog breeds, but has been noted to be over-represented in dogs with white pigmentation. Two pigmentation genes in particular are often associated with deafness in dogs: the merle gene and the piebald gene.

A BAER test (the Brainstem Auditory Evoked Response) is necessary and is the only accepted method to identify dogs with partial or unilateral hearing deficits. Facilities that perform the BAER are usually only available at veterinary schools or specialty practices and are usually performed by a Board-Certified Neurologist.

Testing is done on dogs a minimum of 35 days of age. One test is all that is necessary for the dog's lifetime. Chemical restraint is administered at the discretion of the veterinarian performing the evaluation. Only dogs with bilateral hearing are classified as passing the test. The submission includes a printed copy of the BAER tracing complete with the dog's name or identification, the completed application form, and the appropriate fee.

The decision on how to proceed with a breeding program in which deaf individuals are identified should include researching the inheritance pattern in the breed and the pedigrees of affected individuals.

Screening for inherited liver shunts

Inherited liver shunts are found in 5 of every 1000 dogs. Most are small breed dogs. Breeds affected include Havanese, Yorkshire Terriers, Maltese, Dandie Dinmont Terriers, Pugs, Miniature Standard Schnauzers, Shih Tzus, Bernese Mountain Dogs, and Bichen Frises. Yorkshire Terriers, Cairn Terriers, Irish Wolfhounds, and Maltese have a proven hereditary basis. Research shows it is not a simple autosomal recessive mode of inheritance.

Testing all potential breeding stock of breeds at risk has been proposed. Testing involves paired fasting and 2 hour post prandial bile acids and blood ammonia levels. Not including dogs with elevated levels of either has been proposed as a method to eliminate phenotypically affected dogs from the gene pool.

Radiographic and ultrasound findings
OFA hip dysplasia

Hip dysplasia is a serious genetic disease which has been reported in every dog breed, in mixed-breed dogs and cats. Many veterinarians think that every dog, regardless of breed, should be evaluated radiographically for hip pathology prior to use in a breeding program. By contrast, many breeders consider their breed to be unaffected and do not screen for this. Hip dysplasia manifests as arthritis, pain and debilitation caused by the inherited abnormal biomechanics of an abnormally developed hip joint. Of significance is the lack of correlation between radiographic findings and clinical findings (Figure 2-2).

Radiographs for an OFA (Orthopedic Foundation for Animals) hip study are taken by the breeder's choice of veterinarian. The dog must be in the required dorsally recumbent, hip extended position. The view must include the wings of the ilium and patellas. The properly positioned, identified and exposed radiograph, completed application form, copy of the AKC certificate (or other registry if available) and appropriate fee are submitted to OFA either by mail or electronically. If the radiograph is sent by mail, it is prudent to send it with a tracking number so the film can be located if lost. The application form, detailed instructions on the correct positioning, and required film identification are included on the website: www.offa.org. If the patient is not positioned correctly, the exposure is not correct, or the film is not permanently identified, the radiograph will not be accepted by OFA and it will be necessary to repeat the study.

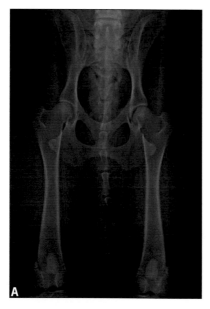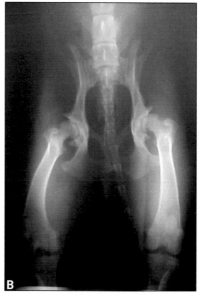

Figure 2-2.
A. VD Pelvis position, OFA excellent hips. Also the position for the first of 3 required PennHip views. Wings of ilium and patellas visible on view, bilateral symmetry, femurs parallel. B. VD Pelvis position- dysplastic hips.

To apply for an OFA number, the dog must be a minimum of 2 years of age. Preliminary evaluations can be submitted from ages 4 months to 2 years of age. Discounts are available if multiple films are submitted together. Results for accepted applicants are available approximately 4 weeks after submission.

As of January 1, 2001, OFA started requiring permanent identification (tattoo or microchip which must be verified by the veterinarian taking the radiograph if they have signed it was verified) for inclusion in their database. These identified animals will have a suffix of "PI" following their OFA number if one is issued. Animals without permanent identification will still be evaluated but will not be listed in the database and their OFA number will have "NOPI" as a suffix.

OFA recommends but does not require sedation or anesthesia to take radiographs. This is left to the discretion of the attending veterinarian and the owner of the dog.

In one small study, it was shown that some females show laxity of the hips around the time of estrus and whelping. It is not recommended to take radiographs of pregnant females. The OFA recommends radiographing three to four weeks before or after the heat cycle, and three to four weeks after weaning a litter of puppies. (See PennHip® study on this in the following section).

Results are provided by a consensus of three veterinary radiologists. Each radiologist will grade the hips with one of seven different physical (phenotypic) hip conformations: normal which includes excellent, good, or fair classifications (which are issued OFA numbers); borderline; or dysplastic which includes mild, moderate, or severe classifications (which are not issued OFA numbers).

OFA suggests the following use of hip dysplasia information for breeders in selecting breeding stock and mates:
- Breed normals to normals
- Breed normals with normal ancestry
- Breed normals from litters (brothers/sisters) with a low incidence of HD
- Select a sire that produces a low incidence of HD
- Replace dogs with dogs that are better than the breed average
- OFA fair dogs with 75% normal siblings are good breeding prospects if other genetic factors support inclusion in a breeding program.

Many breeders and dog handlers find early information of the hip status of puppies to be valuable. Early screening can permit early selection of dogs suited for show, performance, and breeding; this minimizes financial and emotional losses should dogs selected without this data fail to pass OFA ratings as they mature. Preliminary hip evaluations are accepted by OFA as early as 4 months of age. These preliminary films are read only by the OFA staff veterinary radiologists and are given the same hip grades as other OFA cases. As of May 1, 2004 the dog must be at least 12 months of age at the time of the radiograph, and permanently identified via microchip or tattoo before the preliminary results can be published (this should be verified by the veterinarian at the time the radiograph is taken).

Dr. Corley of OFA published a comparison of the reliability of the preliminary evaluation hip grade phenotype with the 2 year old evaluation in dogs. There was 100% reliability for a preliminary grade of excellent being normal at 2 years of age (excellent, good, or fair). There was 97.9% reliability for a preliminary grade of good being normal at 2 years of age, and 76.9% reliability for a preliminary grade of fair being normal at 2 years of age. Reliability of preliminary evaluations increased as age at the time of preliminary evaluation increased, regardless of whether dogs received a preliminary evaluation of normal hip conformation or HD. For normal hip conformations, the reliability was 89.6% at 3 to 6 months, 93.8% at 7 to 12 months, and 95.2% at 13 to 18 months. These results suggest that preliminary evaluations of hip joint status in dogs are generally reliable. However, dogs that receive a preliminary evaluation of fair or mild hip joint conformation should be reevaluated at an older age (24 months). Additional information on hip dysplasia, film submission, hip evaluation, and fees is available at www.offa.org.

OFA Legg-Calve-Perthes

Legg-Calve-Perthes Disease (LCP), also known as avascular necrosis of the femoral head, is seen in the hip of dogs and humans. In dogs, it is seen in young small breed dogs between 4 and 12 months of age. Dogs usually present with unilateral pain and lameness, but can have bilateral disease. LCP is believed to be an inherited disease, although the mode of inheritance is not known.

Radiographs,taken in the standard hip extended ventrodorsal view, show changes in the femoral head and neck. Dogs must be a minimum of 12 months of age on the date of the radiograph to be eligible for an LCP number. The radiographs may be taken by any veterinarian, but must contain the required dog identification as a permanent part of the radiograph, be properly positioned, and must be of sufficient quality for the OFA to reach a diagnosis. The application form, fee and radiographs are submitted for evaluation. Phenotypically normal dogs are assigned an OFA Legg-Calve-Perthes number.

OFA elbows

In 1990, OFA began to provide a service to evaluate elbows. Elbow dysplasia is a general term used to classify inherited pathology of the elbow. Four specific etiologies make up this disease and they can occur independently or in conjunction with one another. These etiologies include:
1. Pathology involving the medial coronoid of the ulna – fragmented coronoid process or FCP.

2. Osteochondritis of the medial humeral condyle in the elbow joint or OCD.

3. Ununited anconeal process or UAP.

4. A fourth cause of elbow pathology is premature ulnar growth plate closure, an inherited disorder in some chondrodysplastic breed. This condition may also be caused by trauma to the open growth plate in a young dog of any breed (Figure 2-3A and B).

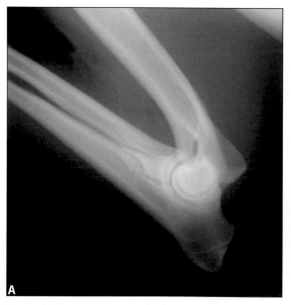 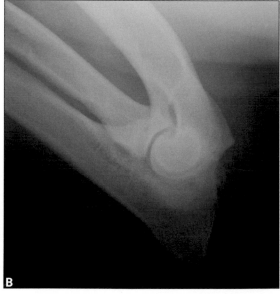

Figure 2-3.
A. Lateral flexed view of elbow, OFA elbow normal. **B.** Lateral flexed view of elbow, OFA dysplatic elbow.

The inherited polygenic traits that cause elbow dysplasia are unrelated to one another. Onset of clinical signs may be related to trauma, severity of the changes, and weight gain. Clinical signs, which may appear at nearly any age, range from slight gait changes, inward deviation of the foot, decreased range of motion of the elbow, to severe lameness.

The view required by OFA to diagnose secondary degenerative changes in the elbow joint is an extreme flexed medio-lateral view of the elbow. When there is instability of the elbow joint due to elbow dysplasia, it leads to a of new bone proliferation (osteophytes) on the anconeal process of the ulna) associated with secondary developmental degenerative joint disease.

For elbow evaluations, there are no grades for a radiographically normal elbow. The only grades assigned are for abnormal elbows with radiographic changes associated with secondary degenerative joint disease. Like the hip certification, the OFA will not certify a normal elbow until the dog is 2 years of age. The appropriate positioning, a well-exposed radiograph with the required permanent identification included on the film, and necessary application form and fee must be submitted to OFA for a rating to be issued. The OFA also accepts preliminary elbow radiographs. To date, there are no long term studies for preliminary elbow examinations like there are for hips. However, preliminary screening for elbows along with hips can also provide valuable information to the breeder.

OFA provides the following rating for abnormal elbow radiographs:
Grade I Elbow Dysplasia shows minimal bone change along the anconeal process of ulna (less than 3 mm).
Grade II Elbow Dysplasia shows additional bone proliferation along the anconeal process (3 to 5 mm) and subchondral bone changes (trochlear notch sclerosis).
Grade III Elbow Dysplasia shows well developed degenerative joint disease with bone proliferation along the anconeal process being greater than 5 mm.

OFA hip and elbow follow-up
OFA has recently begun to offer a new resubmission service. For a small fee, OFA will provide a "Follow-up Study" for hip and elbow studies taken later in a pet's life. The film will be read only by the OFA board-certified in-house veterinary radiologist. Owners will receive a report of the findings. The results from these "Follow-Up Studies" will not alter or risk the earlier official OFA consensus reading on which the dog may have received a hip or elbow number. The primary benefits of this new service are twofold: 1. the OFA will generate additional information on changes in hip status over the lifetime of the animal, and 2. owners will benefit from the same information without risking the earlier rating assigned by the OFA. Specific information on this service is available at www.offa.org.

OFA shoulders
This study is to evaluate for ostoechondrosis (OCD) of the shoulder. OCD is a disruption in the ossification of the cartilage mold under the articular cartilage of the joint. OCD has been reported in many joints, most commonly the shoulder, but also in the elbow, stifle, hock, and spine. It can appear to be unilateral or bilateral. Typically, affected dogs are large breeds, show clinical signs at less than 1 year of age, and males outnumber females. OCD is considered a genetic disease although the mode of inheritance has not yet been established (Figure 2-4).

To receive an OFA number for shoulders, the dog must be a minimum of 12 months of age. Preliminary evaluations are also available. As with other OFA studies, the patient must be appropriately positioned, the film must have the patient identification permanently as part of the radiograph, the film must be properly exposed, and all fees and signed paperwork must be included in the submission.

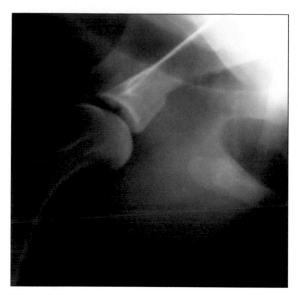

Figure 2-4.
Lateral shoulder view, OFA shoulders normal.

PennHIP®

PennHIP® (University of Pennsylvania Hip Improvement Program) uses a radiographic technique to assess the quality of the canine hip and quantitatively measures canine hip joint laxity. Only PennHIP® trained member veterinarians are qualified to take radiographs to submit for evaluation. Three views of the hip are taken with the patient under general anesthesia. The first view, the standard hip-extended view, is used to evaluate for DJD. The second view is used to evaluate hip joint congruity with the hip in a compression view. The third view is used to make quantitative measurements of the hip joint laxity in a distracted view. This set of 3 films is submitted to the University of Pennsylvania for analysis, providing results in a numeric format called a "distraction index." This is based on the theory that a joint with greater laxity (i.e. a higher distraction index or a number closer to 1) will lead later in life to a higher likelihood that the patient will develop more severe DJD than a patient with less joint laxity (i.e. a lower distraction index or a number closer to 0) (Figure 2-5A and B).

This diagnostic procedure may be done on patients as young as 16 weeks of age to produce reliable results. Unlike OFA, all patients who undergo a PennHIP® evaluation must be under general anesthesia and all radiographs taken must be submitted to PennHIP® for assessment, regardless of how obvious the pathology may be. This is to prevent skewing of the data collected by selectively withholding films to PennHIP® on affected dogs.

In 1997, PennHIP® completed a study to assess for laxity of the hips of female dogs related to estrus. The study showed the rise in hormone levels during the heat cycle does not affect hip laxity as measured by PennHIP®. However, hormones released during the birthing process and during lactation can increase hip laxity and hip evaluation at this time is therefore not recommended. PennHIP® recommends waiting 8 weeks post lactation or 16 weeks post whelping, before a PennHIP® evaluation.

Additional information regarding training to become a PennHIP® certified veterinarian, equipment required, and the research that supports this analysis is available at www.pennhip.org.

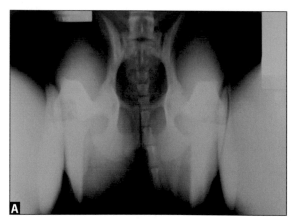
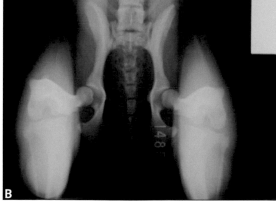

Figure 2-5.
A. *PennHip Compressed view - the second of 3 PennHip views required.* **B.** *PennHip Distracted view – the third of 3 views required.*

Echocardiographic (Echo) exam

There are some breed clubs which recommend an Echo be performed instead of or in addition to Holter monitoring prior to a dog entering the breeding pool.

For most veterinarians, the Echocardiographic exam will be a referral case. Board certification by the American College of Veterinary Internal Medicine, Specialty of Cardiology, is considered by the American College of Veterinary Medical Associations as the benchmark of clinical proficiency for veterinarians in clinical cardiology, and examination by a Diplomate of this Specialty Board is recommended. Other veterinarians may be able to perform these examinations provided they have appropriate equipment and have received advanced training in echocardiography. The examiner must be able to perform two-dimensional, pulsed-wave Doppler, and continuous wave Doppler examinations of the heart. The availability of color Doppler is valuable but not essential for most examinations. Echocardiographic studies should be reported on videotape for subsequent analysis and a written record of abnormal findings should be entered into the medical record.

Laboratory test findings for enzyme or hormone levels
Thyroid testing

Autoimmune thyroiditis is the most common cause of primary hypothyroidism in dogs. If the dog develops autoantibodies at any time in the dog's life, this is an indication that the dog probably has the genetic form of the disease. This disorder tends to appear clinically at 2 to 5 years of age. Prior to the onset of clinical signs, thyroglobulin autoantibody (TGAA) becomes detectable on a blood test.

Since the majority of affected dogs will have autoantibodies by 4 years of age, annual testing for the first 4 years is recommended. The majority of dogs that develop autoantibodies have them by 3 to 4 years of age; however, after age 4, biannual retesting is recommended. A negative test at any one time will not guarantee that the dog will not develop thyroiditis. By knowing the status of the dog and the status of the dogs lineage, breeders and genetic counselors can decide which matings are most appropriate to help reduce the incidence of autoimmune thyroiditis in the offspring.

Dogs being should be examined by a veterinarian and have serum drawn and sent only to an OFA approved laboratory following the testing instructions. Dogs should not receive any type of thyroid supplementation for 3 months prior to thyroid testing. Female dogs should not be tested during an estrus cycle. It is important to use a plain red top tube without a serum barrier for sample collection. Details for sample handling and shipment are available at http://www.offa.org/thyvetinstruct.html. Under separate cover, the OFA application and appropriate fee must be submitted for certification.

Evaluation of dogs under 12 months of age can be performed for private use of the owner since few dogs are already positive at that age. However, certification will not be possible at that age. A breed database number will be issued to all dogs found to be normal at or after 12 months of age. Ages will be used in the certification process since the classification can change as the dog ages and the autoimmune disease progresses. It is recommended that reexamination occur at ages 2,3,4,6, and 8 years.

All data, whether normal or abnormal, should be submitted for purposes of completeness. There is no OFA fee for entering an abnormal evaluation of the thyroid into the data bank. Information on results determined to be positive or equivocal will not be made public without explicit written permission of the owner.

Thyroid abnormalities fall into several categories. Two types will be defined by the registry: 1. autoimmune thyroiditis and 2. idiopathically reduced thyroid function. Autoimmune thyroiditis is classified as a genetic disorder. Dogs with autoimmune thyroiditis may not be considered ideal candidates for breeding stock.

von Willebrand's blood coagulation testing

von Willebrand's disease (vWD) is the most common inherited bleeding disorder of both animals and humans. The cause is a reduction in the amount or function of von Willebrand factor (vWF), the protein necessary for normal platelet function. There are 3 forms of vWD: type I (low concentration of normally structured vWF protein); Type II (low concentration of an abnormal vWF), and Type III (complete absence of vWF). Different breeds exhibit different variations of the disease.

Most dogs, whether carriers or affected, are clinically normal. Affected dogs may present with spontaneous bleeding, usually from the mucosa of the mouth, nose, or gastro-intestinal tract. Injury that is accompanied by bleeding may require administration of a transfusion. A buccal mucosal bleeding time is an easy and quick test to perform in a suspect pre-op patient but is not a definitive diagnostic test to screen for vWD.

There are 2 screening tests currently available. The first test developed was an assay to measure the percentage of vWF protein present in an individual patient. This test was developed by Dr. Jean Dodds and is still run in the lab at Cornell University College of Veterinary Medicine. It is the only test available that will screen dogs of all breeds for vWD. Because the test measures a protein in the dynamic system of the dog's body, it is expected the result will vary from one test to the next in the same patient. Despite this variation of the absolute number of a test result, the typical patient will still be reported in the same category (normal, carrier or affected) on subsequent tests unless the patient has a change in their health status or estrous cycle from one testing date to the next. This variation has caused some confusion in the interpretation for some breeders but this should not undermine the value of the test results.

The second screening test available is a DNA test for vWD. It has been marketed as a test for multiple breeds but this author is not aware of any published reports that support the accuracy of use in breeds other than the Scottish Terrier.

Sebaceous Adenitis skin biopsies

Sebaceous Adenitis (SA) is a hereditary skin disease in which the sebaceous glands become inflamed, often leading to progressive loss of hair. SA symptoms can mimic other diseases including allergies and endocrine disorders. Some dogs affected with SA are asymptomatic. Diagnosis is based on histopathologic evaluation of skin biopsies.

The attending veterinarian examines the dog for clinical symptoms of the disease and notes any findings on the application form. A minimum of two 6mm punch biopsy samples are taken from the skin of the dog's neck between the top of the head and the withers. If there are areas of scaling and hair loss, samples should be taken from those areas.

To collect the sample, a local anesthetic such as lidocaine may be used. General anesthesia may be used as determined by the attending veterinarian. The area should not be scrubbed or otherwise cleaned, however gentle clipping of the area may be necessary. When obtaining the sample with a local anesthetic, use of a colored marker or white liquid correction fluid is helpful in finding the area with the lidocaine block. After the skin punch has removed the skin biopsy specimen, the skin should be closed with 1 to 2 absorbable sutures. The specimen should be placed in a crush proof container with formalin in preparation for shipment to the lab. The samples, the completed OFA application, and both the lab fee and OFA fee are sent only to an approved dermapathology laboratory for evaluation.

The lab results are classified as either:
- No Evidence of Sebaceous Adenitis (at the time of the evaluation)
- Affected
- Affected without Clinical Symptoms
- Equivocal (some inflammation is present, but the cause cannot be determined.

The lab results and final diagnosis are returned to the OFA and to the owner. The minimum age for registration in the OFA SA database is 12 months.

It is believed that SA is inherited as a simple autosomal recessive. There is currently no DNA test to determine a dog's status with regard to SA. As enough phenotypic information on families of dogs is entered into the database, breeders will be able to make educated assumptions about a dog's genotype. This will allow breeders to apply greater selective pressure in controlling and reducing the incidence of the disease.

Two factors make SA particularly difficult for breeders to control: the possible late onset of the disease, and the subclinical state of the disease. With late onset, the dog may have already been bred long before it ever shows clinical signs of the disease. In its subclinical state, an owner may be unaware that the animal is affected since it shows no visible signs of the disease.

OFA certificates

Some of the OFA submission forms include a line for dog owners to initial to allow the release of abnormal findings to a public database. This should be discussed with the client in advance of submission as some owners prefer to limit results to their own use.

Any questions on how to read an OFA certificate can be clarified by visiting http://www.offa.org/numberkey.html.

Genotypic screening

Tests available

Selection based on genotype – there are currently 4 types of DNA tests: parentage tests, mutation-based tests, linked marker tests, and tests to identify the breeds but not the individual parents who contributed genetics to an individual dog. DNA genetic screening is the most rapidly evolving. Although many DNA tests have been available up to now, the completion of the canine genome in 2004 and research at both commercial and non-commercial facilities is expanding the number of DNA tests available exponentially. Because tests are becoming available so quickly, it is not possible to include an all-inclusive list of DNA tests here. It is also not likely that veterinarian will be able to stay current with the available tests. Breed clubs will have recommendations regarding the tests available for screening. Careful and current research into each test should be done to be certain the test was evaluated for the breed in question prior to recommending the test. In some cases, DNA markers for one breed do not necessarily serve as the DNA marker for another breed. The laboratory selected for the analysis should be a university based laboratory, or one with an excellent reputation, have a PhD geneticist on staff and be recommended by the parent breed club.

Samples for DNA tests are usually either provided as a cheek swab on a specifically-produced cytology brush or a whole blood sample. Serum is not a suitable sample as it contains very little DNA. Frozen semen can also be used in some cases by extracting whole cells from the frozen sample. However, it is an expensive way to obtain DNA, both from the actual financial cost of sacrificing the sample and from the aspect of the loss of valuable semen which is usually limited in quantity. Each lab will have very specific sample and paperwork requirements. The most up-to-date information should be used prior to collecting and submitting the sample. A visit to the website or a phone call to the testing facility is recommended to be certain the sample and forms are the most current available as this is likely to change frequently.

General types of DNA tests available

1. Disorders of blood or blood cells: hemophilia A and B, vWD types I, II, and III, factor VII deficiency
2. Storage diseases: copper toxicosis, cystinuria, renal cystadenocarcinoma and nodular dermatofibrosis,
3. CNS and skin: Lafora type epilepsy, narcolepsy, epidermolysis bullosa (two forms)
4. Eye: Collie eye anomaly, progressive retinal atrophy/PRA
5. Drug sensitivities: malignant hyperthermia, multi drug resistence gene (MDR-1)

Parentage DNA tests

These tests have great value in determining if the pup has the parents accurately recorded with their respective registry. The only value in parentage genotypic screening applied to screening for genetic disease is for use when a DNA test used to clear a parent is used to clear offspring as genetically disease-free.

Mutation-based tests or Gene-specific tests

This is the "gold standard" DNA test. Because of accuracy of testing and shorter time needed to develop a DNA test, this test is preferred over the linked-marker test when it is available. The test identifies the actual mutated DNA that produces the defect being evaluated. Often, a canine inherited disease will be identical to a disease in human or mouse (genomes more heavily researched than the canine genome). If the mutant gene has been identified in either of these species, researchers can immediately test whether the same gene is involved in the canine disease. When it is, researchers have a very rapid route to identifying the mutations that cause inherited disease in the dog. However, it must be assessed to be the same gene in each breed of dog as in the mouse, human, or other dog breeds. On occasion, there can be different mutations that cause similar diseases in different breeds. When the scientific literature can show the defect is testing for the correct mutation in a specific breed and the parentage can be confirmed, the test is considered to be 100% accurate.

These gene-based DNA tests can be used to analyze an individual dog's DNA to determine how many copies of the mutant gene it possesses. A dog with two normal versions of the gene is classified as genetically clear; a dog with one normal version and one mutant version will be a carrier; and a dog with two mutant copies will be affected or at risk (for a disease that results from a single recessive mutation).

Examples of this type of test include progressive retinal atrophy in the Irish Setter and cystinuria in the Newfoundland. http://www.thekennelclub.org.uk/item/315.

Linkage or Linked-marker tests

With this type of test, the actual mutated DNA marker has not been identified. Instead, the test uses an identified marker that is always inherited by an affected dog but is not inherited by clinically normal dogs. Using special DNA markers developed by the Canine Genome Research project, researchers can identify unique regions along each and every canine chromosome. This co-inheritance of the DNA marker with the disease signifies that the marker is physically close to the mutant gene that causes the disease on one of the chromosomes. Here, the marker is determined to be linked to the disease gene, thus the terminology linked-marker tests. Since the markers used have all been mapped to their unique location on one or other of the chromosomes, identifying a linked marker will identify a relatively small region of just one chromosome where the mutant gene will be found. Scientists can then scan this region for potential candidate genes that can be screened for their involvement in the disease.

The presence of the linked marker is usually diagnostic for the presence of the associated mutant gene. However, linked-marker tests are rarely 100% accurate (realistically 95 to 99% accurate) because the test does not directly measure the presence or absence of the mutant gene, but rather it's next door neighbor gene. Another cause of error using linkage testing is when a genetic marker recognizes a false allele that is not linked to the disease gene. Therefore, inaccurate diagnoses can be made if, on the rare occasion, the mutant gene and the linked marker become separated during meiosis. As technology allows, this type of test will be replaced by mutation-based tests. Be sure you or your client has checked the internet for the most current and reliable tests available prior to submission of samples.

Current examples of this type of test include renal dysplasia in the Shih Tzu and PRA in the Toy and Miniature poodle. http://www.thekennelclub.org.uk/item/315

Breed identification
Testing is available commercially to identify the breed(s) an individual dog is derived from. This will not identify specific individuals as parents, rather the breeds contributing DNA to an individual. Pet owners can submit blood samples through their veterinarian to this commercially-available service for a fee. This testing is more than a novelty; it is thought this can assist pet owners and veterinarians in identifying breed-specific traits and disorders. This test will also be of value if it is suspected an individual is not the purebred dog the breeder selling the dog represented it to be.

Use of test results
Most DNA tests currently available are tests for single gene, autosomal recessive diseases. This type of test is accurate and affordable.

These tests can distinguish between:
1. Normal (a clear dog, with two normal alleles at gene of interest)(NN).
2. Carrier (a dog with one normal allele, one disease-causing allele but without symptoms of the disorder) (Na).
3. Affected (a dog with two disease causing alleles, clinically affected or at risk of showing clinical signs) (aa).

DNA test results have many applications. First is to detect affected dogs prior to the onset of clinical signs. Second is to predict disease outcome or to prescribe treatment prior to clinical signs developing. Third is to diagnose affected dogs when they become clinically abnormal. Fourth is to detect asymptomatic carriers in the breeding population. This allows clinically normal carrier or affected dogs to be bred to clear mates, leaving these dogs in the gene pool so that their "good" genetics can be perpetuated without compounding the "bad" genetics. In doing so, genetic diversity can be maintained. In genetic diseases with complex inheritance patterns, this can be more difficult.

Counseling the breeder
While DNA testing is useful, it cannot stand alone as a diagnostic tool. Merely finding that a dog carries two abnormal genes does not prove that the dog's disorder is caused by the disease they appear to carry. For instance, a dog with two abnormal genes for degenerative myelopathy may show signs of neurologic disease, but there are other causes such as intervertebral disc disease that may produce a similar clinical picture.

For our uses, mutation-based tests and linked marker tests provide diagnostic insights. Removing all dogs who carry a genetic defect from the breeding pool is neither practical nor recommended. Our purebred dogs have been described as "endangered species" by Dr. Anne Traas. If we eliminate every dog with a defect, we will have no purebred dogs left (or any dogs left as there is no dog, purebred or mixed breed without a defect). Instead, we can apply these test results to breed phenotypically normal genotypically affected carriers to genotypically normal dogs to produce litters with small numbers of genotypically abnormal pups. The affected dogs can then be removed from the breeding pool, allowing breeders to use dogs with valuable genetics in their lines without limiting the gene pool.

There are four modes of inheritance that cause most genetic defects in dogs: simple autosomal recessive; sex-linked recessive; autosomal dominant; and polygenic.

Including a dog with a simple autosomal recessive disease into a breeding program when a genetic test is available

To produce an affected pup (aa), both parents of an affected puppy must be carriers of the abnormal gene that causes the disorder. Frequently, neither parent (both Na) will show the trait. An autosomal or simple recessive trait results when a matched pair of genes is present on any of the dog's 38 pairs of autosomes. An autosome is a non-sex chromosome.

Dogs that carry only one simple autosomal recessive gene (Na) may be used in a breeding program if matched carefully with a genetically screened (NN) mate. Even an affected dog may be included if bred to a genotypically normal dog.

First, a Punnett square should be drawn to illustrate the risks of the planned breeding to the owner.

Second, a diagram of a scientific pedigree of the dogs involved should be constructed, identifying known carriers in the pedigree. There are computer programs and articles written on how to designate male/female and normal/carrier/affected available to assist in this task. Be sure to identify both parents of affected offspring as carriers. (Standard Pedigree key: Males are identified as squares, females as circles; affecteds are colored in; carriers have a small mark through the square or circle; and clears are a clear square or circle). Identify which dogs the breeder would like to incorporate as breeding stock. Start testing with the foundation dogs as this may reduce the number of tests necessary. If all foundation dogs are clear and there is not a recent mutation, no additional tests are necessary. If affected and carrier dogs are found, testing of offspring is necessary.

Third, if indicated, test all potential sires and dams. If only normal/clear (NN) dogs are mated, no affected dog will be produced. When an x-linked gene carried by an (unaffected) male is bred to a clear female, all offspring from this mating must be tested to assess their carrier (male or female) or affected (female) status. When an affected male is bred to a clear female, ALL offspring must be carriers and need not be tested.

Fourth, if any carrier (Na) is included in the breeding, offspring may be tested as very young pups to detect carrier (Na)/affected (aa) status prior to placing pups in homes.

If an affected dog (aa) is to be included as a breeding dog, the breeder should be counseled that the dog must be outstanding in many other ways to merit this. This may include temperament, performance, and physical traits but this should be in line with objective goals established for their breeding program. The disadvantage to including this dog as a breeding dog is it will quickly increase the incidence of the mutant allele (Na) in this population. By design, all offspring of the affected dog will be carriers (Na) and need not be tested (or affected (aa) if the gene is carried by both parents – this is NOT advised). In future generations, the affected (aa) breeding stock can be replaced with their offspring that are clear (NN) or carriers (Na) with outstanding qualities. These carriers (Na) can be replaced by adding new animals to the line that have been tested.

Used correctly, these DNA results will allow veterinarians and breeders to select potential breeders with greater insight.

With all of these test findings available to the breeder, the breeder may look to the veterinarian for input on how to interpret the data and how to put it to use in their breeding program. This is a great challenge for us as veterinarians. There is no genetically perfect dog, whether purebred or hybrid; they all have at least one genotypic or phenotypic defect. Our goal as consultants to our breeder clients is to assist them in making the best genetic choices they can.

Option #1
2 NORMAL PARENTS (NN) → 100% NORMAL OFFSPRING

PARENTS	N	N
N	NN (normal)	NN (normal)
N	NN (normal)	NN (normal)

Option #2
1 normal (NN) and 1 affected (aa) parent = 100% carrier OFFSPRING but 0 affected pups

PARENTS	N	N
a	Na (carrier)	Na (carrier)
a	Na (carrier)	Na (carrier)

Option #3
Both carrier parents (Na) → 25% normal and 50% carrier and 25% affected OFFSPRING

PARENTS	N	a
N	NN (normal)	Na (carrier)
a	Na (carrier)	aa (affected)

Option #4
1 carrier parents (Na) x 1 affected (aa) parent → 50% carrier and 50% affected OFFSPRING (Not recommended)

PARENTS	N	a
a	Na (carrier)	aa (affected)
a	Na (carrier)	aa (affected)

Option #5
Both affected parents (aa) → 100% affected OFFSPRING (Not recommended)

PARENTS	a	a
a	aa (affected)	aa (affected)
a	aa (affected)	aa (affected)

Use of this visual tool with help veterinarians and breeders alike make better decisions on who to include and exclude, or who to combine genetically for breeding when breeding dogs with known traits with known genetic tests when an autosomal recessive gene is believed to be involved.

Incorporating a dog with a simple autosomal recessive disease into a breeding program when a genetic test is NOT available
Known carrier dogs should not be used for breeding. We can only counsel clients by using phenotypic tests – traits visible on examination or by testing using specific criteria. Then we can advise the client using probabilities of inheritance.

Counseling for X-linked recessive diseases
Sex-linked genes can be either dominant or recessive and always appear on the X-chromosome, making the female the carrier. By definition, males cannot be carriers (they have no X chromosome), only affected or normal. In the male, as he has only one X chromosome, the single recessive gene that is part of that chromosome expresses itself, expressing the trait that requires two genes to be expressed in the female. The mothers of all affected males must be either a carrier or affected; they

are never normal. Females can only be affected if their fathers are affected AND their mothers are carriers or affecteds. Only females must be tested for carrier status.

If these dogs are identified early, the disorder can be eliminated before they enter the gene pool of their breed.

An example of an x-linked recessive disease is Ectodermal Dysplasia found in German Shepherds and Border Collies.

Counseling for autosomal dominant diseases

An autosomal dominant trait results when a trait is expressed without a pair of matching genes. Only one parent must have the defective gene for the disorder to cause the trait to occur in the offspring.

This type of disorder is easy to eliminate from the gene pool if the onset is early in life, as it is obvious this dog is not a candidate to join the gene pool. However, if the onset is later in life, the dog or bitch has often already been bred. Typically, only one parent carries the genetics for this type of disorder. It may be necessary to test both parents, but it is reasonable to test one at a time to save money. If a DNA test is available, affected animals should be de-sexed and never included in the gene pool. If a DNA test is unavailable, affected dogs should be de-sexed. If the onset is later in life and there is no DNA test available, dogs with the potential of being affected should NOT be used for breeding until they are past the age of onset. For quality male dogs, semen can be frozen while they are young and reserved for use until they are past the age of onset of the disorder to improve the likelihood they are clear before breeding.

If this type of disorder is found to be a new mutation in the germ line, the mutation may appear for the first time in this generation with neither parent affected. It may be possible to have more than one affected offspring in this generation.

Examples of these diseases are Severe Combined Immuno-deficency (SCID) in Pembroke and Cardigan Welsh Corgis, Ehlers-Danlos Collagen deficiency, and dominant PRA in Mastiffs and Bull Mastiffs.

Decision-making on inclusion in a breeding program is more difficult when a large percentage of a breed population is affected by an autosomal dominant disease. Elimination of all affected dogs will allow a faster decrease in the number of affected puppies produced. However, the trade-off is a loss of genetic diversity in the line, leading to 2 outcomes. One is the chance of uncovering or increasing the incidence of another genetic disease due to increased inbreeding coefficients. The other is the loss of other desirable traits, limiting the opportunities in future generations to maintain or improve the breed in future generations.

The alternative to elimination of all affected breeding dogs is to continue to breed affected dogs. Even if an affected dog is bred to an affected bitch, statistically only 50% of their offspring will be affected. The dilemma is how the breeder is to manage finding homes for affected puppies. The breeder would then be counseled to continue to breed affected animals replacing them with the best quality offspring. Once a DNA test becomes available, testing can be applied to determine which dogs should be maintained in the breeding pool.

Genetic counseling for diseases with suspected genetic basis or multiple gene inheritance

Polygenic traits or complex traits are controlled by multiple genes, each of which adds incrementally to the total phenotype.

There are many diseases suspected to be inherited but either the inheritance pattern has not been established or it is suspected this is inherited on multiple genes. These include hip dysplasia, many forms of cancer, allergies, gastric dilatation and volvulus, and immune-mediated diseases.

Even without DNA tests, progress to reduce the incidence in a population is possible. Using results from OFA or PennHIP® and analyzing not only the results of the proposed breeding pair but also including the information from the grandparents and siblings of the parents, it is possible to lower the incidence of the disorder. It must be remembered to factor the other traits of the dogs to be mated into the decision and not to breed for one trait alone.

The future of DNA testing

Progress in DNA profiling has made testing for genetic disorders a rapidly evolving process. Fortunately, internet research allows us to keep up with the advances. A search by dog breed allows us access to current information on tests available. A search by laboratory will provide testing information to the veterinarians – what samples to collect, how to submit them, the fees, and how and where to ship the samples.

It is possible now to offer DNA banking services, either in your own practice or by referring breeders to a company which provides this service. By banking DNA, clients can access the DNA of dogs and bitches important to their breeding program later and evaluate these dogs as new DNA tests become available in the future.

Soon, tests for polygenetic diseases and DNA profiles including thousands of genes will become available. Using DNA profiles and computer programs, we will not only be able to calculate the probability of individual offspring inheriting desirable or undesirable traits, but we will also be able to predict the effect of changing one or several gene frequencies in a dog population over time. As new mutations arise, they have the potential to be singled out and eliminated from the gene pool efficiently. Until recently, many breeders were advised to "outcross" a dog with an unknown defect. "Instead of controlling a trait when there are one or two dogs, or one or two families involved, we outcross the dogs and spread the trait throughout the breed." "This advice has messed up breeds of dogs from the beginning of time," Padgett says. By doing so, instead of diluting the genetic defect out, they inadvertently spread it throughout their breed, infiltrating many pedigrees with this new mutation. (George Padgett, D.V.M., former professor of pathology at Michigan State.)

The power of this genetic manipulation has yet to be seen. There is great potential to improve the health, appearance, and behavior of an entire population. However, if we err, there is great potential for causing harm. Until we understand this power more thoroughly, we must take great care in how we advise clients.

Line breeding

There are two broad categories of mating schemes: inbreeding and outbreeding (or outcrossing). To some degree, mating any two dogs of the same breed is inbreeding. Mating closely related animals is classified as inbreeding – this includes breeding parent to offspring, or breeding full brother to full sister. Here, the breeding coefficient is 50%. Mating less closely related animals together is outbreeding. There is disagreement on how distant a relationship between the two animals needs to be to classify it as an outbreeding. Line breeding is the term used when individuals to be bred have one or more common ancestors on one or both sides (sire or dam's side) of the pedigree in the last five generations. Computer programs have been developed to calculate the breeding coefficient.

Line-breeding is a technique used in many species by breeders. Although not a new technique, it became well-known in dogs when popularized by Lloyd Brackett, a German Shepherd dog breeder in the 1950's. It is most commonly used to produce a group of individuals with similar characteristics, dogs homozygous for a hopefully desired similar characteristic. The desired outcome is to produce a uniform quality of offspring. To produce consistent quality, this generally requires line-breeding for several generations. The advantage of line breeding, especially of having the same dog on both the sire and dams side of the pedigree, is that genes can then pair up and produce a more uniform litter than when an outcross breeding is done. With careful analysis, many breeders have produced quality offspring when breeding siblings to one another or breeding a female back to her father's father. If the breeding co-efficient becomes too high, the breeder may then look to a less closely related dog and breed to produce an "outcrossed" litter.

The disadvantage of line breeding is, at times, it can uncover or magnify traits that were not foreseen. Inbreeding does not cause a mutation that results in an inherited disease, but once such a mutation has occurred, inbreeding will increase the frequency of the mutant version of the gene in the breed more quickly than other more random breeding programs. Until all genetic diseases have a phenotypic or genotypic test available, there is a degree of risk when line-breeding. To effectively and safely line breed a litter, the breeder must be very familiar with individuals in the preceding five generations. Therefore line breeding is not recommended for the breeder who is not experienced or the weak-at-heart breeder. Should a line breeding lead to an unexpected and unfortunate outcome, difficult decisions may need to be made pertaining to the future of the offspring produced.

Line breeding may be necessary to perpetuate a breed with a very small gene pool. AKC records show that in 2002, there were 44 breeds with fewer than 100 pups produced each year for 5 consecutive years (1997 to 2002).

Most experienced breeders will use some degree of line-breeding to produce consistent appearing or consistent performing dogs.

"Founders effect" or "Matador"

At times, a stud dog is used so frequently he can have a disproportionate effect on the gene pool of a breed. This phenomenon, known as "founder's effect" or the sire known as a "matador", can cause the loss of genetic diversity. The concern is that he not only has a positive influence on the breed, but that he can concentrate undesirable traits in the breed. To minimize this possibility, some people have suggested a stud dog should not sire more pups in his lifetime than a bitch could produce.

The advantage of breeding to a frequently used stud dog is that a great deal is known about the offspring he produces. If a stud dog has been used heavily and has produced few pups with undesirable traits, this dog is likely to be more valuable to include in a breeding program than a unknown or unused stud dog with no track record of what they produce.

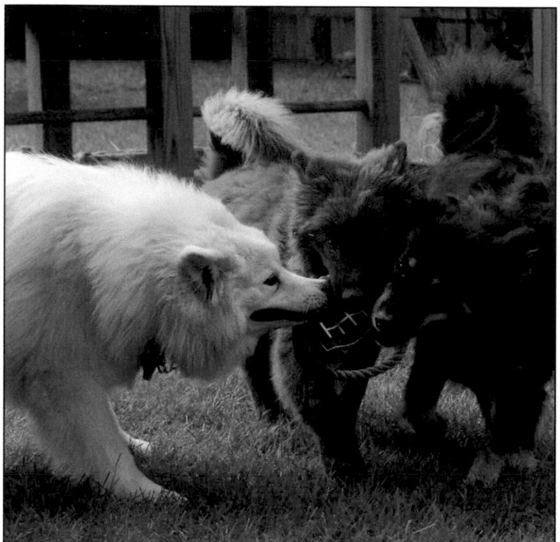

The breeding program

A great challenge, but great tool, in selecting dogs to be used in a breeding program is to follow the pups produced for their lifetime. Encourage your breeder clients to do the following:

Have "puppy parties" where the pups they have bred have reunions. At these events, have someone (not the breeder) videotape the dogs in attendance. With this method, the breeder can speak to the owners of the pups to learn of health histories, temperaments, and accomplishments, and later view video showing their conformation, movement, and behavior (Figure 2-6).

Figure 2-6.
At a puppy party, the breeder has an opportunity to assess offspring for breed type, soundness, temperament, and overall what their breeding program is producing.

On a weekly to yearly basis, suggest the breeder write, e mail or call owners of their pups just to stay in touch. Christmas cards with photos from puppies sold to families can be an invaluable source of information to the breeder.

Arrange to have the offspring's hips (and other joints as indicated) radiographed and have eyes examined, as well as have other screening tests done as dictated by the prevalence of disorders in the breed. Arrangements may be made to do them as a group if the pups live in close proximity to the breeder, when a group discount may be negotiated. OFA offers a significantly reduced fee to read films when they are submitted (not taken) together. This will provide valuable data to the breeder. Some breeders provide a financial incentive such as a reimbursement if the pet owner has these tests or examinations completed. This is usually a fee included in the purchase price of the dog, and terms of the reimbursement and testing required are written into the contract at the time of purchase. It is not enough to know the results of the tests from only the dogs kept by the breeder. Dogs sold as "pets" should be included in the analysis by the breeder to permit a comprehensive assessment of the breeding program.

The perfect dog
Should you use this dog or bitch in your breeding program?
There is no perfect dog! All dogs in breeding programs carry one or more undesirable traits. Yet, to prevent extinction of the breeds we know today, some of these dogs need to be included as breeding stock.

It is critical to recall that dog and cat breeds are closed populations with no new genetics available. Of course, the goal of breeders is to plan matings to avoid the "production" of an affected dog. However, selection based upon only one trait will limit genetic diversity and ultimately will be detrimental to a breeding program. Therefore, harsh elimination of individuals from a breeding pool must be avoided and should not be recommended without discussion of the pros and cons. Instead, with careful selection, carriers can be bred to other carriers or clears, the offspring tested and breeding stock can be replaced with clears.

Summary for counseling clients in genetic selection

1. Do not breed affected dogs unless they carry only a mild or curable disorder. Examples are umbilical hernias and disticihia.
2. Screen all breeding stock for as many disorders as is feasible, based on the tests available and the associated costs.
3. Breed clear to clear whenever possible.
4. Breed clear to carrier when there is a 30% or less incidence of disorder or if this is otherwise a very desirable dog.
5. Test all offspring, not just breeding stock.
6. Select clear in next generation.
7. Do not select only against one disease as this ignores other diseases and will limit the gene pool.

There are many highly qualified breeders who are skilled at evaluating pedigrees and genetic testing, then applying it to develop breeding plans. However, as veterinarians, we must continue to offer this counseling service to our clients or aid them in locating a qualified geneticist to advise them in planning their breeding programs. If we fail to provide this testing and fail to advise our clients on how to use genotype and phenotype results, they will rely on others who may be less able to assist them in collecting data, interpreting test results and applying it to their breeding program. The power of genetic insight has yet to be realized. Used inappropriately, we could do great harm to the genetic diversity of the canine population. Used well, we have great potential to improve the health of the canine population. Our clients depend on us to help them make ethical and scientifically-based decisions. Understanding the basics of genetic selection is an invaluable service we can provide to breeder-clients.

CHAPTER 3
Preparing to Breed

Preparing to breed
Planning the breeding
To successfully orchestrate a breeding, the breeder and the veterinarian must achieve a delicate balance of advance planning for months to years in advance of the breeding and yet retain the ability to be incredibly flexible in thinking and acting at the last possible moment. Additionally, both the breeder and their veterinary staff needs to pay great attention to detail and communicate well.

Most commonly, the breeding is planned by the bitch owner. The bitch owner will approach the stud dog owner to ask for permission to use the dog or his semen for the breeding. The typical breeder has spent untold hours at competitive dog events discussing potential mates for their bitch with his or her colleagues. She or he has pored over breed magazines, visited websites, and scrutinized pedigrees. The breeder has watched the pups produced by the potential stud dog. They have researched and evaluated the health clearances of the stud dog, his get, and other relatives.

The veterinarian's and their staff's role in planning
Clients will find that using a veterinarian who is experienced in handling breedings or one who is willing to learn canine reproduction and is willing to be available outside regular office hours is crucial in making a breeding successful.

It is helpful to train your clients to alert you to their potential needs for your reproductive services so they will notify you and your staff well in advance. This allows staffing arrangements to be made. Very few emergency and referral veterinary hospitals (unless they have a theriogenologist on staff) are in a position to assist with weekend breedings.

If you plan to offer reproductive services to your clients, you must also plan to be available for evening, weekend and holiday calls. This will endear you to your clients, but there is a trade-off in personal time. Therefore, you should charge a fair, but increased fee for after-hours reproductive services. It is appropriate to charge an additional fee for services offered outside of regular hours. This will probably remind clients not to wait till evening hours to call if they are unsuccessful in achieving a natural breeding and need an emergency artificial insemination. Most clients would prefer to pay a slightly higher fee for weekend services than to miss a breeding opportunity that only rolls around twice a year.

If you anticipate offering client services for breedings, there are some special supplies and services you will need to purchase or arrange for in advance:
1. Artificial insemination sleeves, pipettes, and semen extender.
2. Boxes and media for fresh chilled semen shipments.
3. A laboratory with rapid turn-around times for progesterone testing.
4. Method to evaluate semen for morphology, motility, and sperm counts (Hemocytometer and Unopette) or sperm counter.
5. Brucellosis test kit or reference laboratory support.
6. Veterinary assistant to aid in blood and semen collection and inseminations.

The breeder's role in planning
Well in advance, often years, the breeder has been evaluating the line or individual dog that will best suit the line or individual bitch to be bred. If the breeder owns or co-owns the stud dog, the process may be much less complicated. Of course, if they own the stud dog, there is no need to ask consent to use him. However, there are still responsibilities the breeder must bear. The stud dog must still be available (not living elsewhere or at a show/event when he is needed), in good health, and be reproductively sound.

If the stud dog is owned by another breeder, the bitch owner must be in contact with the owner, preferably in advance of her estrous cycle, to alert them that the bitch is going to be ready to breed soon. Of course, they first must agree to allow the stud dog to be used for this bitch. All necessary contracts, health screenings, and other arrangements should be made in advance. The prospective stud must be available, in good health, and still reproductively sound. If he is not available, frozen semen is a great option.

The stud dog owner should be available to receive the bitch for breeding if she will be traveling to the stud dog. If the stud dog is to travel to the bitch, these arrangements must also be planned. In some cases, both the stud dog and bitch will travel to a mutually agreed-upon location for the breeding. Veterinary assistance should be arranged for in advance if intervention is anticipated.

If frozen semen is to be used, paperwork for this must be signed by the stud dog owner and shipping arrangements made. If semen is to be collected and shipped as fresh chilled semen, appropriate shipping and extending supplies must be available in advance. The veterinary staff that will be collecting and shipping the semen should be alerted in advance to allow for staffing arrangements. If a holiday or weekend shipping and/or breeding are anticipated, these arrangements must be planned.

In most cases, progesterone results will require a 24 hour turn-around time. Arrangements for receiving and communicating results should be made so there is no delay in arranging travel of the dogs or shipment of the semen. Invariably, some of this must take place over weekends. Exchanging cell phone numbers and e mail addresses with the veterinary staff, stud dog owner and bitch owner will expedite communication.

All three parties involved, the veterinary staff, the stud dog owner, and the bitch owner need to pay great attention to detail and arrange for communication to occur on short notice, sometimes after routine veterinary hours. As little as a 1 day delay in receiving progesterone results or a semen shipment can jeopardize years of careful planning.

In spite of careful advance planning, bitches ovulate when they find it convenient, lab results get delayed, and shipments get lost. Sometimes stud dogs fail to "perform" as expected. With all the players and variables involved in a breeding, there are times that carefully made plans need to be altered and last minute arrangements made. Breeders and veterinarians alike must be prepared to think on their feet and develop back-up plans when necessary. Changes of plans may be as simple as rescheduling an appointment to another day if the bitch is slow to ovulate. But changes may be more complex, such as changing shipping plans from delivery of the semen to the office to making a dash to the airport to pick up a counter-to-counter shipment, or changing to an alternative stud dog.

Stud dog selection

Ordinarily, stud dog owners will have completed most or all health clearances prior to being contacted by the bitch owner. At the time they are contacted, their role is to:

1. Have a **complete breeding soundness examination** (see Appendix D-6) completed by their veterinarian. This should include palpation of the prostate and testes, evaluation of the penis and external genitalia, and include an ejaculation with sperm count, morphology and motility. He should also be evaluated for his physical ability to mount a bitch if a natural breeding is planned. Any reproductive concerns should be addressed at this visit. If he is over the age of 12 and the litter will be registered with AKC, the examining veterinarian must issue a letter stating he is capable of siring the litter. He should have a health history taken. Any medications such as steroids (oral or topical) that could interfere with his sperm production should be discontinued if medically appropriate.
2. Complete any **health clearances** not current or completed to date. Each breed and family of dogs within a breed has a different set of potential inherited disorders. The attending

veterinarian and breeder should identify which genetic disorders should be screened for. Proper genetic screening for selection of breeding stock can minimize inherited congenital defects. See Chapter 2 for a detailed description of screening tests.

Hips and Other joints: Regardless of size or breed of the dog, there are a variety of joint problems found in most breeds. Hip dysplasia is probably the best known problem. This is a malformation of the ball and socket of the hip joint, found primarily in large breed dogs, which leads to premature development of arthritis in the hips. In many breeds, 30% and up of individuals may be affected. Either OFA hip screening or PennHIP® evaluation should be done prior to breeding. Results are usually not available for up to 4 weeks, so this should be scheduled well in advance of the time semen is needed. Shoulders, elbows, and stifles are other joints frequently evaluated for abnormalities.

Other Genetic Testing: Some breeds may be candidates for other health screens. These include testing for thyroid disease, von Willebrand's disease (a bleeding disorder), heart disease, and deafness to name a few. In addition, dogs exhibiting or carrying genes for certain health problems felt to be inherited such as epilepsy, should not be bred (see Chapter 2).

Temperament: We feel it is important to advise breeders to only include dogs in breeding programs that are happy, confident, well-suited to their function, and obedient, as research indicates temperament is a highly inherited trait. Suggest that the breeders be honest with themselves. Ask them "is this the type of dog YOU like to live with"? "Is the temperament suitable for a dog to be placed in a "pet" household?"

The BIG Picture: No stud dog is perfect. Assist the client in determining selection of the genetics they want to include in their breeding program. Guide them in assessing if the potential inherited health problems may be life-threatening, difficult to live with, or expensive to control or correct. The puppies produced will be the responsibility of the bitch owner, not the stud dog owner and the breeder should be counseled on this prior to the "production" of a litter.

3. Have a **current negative Brucella test report**. Brucellosis is a bacterial disease which is most frequently transmitted between dogs by sexual contact. There are still active cases of <u>Brucella canis</u> in many parts of the United States. This disease has not been eradicated. It is easily screened for on a blood test. Both the male and female dog should be tested prior to EVERY breeding. Brucellosis not only can cause health problems for the adult dogs, but it can also cause sterility, abortion and early puppy death. Of highest concern is that this incurable canine disease is transmissible to humans. In most cases of Brucellosis, euthanasia of all affected dogs is still recommended. Our responsibility to our clients is to educate and inform them that this infection would devastate their breeding programs and could pose a threat to human health (See chapter 9).

4. **Vaginal cultures** are not indicated for routine breedings of healthy bitches with normal vaginal cytology and no history of infertility. It is normal for all bitches to have bacteria in the vagina. A study done by Patricia Olson published in 1978 showed the following microorganisms were commonly isolated from the caudal vagina of adult bitches: staphylococci spp., streptococci spp., <u>E. coli</u>, <u>Pasteurella</u>, <u>Proteus</u>, and Mycoplasma spp.

This study suggests that these bacteria are normal flora of the vagina of the bitch. General consensus is that these bacteria are expected to be found in the reproductive tract of the bitch and serve as a barrier to pathogenic bacterial infections. Routinely administering antibiotics to bitches prior to breeding has been proposed to be harmful, as eliminating normal flora may allow pathogenic bacteria to establish themselves and may allow infections that cannot be treated successfully with antibiotics.

Also to be discussed with the owner of the bitch, if a vaginal culture is mandated by the stud dog owner, is that the stud dog's prepuce is not a sterile environment; normal flora resides there too. There are only rare reports suggesting venereal transmission of bacteria, other than Brucella canis, that caused disease in the dog or bitch.

If the stud dog owner requires vaginal culture pre-breeding, 2 approaches can be made in response. One is to also require culture of the prepuce of the stud dog prior to breeding.

The other is to proceed with the culture and include the results of the vaginal cytology in the culture report, with the interpretation that "a culture of normal bacteria without evidence on cytology of infection or inflammation is a normal finding and does not merit treatment of the bitch with antibiotics prior to breeding".

Should the bitch have a history of infertility, it may be appropriate to do a guarded cranial vaginal culture in early proestrus. If one bacteria cultured is found to predominate over normal flora, suggesting a uterine or vaginal infection, appropriate antibiotic therapy can be initiated in time to breed the bitch on this cycle. Culture only during proestrus. Cultures collected during proestrus allows the culture collected from the vagina to include bacteria from the uterus. Following this protocol allows you to culture material from the uterus without using a surgical or TCI approach.

Anytime the owner is concerned about transmission of any disease or injury to the bitch or stud dog, artificial insemination (vaginal AI) is a reasonable alternative. This will protect only the stud dog, not the bitch, from bacterial disease transmission, but may be sufficient to satisfy a stud dog owner that is adamant about having a "negative" vaginal culture prior to use for natural breeding.

5. Issue a **contract to the bitch owner** – A complete legal discussion of contracts is beyond the scope of the veterinary relationship and this book. However, a few words of advice can be useful for a novice breeder and help assure that you receive payment for your veterinary services. It is recommended that the stud and bitch owners have a written agreement defining the details of the breeding, especially if they are friends! For example, stud fees, which client pays the veterinary fees, and the number of pups guaranteed, are a sampling of topics that need to be defined prior to breeding to avoid any misunderstandings. A contract with the stud dog owner usually will include health clearances the bitch must have completed prior to allowing her to be bred to the chosen stud dog.

6. Arrange for a **veterinary appointment** or for frozen semen to be released.

7. **DNA** will need to be on file or collected if the stud dog is a frequently used sire or if fresh chilled or frozen semen is to be used.

Preparing the bitch for breeding

Ordinarily, the bitch owner has completed all of her health clearances prior to the start of her estrus cycle.

The role of the bitch owner in most cases consists of:

1. Scheduling a **breeding soundness examination** (See Appendix D-6) with her veterinarian.
   Several weeks to months prior to the bitch's heat cycle during which the breeder intends to breed her, the bitch should be examined by her veterinarian. She should be in good general health, current on core vaccines, have good parasite control, and be free from orthopedic problems. Her dental health should be addressed by dental procedures as indicated. Particular attention should be paid to her external genitalia. Mammary glands should be palpated and counted. Mammary tumors, if found, should be removed without removal of the associated nipple if possible. Bitches can still lactate and raise a normal litter if most of their mammary tissue can be retained. If she appears to have a vulva that is small or tips forward, artificial insemination should be discussed. A vaginal digital examination should be attempted at this time. However, anestrous bitches tend to be uncooperative about a thorough evaluation and it can be difficult to fully assess them for strictures or septa at this time. A more complete vaginal examination can be done digitally or with a scope during proestrus. She should not be overweight and should be on a moderate exercise program.

2. Complete any **health clearances** not current or completed to date. Each breed and family of dogs within a breed has a different set of potential inherited disorders. The attending veterinarian and breeder should identify which genetic disorders should be screened for. Proper genetic screening for selection of breeding stock can minimize inherited congenital defects (See Chapter 2).

Hips and other joints. Radiographs of the hips to screen for hip dysplasia should not be taken near the onset of estrus as some females show laxity of the hips around the time of estrus and whelping. It is not recommended to take radiographs of pregnant females during the first trimester (3 weeks of pregnancy). The OFA recommends radiographing three to four weeks before or after the heat cycle, and three to four weeks after weaning a litter of puppies.

Regardless of size or breed of the dog, there are a variety of joint problems found in most breeds. Hip dysplasia is probably the best known problem. This is a malformation of the ball and socket of the hip joint, found primarily in large breed dogs, which leads to premature development of arthritis in the hips. In many breeds, 30% and up of individuals may be affected. Either OFA hip screening or PennHIP® evaluation should be done prior to breeding. Results are usually not available for up to 4 weeks, so this should be scheduled well in advance of the time semen is anticipated to be needed. Shoulders, elbows, and stifles are other joints frequently evaluated for abnormalities.

Other genetic testing: Some breeds may be candidates for other health screens. These include testing for thyroid disease, von Willebrand's disease (a bleeding disorder), heart disease, deafness, eye disorders and so on. Testing for thyroid disease and von Willebrand's disease should not be done during estrus as these test results may be altered during this time. In addition, dogs exhibiting or carrying genes for certain health problems felt to be inherited such as epilepsy, should not be bred. For a complete discussion on health screening (see Chapter 2).

Temperament: It is important to advise breeders to only include dogs in breeding programs that are happy, confident, well-suited to their function, and obedient as new research indicates temperament is a highly inherited trait. Suggest to the breeder to be honest with themselves. Ask them "is this the type of dog YOU like to live with"? "Is the temperament suitable for a dog to be placed in a "pet" household?"

The BIG picture: No bitch or stud dog is perfect. Assist the client in determining selection of the genetics they want to include in their breeding program. Guide them in assessing if the potential inherited health problems may be life-threatening, difficult to live with, or expensive to control or correct. The puppies produced will be the responsibility of the bitch owner, not the stud dog owner and the breeder should be counseled on this prior to the "production" of a litter.

3. **Brucella testing:** Both the dog and bitch should have a **current negative Brucella test report**. Brucellosis is a bacterial disease which is most frequently transmitted between dogs by sexual contact. There are still active cases of Brucella canis in many parts of the United States. This disease has not been eradicated. It is easily screened for on a blood test. Both the male and female dog should be tested prior to EVERY breeding. Brucellosis not only causes health problems for the adult dog, but it can also cause sterility, abortion and early puppy death. Of highest concern is that this incurable canine disease is transmissible to humans. In most cases of Brucellosis, euthanasia of all affected dogs is still recommended. Our responsibility to our clients is to educate and inform them that this infection would devastate their breeding programs and pose a potential threat to human heath.

4. **Health care:** All necessary upcoming (within the next 4 months) core vaccines should be given prior to the start of her estrous cycle. No vaccinations should be administered near the time of the breeding. She should have a negative fecal analysis or be treated if positive. Good parasite control measures (both individual and environmental) should be discussed. Most heartworm preventives and topical/oral flea control products currently on the market are labeled as safe during lactation and pregnancy. Permethrin containing products should not be used during late pregnancy or any time during lactation as the product may translocate on to the pups. However, the label on all products should be evaluated prior to prescribing.

5. Locate a **stud dog** or contact the owner of the dog you plan to use, and arrange the breeding or semen shipment: locating an eligible stud dog with all desired health clearances, Brucella testing, current semen evaluation, and is available when needed for breeding, is the full responsibility of the owner of the bitch. If fresh chilled semen is to be used, the bitch

owner will need to arrange for the availability of the stud dog, make shipping arrangements for the semen, assure there is someone available to receive the shipped semen, arrange appointments to time the bitch, and arrange for the inseminating veterinary clinic to be available and capable of managing the fresh chilled semen shipment and breeding.

If frozen semen is to be used, the bitch owner will need to be certain the semen release forms have been signed by the stud dog owner, the semen shipment has been arranged, the receiving veterinary clinic is aware of the semen shipment, the receiving veterinary clinic is available and capable of handling the frozen semen. Additionally the semen shipping tank needs to be returned in a timely manner to the shipping veterinary clinic, appointments made to time the breeding of the bitch, and ensure that the inseminating clinic is available and capable of managing the frozen semen breeding.

The owner of the bitch is also responsible for completing AKC or other registry forms and arranging for signatures of the stud dog owner(s) and veterinarian to be included.

6. Sign a **contract** with the stud dog owner. A complete legal discussion of contracts is beyond the scope of the veterinary relationship and this book. However, a few words of advice can be useful for a novice breeder and help assure that you receive payment for your veterinary services. It is recommended that the stud and bitch owners have a written agreement defining the details of the breeding, especially if they are friends! For example, stud fees, which client pays the veterinary fees, the number of pups guaranteed, and the health clearances the bitch must have completed prior to considering her for breeding are a sampling of topics that need to be defined prior to breeding to avoid any misunderstandings.

7. Arrange **veterinary appointments** for timing the breeding and breeding assistance. Many natural breedings require little or no veterinary intervention. However, if the stud dog or bitch have a history of reproductive problems, or if the breeding will be done with shipped or frozen semen, veterinary appointments to time the bitch, evaluate semen quality and provide insemination services will be necessary.

8. **Medications during pregnancy:** Pregnancy should be as drug-free as possible but there are a few exceptions.

In a life-threatening situation, medications may be indicated. The risks versus the benefits must be determined on an individual basis. There are a few notable exceptions in the use of medications and vaccines. Panacur® to control parasite migration in the bitch and minimize the exposure of her pups will be discussed in chapter 5. Canine Herpes Virus vaccine, if available, is used during pregnancy to be effective (See chapter 9).

All medications should be handled on a case by case basis. Resources such as Plumb's Veterinary Drug Handbook, The Harriet Lane Handbook (a human book published by Johns Hopkins Hospital), VIN.com, the internet, and package inserts from the pharmaceutical companies are available. In general, if the package insert doesn't say you cannot use a product safely during pregnancy, it means you can use it. If there is a doubt, contact the manufacturer's technical services department. Even over-the-counter and topical medications can affect fetal development and well-being and should be researched before use.

Although most heartworm preventives and some topical/oral flea control products currently on the market are labeled as safe during pregnancy and lactation, all labels should be evaluated prior to prescribing. As the first trimester in the bitch is 3 weeks long (this is the stage of fetal cell differentiation – the period where a teratogenic drug would generally have most of its effects) and heartworm and flea control products only need to be administered every 4 weeks, with a little manipulation, even these medications do not need to be administered during this important phase of tissue differentiation. Imidacloprid (Advantage®) according to the label should NOT be used during pregnancy and praziquantel (Drontal®, IverhartMax®) is labeled as unknown.

If the bitch develops a life-threatening condition and medications are necessary that may threaten the pregnancy, the owner should be consulted on treatment choices before proceeding. In most cases, the owner will elect to treat the bitch and gamble on the pups.

In particular, preparations containing corticosteroids should be avoided. This includes injectable and oral steroids as well as topical medications such as ear and eye medications. In some individuals, sufficient amounts of topical medications including steroids can be absorbed through the skin, eye, or ear to lead to teratogenic effects or abortion. Hydrocortisone is the only corticosteroid documented to be safe during pregnancy. Dogs are more resistant to the pregnancy-termination effects of steroids in the last 2 trimesters of pregnancy than ruminants. Other products to be avoided, unless the bitch's life is at risk are (See also Table 9-1):

Anesthetic agents of all kinds;

Antibiotics: metronidazole, aminoglycosides, chloramphenicol, tetracycline and doxycycline;

Anti-convulsants: primidone and diazepam;

Antifungals: griseofulvin and ketoconazole;

Anti-inflammatory agents: aspirin, DMSO, corticosteroids

Anti-neoplastic agents of all kinds;

Anti-parasiticides: Imidacloprid (Advantage®)

Hormones: mibolerone and other testosterones, progestins such as megestrol acetate, prostaglandins such as Lutalyse® and Estrumate® (cloprostenol), progesterones, estrogens such as DES; *Nutritional supplements:* Excess Vitamin A and Vitamin D, any raspberry tea leaf preparations; other products not approved by the FDA.

9. **Nutrition and dietary supplements:** The bitch should not be overweight and should be on a moderate exercise program. She should also be on a high quality Pregnancy or Performance diet prior to breeding. Research has shown that it requires a minimum of 8 months for a post-partum bitch to return to her pre-pregnancy nutritional status. For bitches that will be bred on back-to-back heat cycles (See Chapter 9), a performance diet can be fed continuously.

Nutritional supplements are generally not necessary for dogs eating a high quality diet. Calcium in particular should NOT be supplemented during pregnancy as it will produce negative feedback to the parathyroid glands and limit calcium mobilization during lactation. Vitamin A should also be avoided in large quantities as it can have a teratogenic effect by producing mid-line defects.

There are conflicting reports on the use of products containing raspberry tea leaves. These products are marketed to increase fertility and ease labor and delivery. However, there are anecdotal reports suggesting some of these products can cause premature labor and abortion. When in doubt, it is better to avoid the use of products without FDA approval for use in the pregnant bitch.

Homemade and raw meat diets are a particular challenge. The concerns are multiple. First is the increased risk of food-born bacterial and parasitic diseases that can affect not only the bitch but also the fetuses. Second is the concern that the diet may be unbalanced – excesses of some nutrients and deficiencies of others; deficiency of Vitamin D is of particular concern. There are anecdotal reports of increased rate of dystocias associated with non-commercial diets. Zoonotic diseases pose a risk to humans handling the food and dogs. Many clients who are devoted to these diets cannot be swayed to feed commercially prepared diets. If however, your client is open to discussing diets, a high quality commercially-prepared pregnancy, performance or puppy diet should be recommended.

Dietary modifications can be made mid-pregnancy at the time an ultrasound confirmation of pregnancy is made.

The most reliable clinical indicator of pregnancy in the bitch is appetite loss between the 3rd and 5th weeks of pregnancy. Most bitches miss a few meals or pick at their food; few vomit so this is seldom severe enough to require veterinary intervention. At this time, the owner can feed canned dog food or add yogurt, cooked meat or eggs to the diet until her appetite returns. Unless the appetite loss is long-standing or she vomits to the extent that she may dehydrate or suffer from nutritional insufficiency, no intervention is necessary.

10. **Exercise:** For bitches bred naturally, or by vaginal or transcervical inseminations, during the first 5 weeks after breeding, no significant changes need to be made in their activity level. The primary limitation should be to keep them from overheating. Sometimes even light work in the field on moderately warm days can lead to higher-than-normal body temperatures so this is to be avoided.

    During the last 3 to 4 weeks of pregnancy, exercise should be more restricted as the uterus is heavy, most bitches will be mildly anemic, her lung capacity diminished and the blood supply is diverted to the uterus. Swimming should be avoided close to term to reduce the chance of introducing organisms into the reproductive tract. Avoid activity that may cause overheating or potential abdominal trauma.

    If the bitch has been surgically bred, she should rest for 3 to 5 days post-op and should not swim for 14 days post-op.
11. **DNA:** There are no dog registries in the United States requiring DNA on bitches.
12. **Pregnancy diagnosis:** Even prior to the breeding, the owner of the bitch should be advised to look ahead to their schedule and that of the veterinary team to assure services can be performed when needed.

    Ultrasound: Early diagnosis of pregnancy is best achieved via ultrasound. The earliest time for this to be performed is approximately 4 weeks after ovulation. This can vary with the ultrasound equipment and veterinarian performing the diagnostics and should be scheduled according to each veterinarian's preferences. Ultrasound can be performed from the 4th week of pregnancy until the date of delivery.

    Radiographs prior to whelping: This is the single most accurate way to assess litter size and predict dystocias. These should be performed 55 to 59 days after ovulation.
13. Veterinary care at the time of **whelping**. Although it sounds like there is plenty of time to arrange this between the time of the breeding and the whelping, the breeder is well-advised to make arrangements for possible or necessary veterinary intervention prior to the breeding.
14. Veterinary care in the **immediate post-partum period**. Many whelpings and neonatal care require little veterinary intervention. However, the veterinarian and the client may wish to arrange for a contingency plan well in advance of the time of the whelping.
15. **Veterinary care of the litter prior to sale.** Pups should have individual physical examinations with complete written reports of findings, vaccinations, and parasite control prior to their placement in new homes. This appointment can take an hour or more and it may be helpful to the veterinary staff and client to schedule this appointment well in advance.

    If pups are being sold out of state or out of the country, government issued health certificates may be required. If the pup will be transported by air cargo, a letter of acclimation should be provided.

Timing the bitch for breeding

Bitches usually reach puberty between 6 and 9 months of age, but this may occur as early as 4 months in small breeds and as late as 24 months in giant breeds. It is often recommended that a female not be bred until her second or third heat cycle, and older than 2 years if OFA certification is expected. Waiting until the bitch has had several heat cycles assures she has reached her full size and maturity prior to breeding. Most dogs have two heats or estrous cycles a year, approximately 6 months apart, usually in spring and fall.

The estrous cycle can be divided into 4 parts. The first, called proestrus, is the part where the vulva swells and a bloody vaginal discharge occurs. It lasts approximately 7 to 12 days and the bitch is neither fertile nor will she accept the male during this time. However, males, especially those without experience, are frequently attracted to the bitch at this time. The second part, called estrus, lasts 5 to 7 days. During this stage, there is usually a straw colored discharge (sometimes with blood). Ovulation occurs at this time, the bitch is fertile and will usually accept the male for breeding. The third and fourth parts are called metestrus and diestrus respectively. During this time, the bitch is not fertile and is not interested in the male.

The usual protocol for breeding a female without progesterone timing is to breed her on days 12 and 14 after the onset of vaginal bleeding. At this time, the vaginal discharge is straw colored and the vulva lips are softer. Two or possibly 3 natural breedings are ideal and adequate for a good conception rate.

When is it necessary to time the breeding?

It is often important to evaluate the bitch in order to estimate the ideal time for breeding. This is necessary if the dog or bitch will be traveling a long distance for breeding, if fresh chilled or frozen semen is to be used, or in dogs that have a history of being difficult to breed. Accurate timing of ovulation is essential when a C-section is planned. Testing at the time of ovulation can increase conception rates and save time, money and puppies at the end of the pregnancy.

Vaginal cytology

A vaginal cytology is an evaluation commonly done. For many years, this was our only practical tool with which to time breedings.

To do this procedure;
1. A 6 inch clean cotton swab (this does not need to be sterile) moistened with saline is gently placed dorsally well up into the vagina while the bitch is being restrained,
2. the cells are carefully rolled onto a microscope slide,
3. the slide is stained with a Dif-Quik® type stain, and
4. the slide is examined microscopically for cell types in the vaginal fluid.

The cells seen at the ideal time for breeding are a high percentage of cornified epithelial cells, with few red blood cells (RBC's), white blood cells (WBC's) or debris. The vaginal smear may also indicate the presence of other problems such as vaginitis. The test is simple, safe, inexpensive, well tolerated by the bitch approaching estrus, and very helpful in timing breedings.

Examination of a single smear can provide useful information, but can also be misleading. For example, it is often difficult to differentiate proestrus and diestrus from an isolated smear. It is most useful to evaluate multiple smears taken of the same bitch. These slides can be labeled with the date collected and stored for evaluation sequentially as she moves through her estrus cycle to monitor trends in cellular cornification.

Proestrus

The bitch develops swelling of the vulva with variable blood-tinged vaginal discharge. Males may become interested, but she is usually not receptive to mounting at this time.

As serum concentrations of estrogen rise during proestrus, red blood cells leak through uterine epithelium and appear in the vaginal discharge. The vaginal epithelium proliferates which leads to a change of epithelial cells from round faintly staining epithelial cells to intermediate and parabasal cells which stain more intensely and are more angular on the edges. Typically, red blood cells are present in large numbers and few neutrophils should be seen. Large numbers of extracellular bacteria are also often present.

Estrus

The period of behavioral estrus is variable; it may last several days before and after cytologic estrus or it may never occur. Typically, the bitch will have a softer vulva with a straw colored discharge, and she will probably flag (hold her tail to one side, if she has one) and stand solidly when pressure is applied over her rump.

As estrogen levels begin to drop and progesterone levels begin to rise above 2 ng/dl, the vaginal cytology is predominated by cornified epithelial cells, large darkly staining angular epithelial cells without an identifiable nucleus. Some bitches will undergo full cornification, that is 100% of the cells present are of this type. However, some bitches will not exceed 70% and some will continue to show red blood cells on the cytology throughout estrus. This is one reason vaginal cytology is not specific enough to be used exclusively for challenging cases. The other reason vaginal cytology alone is insufficient for timing breedings is that the cytology will remain cornified for up to 7 days, but the bitch's peak fertility lasts only 2 to 3 days, and fragile semen is viable for 12 to 24 hours. No white blood cells should be seen.

If the bitch has been bred within a day of preparing a vaginal smear, it is possible that sperm will be observed among the epithelial cells. Indeed, careful examination for sperm in a smear taken within a few hours of an alleged breeding is a fairly reliable means of confirming such an incident. However, not identifying sperm on a vaginal cytology cannot be used to assure a breeding did not take place.

As estrus progresses, progesterone levels rise from a baseline of to <2 ng/dl to 5 ng/dl at ovulation and continue to rise.

Metestrus I
The onset of metestrus is marked by a rapid decline in the number of superficial angular cells and reappearance of rounder nucleated intermediate and parabasal cells. White blood cells may appear in large numbers but do not look active. There are usually no red blood cells present. Most commonly, the cellular profile changes within a single day from essentially 100% superficial cells to less than 20% superficial cells. However, it is best to confirm the onset of metestrus by examining a smear prepared on metestrus day 2. Identifying the onset of metestrus is a considerably more accurate predictor of the time of ovulation than the onset of cornification, and hence gestation length. Dogs ovulate 5 to 7 days before the onset of metestrus so gestation length is calculated to be 57 days ± 1 day from the onset of metestrus day 1. At this time, progesterone levels are high, usually 20 ng/dl or higher.

However, this change is not helpful in determining the ideal time to breed because it only provides historical information. Breedings done during metestrus are rarely fertile as the cervix is usually closed.

Diestrus or Metestrus II
Diestrus lasts approximately 60 days. On vaginal cytology, there are few cells, but the cells present are noncornified with some white blood cells, bacteria and debris, similar to those seen in anestrus. Progesterone levels are high, usually 20 ng/dl or above and stay high for approximately the entire 60 days.

Anestrus
The bitch should not be attractive to male dogs and typically is not receptive to his advances. Non-cornified cells are the predominant cell type present. Other cell types are present in small numbers. There is typically no vaginal swelling, odor, or discharge. Progesterone levels during anestrus should be less than 1 ng/dl.

Progesterone testing
A quantitative progesterone blood test is the single <u>most accurate</u> method for timing breedings. The test is reported as a numeric result, usually in ng/dl. Combined with observing the behavior of the dog and the bitch, vaginal cytology, LH testing and vaginoscopy, ovulation can be pinpointed with great accuracy in most bitches (Figure 3-1).

Progesterone levels are the preferred assay for detecting ovulation. They are commercially available. Human assays can be used. The progesterone results are highly reproducible when run at different reference labs. The results are very accurate and easily interpreted.

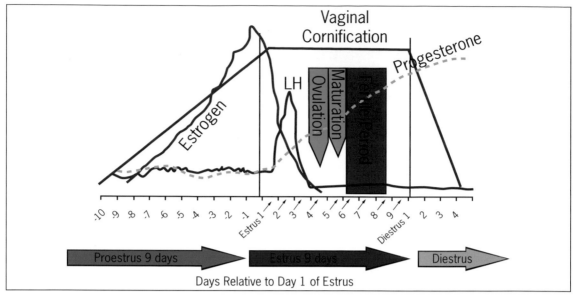

Figure 3-1.
Progesterone Graph, courtesy of Dr. Bruce Eilts.

An exact progesterone level is also needed when the dog or bitch will be traveling a long distance for breeding, when fresh chilled or frozen semen is to be used, or when breeding dogs or bitches that have a history of being difficult to breed. In addition, an exact progesterone level for timing ovulation is necessary when a C-section is anticipated or when the bitch is near term and fetal survivability needs to be assessed.

It is generally thought that most missed breedings or small litters are due to poorly timed breedings. Therefore, to maximize fertility, accurate timing is essential. There are many reasons why accuracy in timing bitches for breeding is essential.

They include:
1. Availability of semen, particularly frozen semen, is often very limited.
2. Frozen semen has a short life-expectancy once thawed – probably 12 to 24 hours or less.
3. If a breeding is unsuccessful, the stud dog and bitch will be at least 6 months older by the next opportunity to breed. Both the bitch and stud dog's fertility diminishes every year.
4. Bitches normally cycle twice a year, not as frequently as other domestic species such as cats.
5. Bitches often have only 4 to 8 available fertile cycles in their reproductive lifetime.
6. Every breeding and pregnancy carries with it some risk to the bitch so we need to make every breeding count by producing as many pups per litter as physiologically possible.
7. Breedings can be expensive when calculating shipping dogs or semen, paying stud fees, paying for inseminations and veterinary consultations.
8. Veterinarians and breeders prefer to be successful in their breeding attempts.

A serum sample from the bitch to be timed can be sent to many reference laboratories for quantitative progesterone testing throughout the United States and other countries. **(See appendix A-4)** Many of these commercial labs have courier services. If this service is not available, the veterinary clinic or the client can ship the serum sample in a padded envelope overnight to a referral lab. In some cases, local human hospital laboratories may be available to run these samples as progesterone is not a canine-specific assay. There are some veterinary clinics that have a high enough volume of progesterone samples that they have purchased equipment (Immulite, Tosoh, or Mini-Vidas) to run quantitative progesterone samples in their veterinary clinics. In these veterinary hospitals, results are typically available within a few hours. This service is valuable when courier service is unavailable (weather or holidays) or waiting for results the following day is unacceptable.

The sample should be placed in a plain red top non-barrier tube (not an SST tube), spun down within 30 minutes of clotting, and the serum transferred into a labeled transport tube. The serum should be refrigerated and kept chilled until it is received by the lab. If the sample is not going to be run immediately, the sample can be kept stable by freezing. Progesterone appears to be stable during shipping. (Personal conversation with Dr. Fran Moore at Marshfield Veterinary Laboratory)

A semi-quantitative test to estimate progesterone levels can be done in many veterinary offices. These commercially available test kits are run on serum in wells or on membranes. Unlike the quantitative results from reference labs, they are read as a color change, not as a number. They are useful for estimating breeding and whelping, but are not specific enough to use for frozen semen breedings and more challenging cases (Figure 3-2).

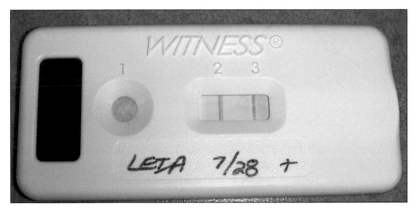

Figure 3-2.
LH test showing a line in the "positive" position.

A **LH** (Luteinizing Hormone) (See Figure 3-2) peak test can also be run if it is necessary to specifically pinpoint the time of ovulation. Unlike progesterone which can be run as a human sample, this is a canine-specific test and can only be run on the commercially available canine LH kit. In the dog, LH is the hormone that causes ovulation. However, this peak is very short-lived. Because of this, the test requires daily testing with the blood sample drawn at the same time every day. Although this is the most specific way to determine the date of ovulation, for many dogs and many clients, this becomes impractical. Some veterinarians use them in conjunction with vaginal cytology and progesterone testing. In some veterinary clinics, each serum sample that is drawn for progesterone testing is frozen, and when ovulation is detected based on progesterone rise, the serum from 48 hours prior is thawed and the LH peak test is run. If this sample pinpoints ovulation, the breeding is done 5 to 6 days AFTER the LH surge, if the progesterone level is also high enough (over 20 ng/ml). If the first LH test does not pinpoint ovulation, the samples drawn at 24 and 72 hours prior to the progesterone rise are run one at a time in an effort to determine the ideal time to breed.

Progesterone interpretation

(See figure 3-1)
The canine's reproductive cycle is unlike any other species. This is probably the most confusing part of canine reproduction. Many breeders and many veterinarians do not understand the cycle well until they see it graphed. Once you understand that progesterone rises slowly and stays high throughout the cycle, it all becomes clear. The letter in Appendix C-9 can be used to communicate to veterinarians when the progesterone testing and breedings are not being done at the same hospital.

At the start of the estrous cycle, proestrus, the estrogen levels are rising. The hormone of interest, progesterone, of the bitch is at a very low level, less than 2 ng/ml. This is often referred to as "baseline." During proestrus in a normal bitch that has started estrus spontaneously (without drug or hormone intervention), the first progesterone level should be run on day 5 to day 6 of her cycle.

For bitches who have had their cycles initiated with drugs or hormones (see Chapter 8) or those with a history of infertility, it is recommended to start progesterone testing on day 3 of the cycle. The progesterone level should be repeated approximately every 3 days when it is below 3.0 ng/ml. It is common to see the level rise and fall in the range of 0.4 ng/ml and 3.0 ng/ml. This does not indicate that you have missed her progesterone rise. (Once the progesterone reaches 5, it will continue to rise into double digits so don't worry yet).

As the bitch enters estrus, she approaches her fertile period and her progesterone level will rise above 2 ng/ml. She will become increasingly attractive to the male and receptive to his advances. This slight rise is often called the initial rise. Its only significance is that you will want to monitor her progesterone levels more closely now as she is about to ovulate. Bitches are only fertile for a few short days during estrus, not for the entire time they are in estrus.

As the progesterone rises above 2 ng/ml, continue to draw serial serum samples for testing, usually every 1 to 3 days.

Ovulation is thought to occur when the progesterone level reaches 5 ng/ml. **This may be the single most important concept regarding breeding in this book.** The bitch's ovary responds to LH from the pituitary, which allows the release of one egg from each of many multiple mature follicles.

But stop: it is too early to breed if you are using fresh chilled or frozen semen. When the bitch ovulates, the eggs are not yet mature and ready to fertilize. Unlike in other species, the eggs mature over next 48 hours before they are ready to fertilize. The timing of the breeding must occur when when the eggs are mature and ready to fertilize and viable semen is in the oviduct, estimating how long the semen is anticipated to survive in the reproductive tract (Figure 3-3).

Breeding with fresh semen, by either natural breeding or vaginal AI with fresh semen, can be done on the day of ovulation, when the progesterone level reaches 5 ng/ml. Although the eggs are not mature yet, most fresh semen is viable enough to survive in the bitch's reproductive tract until the eggs are ready.

Breeding with fresh chilled semen should be delayed until approximately 48 hours after ovulation. Fresh chilled semen usually will not survive as long in the reproductive tract as fresh semen. If the fresh chilled semen is deposited vaginally or directly into the uterus 2 days post-ovulation, the eggs should be fertile when the semen appears in the oviduct.

Breeding with frozen semen should be delayed even longer, 60 to 80 hours after ovulation (Ovulation occurs when the progesterone is at 5 ng/ml). It is thought most frozen semen will only live 12 to 24 hours (or less) in the reproductive tract. For this reason, the semen should arrive in the oviduct when the eggs are mature and ready to fertilize. If necessary to choose, it is better to breed slightly too late than slightly too early. Most breedings with frozen semen are done by depositing the semen directly

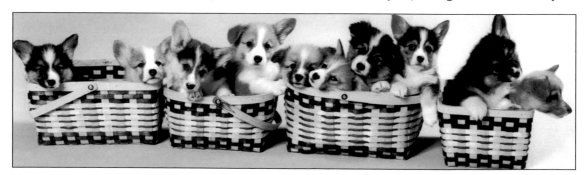

Figure 3-3.
Timing is everything – 10 pups from one well timed vaginal insemination.

into the uterus, usually by surgical insemination but in some cases by transcervical insemination.

Once the progesterone level is 5 ng/dl we are still not done testing. Although it is believed that ovulation occurs around the time the bitch's progesterone level reaches 5 ng/ml, we still need to keep our eye on one more number; that number is a progesterone level of 20 ng/ml. To assure that ovulation is complete and the progesterone level is high enough to maintain a pregnancy, delay either the final or the surgical insemination until the progesterone level has reached or exceeded 20 ng/ml.

After ovulation and breeding are completed, the progesterone level will continue to rise. The level typically rises to 40 to 50 ng/ml (the normal range can be 10 to 90) whether the bitch is bred, pregnant, or not. An elevated progesterone level only indicates that the corpus lutea in the ovaries can support a pregnancy, not that the bitch is pregnant. Bitches maintain this level unless they have ovarian or uterine pathology.

Vaginoscopy

Vaginoscopy is the visual evaluation of the lining of the vagina with a lighted scope. This can be done with either an otoscope (clean otoscope tip please), a rigid pediatric proctoscope or with an endoscope, either rigid or flexible.

Anestrus: There are few folds at this time–the mucosa is thin, red and relatively flat, with no discharge normally noted.

Proestrus: The vaginal lining is pink, puffy, round, and edematous and there is red clear fluid present.

Estrus: The vaginal lining is white to pale and deeply wrinkled. A smaller quantities of red fluid is still present.

Metestrus and Diestrus: The vaginal lining returns to a smoother, less wrinkled, thinner look, with a more pink color. There is little fluid present.

Vaginoscopy is useful both in timing the bitch for breeding and for assessing for vaginal pathology, such as strictures.

CHAPTER 4
Orchestrating the Breeding
Natural and Special Breeding

Scheduling the breeding appointment
(Appendix B-1)

Table 4-1 Important scheduling considerations	
Reason for Appointment	Request for assisted breeding or unsuccessful attempts to breed male and female
Ask client and pet name	Name of both male and female owners – including co-owners who may need permission to access information.
How soon to schedule Appt/**Urgency**	Often need to schedule for same day, at least to test female's progesterone level so the breeding is not missed.
Length of Appointment	Advise the client that they may be at the hospital for a long appointment – if in-house progesterone testing or surgical breeding is to be done the day of the appointment.
Time to Schedule	If a progesterone level is needed, schedule accordingly to allow for test results and breeding is to be done prior to the end of the day.
Dr to Schedule With	
Request Client to **Bring** with them to Appt	IF THEY ARE PLANNING TO BREED THE DAY OF THE APPOINTMENT, THEY MUST BRING BOTH THE MALE AND FEMALE WITH THEM. Recent Progesterone and Brucella test results. History of past breedings for both male and female
To **Ask** Client Before Appt	
Special **Instructions** Client Should Know About Their Appt	If we are unable to collect the stud dog's semen, the stud dog owner must give us consent to administer medication to aid him. If the stud dog proves to be unsuitable, do they have a "back-up" stud dog they can access or bring along?
New Client	10 minutes in advance to complete paper work.
Finalizing	Repeat time, date, phone number, and doctor.

The "Normal" breeding
The "normal" breeding generally takes place outside of the hospital with no veterinary intervention. Most veterinarians and veterinary staff have never seen a breeding and its associated tie unless they are personally involved in breeding dogs. Nevertheless, it is important to know something about this so that you are in a position to assist clients if veterinary intervention is indicated.

Timing the breeding without veterinary intervention and progesterone testing
The usual recommendation for breeding the female is to breed her on days 12 and 14 after the onset of vaginal bleeding. At this time, the vaginal discharge changes from blood-tinged to straw colored and the vulva lips soften. Two or possibly 3 breedings are considered to be ideal and adequate for a good conception rate when breeding a young healthy bitch to a young healthy stud dog.

The best guideline based on observed behavior (without using timing tests) is to introduce the male to the female daily starting day 9 after the onset of bleeding. Allow them to breed as soon as the female will accept the male and repeat at 24 to 48 hour intervals until the female will no longer accept the male. The most challenging aspect of this untimed approach is to calculate a whelping date or to know when to intervene at the end of a pregnancy when precise ovulation dates are not documented with progesterone testing.

When selecting a male for an inexperienced female, it is best that he be experienced but not overly aggressive, and vice versa. It is a good idea to introduce the dog and bitch to one another prior to breeding, but not to allow them to become too familiar as this may diminish the chance that they will breed.

When initially introduced, the male and female will usually check each other out, sometimes with caution and sometimes with great enthusiasm. This should be supervised to protect either from harm. However, it may be necessary for one or more owners to leave. If the dog or bitch may have been told "no" too many times by that individual, the result will be a reluctance to relax and interact with the other dog appropriately.

Conventional wisdom told us the male did all the approaching and all of the "work" of breeding. However, Ian Dunbar and others have shown us that in addition to being receptive, the female plays a critical role in foreplay, positioning herself, and intromission.

After some introductions and attempts of the female mounting the male and the male mounting the wrong end of the female, Mother Nature usually takes over and the stud dog at least finds the right position. He should mount the bitch, hold her at the hips with his front legs, she should flag (move her tail off to one side, if she has one), she should stand steady, and he should attempt to insert his penis into her vulva. This may take several attempts. Some stud dogs will allow a handler (owner or veterinary staff) to assist them, others will quickly dismount or even become aggressive if approached.

The tie

Observing a "tie" between the male and female is the best indication that a successful breeding occurred. The tie occurs because the bulb of the male's penis engorges with blood once inside the female's vagina and remains enlarged for approximately 15 to 30 minutes. A tie is normal and should not be misinterpreted that the dogs are stuck together. No attempt should be made to separate the dog and bitch as this could harm both the male and female physically and psychologically for future breedings. Although a tie is normal and occurs with most natural breedings, an "outside tie", when the male ejaculates and does not maintain a tie, can still be a fertile breeding.

Problems with natural breedings

If the stud dog is incapable of intromission or is tiring, is at risk from an aggressive bitch, or the bitch seems to exhibit pain when he is attempting to insert his penis, the handler should intervene. Intervention should occur before the stud dog is too exhausted to use for an AI, before one of the dogs is injured, or before the only sample you might get is ejaculated onto the floor.

Several possibilities exist for difficulty in achieving a tie:
1. **Incorrect timing:** Either too early or too late – this is the most common cause of breeding failure.
2. **Incompatibility of size:** The stud dog is mismatched in size to the bitch, even when both are the same breed.
3. **Incompatibility of temperament:** Sometimes one doesn't like the other.
4. **Physical limitations:** Back pain, other orthopedic pain, phimosis, prostate or other male genital pain, penile frenulum, small vulva, vaginal stricture, vaginal septum, vaginal hyperplasia, vaginal tumor, or other vaginal disorder.
5. **Low libido:** Low libido of either the stud dog or bitch.
6. A bitch or stud dog who has been **trained to overcome** their natural tendency to breed.

When to intervene to assist in breeding or "The phone call from a desperate client"

Often, the first contact your receptionist will have with a client is after they have made several unsuccessful attempts to do a natural mating. At this point, the dogs and owners are usually frustrated and tired.

The best recommendation your staff can make is to schedule an appointment to bring both the bitch and stud dog in to your office for evaluation, on the day of the call whenever possible. This situation may not sound like an emergency, but if you fail to schedule the appointment ASAP, the breeding may be missed on this heat cycle. Breeder clients will know they are running out of time when they make the phone call. Both the dog and bitch will need an evaluation to assess the reason for the failed attempts to breed, so should both be presented at the appointment.

The bitch
(Appendix A-10)
1. Complete physical examination (Appendix D-6) including visual, which could include scoping, and digital examination of the vagina to assess for size of the vulva, position of the vulva and for vaginal strictures or septa. If an abnormality is present, a vaginal AI can be performed. If there is a structural abnormality, the client should be advised that a C-section may be necessary – this should be discussed BEFORE the AI is completed.
2. Comparative size of the bitch to the stud dog – she may be too tall or too short. If so, a vaginal AI may be all that is necessary to complete the breeding.
3. Vaginal cytology to assess the stage of her estrus cycle.
4. Progesterone testing
   If the vaginal cytology suggests she is in proestrus and this is supported by a progesterone level of less than 5 ng/ml, simple patience and perhaps another visit for progesterone testing may be all that is necessary.
   If the vaginal cytology suggests she is in estrus and the progesterone is between 5 ng/ml and 25 ng/ml, a vaginal AI is indicated soon to be certain the breeding is completed.
   If the vaginal cytology suggests she is in anestrus, you can assess if she has been in estrus in the last 60 to 90 days. If so, the client can relax until she starts her next cycle. At that time, she should be presented early in her cycle for timing.
   Breeding without a progesterone result or vaginal cytology can lead to late breedings, resulting in an abnormally small litter. This concern should be discussed with the client prior to the insemination to be certain they are willing to cope with a one puppy litter.
5. Some bitches, regardless of their physical structure and phase of their heat cycle, will not breed with the selected stud dog. This can be due to her temperament, or caused by her particular dislike for the individual male selected by a human to be her mate. In this case, unless it is too late in her cycle to do the breeding, a vaginal AI is an easy solution to this situation.

The stud dog
(Appendix A-9)
1. Complete physical examination (Appendix D-6) including a visual examination of the penis, palpation of the prostate, and palpation of the testes and scrotum. (See chapter 10 for a complete discussion of these abnormalities.) The male should also have an orthopedic evaluation to determine if his back and rear limbs are capable of supporting his weight to allow mounting the bitch.
2. Comparative size of the bitch to the stud dog – she may too tall or too short relative to the male. If so, a vaginal AI may be all that is necessary to complete the breeding.
3. Some stud dogs, regardless of their physical structure and phase of the bitch's heat cycle, are not willing to breed the selected bitch. This can be due to low libido, a fearful temperament, a previous negative experience when bred or with this individual female, or his particular dislike for

the individual female selected by a human to be his mate. In this case, unless it is too late in her cycle to do the breeding, a vaginal AI may be the solution IF he can be collected. If the individual female is the limitation to the collection, finding a different female to use as a teaser bitch, in estrus if possible, may allow the stud dog to relax and allow semen collection (Figure 4-1).

Some of your clients have a microscope and the skills to accurately evaluate semen and vaginal cytologies. The information they gain may be of great value to your ability to assist them. Even without a microscope, you may have clients make their own vaginal cytology slides and deliver them to your office every 3 or 4 days for evaluation. This allows you to follow the estrous cycles on bitches who have been historically difficult to breed.

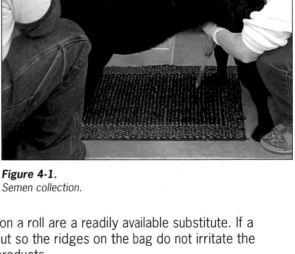

Vaginal artificial inseminations
(See chapter 10)
Vaginal insemination of the bitch in standing heat is a relatively easy procedure to perform. All that is required is a stud dog that is cooperative to collect, a few simple pieces of equipment, and a willing assistant to aid in positioning the bitch (Figure 4-2).

Figure 4-1.
Semen collection.

Supplies and equipment
1. **AI sleeve and labeled tube,** preferably disposable. If this is not available, a clean plastic bag will do. Plastic baby bottle liners on a roll are a readily available substitute. If a Ziploc bag is to be used, turn it wrong-side out so the ridges on the bag do not irritate the penis. Avoid the use of any latex-containing products.
2. **6 to 12 cc syringe,** preferably one without a latex stopper.
3. **AI pipette,** small animal size for most dogs. These are approximately 6 inches long. They should be clean, and disposed of after each use, but do not need to be sterilized. If this is not available, a large animal pipette can be used and not fully inserted. The longer version should not be cut off as it will leave a sharp edge. As a third choice, a soft tube such as a new sterile red rubber feeding tube can be substituted.
4. **Semen extender** – not essential but helpful for compromised semen.
5. **Microscope slide,** cover slip and microscope – to evaluate semen motility, morphology, and to estimate numbers.
6. **Exam gloves** – non-latex gloves, with the outer surface rinsed free of glove powder before use.
7. **A non-slip surface** – for good footing for the bitch and stud dog.
8. **A short flight of stairs or stool** – to keep the bitch's rear quarters elevated.
9. **A unopette** (or other suitable diluent) and **hemocytometer** – if a sperm count is to be performed.

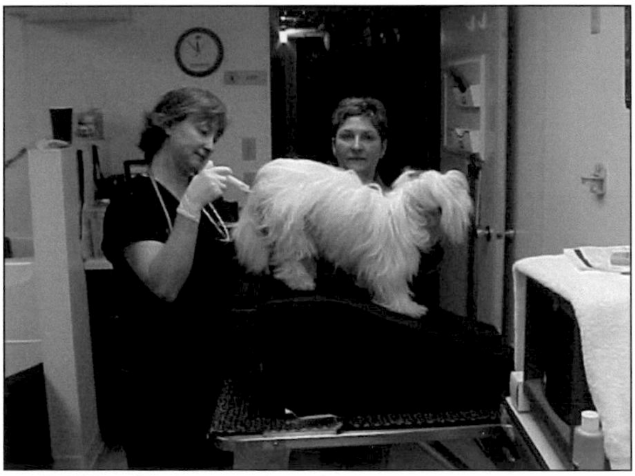

Figure 4-2.
Vaginal artificial insemination with hind quarters elevated.

Step by step vaginal insemination in the bitch
(Appendix D-1)

1. Allow the bitch to urinate before beginning.
2. After the semen is collected, with as little prostatic fluid collected as possible, the volume should be measured. The semen should be examined shortly after collection on a warm slide with a warm coverslip. The semen sample should be evaluated for motility while warm. After the semen has cooled, and before it dries out, morphology is easier to perform.
3. Add the semen extender in a 2 to 1 ratio of extender to semen, not to exceed 4 cc in a small bitch and 8 cc in a large bitch.
4. Aspirate the semen into the syringe through the pipette. Avoid bubbling air through the semen while handling.
5. Position the bitch on a short flight of stairs, stool, ramp, or an assistant's lap while the assistant is seated, to elevate the hindquarters of the bitch while allowing no pressure on her ventral abdomen.
6. The veterinarian or veterinary technician handling the semen should wear non-latex gloves that have been rinsed with tap water and dried.
7. Cleanse the vulvar lips with a small amount of chlorhexidine, then rinse, only if there is obvious contamination. No lubrication is normally needed for a bitch in standing heat. Only if needed, use non-spermicial lubricant.
8. With one hand, part the lips of the vulva. Hold the syringe with the pipette attached with the opposite hand. Slip the pipette between the lips of the vulva at the dorsal commissure, directing the pipette upward at approximately a 45 degree angle. Gently advance the pipette in an upward direction, then when the pipette is approximately half-way in, redirect the pipette more parallel with the floor. In all but very small bitches, the pipette should advance nearly its full length into the vagina. Stop and redirect if resistance is met or the bitch seems uncomfortable. It is important to enter the vagina dorsally to avoid placing the semen in the urethra (you would never hit the urethra if you needed to, but of course you will if you are inseminating.)
9. Slowly depress the syringe plunger to deliver the semen into the cranial vagina. If the semen flows out around the pipette, stop and reposition the pipette.
10. Maintain the bitch in the rear quarters elevated position for approximately 5 minutes. While she is in this position, stimulate her around the perineum by rubbing the area with a gloved hand. Avoid latex contact with semen. An Osiris Catheter may be used to aid in blocking retrograde flow of semen after insemination. These are now available in the U.S.
11. Have the owner return the bitch directly to the car without allowing her to stop to urinate and without lifting her with pressure under her abdomen.

Handling fresh chilled semen
Step by step fresh chilled semen collected at your veterinary clinic to be shipped to a recipient veterinary clinic
(This is available as a client handout in Appendix C-1)

1. Remind your client to contact both the shipping and receiving veterinary clinics as early in the bitch's estrus as possible to assure that staff, supplies, and shipping methods are available when needed. Be sure the recipient veterinary clinic's address is available and accurate.
2. Confirm that the dog and bitch are both in good health, have had health screening, such as OFA and eye exams, completed in advance, negative Brucella tests in the past 3 months, and are current on immunizations and preventive worming. Consider having a semen analysis with test chill done on the male to be used to assure he is currently fertile and his semen ships well.
3. Upon confirmation of the date(s) the semen is to be shipped, call to schedule an appointment. Collections for shipment are best done early in the day to allow adequate time for the courier service to arrange for pickup. This will help assure timely delivery of the semen. The semen, once collected, is typically viable for 24 hours or longer, depending on the semen

health and extender used; delayed insemination reduces the chance of a breeding resulting in a pregnancy. The inseminating veterinarian also needs time to schedule the bitch for insemination.

4. Inform the receiving veterinarian if additional semen shipments are requested. Frequently when using fresh chilled semen, two collections are made and shipped.

5. DNA testing of the stud dog is required (if not previously done) to register the litter with the AKC. This test is a simple cheek swab, collected at the appointment. The owners signature and payment are required for submission to the AKC. A color DNA certificate, which includes the dog's DNA profile number, will be mailed directly to the owner of the stud dog.

6. The collecting veterinarian may sign the AKC paperwork (should be completed prior to this by the stud dog owner) for insemination with fresh chilled semen at the first shipment. The stud dog owner will need the dog's registered name and AKC number and, if previously DNA profiled, his DNA profile number. The stud dog owner should also provide the AKC registered name and number of the bitch.

7. The owner of the bitch usually pays fees for the service of collecting and shipping the semen. This is best handled by credit card and should be paid prior to shipping the semen. Charges are as follows:

   Fee to collect the stud dog, handle and evaluate the ejaculate;

   Fee for specialized packaging and shipping media;

   Fee for shipping, usually FedEx, UPS, or U.S. Postal Service overnight shipping. If the owner of the bitch requests an alternative courier, they will need to make arrangements. If same day service is required or necessary, such as on weekends or holidays, the owner of the dog or bitch must make arrangements to transport the semen to the airport and select the airline and flight to be used. Known shipper status is required. The airline should be aware that the box contains canine semen and ice packs (not dry ice), as not all airlines will accept these contents. The stud dog owner and the owner of the bitch are responsible for travel to and from the airport. This is the least expensive and fastest way to transport semen. Other same-day courier services may be available but are usually very costly and may not be as reliable.

   Fee for the teaser bitch if available and if the stud dog owner does not provide one.

8. **Collecting and Packaging Semen (See Appendices A-2 and C-1)**

   Collect only the sperm-rich fraction, the second fraction, if possible. If fractionation cannot be accomplished, the semen can be centrifuged at 2500 rpm maximum for 5 minutes. The prostatic fluid can be carefully pipetted off and discarded. The semen pellet can be resuspended and 2 to 5 ml of extender added.

   The semen should be placed in a tube that seals securely. The top of the tube should be wrapped with 2 pieces of Parafilm® to prevent leaking. The tube should be labeled with the donor dog's name, dog's owners name, AKC number, breed, date, and time of collection. The tube should be placed in a sealed plastic bag – such as a Whirl-Pak® or zip-top bag.

   The shipping box, produced specifically for this purpose, is a cardboard box with a Styrofoam liner. The box should be packed with a frozen gel pack in the bottom (this gel pack is specifically manufactured for this purpose; those from other shipments may not be suitable for this use). Next layer is a chilled but unfrozen gel pack. The third layer from the bottom should be several sheets of newspaper folded. The fourth layer from the bottom is the bagged tube containing the semen, laid on its side in the box. The top layer is crumpled newspaper, in a quantity adequate to keep the packing from shifting in the box. The top of the Styrofoam box should be placed securely on top. In extreme temperatures, a stainless steel thermos (pre-chilled with damp cotton balls in the bottom) may be used to protect the semen from temperature extremes during shipment (Figure 4-3).

   AKC papers and information regarding the semen shipment and use should be placed on top of the Styrofoam.

   The box should be taped closed.

   The appropriate courier information should be applied to the outside of the box. This includes the shipping label and any special delivery instructions.

The package should be sent with the client to deliver to the shipper (DO NOT use a drop box for the shipper) or the shipping service should be contacted for a pick-up at the veterinary hospital.

The recipient should be contacted by phone or email with the tracking number of the package. This is especially important if your hospital staff will not be available at the time of the anticipated delivery.

9. Delays in receiving the semen can occur due to problems with inclement weather, lost or misdirected shipments. This is an inconvenience and may interfere with a successful pregnancy, but at least it is only a box and not your valued dog which was lost or delayed. It is always possible to arrange for an additional shipment. If a replacement shipment is by counter-to-counter service, you can often make up for the lost time of the original next day air shipment. It is the responsibility of the stud dog or brood bitch owner to track the shipment and make sure it arrives on time. The veterinary clinic shipping should provide the clients (both shipping and receiving) with the tracking number at the time of the outgoing shipment.

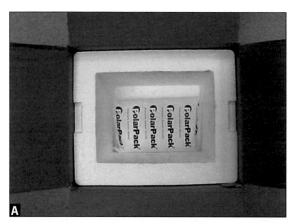
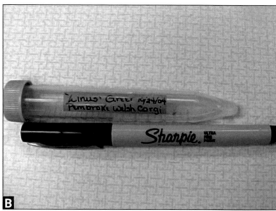
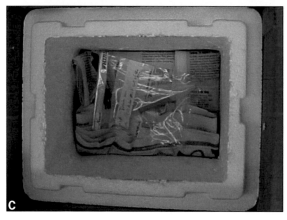

Figure 4-3.
A. Shipping box for semen. B. Labeled tube reduce errors on receipt of semen. C. Semen packaged for shipment.

Step by step fresh chilled semen collection to be shipped to your veterinary clinic

1. Prior to the expected estrus, the bitch owner should have the bitch's vaccinations updated, worming completed, and a complete physical examination. A breeding history should be taken, and vaginal exams and cultures done if indicated. A <u>Brucella</u> test should be run within the 3 months prior to breeding. Health screening tests such as OFA and eye exams should have been completed in advance. At the time estrus begins, it is too late to initiate testing and receive results in time for a breeding.

The same should hold true for the stud dog – <u>Brucella</u> testing, OFA and eye exams. If he has not recently had semen shipped successfully, a semen analysis and test chill should be performed.

2. The bitch or stud dog owner should contact both the shipping and receiving veterinary clinic at the first sign that the bitch is in estrus. The receiving veterinary clinic will often recommend an appointment in the first 5 days for a vaginal cytology to assess that she is truly early in her cycle and has not come into estrus silently. They will plan sequential vaginal cytologies and progesterone testing based on this cytology and her reproductive history.

3. Either the receiving veterinarian or owner of the female can contact the collecting veterinarian to plan how the semen will be shipped, received and stored and provide them with your veterinary clinic's address and phone number for shipping. In some cases, the shipping veterinary clinic will have supplies (specially made shipping box, ice packs, and extender) in stock at their hospital. In other cases, you may prefer to have the receiving veterinarian or a semen shipping company send out a shipping pack to the stud dog owner's veterinarian. These charges will be put on the bitch owner's credit card.

4. Inquire if the collecting veterinarian has experience in collecting semen. If they are inexperienced, request the receiving veterinarian to contact them with detailed information on semen collection and handling. **Be sure the stud dog owner's collecting veterinarian labels the TUBE with their name, the dog's name, AKC number, and date and time of collection. Veterinary clinics receive a number of samples unlabeled and when multiple semen shipments are received on the same day, the recipient veterinarian will need to be able to identify that the correct semen is being used on the correct bitch.**

5. At the time ovulation is about to occur (based on a progesterone level of 4 to 8 ng/ml), the owner of the recipient bitch or receiving veterinary clinic will advise the owner of the stud dog to arrange for collection and shipment. On weekdays, an overnight courier service such as FedEx, UPS, or U.S. Postal Service can be used. On holidays and weekends, airline counter-to-counter or the U.S. Postal Service needs to be used. At shipment, you should request the air bill or tracking numbers in case a shipment needs to be tracked.

6. The receiving veterinary clinic will arrange an appointment for the bitch to come in for insemination. **BE CERTAIN THE STAFF IS EXPECTING THE PACKAGE AND HANDLES IT TO KEEP THE SEMEN COOL BUT NOT FROZEN UNTIL USE.** The semen usually arrives at mid-day. The insemination is usually done vaginally or by TCI (or surgically in some cases) and is best repeated in 24 to 48 hours to improve the chances of conception. The inseminated bitch should be encouraged to urinate prior to insemination and kept quiet/crated for 2 hours post-insemination.

7. The collecting veterinarian may have a regular courier service they prefer for overnight delivery. If so, it is probably easiest to use their preferred service. If they do not routinely use one courier, you may wish to contact several to determine fees, pick-up and delivery times. Some to consider are FedEx (1-800-463-3339), UPS (1-800-742-5877), or the US Postal Service (local numbers). On holidays or weekends, counter-to-counter at the airlines may be an option. The stud dog or bitch owner will need to arrange to have the shipment at the airport at least 2 hours prior to departure to get the shipment loaded. Some airlines will not accept canine semen, so each airline needs to be individually checked. The shipper must have a known shipper status with any airline you use. The bitch owner and the owner of the stud dog are responsible for travel to and from the airport unless alternative arrangements are made in advance.

    Be sure to state, if you are questioned, that you are shipping canine semen in a Styrofoam shipper on ice packs (no dry ice is used – this is a hazardous material). In some situations, the USPS will do weekend and holiday pickups and deliveries, but this is not available at all locations, so you need to call ahead to assess service availability.

8. Twenty four to 28 days post-insemination, palpate or ultrasound the bitch to establish if she has become pregnant. This is an important piece of medical information for establishing a reproductive history. If she is pregnant, this is the time to change her diet to a high quality puppy, performance or pregnancy diet, line up supplies for whelping and arrange for someone to be available for whelping assistance.

9. Fees for the services may be structured as follows:
   Serial vaginal cytologies and progesterone levels per sample.
   Fee for insemination(s) of the bitch for the first and subsequent OR
   Fee for transcervical insemination (TCI) per insemination or surgical insemination.
   Fee for palpation/ultrasound/x-rays to confirm pregnancy.
   Fee to the collecting veterinarian for collection, shipping medium and packaging, and shipment.
   <u>Brucella</u> test to draw and run the sample.
10. The semen should be evaluated upon receipt if possible to assess motility and quality. If the semen evaluation is not of the quality the shipping veterinarian represented it to be, call as soon as possible for an additional shipment.
11. Vaginal insemination, TCI, or surgical insemination can be performed as detailed in this chapter. The semen should be handled according to the information the shipping veterinarian included in the package. Different extenders are handled differently at receipt and insemination. Some require warming all or part of the extender, others are inseminated without warming.
12. Remember, at times, delays in receiving the semen can occur due to problems with inclement weather or lost or misdirected shipments. This is an inconvenience and may interfere with a successful pregnancy as the outcome, but keep in mind it was only a lost box and not a valued dog, which was lost or delayed. It may be possible to arrange for an additional shipment if notified of this minor catastrophe. If the replacement is shipped counter-to-counter, lost time may be regained. It is the responsibility of the stud dog or brood bitch owner to track the shipment and contact the courier if it is delayed or lost. The shipping veterinarian can provide the stud dog and bitch owners with the tracking number at the time of the outgoing shipment.

Frozen semen handling and use

Frozen semen to be used for breeding has very specific shipping and storage requirements. The semen must be maintained in liquid nitrogen or the vapor of liquid nitrogen to be viable at the time of use. If the dry shipper will also be used for storage of the semen until use, arrange for additional liquid nitrogen in advance. There is no alternative – freezers or dry ice cannot be substituted.

Carefully check the identification of the semen **on the straw or vial** to be used (not just the goblet and paperwork enclosed) to be certain the semen is from the stud dog intended. Each unit of sperm – vial or straw – should include the stud dog's breed and registration number. Use of the wrong dog's semen can be a very distressing event for all parties involved.

The semen should NOT be thawed until ready to use immediately. If using for a surgical AI, the uterus should be exteriorized prior to thawing. If using for TCI, the cervix should be canulated with the catheter prior to thawing.

Each freezing center has their own specific techniques for thawing and resuspending frozen semen. The instructions from each freezing center should be followed precisely.

Equipment
1. A water bath that can maintain temperature from 90° to 95° F.
2. A thermometer to monitor the temperature of the water bath.
3. A microscope.
4. A slide warmer or way to warm slides.
5. Microscope slides and cover slips.
6. Disposable pipettes.
7. WhirlPaks® to thaw semen in – a sterile tube or zip top bag can be used as an alternative.
8. Pair of sponge forceps for handling the vials.
9. Pair of leather gloves with good flexibility (not too stiff).

10. Thaw media as specified by the freezing center OR Sterile saline, freshly opened bag.
11. Tom cat catheter.
12. 20 g IV catheter 1-2".
13. 20 g needle 1".
14. 2 10cc syringes (without black plunger).

Surgical insemination

Surgical insemination of the bitch is an elective, frequently used, valuable, very successful but invasive approach to breeding, allowing intrauterine deposition of the semen, which requires general anesthesia. It has value when breeding a bitch with a history of infertility or using semen that is compromised (frozen, fresh chilled shipped semen that arrives late or in marginal condition, or semen from a stud dog with poor fertility.) In some veterinary hospitals, laparoscopic insemination or transcervical insemination (TCI) is preferred.

Prior to anesthesia, the bitch should be appropriately timed using progesterone levels as described in Chapter 3. She should also have appropriate pre-surgical screening as done routinely in the practice. This may include CBC, chemistry profile, coagulation testing, and EKG.

The sequence of events:
1. Receipt of Semen: Log in, contact owner of bitch. Bill for storage.
2. Confirm time and date of insemination based on progesterone levels.
3. Owner signs consent form for procedure after informed consent is done with the attending veterinarian. Have the owner contact information available if the owner is not staying, in case questions arise.
4. Pre-op physical exam on bitch.
5. +/– Pre-surgical blood work and EKG; may include Brucella test on bitch.
6. Pre-med bitch with sedative and post-op pain medication.
7. Place IV Catheter.
8. Anesthetize with propofol or preferred agent, intubate.
9. Surgically prep abdomen.
10. Move to surgery table and prop up rear quarters with towels, position on v-tray.
11. Hook up to monitors and anesthetic machine.
12. Make incision, EVALUATE UTERUS.
13. Thaw semen and inseminate bitch OR thaw semen immediately prior to anesthesia based on owner and surgeon's preferences. Use thaw instructions from freezing center.
14. Complete the surgery.
15. Recover bitch from anesthesia, remove IV catheter when ambulatory.
16. Discharge instructions, medications, staple remover, recheck appointment.

Surgical procedure
(Appendix D-10)
The bitch receives pre-operative medication for sedation and pain management. An IV catheter is placed. General anesthesia is induced, using a short-acting anesthestic agent such as Propofol®. Anesthetic monitoring and IV fluid support is initiated. She should be prepped by clipping the hair over her caudal abdomen with a 40 clipper blade from the vulva forward as the surgeon prefers. She should be moved to the surgical suite. She should be positioned on the surgical table with thermal support, in dorsal recumbency with her caudal end elevated slightly above her cranial end. A sterile prep is applied. The surgeon, scrubbed, gowned and gloved, places a sterile drape over the abdomen. A ventral midline abdominal skin incision is made between the 3rd and 4th or 4th and 5th nipples 3 to 6 cm long with a #15 scalpel blade or laser. The subcutaneous fat is dissected off the abdominal muscle wall. The linea is incised. The uterine body is identified and exteriorized, and both uterine horns were partially exteriorized so as to visualize them. The ovaries can be palpated for

cystic structures but should not be exteriorized or otherwise disturbed. The uterus should be gently palpated to assess for cysts or other abnormalities. If the uterus appears normal, the semen may be thawed. (In some cases, the semen or a portion of the semen may be thawed prior to anesthesia to determine if the semen quality merited the anesthesia and surgical incision) (Figure 4-4).

If using frozen semen, the semen should be thawed according to the freezing centers enclosed guidelines. The semen should be evaluated and the motility recorded. If using fresh, fresh chilled, or frozen semen, it should be handled so the surgeon can remain sterile but have the semen in a sterile syringe for insemination.

While the semen is being thawed by one technician, the surgical technician who is monitoring the patient can open the sterile supplies the surgeon will need to do the insemination. The supplies are: (1) tom cat catheter, (1) 20 gauge needle, (2) 10 ml syringes without black latex plunger, (1) 20 g IV catheter, access to a freshly opened bottle of sterile saline and suture to close the abdomen.

The fresh/fresh chilled semen or the thawed semen should be in a sterile tube or sterile Whirl-Pak® bag. The surgeon should place the tom cat catheter on the syringe, and aspirate the semen from the tube or bag into the syringe, taking care to avoid excessive air exposure. When using a bag to handle semen, avoid using a sharp needle or catheter to retrieve the semen as puncturing the bag will risk loss of the contents. This should be set aside with the tip of the syringe in a location that will not lead to contamination of the patient or instruments as the semen and extender are not sterile. The second syringe should be filled with FRESH sterile saline and also set aside. The total volume of extended semen to be injected into the uterus should not exceed 0.5 ml for toy breeds and up to 4 ml for giant breed dogs or dogs who have previously had successful pregnancies.

The uterine body should be held off with digital pressure encircling the cervix distal to the puncture site. No incision is made into the uterus. The IV catheter should be inserted into the lumen of either the uterine body or each uterine horn, with the bevel up and tip aimed cranially toward the ovary. The uterus should be reflected to assure that the catheter is in the lumen and did not puncture through to the opposite side. The area around the catheter should be packed with moistened sterile gauze to protect against the extended semen contaminating the abdominal contents. The extended semen should be slowly injected into the uterine body as one dose or divided into two doses and injected into each horn near the ovary. The syringe may be removed from the IV catheter and replaced by a syringe containing only sterile saline if the surgeon believes a small volume to flush the semen cranially into the uterus would be beneficial and not lead to excessive uterine volume. The catheter should be removed from the uterus, taking care to avoid any excess from causing abdominal contamination of the site. Digital pressure with gauze should be held over the puncture site for 3 minutes. The area should be carefully wiped with gauze moistened with sterile saline. While maintaining a digital barrier around the cervix, the uterus should carefully be repositioned into the abdomen, taking care to avoid excessive pressure on the uterus as the cervix is patent and semen can easily be lost if excessive pressure is placed on the uterus.

The abdominal wall should be closed using absorbable suture of the surgeon's preference in a simple interrupted pattern in the linea. The subcutaneous layer should be closed using absorbable suture in a simple continuous pattern. The subcuticular layer should be closed using absorbable suture in a simple continuous pattern. The skin should be closed using staples or non-absorbable suture. A staple remover may be sent home with the client if this is acceptable practice for the hospital.

In general, the patient may be discharged from the hospital the same day as the surgical procedure is done. The patient should be ambulatory prior to discharge. Post-op pain medication should be sent with the owner to administer for several days along with discharge instructions including immediate post-op care. Appropriate pre-natal care instructions should also be prepared for the owner (Appendix C-14).

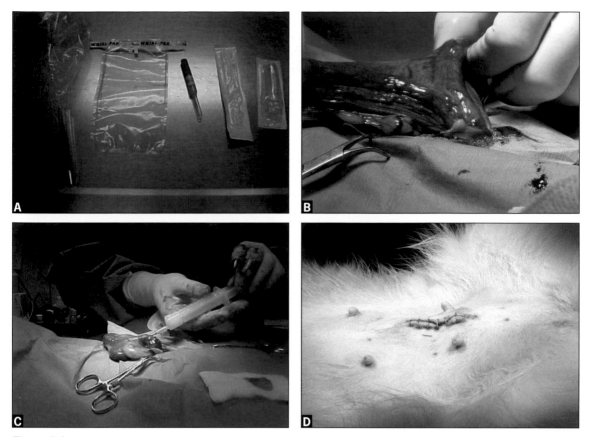

Figure 4-4.
*A. Surgical insemination supplies. **B.** Surgical insemination with uterus exteriorized for evaluation and insemination. **C.** Surgical insemination: catheter and syringe positioned for insemination. **D.** Surgical insemination post op with incision closed.*

Transcervical insemination

Transcervical insemination (TCI) describes the use of a rigid endoscope to deposit semen into the uterine body, proximal to the cervix. The same endoscopic equipment can also be use for vaginoscopy to assess the stage of the bitch's estrus cycle, to look for strictures, masses, and other anatomical abnormalities, and to flush the uterus when affected by pyometra (TECT procedure as described by Dr. Verstegen).

Intrauterine insemination is recommended when using frozen semen, other semen with compromised motility, when the breeding is delayed past the ideal date, or the bitch has a history of infertility. The main advantages of TCI over surgical insemination is that general anesthesia and abdominal surgery is not necessary. TCI also allows for multiple inseminations to be performed on the same estrus cycle.

The main disadvantages of TCI over surgical insemination is that it requires expensive equipment with specialized training to become proficient, the bitch must be cooperative when the rigid endoscope is passed into the cranial vagina and the appearance of the uterus cannot be assessed.

Minimum equipment needed
1. (1) Hopkins telescope, 3.5 mm x 36 to 43 cm working length, 30 degrees or Minitube scope.
2. (1) cystoscopy/reproductive sheath with obturator, 22 Fr.
3. (1) bridge with instrument channel.
4. (1) light source, halogen or xenon.
5. (1) light guide cable.
6. (6 and 8) French urinary or TCI catheters (disposables) or Minitube TCI catheters.

In addition, a video camera, medical grade monitor, and insufflation can be added to aid the operator and to allow staff and clients to also visualize the procedure. The total purchase price for new equipment is typically well over $10,000.00. Several vendors have packages available for purchase for this specific use. TCI training is available by videotape and at seminars held by the manufacturers and distributors of the endoscopic equipment.

There is a small risk to the bitch of uterine or vaginal perforation or other trauma, so care must be taken. The bitch must be adequately restrained on a table of appropriate working height. During the learning phase, this procedure can take some time, so the operator, bitch, owner of the bitch, and staff should be advised to be patient (Figure 4-5).

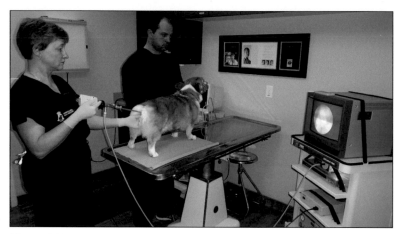

Figure 4-5.
Transcervical insemination.

Procedure for TCI

1. While preparing for the TCI, have the owner walk the bitch to allow her to relieve herself.
2. Have all of the endoscopic equipment assembled, with the light source on including the sheath, obturator, endoscope, light source, bridge and camera.
3. The fresh or shipped (do not thaw frozen until the catheter is positioned in the cervix) semen should be prepared for insemination, with a 2 cc maximum volume in a 5 cc syringe.
4. The bitch should be held in standing position, with her back feet near the edge of the table, on a non-slip surface. The table should be at a comfortable working height.
5. With the operator wearing gloves, the lips of the vulva are gently cleansed and parted.
6. If using the MiniTube TCI Shunt System, this should be inserted and the balloon inflated prior to inserting the scope.
7. The assembled equipment should be introduced through the lips of the vulva and gently advanced dorso-cranially, avoiding the opening to the urethra. The dorsal median fold of the vagina should be followed cranially until the cervical os is located. Locating and canulating the cervical os is the most technically difficult aspect of the procedure.
8. If using the MiniTube TCI Shunt System, the vagina should be insufflated.
9. The catheter should be introduced.
10. The cervix should be canulated with the catheter.
11. If using frozen semen, thaw the semen now, with the volume not to exceed 2 ml.
12. The fresh, shipped, or frozen semen should be gently and slowly deposited into the uterus.
13. The semen should be followed with 1 cc of saline or extender to flush the semen into the uterus, so it is not retained in the lumen of the catheter.
14. The equipment should be removed from the cervix and vagina and the bitch carefully placed on the floor, avoiding excess pressure on the abdomen during lifting.
15. The equipment should be cleaned in an appropriate solution such as CidexPlus®. The equipment should be rinsed in sterile water, dried well with a soft sterile cloth and stored carefully.

CHAPTER 5
Managing the Pregnancy

Managing the pregnancy
(Appendix C-13)

As soon as a bitch is bred, she should be treated as if she is pregnant unless proven otherwise. This includes management at home as well as medical care provided by the attending veterinarian.

She should be fed a commercially available high quality performance or pregnancy diet at a quantity to maintain her weight.

Her exercise level should be moderate. Bitches should be kept in good physical condition to reduce the likelihood of excess weight gain, poor muscle condition, and dystocia. Avoid overheating, swimming, or situations that could cause trauma to her abdomen.

Environmental management and housing the pregnant bitch

Many of the bitches in breeding programs are housed in homes or kennels with other dogs. Frequently, these other dogs are in and out of the home or kennel to attend training classes, dog shows, and other dog events. This can result in the introduction of infectious diseases to the environment of the pregnant bitch. In some cases, even the pregnant dog is attending dog-related events. One of the most feared contagious diseases for pregnant bitches is Canine Herpes Virus (CHV). CHV has been shown to cause no symptoms or only mild symptoms of upper respiratory disease in the nonpregnant adult dog. CHV infection often mimics kennel cough in adult dogs. However, infection with CHV during pregnancy attacks the placenta, and can lead to abortion, stillbirth and/or resorption of the fetus. Because this can occur in early pregnancy, before a pregnancy can be diagnosed with palpation or ultrasound, it may appear only as infertility, not fetal loss. The only preventive is through vaccination, but the vaccine is not currently available in the United States.

As a result, the owner or handler of these bitches may question how to manage her environmental exposures. Ideally, the pregnant bitch should not be exposed to other dogs during the pregnancy. This would preclude not only dog events for the pregnant bitch, but also for her house or kennel mates. Strict isolation of one or more dogs in most homes or kennels is not practical. Even a visit to the veterinary clinic could be interpreted as a risk to the bitch.

Common sense comes into play here. Several months prior to breeding, all necessary vaccines should be updated. Many breeders are familiar with the newer less-frequently administered vaccine protocols. Each household or kennel should be evaluated and the principles of risk assessment applied on an individual basis when developing a vaccine protocol. Should there be a report of an infectious disease outbreak, the breeder or handler would be well-advised to avoid large-scale dog events. A short period of isolation of the pregnant bitch from others in the household or kennel after return from a dog event should be instituted if feasible. Good hygiene should be practiced in parasite and feces management. Most infectious diseases are carried in feces or other body fluids, not on the skin surface, so disinfection of the dog by bathing is not likely to aid in disease control.

As a practical matter, a bred bitch cannot be maintained in isolation throughout her pregnancy any more than a pregnant woman can be. If the kennel has multiple bitches being bred throughout the year, it could mean months of restricting dog-related activities. Even the most careful breeder will take precautions to protect their bred bitch, but will probably still participate in dog events throughout her pregnancy.

Drugs and vaccines during pregnancy

No vaccines should be given during pregnancy. The only exception to this is the vaccine for Canine Herpes Virus (CHV). If this vaccine is available to you and indicated for the bitch, it may be helpful as it has been shown to improve weaning rates, increase puppy birth weights and reduce early puppy death. There appears to be a trend to larger litter sizes, indicating a protective effect on the unborn pup. Bitches that already have the virus can be vaccinated. **Two** doses of the vaccine are given to the bitch, the **first dose at or soon after mating** followed by a **second dose six to seven weeks later,** i.e. mid to late pregnancy. This stimulates the bitch to produce high levels of protective antibody to CHV, which she then passes to the puppies in their first feeding of colostrum. Because immunity to CHV is not life-long, the vaccination series should be repeated at each pregnancy. (Merial product literature.)

Pregnancy should be as drug-free as possible. That being said, if the bitch was surgically inseminated, she will benefit from post-op pain medications for the first 2 to 3 days. There are no veterinary non-steroidal medications labeled for use in the pregnant bitch. The author has used meloxicam (Metacam®) and others have used Tramadol safely. See the appendix for drug information resources. Other prescription and over-the-counter medications should be researched and prescribed on a case by case basis. Exceptions should be made if the bitch has a life-threatening condition (see Chapter 4).

There are conflicting reports on the use of products containing raspberry tea leaves. These are marketed to increase fertility and ease labor and delivery. However, there are reports suggesting that some of these products can cause premature labor and abortion. When in doubt, it is better to avoid products without FDA approval for use in the pregnant bitch.

Avoid supplements or food containing excessive levels of calcium, vitamin D and vitamin A.

> **Plumb's Pharmacotherapy Pontifications:**
> 1. Avoid drugs in pregnancy, and non-pregnancy too as all drugs have side effects.
> 2. Be particularly cautious using drugs with a narrow therapeutic index – if you can't avoid drugs, watch them carefully.
> 3. There is no such thing as a 100% safe drug – anything can cause anything.
> 4. Drugs which are more toxic in adults are also more toxic in fetuses.
> 5. Drug therapy comes with no guarantees.

Antiparasiticides during pregnancy

One exception to this drug-free proposal is the use of anthelmintics. There are several published protocols using anthelmintics in late pregnancy and early lactation that have been proven effective in reducing transplacental and transmammary transmission of T. canis and A. caninum. The Toxocara canis larvae which are encysted in the pregnant bitch's muscles are reactivated during the last 3 weeks of pregnancy and migrate transplacentally to the pups. The larvae then enter the lungs of the fetus. After birth, the pup can cough up and swallow larvae, which then become mature in the pup's intestine. In addition, the larvae enter the bitch's mammary glands and pass through the milk and into the pup's intestine. These parasites are then ingested by the bitch when she is licking the pups, completing the life cycle. The roundworms mature in the intestines of the pups and bitch within about 4 weeks. Prepatent infections in the pups are common, meaning the pup can have an active parasite load but have no eggs present on the fecal sample.

The Center for Disease Control and Companion Animal Parasite Council recommends the protocols below as well as beginning worming pups and mothers starting every 2 weeks when the pups are 2 weeks old (3 weeks for kittens). This should be repeated until the dogs are placed on a monthly control product with efficacy against ascarids. This is to reduce environmental contamination with parasite eggs to protect the pets as well as humans from zoonotic diseases. Veterinarians and breeders both should attempt to minimize their liability by following these protocols that reduce the possibility a zoonotic transmission may occur. Current guidelines can be reviewed at www.capcvet.org.

There are 4 established protocols that can be used to reduce parasite transmission from mother to puppy or kitten. All the following protocols are off-label uses. 1. Fenbendazole (Panacur) dosed at 50 mg/kg PO once daily from the 40th day of gestation to the 14th day of lactation is the most commonly used protocol. (37 consecutive days total) 2. The use of ivermectin weekly at 200 mcg/kg once a week from week 5 of pregnancy to week 3 of lactation has been shown to reduce roundworm and hookworm infections by 98 to 100% in the neonate. 3. For Ancylostoma caninum, two treatments with ivermectin at 500 mcg/kg, with one given 4 to 9 days before whelping and one treatment 10 days later. Although considered safe during pregnancy, dogs who carry the MDR-1 gene should not be treated with these ivermectin protocols. 4. The use of selamectin topically at 6 mg/kg applied to pregnant bitches and queens 6 weeks and 2 weeks before delivery and 2 weeks and 6 weeks after delivery reduced roundworm burdens in the offspring and egg shedding in the mothers.

By carefully calculating timing, heartworm preventive and flea control products can be used shortly before the breeding and not need to be repeated for 4 weeks, which will fall just past the first trimester of the bitch. In some areas, heartworm, fleas, and other internal and external parasites are a great risk so these preventive medications should be continued throughout pregnancy and lactation. Most manufacturers have studies showing if their products can be used safely during pregnancy and lactation. Some topical products translocate onto the pups, so these products should not be used during lactation (Table 5-1).

Nutrition
(See Chapter 9)
The pregnant bitch should be fed a high quality pregnancy or performance commercially available diet at a quantity to maintain her weight. This is not the time to reduce her caloric intake if she is overweight. She also should not gain weight during the first 4 weeks of pregnancy unless she is underweight (Body condition score should be 3 out of 5, allow her to gain only if she is a 1 or a 2 on a scale of 1-5).

Changes to expect during a normal pregnancy
There are several changes to expect during pregnancy. During the first several weeks, there are generally no visible physical changes Approximately 3 to 5 weeks after breeding, many bitches lose their appetites, and some will vomit. This is usually a short term change and does not need treatment. After the 5th week, the bitch's appetite will usually increase. At this time, her food intake can be increased by approximately 20%, but should be tailored to her nutritional needs based on her body condition and size of her litter. As the bitch approaches whelping, her appetite will often diminish. She may still have an appetite, but her stomach capacity may not allow her to eat normal size meals. Additionally, the pregnant bitch has a lower pH in her stomach contents than the non-pregnant bitch. The use of antacids and smaller more frequent meals are indicated. Every effort should be made to encourage her to eat until the day she is expected to whelp. If the litter is exceptionally large, some bitches may eat very little and need to be monitored for ketosis. Another common finding in a normal pregnancy is a clear mucoid vaginal discharge.

By about the 5th week, past the time she could first be ultrasounded, she will start to look fuller behind the ribcage on both sides. During the last 3 weeks of the pregnancy, she will have obvious abdominal expansion.

Near the time of whelping, the mammary glands will enlarge and fill with milk. There is variation on how close to whelping this will occur. Although this alone cannot be used to predict whelping, it is preferred to delay a C-section if possible until after the bitch is ready to lactate.

Temperament can change during pregnancy. Many owners note that their bitches become more affectionate, some clingy, when pregnant. Late in pregnancy, they may become aloof and can become aggressive toward other dogs, particularly other bitches.

Table 5-1 Drugs that can be used or should be avoided during pregnancy

Drugs considered safe during pregnancy	Drugs considered unsafe or of unknown safety during pregnancy-avoid if bitch is not in a life-threatening state and owner does not approve of use
Amoxicillin	Acepromazine
Amoxicillin with Clavulanic Acid and other beta lactams	Aminoglycosides given systemically – i.e. gentamycin, amikacin, kanmycin
Azithromycin	
Cephalosporins	Anesthestic agents of any kind
Clindamycin	Anti-neoplastic agents of all kinds
Erythromycin	Aspirin
Famotidine	Barbiturates and primidone
Fenbendazole	Bromocriptine
Fluorquinolones while pregnant and lactating to 4 weeks of age	Cabergoline
Ivermectin	Chloramphenicol
Metoclopramide	Cyclosporine
Milbemycin	Oxime Diazepam
Nystatin	DMSO
Penicillins	Enalapril, benzepril, captopril & other ACE inhibitors
PyrantelPamoate (Nemex®)	Glucocorticoids, including topical (eye and ear drops, skin preparations)
Praziquantel (Drontal®)	Griseofulvin
Selemectin	Hormones including mibolerone and other testosterones, pro-gestins, prostaglandins including Lutalyse® and Estrumate®, progesterone, estrogens including diethylstilbestrol
Sucralfate	Ketamine
Thyroid supplements	Ketoconazole, Itraconazole, Fluconazole
	Metronidazole
	Misoprostol
	Mitotane, o'DDD
	Omeprazole
	Organophosphates
	Phenobarbital
	Raspberry tea leaves and other non-FDA approved preparations
	Salicylates (aspirin) and products including salicylates such as PeptoBismol®
	Sulfonamides
	Tetracyclines including doxycycline
	Theophylline
	Vitamin A analogs
	Vitamin D supplements

Near term, many bitches become exercise intolerant: they are both anemic and have decreased thoracic capacity as the uterus expands. Most bitches become uncomfortable and restless when resting or sleeping as they near term. Bitches with very large litters may have difficulty breathing even when they are resting. It is advisable to minimize stress and keep mandatory activity to a minimum in near-term bitches.

As the uterus expands, there is increasing compression of the bladder. Most bitches will need to urinate more frequently.

Diagnostic lab work may be indicated during pregnancy or prior to C-section. Pregnancy may cause laboratory values to change significantly. The following changes are "typical" during pregnancy:
1. The **WBC** often increases moderately. The change is important to distinguish from the elevation seen in pyometra. It tends to be a more subtle elevation and tends not to have a left shift. Remember a pregnancy can co-exist with a pyometra.
2. The platelet count tends to increase.
3. The **RBC** will tend to decrease. The bitch's blood volume expands, but the RBC tends not to increase rapidly enough to prevent mild anemia. The anemia is usually a progressive normochromic, normocytic form starting at day 25 and lasting throughout the pregnancy. (Physiology and Clinical Parameters of Pregnancy in Dogs WSAVA 2002 Congress Patrick W. Concannon, PhD, Dipl ACT (Hon) Department of Biomedical Sciences, Cornell University Ithaca, NY, USA)
4. The **cholesterol** tends to increase.
5. The **total protein** increases early in pregnancy, but tends to be lower as does the albumin in late pregnancy.
6. The **calcium** tends to be slightly lower late in pregnancy, but this may reflect a decrease in the albumin.
7. **SAP (serum alkaline phosphatase)** frequently increases for many reasons. If the other liver enzymes are normal, this is not reason for concern.
8. **Progesterone** is elevated after ovulation in the range of 15 to 80 ng/ml, whether she is pregnant or not, so cannot be used to distinguish pregnancy from other disorders.
9. **Other lab values should remain normal.** This includes RBC and WBC morphology, and other chemistries not noted above. If changes are seen in the other chemistries (BUN, creatinine, glucose, liver enzymes) or electrolytes (including calcium), this should be considered a disorder and pursued diagnostically.

Diagnosing the pregnancy
Palpation
Careful and thorough palpation of the uterus through the abdominal wall between days 28 to 35 remains the most frequently utilized pregnancy diagnostic tool.

There are several limitations on palpation as a diagnostic tool:
1. The body type and level of relaxation of the bitch can make diagnosis difficult. If the bitch is short-bodied or thick-bodied, or is tense, this procedure may not be reliable.
2. Experience is required to develop a "feel" for this procedure.
3. Clients may be anxious because they may have been told there is a risk to the pregnancy from this procedure.
4. This is an all-or-none answer; pregnancy can be confirmed, but cannot be ruled out.
5. An approximation of litter size cannot be determined by this procedure.
6. Viability of the pregnancy cannot be assessed, nor can other uterine pathology such as a unilateral pyometra.
7. The accuracy and repeatability are low; so if a bitch fails to carry a litter to term, there is no way to go backwards in time to assess whether she was really pregnant or if the pregnancy was one without viable fetuses.

The advantages are also multiple. Palpation requires no specialized equipment; the procedure can be done economically. The procedure is as portable as the veterinarian – it can be done in the office or at a house call. Many breeders are quite skilled in the art of pregnancy palpation.

The technique is simple but requires practice to distinguish fecoliths, segmental pyometra, and the bladder from amniotic vesicles. There are several approaches to palpation and each veterinarian will develop their own technique. It is commonly done with the bitch standing on the floor or table. In all but very small bitches, both hands are used. With the bitch facing away from the person palpating, one hand is placed on each side of the abdomen, starting just below the lateral spinous processes. As you allow your opposed hands to travel ventrally across the dog's abdomen, you can feel the "slip" of the amniotic vesicle, a round to oblong turgid structure. This can be done several times in rapid succession, but no pressure should be put on the vesicles. The size of the vesicle varies with the size of the dog. Some have described this as "a string of pearls." Often, you can feel several, but an accurate count cannot be done. After day 35, the amniotic vesicles enlarge and become too confluent to distinguish so diagnosis of pregnancy based on palpation from day 35 until late pregnancy is not possible. Close to term, the fetuses become palpable and with patience, movement of the fetus can often be felt or seen.

Ultrasound

Ultrasound is the most useful method of pregnancy diagnosis. It is useful for assessing the uterus for many conditions. If your practice will be seeing reproduction cases, you should consider the purchase of ultrasound equipment. Affordable used ultrasound equipment is available through many vendors. If possible, ask to use it on a confirmed pregnancy before you make the purchase. Additionally, there are several companies now manufacturing portable ultrasound machines.

B mode ultrasound is done transabdominally in the bitch using either a sector or linear transducer with a frequency of 5.0 or 7.5 MHz. Positioning is at the discretion of the attending veterinarian taking the size and temperament of the bitch into account. Most are done in lateral or dorsal recumbency, but can be done standing if necessary. Positioning in dorsal recumbency will reduce the likelihood of counting the same fetus more than once. At best, ultrasound provides an estimation of litter size. Even the most accurate ultrasound cannot be used to assure there is an accurate count of fetuses. Approximate counts can be useful in detecting evidence of fetal death or fetal resorption. Clipping the hair is preferred but not allowed by many clients of bitches being actively shown. In this case, use of rubbing alcohol and ultrasound gel in enough volume to remove air pockets from the hair will allow assessment but not as accurate a count as bitches that have hair clipped. Ultrasound is considered 94 to 98% accurate for diagnosis of pregnancy from day 24 post-ovulation. Accuracy in counting the number of fetuses present is far lower. Fetal viability can be monitored from day 24 post-ovulation to term.

The urinary bladder can be a useful landmark and helpful in assuring that the ultrasound machine is set up correctly. First, the ultrasound probe is placed on the midline, over the 4th and 5th pair of mammary glands. The black fluid in the bladder helps the veterinarian and client visualize the fluid they will see if fetal vesicles are present. The non-pregnant normal uterus is difficult to identify and follow on ultrasound. Once the bladder is identified, the probe can be moved cranially just off the midline to the right and left to identify embryonic vesicles. The vesicles appear as discrete anechoic (black) round structures. The perimeter of the fluid is a hyperechoic (white to light gray) ring, the fetal membranes. In some views in early pregnancy, the fetus can be identified as a small wisp of hyperechoic tissue (white to light gray). Early in pregnancy, some amniotic vesicles may be identified without central tissue – this is not typically reason for concern, as it usually means nothing more than the plane of the beam missed the fetal structures. By following each of the 2 horns, an approximate count of embryonic vesicles can be made. In early pregnancy, the flutter of the fetal heart may be difficult to note on ultrasound. Often, the first indication of abnormal fetal development is the lack of a uniformly round vesicle. If the vesicle appears misshapen or collapsed, there may be an arrest of fetal development with resorption occurring. Typically, the ultrasound of a pregnant bitch past day 28 allows for very rapid and easy identification of fetal vesicles. As soon as the probe is placed on the abdomen, with correct positioning and adequate equipment, the fetuses will almost jump onto the screen. If this is not the case, look thoroughly and consider a repeat ultrasound in 7 to 10 days to assure that an early pregnancy or small number of fetuses is not misdiagnosed as a non-pregnant bitch.

As the pregnancy advances, the fetuses become larger and easier to identify on ultrasound. Crown-rump length or diameter of the fetal membranes in two dimensions is measured by some operators as an estimate of fetal age. The heart beating in each pup and increasing size, progressive development and activity indicate normal fetal development is progressing. As this occurs, crowding makes it more difficult to accurately count the number of fetuses present. Changing the magnification on the ultrasound machine can make seeing individual fetuses easier. At this time, assessment of fetuses on ultrasound has not progressed to the point that fetal sexing or fetal defects can be determined.

The only techniques that can be used to assess for fetal viability are audibly by fetal Doppler and visually by abdominal ultrasound. Ultrasound allows each fetus to be visualized for general size and shape of the fetal vesicle, a heartbeat, or fetal movement. Fetal Doppler can be more difficult to use as the signal is audio only and distinguishing that every fetus has been assessed can be very difficult even for an experienced operator. Normal fetal heart rates are typically in the range of 200 to 220 beats per minute. Heart rates in the range of 160 to 180 beats per minute may indicate normal quiet fetuses. Heart rates consistently below 140 to 160 beats per minute indicate fetal distress.

Additionally, with ultrasound, the uterus can be monitored for evidence of pyometra. In some cases, pregnancy can co-exist with pyometra. Radiographs are of little use in distinguishing pyometra from pregnancy until day 45 when the fetal skeleton becomes visible radiographically. Radiographs are also not useful in assessing for fetal distress, for recent fetal death, or other signs of uterine or ovarian pathology.

Other than pyometra, most ovarian and uterine pathology is below the resolution of the ultrasound equipment available in general veterinary hospitals or expertise of the general practitioner. More prominent lesions or equipment at specialty or referral hospitals used by veterinary specialists may detect other pathology.

Blood tests

Two blood tests are used to diagnose pregnancy. The tests are for fibrinogen and relaxin. Fibrinogen is a protein that is released during many kinds of inflammation. Although the level increases during implantation and placental formation, there are many other causes for it to increase including pyometra. An elevated fibrinogen level only indicates that an inflammatory process is occurring, but does not specifically indicate pregnancy. Relaxin is a hormone produced by the canine feto-placental unit. The test is available as a commercially available in-house assay. The test is most accurate when used 28 or more days after breeding, particularly when the bitch is pregnant with a small litter. The results are read as positive (pregnant) and negative (not pregnant). Although this hormone is produced by the placenta, it is unknown how long the test will remain positive after fetal death, resorption, or abortion. The relaxin test's primary value is for use when ultrasound is not available. Since neither of these tests can assess for fetal viability, ultrasound remains the most valuable method of assessing for the presence of fetuses and their viability.

Neither progesterone nor human early pregnancy tests can be used to diagnose pregnancy in the dog. Progesterone levels rise at ovulation and remain high (between 10 and 80 ng/ml) for 60 days after ovulation regardless if the bitch is pregnant or not. The human early pregnancy test detects human chorionic gonadotropin (HCG). HCG is species specific to the human. Dogs do not produce any form of chorionic gonadotropin during pregnancy.

Radiography

Pups are visible after day 42 to 45 from ovulation on radiographs as their skeletons mineralize. Prior to this time, the enlarged uterus is visible radiographically, but it is not possible to distinguish pyometra from pregnancy. Prior to day 45, ultrasound is recommended for this purpose (Table 5-2).

Radiographs from day 55 to 61 from ovulation are very useful in determining fetal maturation, fetal size, fetal position, and number of fetuses present. The one or two radiographs needed to count puppies will not harm the fetuses. The fee to the client for a puppy count radiograph is money well spent to assure them that all the puppies have been born and no veterinary attention is required. It is also invaluable information if labor stops with pups left behind. The client will know that veterinary assistance is needed before it is too late to save the pups. If a particularly small or large litter is detected, or if a fetal mal-presentation or oversized fetus(es) are found, a C-section can be scheduled during hours that are convenient.

Fetal death will appear on a radiograph as failure of the fetus to grow or calcify, skeletal collapse, or gas in or around the fetus. Fetal distress can be detected prior to fetal death if ultrasound or fetal Doppler (hand held unit available through Whelpwise™) is used to monitor the bitch daily or if she shows signs of not feeling well.

Table 5-2 Radiographic findings two to thirty five days following whelping		
Number of days prior to whelping	Structures visible	Comments
35 days	General uterine enlargement	No mineralization of fetuses visible
24 days	Uterus changes from circular to tubular shape	No mineralization of fetuses visible
20 days	Faint mineralization of fetal skull and backbone	
14 days	Skull	
7-10 days	Skull and backbone	
5-7 days	Skull, backbone, and ribcage	
3-5 days	Skull, backbone, ribcage, femur, shoulder blades, and teeth	
48 hours	Skull, backbone, ribcage, femur, humerus, shoulder blades, tibia, ulna, teeth, and toes	Teeth and toes can be difficult to see in large litters and large bitches due to scatter of the x-ray beam.

Although correctly exposed radiographs are 100% accurate in diagnosing pregnancy after day 50 from ovulation, it can be difficult to determine with 100% accuracy a "puppy count" when the litter is larger than 8 to 9 puppies. Not feeding a large meal prior to the appointment and allowing the bitch to relieve herself prior to taking the radiographs can be helpful in minimizing loss of detail. A lateral abdominal radiograph from the diaphragm caudal to the pubis is the preferred view. The KVP should be increased 10% to allow for the increased density. In very large bitches, the scatter can make interpretation difficult. Use of a grid if she measures over 10 cm at the 12th rib will reduce scatter.

Radiographs can help determine fetal maturation when exact ovulation dates are unknown. Skeletal maturity, presence of colostrum in the mammary gland, progesterone level as the bitch nears term (if she has a typical progesterone drop, less than 3 ng/dl = safe to deliver pups, less than 1 ng/dl = pups must be delivered within 24 hours to improve viability), the bitch's rectal temperature (variably reliable) and the bitch's behavior and appetite are all factored in to predicting parturition. When the ovulation date is known based on progesterone testing at breeding, this process is simplified (Figure 5-1).

Remember to assess the integrity of the diaphragm. On rare occasions, trauma or congenital defect can lead to a diaphragmatic hernia, and the uterine horn and contents may slip into the thorax during pregnancy. This is a serious complication and needs to be addressed.

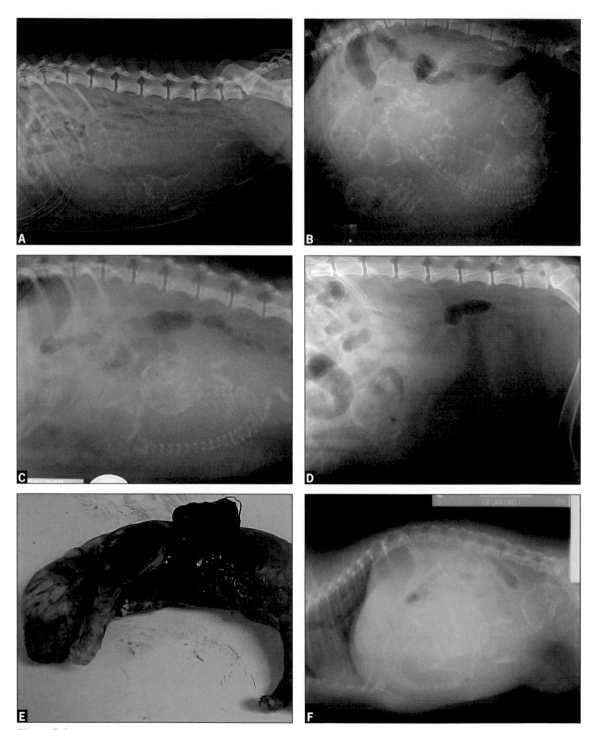

Figure 5-1.
A and B. Puppy count. Accuracy is essential and walking and fasting before radiography helps. **C.** *Dystocia radiograph – malpresentation.* **D.** *Emphysematus fetus on radiograph – note the air around the head of the deceased fetus.* **E.** *Emphysematus fetus shown on previous radiograph when delivered surgically.* **F.** *Dystocia radiograph fetal-maternal size mismatch.*

Managing the abnormal pregnancy
Illness in the bitch
There are 2 major categories of illness in the pregnant bitch. One is illness unrelated to pregnancy; the other is illness related to pregnancy. Almost any infectious or metabolic diseases that occur in the non-pregnant bitch can occur in the pregnant bitch, including pyometra. Probably the most difficult part of managing a sick pregnant bitch is determining if her illness is related or unrelated to pregnancy. Look for both – look at her first as a sick dog that is also pregnant, then as a pregnant dog that is sick to avoid overlooking a disorder unrelated to her pregnancy.

When presented with an intact bitch, before proceeding with any diagnostics, take a good history including her reproductive history or possible exposure to male dogs. Early pregnancy can be confused with many disorders including pyometra. Missing the diagnosis of possible pregnancy and proceeding with treatment for pyometra can be disastrous. It is also advisable to consider a possible early pregnancy before prescribing drugs that could potentially harm fetuses or terminate a pregnancy.

A diagnostic work-up on a pregnant bitch should vary little from a diagnostic work-up on a non-pregnant bitch. Although you should include pregnancy-related disorders in your differential list, don't allow the pregnancy to paralyze your thought process. Pregnant dogs eat things they shouldn't and get exposed to diseases just like the non-pregnant bitch.

Possible diagnostic work-up on the pregnant or bred (potentially pregnant) bitch based on history and clinical signs can include:
1. CBC.
2. Chemistry panel including electrolytes.
3. Progesterone level.
4. Urinalysis – DO NOT collecte by cystocentesis.
5. Ultrasound.
6. Radiographs.

Test results will be the same as for a non-pregnant bitch with a few exceptions. There are a few minor changes in the CBC and chemistry results that should be included in the interpretation (see "Changes to expect" earlier in this chapter). A CBC and chemistry panel +/– a urinalysis should be included if you would ordinarily run these tests. However, collecting the urine by cystocentesis should be avoided. An ultrasound to assess fetal presence, viability and development is recommended. Additionally, a quantitative progesterone level should be run as soon as possible. Progesterone levels can drop either because of luteal failure (primary hypoluteoidism) or as a result of illness in the bitch (secondary hypoluteoidism) and it should be monitored in a bitch that is ill or with a history of infertility.

Illness not related to pregnancy
Pregnant bitches often present with all the typical illnesses and traumas of the non-pregnant young to middle-aged dog. Most common is a mild gastroenteritis, with varying degrees of vomiting and diarrhea. Causes include hormonal changes and physical alterations related to pregnancy; dietary indiscretion; foreign body ingestion; parasites; and bacterial and viral causes. Also common are upper respiratory symptoms – primarily a concern if there is possible exposure to Canine Herpes Virus (CHV), which will be discussed later in this section. Skin and allergic disorders can be seen. Renal,hepatic and endocrine disorders can be seen, although possibly pre-existing but aggravated by the additional metabolic load of the fetuses. Neoplasia of nearly every kind seen in adult dogs can develop during pregnancy. No organ, system, or disease is exempt.

Once a diagnosis is made, a treatment plan must be developed. Investigation of which drugs are safe during pregnancy can be done on www.vin.com, in Plumb or in the Harriet Lane handbook. Whenever possible, avoid the use of medications. Other treatment such as dietary manipulation can be used. When not possible, drugs known to be safe during pregnancy should be used. Even over-the-counter medications and nutritional supplements can be harmful to the pups and should only be used when researched and found to be safe. Medications and other treatments that may harm the puppies or duration of the pregnancy should only be used when the bitch has a life-threatening condition and the client has given informed consent.

Illness related to pregnancy
Hypoglycemia
Hypoglycemia or pregnancy toxemia is typically seen only in underweight pregnant bitches. They generally do not have the body resources of fat, muscle, and carbohydrates necessary to support a pregnancy. Hypoglycemia can also occur in pregnant bitches that start in good body condition but cannot eat enough or are not fed enough to support pregnancy. A bitch with hypoadrenocorticism (Addison's disease) can become stressed and profoundly hypoglycemic during pregnancy.

Presenting signs may be vague; GI distress, or seizures may be noted if the hypoglycemia is profound. Diagnosis is made on laboratory testing: hypoglycemia, ketonuria without glucosuria, and if Addisonian, with an abnormal sodium/potassium ratio. Differentials include hypocalcemia. Short-term treatment requires IV fluids containing dextrose; long-term treatment requires nutritional support. Treatment with mineral and/or glucocorticoids are indicated if she is Addisonian. Many bitches pregnant with large litters have difficulty eating in late pregnancy – care must be taken to prevent the development of this serious disorder that can significantly affect neonatal survival. In rare circumstances, termination of the pregnancy may be necessary to save the bitch.

Hyperglycemia
Although common in human pregnancy, gestational diabetes, or hyperglycemia due to insulin resistance during pregnancy is rare in the dog. This can manifest as a transient disorder that resolves with the resolution (termination) of the pregnancy, or pre-existing subclinical diabetes mellitus may be aggravated by pregnancy. Diagnosis is made on laboratory testing. Differentials include any disorder that can cause PU/PD including renal disease, pyometra, leptospirosis, and many other disorders. Treatment consists of insulin administration with the dose determined by monitoring glucose levels to assess response. The stresses of pregnancy make regulation of gestational diabetes difficult. If the bitch develops this condition during one pregnancy, it is likely to be recurrent, so repeat breeding is not recommended. Finding a surrogate bitch to raise the pups or hand-raising the puppies may be necessary.

Fetal resorption, abortion, and late term fetal death
Fetal loss can occur anytime from conception to delivery. In most cases, the bitch will show no symptoms or may have a vaginal discharge but feel and act clinically normal.

Before ultrasound was widely available, early pregnancy could only be diagnosed by palpation. With palpation, diagnosis was either pregnant or non-pregnant. Partial loss of a pregnancy could not be determined. Ultrasound is now used routinely, and we are increasingly aware of fetal loss after 28 days of pregnancy, with up to 33% of fetuses lost between pregnancy diagnosis and whelping.

It is not uncommon to see many pups on ultrasound (although exact counts are difficult to do accurately) only to find a small litter at term. C-section can confirm partial loss of a litter when resorption sites are found in the uterus. These sites can vary in appearance but look like either a raised yellow plaque of solid tissue or a non-descript mucoid fluid found inside the uterus.

Pregnancy loss may manifest as one of the following:
1. Embryonic death and resorption
2. Abortion of a live or dead fetus
3. Stillborn pups that appear to be full term
4. Fetal death, mummification, and retention of the pup inside the uterus or abdominal cavity after term.

If fetal loss occurs early in the pregnancy, prior to diagnosis with ultrasound, abortion or resorption is the usual result. If fetal loss occurs in the latter half of the pregnancy, either the pup(s) are aborted spontaneously or carried to term and delivered as stillborn or underdeveloped pups. The time at which the insult occurred will be reflected by the maturity and degree of degradation of the stillborn pup. In some cases, a bitch may expel one or more pups and carry the remainder to term. At times, the bitch may consume the fetuses and membranes, and the owner to be unaware of the loss. Some pups will be nearly normal with little degradation, whereas some may be necrotic, emphysematous or mummified. Some bitches show no ill effects from this and others may have a foul discharge and become ill.

Fetal loss can result from infectious and noninfectious causes. Determining the etiology can be difficult, even when diagnostics are completed. Diagnostics require submission of fetal, placental and if a Caesarean was done, uterine tissues, for histopathology and culture (aerobic, anaerobic and mycoplasma). Collecting sterile samples can be very difficult if the bitch has delivered the pups vaginally because the fetuses are probably already contaminated by the time it is determined that samples should be submitted. The fetal stomach contents can be a good uncontaminated sample source for bacterial culture. Tissues should be refrigerated, not frozen, and placed in formalin. Refrigerated samples should be delivered to the diagnostic lab within 24 hours if possible.

Bacterial causes of fetal loss

Brucellosis – this disease is caused by <u>Brucella canis</u>, a zoonotic bacterial infection that can cause infertility in the dog and bitch, as well as loss of pups close to term and puppies that do poorly after birth. Any bitch with unexplained fetal loss or neonatal death should be tested for brucellosis. This disease should be tested for in males and females prior to all breedings because of its zoonotic potential and the general recommendation of euthanasia for all infected dogs. Dogs and bitches with infertility should be tested for brucellosis. Brucellosis is still seen in many regions of the United States (Figure 5-2).

In-office screening may be done quickly and with great sensitivity, if the rapid card/slide agglutination test (RSAT) is available. Because of the sensitivity of the test, any dog that tests negative is negative unless in the early stages of the disease. There is a relatively high incidence of false positive results. A second test is in the Brucella test kit using 2-ME – this screening can be done if the RSAT is positive. Any dog testing positive on both the RSAT and 2-ME tests should have a definitive diagnosis made at the Cornell Diagnostic Laboratory on the AGID test or Iowa State on the PCR Brucella test. The gold standard is multiple blood cultures, but a negative culture does not rule out the possibility of disease.

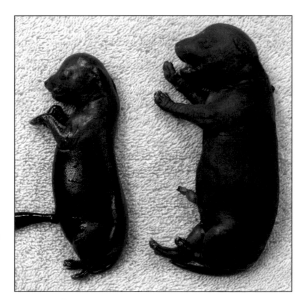

Figure 5-2.
Pups aborted due to a bacterial infection in the uterus during pregnancy.

A number of other bacterial diseases have been found associated with spontaneous abortion and stillborn births in the dog. These include Campylobacter, Beta-hemolytic Streptococci, Escherichia coli, and many other bacteria. It is challenging to determine if bacteria normally found in the lower reproductive tract are a significant cause of fetal loss in an individual bitch.

Good hygiene in the kennel and care in handling food, especially raw food diets, are important in minimizing bacterial diseases.

It is inappropriate to routinely use broad-spectrum antibiotics without supporting evidence based on culture prior to breeding. Pre-breeding antibiotics should only be used when there is a history of infertility, a cranial vaginal guarded culture was done in early pro-estrus (with the culture suggesting a bacterial cause of infertility) when there is one predominant bacteria, and the antibiotic choice is based on sensitivity testing.

Viral causes of fetal loss

Canine Herpes Virus: CHV can cause fetal resorption, stillborns, and the birth of weak or sick puppies. It is possible to have an assortment of these conditions in the same litter. Some pups will be born healthy, contract CHV in the first few weeks of life, and succumb to it quickly. The only treatment currently available for affected or exposed pups is to keep the ambient temperature high enough to keep the pup's rectal temperatures above 101° F. CHV replicates in tissues that are cooler than 101° such as the oral and vaginal areas and neonates. The use of commercially available fresh frozen plasma (Hemopet) or serum collected from dogs in the affected household with a CHV positive titer may support the pups through the disease.

Adult dogs with CHV may be asymptomatic or may have signs of upper respiratory disease (kennel cough). Some may have vesicles visible on the mucus membranes of the oral cavity, vagina or preputial muscosa. Dogs exposed to groups of dogs at events may develop the disease. At one time, it was thought that a bitch would only have one litter of pups susceptible to CHV and that subsequent litters would be protected. This is no longer felt to be the case. It has been suggested that if a bitch is suspected of having CHV during her pregnancy, the pups be taken by C-section and hand-raised to minimize their exposure when passing by the vaginal lesions during the birth process.

A CHV vaccine is available in some countries. The vaccine (Eurican® Herpes 205) is administered at breeding and a second time at the 6th to 7th week of each pregnancy. Merial, the manufacturer, has no reported plans to apply for approval of this product for use in the United States.

Diagnosis in the bitch is based on a positive titer (suggesting recent exposure) or a positive PCR or DNA test (showing evidence of the organism actively present in her body). Presumptive diagnosis in pups is based on a description of their illness and acute death – when ill the pups cry incessantly, show gasping respirations, and die suddenly. Characteristic lesions at post mortem are petecchial hemorrhages on the surface of the liver, intestines and kidneys. Definitive diagnosis is based on viral testing for CHV by a pathologist at a reference laboratory.

Mycoplasma and ureaplasma causes of fetal loss

Mycoplasma is considered to be a normal organism in the reproductive tract of the bitch. Ureaplasma and mycoplasma cultured from inside the bitch's uterus or the stomach contents of the deceased fetus suggests these organisms as a possible cause of pregnancy loss.

Parasitic causes of fetal loss

Neospora caninum is a protozoan proven to be transmitted to fetuses by crossing the placenta. Little is known about the incidence in naturally occurring infections. The organism causes an ascending neurologic disorder in affected pups. The increasing popularity of raw meat diets may cause an increased exposure to this parasite. This parasitism may be detected with serology testing.

Premature labor and hypoluteoidism

Hypoluteoidism is the inability to maintain an appropriate progesterone level needed for pregnancy. There are 2 causes: 1. a primary inability to maintain adequate progesterone levels due to inadequate progesterone production by the bitch and 2. a secondary inability to maintain progesterone levels, initiated by fetal distress or death. It is rare in dogs. The primary cause is treatable with hormonal support. The secondary cause may be treatable with a combination of hormonal support, antibiotics and tocolytics (Figure 5-3).

Diagnosis is based on quantitative serum progesterone levels. A minimum serum progesterone level required to maintain late stage pregnancy is 2 ng/ml. Progesterone levels during a normal pregnancy in the 2nd trimester (or post-estrus in the non-pregnant bitch) range from 15 to 90 ng/ml. Prior to the start of the 3rd trimester, a progesterone level below 15 ng/ml is typical. During the 3rd trimester, progesterone levels normally decrease to 4 to 16 ng/ml. The progesterone level should remain above 5 ng/ml with more than 5 days to go. Just prior to labor and coinciding with the rectal temperature drop, the progesterone level drops to 2 to 3 ng/ml.

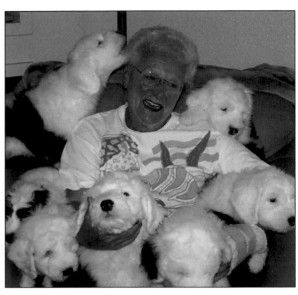

Figure 5-3.
Hypoluteoidism – litter resulting from careful management of a bitch who had previously lost a litter due to hypoluteoidism.

Serial serum progesterone levels should be recommended for bitches with a history of late term pregnancy loss, infertility, or symptoms of the early onset of labor. These symptoms will include an assortment of but perhaps not all of the following: appetite loss, bloody or atypical vaginal discharge, excessive lactation or illness, early nesting and panting, fetal heart rates of less than 160 bpm, decreased fetal movement on ultrasound or premature fetal expulsion. Many experienced breeders will detect subtle changes in activity level and behavior and will present the bitch with these symptoms. Early onset of lactation may indicate the progesterone level is dropping prematurely. Progesterone testing should be performed every 4 to 7 days if the progesterone levels are above 20 ng/ml. Progesterone testing should be done daily if the progesterone levels are 5 to 10 ng/ml.

Endogenous progesterone support for pregnancy is maintained exclusively by the corpus luteum, not the placenta as in other species. The cause of primary hypoluteodism in the bitch has not been determined. It is more prominent in some breeds or lines of dogs, suggesting a genetic component. One theory is that this may be an immune-mediated disorder. Secondary causes of progesterone levels that are too low to support pregnancy include fetal death; trauma and stress; drugs and supplements (steroids and raspberry tea leaves); cystic endometrial hyperplasia and other uterine disease; genetic mistakes or mismatches; placentitis; and infectious diseases that affect the bitch and/or the pups (brucellosis, CHV, CPV).

If the bitch's progesterone level is under 5 ng/ml with more than 5 days until she is due to whelp, treatment can be initiated. Progesterone in oil is dosed at 2 to 3 mg/kg IM every 1 to 3 days, with dosage frequency based on response to therapy. When progesterone in oil is used, progesterone testing can be used to assess response to therapy. The alternative drug, altrenogest (Regumate) can be dosed at 0.088 mg/kg PO daily. However, because this product is synthetic, it will not show up on progesterone testing, making it more difficult to monitor response but easier to assess the bitch's actual need. One challenge in documentation and treatment of this disorder is the 24 hour turn-around time for progesterone results that limits the fast response needed for diagnosis and initiation of treatment. In these cases, a slightly higher progesterone level may need to be considered the cut-off to allow for the lag time from testing to results. Referral to a clinic with a strong reproductive emphasis and same-day progesterone results may be indicated in these cases.

These products (progesterone in oil and altrenogest) should only be used when proof of a low progesterone level is documented. Both feminization of the male fetus and masculinization of the female fetus have been reported with their use. An additional concern is that progesterone supplementation may perpetuate an unhealthy pregnancy: fetuses with primary abnormalities; bitches with placentitis; or bitches with uterine infections, pyometra and septicemia.

When used, the last dose of progesterone should be administered 2 to 3 days prior to the puppy's due date to allow for normal parturition and lactation. Metoclopramide can be started at the time of the discontinuation of progesterone supplementation to aid in initiating the bitch's lactation. Supplemental feeding or surrogate care of the pups may also be indicated.

To effectively monitor progesterone levels and predict parturition, the bitch must have been timed with progesterone levels and/or LH peak to know the exact date of ovulation and thus accurately know the date the pregnancy should end. Use of progesterone levels late in the pregnancy as the only predictor of parturition will not be accurate in either bitches with small litters (1 to 2 pups) or bitches who have hypoluteodism.

When faced with a bitch showing evidence of premature labor, there are limited treatments available:
1. Progesterone level monitoring and pharmaceutical and hormonal support as indicated by blood testing.
2. Antibiotic therapy for the bitch (Amoxicillin, enrofloxacins, Cephalexin or Clavamox® are safe) and should be used until delivery of the pups. Antibiotics should be used if bacterial disease is suspected or the cervix is suspected to be open. Digital vaginal examination cannot detect an open cervix.
3. Tocolytics such as terbutaline to inhibit premature uterine activity. Terbutaline and other drug doses can be titrated using uterine contraction monitoring. This drug must be discontinued prior to the expected delivery date to permit normal labor and delivery to occur.

When presented with a bitch showing signs of premature labor or fetal distress, clinical judgment must be used. This can be a true reproductive emergency, threatening the outcome of the pregnancy. It may be necessary to initiate all 3 therapies in an emergency, pending progesterone results and the arrival of tocodynamometry equipment.

CHAPTER 6
Managing the Whelping and C-section

Managing the whelping

The whelping at home

Pregnancy in the bitch is relatively short. By the time it is confirmed, your client will have only a few weeks to prepare for whelping; by the time the number of pups is confirmed, they will only have a few days.

Therefore, it is recommended that they plan for whelping PRIOR to the breeding.

There are 2 things that require time to plan:
1. Building a whelping box and arranging an area to house the mother and puppies. Having a good whelping box in an appropriate area makes an enormous difference in the husbandry, and the amount of work the breeder must put into the whelping. A well-built box that keeps the pups at the correct temperature, keeps them safe, and allows for good hygiene makes the veterinarian's and breeder's job easier. Whelping boxes are also available commercially.
2. Arranging to be present or have an assistant present for whelping and the early post-natal period. It is strongly recommended that there be an experienced person with the bitch during the time she whelps and in the early post-natal period. Many breeders mentor new people in their breed or have a network of friends to assist them during this period.

There are items that clients should have on hand for whelping (Appendix C-3 and C-9). Many are items, like a whelping box and stethoscope that they will use for each litter. Others are supplies that need to be replenished. It is ideal to have the veterinary technician or assistant spend a few minutes with the client at the appointment used to confirm the pregnancy reviewing the clients whelping skills and addressing their equipment and supply needs. This is time well spent so that when the client's bitch is whelping or they have a health concern, they are well equipped to handle immediate care at home and know when veterinary intervention is needed.

The whelping room and puppy nursery

This room should be quiet, away from the activity of other dogs in the household. This will significantly reduce the stress level of the new mother. It is very upsetting to many bitches to have other dogs, even dogs that are familiar, approaching newborn pups. In many breeds, the new mothers are so protective that it is not advised to have more than one bitch and litter in each area.

This room should be part of the house or in a heated kennel. A basement or garage, even in warm climates and warm times of the year, can still be cold and drafty. Newborn pups cannot raise their own body temperature for the first 3 to 4 weeks of life – they are at the mercy of the temperature in the room around them. Cold floors and drafty areas are not suitable areas in which to raise puppies.

There are products designed to keep puppies and adult dogs warm with electric heat that radiates from a specially designed heated surface. The author's preferred product is Lovett's Electronics Heated Whelping Nest (formerly T.E. Scott). This item can be purchased with instructions to build it into a whelping box. Once built, it can be used for many years. Purchasing and assembling the nest needs to be done prior to the whelping. When built from or sealed with impermeable material, it is easy to clean and disinfect between litters. There are as many whelping box designs as there are breeders. Larger dogs require larger boxes. Some breeders include rails (pig rails) along the sides to protect the pups from clumsy mothers. Some are built with clear sides so pups can be monitored from across the room. Some tear down for storage. Some have sides that can be added on as the pups start to escape. Some have an area for the pups to use to eliminate when they are a few weeks old. Some breeders use a round flat-bottomed rigid plastic children's wading pool. Some unheated boxes can be purchased commercially. The whelping box needs to keep the pups warm, safe, and clean and the mother comfortable so she can be the mother she was meant to be.

Breeders tend to be resourceful and many try using heat lamps or other heat sources or substandard areas for raising puppies. Heat lamps risk starting fires (the author has first-hand experience - don't try it) and can dehydrate puppies. Other heat sources can cause thermal burns, even when used carefully. Substandard puppy nurseries and inappropriate heat sources may seem like an economical way to raise puppies, but in the long run they lead to high puppy morbidity, mortality and/or veterinary costs.

A small room, bedroom, office, den, or area of a larger room can easily be converted temporarily into a nursery in many client homes. Flooring and walls can be protected with temporary floors (vinyl flooring) or impermeable sheeting (vinyl tarps, shower curtains, and flannel-backed vinyl tablecloths.). Another great advantage of housing the pups in the breeder's home is the social experiences they receive from this. Pups need to see and hear normal household activities, they need to be looked in on many times a day, and they need to be handled by lots of different people. When isolated in a remote room or kennel, their social experiences are limited and they are more difficult to integrate as beloved pets into the puppy buyer's household.

There are a few items you may want to stock or know where to purchase to be sure that clients have them on hand (Figure 6-1) (Appendix C-7). These include:

1. Bulb syringe – to suction mouths of newborns – available at most stores with a pharmacy department.
2. DeLee Mucus Trap – to suction newborns' airways - available on-line from suppliers of midwives or from WhelpWise™.
3. Exam gloves, latex or vinyl – to protect breeders from vaginal discharges and placental fluids and the bitch from ascending infections– available OTC in many places.
4. K-Y Jelly® – to lubricate gloves if vaginal examination is indicated – available OTC in many places.
5. Hemostats – to clamp off umbilical cords – available from your suppliers or on-line.
6. Suture or dental floss – to tie off umbilical cords – available from your suppliers (suture) or OTC in many places.
7. Tincture of Iodine - to treat the umbilicus at birth, 2 and 8 hours post partum – available from your suppliers.
8. Chlorhexidine disinfectant solution – to disinfect surfaces in the whelping and nursery areas - available through your veterinary suppliers or local farm stores.
9. Heating pads, rice bags, or Snuggle Safe® – to keep pups warm during transport – heating pads often either overheat or have safety shut-offs so are difficult to keep the correct temperature range. Rice bags made of stockinette or socks filled with cooking rice can be microwaved to warm pups. Snuggle Safe® – a microwaveable disc made to warm puppies, available on-line.
10. Puppy formula – if supplemental feeding is indicated - there are many good ones on the market – available through your veterinary suppliers or on-line.
11. Feeding tube – for tube feeding puppies – there are red rubber feeding tubes and silicone tubes - available through your veterinary suppliers.
12. 25 gauge hypodermic needles – used to perform acupuncture for pups that do not breathe spontaneously at birth - available through your veterinary suppliers.
13. Dopram® injections pre-drawn into syringes 1 per anticipated puppy (controversial but better than losing a pup) – to administer to pups that cannot be resuscitated by clearing airways and with mechanical stimulation - available through your veterinary suppliers.
14. Pyrantel Pamoate – to deworm the bitch and pups at 2, 4, 6, and 8 weeks post-partum as recommended by CAPC - available through your veterinary suppliers.
15. Stethoscope – to assess newborns for a heartbeat - available through your veterinary suppliers or on-line.
16. Fetal Doppler – to monitor fetal heart rates during late pregnancy and whelping - available on-line at Whelpwise™ or some clients have their own.

17. Hair blow-dryer to aid in drying wet puppies.
18. Ice cream – vanilla for the dog, any other flavor for your friends
19. Friends with common sense, and have the ability to drive anywhere under any conditions.

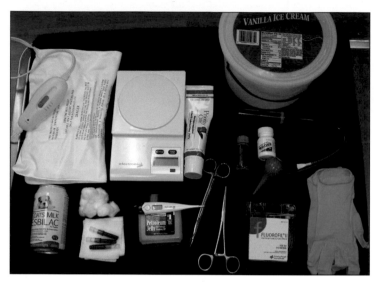

Figure 6-1.
Whelping supplies.

The remaining items, kitchen scale, towels, and thermometers are easy for clients to purchase on their own. They should be reminded to have these supplies readily available and organized. The clients will be ready to start care at home if they are able to monitor temperatures, weights and urine color, while arranging veterinary assistance.

The breeder should be shown how to keep good records on each pup. Each puppy should be permanently identified by color (permanent markers, fabric paint and nail polish – not neck bands please) and have their temperature, weight, and urine color evaluated and recorded at least once daily at the same time every day to allow for objective assessment of each newborn.

Labor and delivery
The normal delivery
So few clients call for assistance when they have a normal whelping that many veterinarians and veterinary staff have never seen a normal whelping. So how do you help your clients when they call to ask if what they are seeing is normal? A checklist for you and your front desk staff will be very helpful. After all, you don't want to have them run to your office with a whelping bitch if it isn't necessary. A puppy born in the car on the freeway is stressful for everyone. But waiting at home too long is a problem too. Veterinarians too often tell clients just to wait it out, but in doing so, puppies are born dead or too weak to survive. The list in the following section should assist you and your staff in making a decision about what is normal and what is not (Follow section called "How to determineif a bitch has a dystocia") (Appendix B-4).

A normal whelping may look different in every bitch. If you or your staff have the opportunity to visit a breeder with a bitch in whelp, you can learn a great deal about "normal" (Figure 6-2).

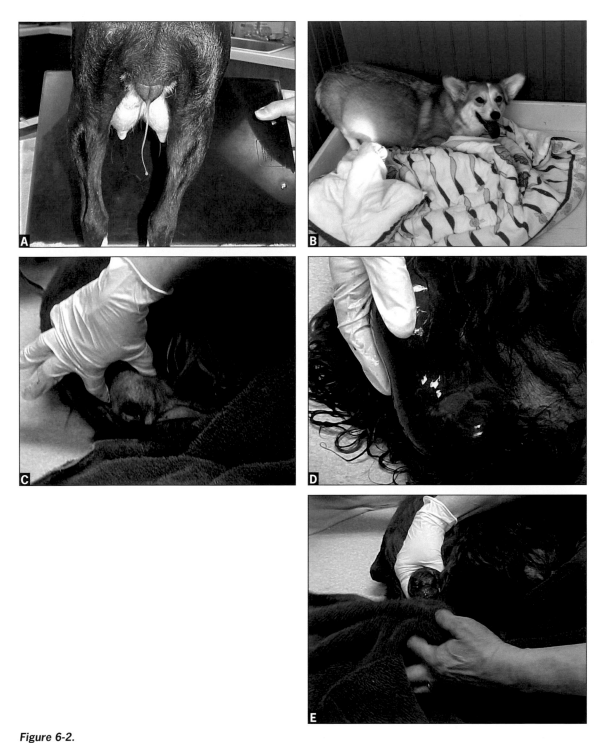

Figure 6-2.
A. Cervical plug passing spontaneously – a sign of impending delivery. **B.** Labor – a Pembroke Welsh corgi bitch nesting in stage 1 labor. **C.** Vaginal presentation of fetal membranes. Stage 2 of labor. **D.** Pup delivered vaginally in membranes. Stage 2 labor. **E.** Clearing membranes from the face so the pup can begin breathing.

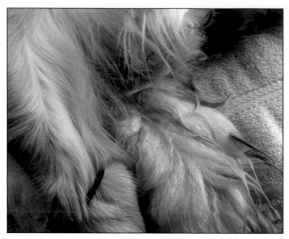

Figure 6-3.
Green colored vaginal discharge indicates placental separation. Discharge is normal if one or more pups have been delivered but a sign of impending fetal distress prior to delivery of any pups.

When the bitch is having puppies normally she:

1. Should have the first puppy in less than 2 hours from the start of labor (pushing). If the bitch is not yet pushing or has been pushing for less than 2 hours, she is probably OK unless there is a green vaginal discharge or excessive blood. If the owner and bitch are calm, she is probably OK (Figure 6-3).

2. Should not be in hard labor (pushing) for more than 1 hour before delivering each subsequent puppy.

3. Can go up to a maximum of 3 hours between puppies if she is resting and not in hard labor (pushing).

4. Should go into labor (pushing) within 4 hours of a rectal temp rise from the pre-labor (under 100°F) to normal (101°F to 103°F)

5. Should whelp on schedule. A normal pregnancy should be 63 days (+/− 1 day) from a progesterone rise over 5 ng/dl, signaling ovulation. When calculated from the breeding date, without the benefit of ovulation timing, the pregnancy can appear to be 58 to 65 days long. If the pregnancy exceeds 65 days from the ovulation date or breeding date, the bitch should be seen that day at the veterinary clinic for evaluation.

6. Should have vigorous puppies that actively attempt to nurse.

There are 3 stages classically described for a bitch in labor: Stage I or pre-labor, Stage II or delivery of the pups and Stage III or delivery of the placentae.

In stage I, the uterus begins to contract, but there is little evidence of this unless the bitch is on a uterine contraction monitoring service. She may start to pant, her rectal temperature may drop (found only in 33% of monitored bitches) from normal to 98 to 99 degrees F. She may begin to nest, be reluctant to eat and/or vomit, and seek seclusion. Some have a faraway look in their eyes or look frequently at their own flank, and some become "clingy". When evaluated on visual observations alone, this stage can appear to last a few hours to a full day. Sometimes the breeder will see the cervical plug, which consists of a thick plug of mucus, pass vaginally. Typically, pups should start arriving within 9 to 14 hours after first stage labor is detected on the tocodynomometer. When labor extends beyond 14 to 16 hours, fetal mortality and C-section rates increase significantly. With careful whelping management, rates as low as 1.5% fetal loss have been reported.

In stage II, the bitch will deliver her pups. She will often show signs of external abdominal wall contractions. She may appear to push and/or hold her breath. Bitches will show their own preference for positioning to deliver the pups – some will stand and squat, some will lay on their side and some push up against a hard surface like the side of the whelping box. Most wish to have their owner with them or even want to be held in their owner's lap.

Stage III is the expulsion of the placentas. Most bitches alternate back and forth between Stage II and Stage III. However, most bitches do not alternate puppy-placenta-puppy-placenta in neat order. This is normal and is not reason for concern. If it is possible to count one placenta per pup, this is ideal. However, the bitch may have one or more unaccounted-for placentas; retained placentas are rarely a cause of clinical disease in the bitch.

Managing a whelping at the veterinary hospital
(Appendix D-12)

In general, assume that the client will put saving the bitch ahead of saving the pups if a decision between the two needs to be made. Fortunately, this decision rarely needs to be made because care that is good for the mother is usually also good for the pups. Also assume that you have at least 1 viable pup when making medical decisions (Figure 6-4).

A radiograph upon arrival of the bitch with dystocia should be the second procedure when she walks in the door – the first is a vaginal evaluation to be certain a pup is not presenting in the vagina and is tragically forgotten while paperwork, history, and radiographs are handled.

The breeder-client should be consulted early on regarding how they prefer to proceed. Some will be very willing to move to C-section if the first pup is not easily delivered upon arrival at the veterinary hospital. Some clients will be reluctant to proceed to C-section regardless of the higher

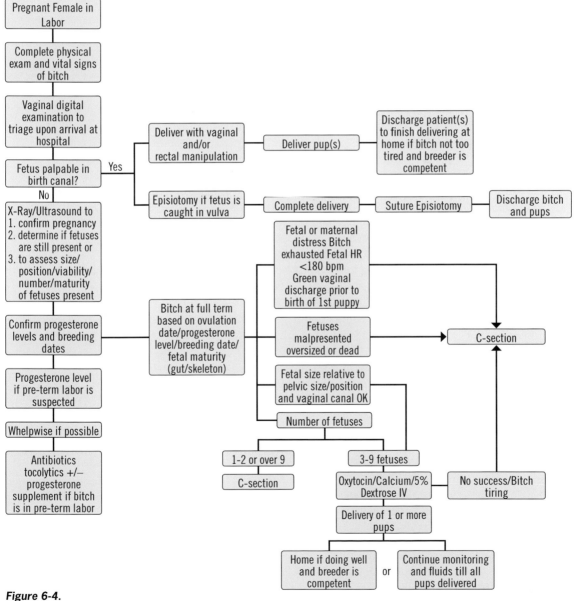

Figure 6-4.
Dystocia algorithm.

puppy survival rate of Caesarian over vaginal delivery. There will come a point at which a C-section may become the ONLY option if pups cannot be delivered vaginally. Sending a bitch home that has retained pups with no hope of vaginal delivery is inappropriate and may be a difficult financial and ethical problem to deal with.

If the bitch is showing productive contractions and the pup is advancing quickly, there may be no need to intervene. When the bitch is delivering a pup, in most cases the chorioallantoic membrane becomes visible as a bubble through the lips of the vulva. It may rupture spontaneously or may be delivered intact. If the pup does not seem to be presenting or the bitch is tired or painful, some gentle assistance can help both the bitch and the puppy.

If time permits, prior to performing a vaginal exam, the lips of the vulva should be cleansed with a disinfectant such as chlorhexidine. If there is excessive hair on the perineum the hair can be clipped. If the tail is heavily haired, the tail can be temporarily wrapped with gauze or tape. Either exam gloves or sterile gloves should be worn, both to protect the bitch from an ascending metritis and to protect the examiner from possible zoonotic diseases such as Brucellosis or Q fever.

If the owner is reluctant to proceed to C-section without first attempting vaginal delivery, there are several "tricks" you can use to aid in the delivery of a litter. There are maneuvers that can be done along with calcium, oxytocin, and IV D5W to assist the delivery of pups.

1. To assist with vaginal delivery, position the bitch either standing or laying on her side with an assistant holding her head as she may resist vaginal examination. Try to do this where the flooring surface and surrounding walls are easy to clean (the green of the placenta stains), there is good footing, and where the examiner and assistant will be comfortable for several minutes. Placing a large blanket or rug under the bitch is very useful. Once the vulva is prepped and gloves are on, the lips of the vulva should be gently parted and one or two fingers inserted carefully into the vagina, sliding upward. If a pup is easily grasped, with gauze or a towel, apply steady gentle traction in a ventral direction (toward the bitch's feet, not straight back). Try to pull gently in coordination with the bitch's pushes to maximize your efforts. Attempt to grasp the neck behind the head, the pelvis, or a pair of feet. Traction on only the tail or one foot or leg can lead to severe damage to the puppy. Rupturing the chorioallantoic membrane does not speed the delivery of the pup. However, it is easier to grasp the puppy and assist the delivery if the membranes are ruptured.
2. If only the tip of a pup can be reached, one of two maneuvers can be attempted. First is to rotate the examiner's hand and stroke the underside of the sacrum from inside the vagina – this is a
3. Ferguson maneuver and many bitches will push with this stimulation.
4. If this is not successful and the pup cannot be palpated, have the examiner insert their gloved fingers into the rectum and by directing their hand ventrally, gently direct the pup through the rectal tissues and slide it caudally. With the other hand, another person's assistance, or a freshly changed glove on the examiner's hand, grasp the now accessible pup and attempt to deliver it.
5. In some cases, the pup is just a little too far up inside the vagina to reach vaginally or rectally. When this occurs, if the forequarters of the bitch can be elevated on a chair or by an assistant; gravity may assist moving the pup outward enough to be grasped and delivered.
6. If the pup cannot be reached, taking the bitch out for a walk to urinate and move can assist moving the pup. In the dark, a flashlight and towel should be taken along as some bitches will deliver a pup while squatting.
7. At home or at the veterinary clinic, vanilla ice cream (orally administered) can improve the hydration, energy and calcium balance of the bitch. The bitch should not be allowed to ingest any other food or placentas in the event she needs a C-section.

8. If no progress is being made, IV 5% dextrose in water, oxytocin administered by SQ or IM route in low doses, and SQ 10% calcium gluconate can aid in coordinating and strengthening uterine contractions. The IV 5% dextrose in water can be given at an appropriate dose based on the patient's condition. The minimum dose would be her maintenance level, and can be increased as indicated. This will improve her energy balance (not a complete replacement, but it helps), and improve her hydration status. Most bitches in labor have gone many hours with little to eat or drink and simple fluid replacement therapy boosts their efforts to labor. Other fluid therapy may be indicated based on the bitch's condition. For instance, if her blood pressure or physical findings suggest she is showing signs of shock, colloidal or crystalloid therapy should be administered according to your veterinary hospital's protocol.

9. Calcium gluconate 10% can be administered at a range of 0.5 to 1.0 ml per 10 pounds body weight SQ only. The calcium preparation MUST be 10% calcium gluconate to administer SQ and should be split into at least 2 injection sites to reduce the risk of a skin slough. IV administration is risky and should be reserved for bitches with eclampsia (see Chapter 7).

10. Oxytocin can be administered on a conservative basis (most published or label doses are too high so check for current dosage recommendations) at 0.5 to 2 IU/bitch (not per pound) of body weight SQ or IM, 2 doses maximum per pup delivered.

This should not be done without first assuring that there is no obstruction to delivery (radiography and palpation), making certain the bitch is not already having strong contractions, and discussing the risks of administering oxytocin and of delaying a C-section with the owner.

Oxytocin is an amazing and powerful hormone. It is the natural hormone that creates both uterine contractions and release of milk from the mammary gland. But it must be treated with a healthy respect. Recent research shows that most of the published doses of oxytocin are too high, putting the pups and bitch at risk. Smaller doses create more effective waves of contraction, and are safer.

When the bitch is strong and healthy, the uterus is correctly positioned, the pups are small enough to be delivered, there is no pup obstructing the way, and her cervix is open, oxytocin administration with caution is appropriate.

Ideally, uterine contraction monitoring (tocodynamometry) is used to assess the safe use of oxytocin. However, this equipment is available only on a limited basis (WhelpWise™) and must be ordered in advance of the delivery. If this is not available, a radiograph and clinical judgment can help determine if presentation of the pups suggests the use of oxytocin is probably safe.

Oxytocin should not be used in certain situations. If uterine contractions are too forceful, this will create several risks to the bitch and the pups. The bitch may experience such forceful contractions that her uterus can rupture, leading to the development of the life-threatening conditions of shock and peritonitis. The risks to the pups are restricted blood supply to the placenta and premature disruption of the placental attachment to the uterus, increasing the risk of fetal death.

The situations in which to avoid the use of oxytocin are:
1. Prior to the delivery of the first pup – if the cervix is closed or there is a mal-presentation of a pup.
2. The bitch is already in hard labor.
3. When 2 doses in 20 minutes have already been administered.
4. When 2 doses do not succeed in delivering a pup, C-section should be recommended to the client.

The lower doses shown above are more effective and safer for the pups and bitch.

Some but not all veterinary clinics are comfortable dispensing oxytocin to their clients. This is best done in combination with uterine contraction monitoring using titrated doses based on the existing uterine activity pattern. Again, oxytocin is contraindicated in the presence of fetal distress or in the presence of existing strong uterine contractions. Oxytocin is a prescription item and must only be dispensed and used under the veterinarian's supervision. Some clients have oxytocin in their possession and would benefit from instruction in its use. The following guidelines can be included with the oxytocin dispensed. It is also a good idea to dispense only small quantities pre-measured and labeled in syringes to minimize the use of the drug and reduce the likelihood of client error. A valid-client-patient-veterinary relationship should be in place for the veterinarian to dispense oxytocin.

Summary – Oxytocin rules
- **When and How can I use Oxytocin? With GREAT care**
- **The correct maximum dose is 0.1 cc per 10 pounds of body weight SQ or IM only – start low and increase if necessary**
- **Maximum 1 cc regardless of size of the bitch**
- **Do not exceed 2 doses in 20 minutes**
- **If 2 doses are unsuccessful, proceed to C-section**
- **Do NOT use if the bitch is in hard labor or no pups have been delivered**
- **Risks include uterine rupture and "shrink wrapping" the pups**
- **In conjunction with oxytocin, IV fluids with 5% dextrose (for fluid, energy, and electrolyte replacement) and SQ calcium injections can be used along with attempts to manually deliver the pups (Table 6-1).**

Table 6-1 Drug doses	
Oxytocin	0.1 ml per 10 pounds of body weight SQ (Hutchison) or 0.25 to 4.0 USP U per dog SQ or IM, repeated in 45 to 60 minutes (Copley) . Best used with uterine contraction monitoring. Without monitoring, limit to 2 doses and proceed to C-section.
Calcium: Calphosan SOLUTION (not Calphosan suspension) or 10% Calcium Gluconate ONLY	0.5 to 1.0 cc per 10 pounds of body weight every 4 to 6 hours. SQ divided into 2 locations, not to exceed 5 cc per location.
IV fluids: D5W	Maintenance fluids: 50 ml/kg daily maintenance plus additional for deficit and ongoing loss.

Oxytocin: (Hutchison, Robert: "Canine Reproduction, Whelping and Neonatal Care." Lakeshore Pembroke Welsh Corgi Club. Crystal Lake, IL. 25 March 2005)
Oxytocin and Calcium: (Copley K: Parturition management: 15,000 whelpings later: An outcome based analysis. Theriogenology 2009; Vol. 1, Number 2: 297-307.)

Episiotomy
Anatomically, the vagina or lips of the vulva may be so restrictive that it is obvious the head or hips of the pup will not pass through. If a specific area of restriction can be palpated vaginally, an episiotomy may facilitate the delivery of the pup. In most cases, if the pup is already in the vagina, it will need to be delivered vaginally, not by C-section. This will need to be done quickly enough to save the pup. Oxytocin and calcium are contraindicated and should NOT be given to a bitch with a puppy lodged vaginally.

This procedure can usually be done with a local anesthetic. If it appears this is indicated, the bitch should be shaved in the perineal area (from the top of the vulva to the rectum) in a 2 to 4 inch wide strip. This area should be prepped with your routine surgical scrub. Lidocaine with sodium bicarbonate should be infused into the area above the vulva. An assistant should be prepared to adequately restrain the bitch, probably muzzled. The doctor should don sterile surgical gloves and use a sterile large pair of straight Mayo scissors, serrated if possible. With the bitch in a standing position, and with the non-dominant hand with one finger on the pup for shielding it from the scissors, one open blade of the Mayo should be gently slipped into the vulva at the dorsal commissure with the tip of the blade directed upward toward the rectum. The technician doing restraint should be advised the procedure is about to start, the scissors in one stroke firmly closed, and incision made. The incision should not exceed 50% of the distance between the vulva and rectum. Care should be taken to avoid damaging the rectum. With this in mind, extend the incision as necessary to release the puppy. To avoid injuring the pup while making the incision, the pup should be gently repelled. There will be some bleeding but it should be minimal if the incision is on the midline. The pup should be delivered and resuscitated as indicated.

The incision should not be sutured until the entire litter is delivered. If this procedure has allowed her to proceed with delivery without a caesarian, suturing can be done with local anesthesia and gentle restraint. It should be a 2 layer closure – with absorbable suture in the mucosa and non-absorbable (not staples) in the skin. If the bitch is to deliver the rest of her pups at home, she can return for closure – the local anesthetic should be re-infused, prep repeated and a new pack of sterile instruments used. If she is anesthetized for a caesarian, it is clear that this is the most comfortable time for the bitch and the attending veterinarian to complete the process. The suturing can be done at the conclusion of the Caesarean, prior to ending the general anesthetic period used for the abdominal procedure.

Oral antibiotics (known to be safe during lactation such as amoxicillin or amoxicillin and clavulanic acid) may be indicated after either extensive vaginal manipulation to deliver the pups or performing an episiotomy. Routine use of antibiotics is not indicated for most vaginal deliveries or after an uncomplicated C-section.

Knowing when to intervene

If the owner is concerned enough to call, the best practice is to have the owner bring the bitch (and puppies already delivered in a warm box) in for an evaluation. In a practice that takes its own calls or is an emergency clinic, it is better to have the client arrive during hours when staff is readiliy available rather than to wait until after-hours. Encouraging the client to "wait it out" often means waiting too long to allow for safe delivery of the pups.

Determining if the bitch has a dystocia is useful in assisting the client and doctor in determine if there is an emergency. Using the guidelines in Table 6-7, the client, staff and doctors can use their best judgment to determine the likelihood that the bitch has dystocia.

The obvious answer as to when to intervene is before it is too late, but not so early as to interfere with the normal whelping. This is always a tough call to make. Most experienced breeder-clients are intuitive and just seem to know when something isn't going as it should. If they call, they are usually asking for intervention, so offer them an appointment at the earliest possible time. If an inexperienced client calls and fulfills the above criteria or calls more than once, they also should be scheduled for an appointment at the earliest possible time. To adequately suit the needs of breeder-clients, the hospital's schedule must allow for appointments on short-notice for this type of urgent problem. When there is a bitch in whelp, you are treating a group of patients with a potentially life-threatening concern, not just one patient. In a practice with a large breeder-client base, most of these other clients are willing to reschedule a non-urgent appointment when the dystocia appointment is explained, because they would want you to do the same for them.

Stillborn puppies

Many puppies that are stillborn were viable until shortly before the delivery. Neonatal death is caused by a prolonged time from placental separation to the first opportunity to take a breath outside of the fetal fluids. Other pups have had their fetal development arrested prior to birth due to infection, genetic defects, or other causes of fetal death. These pups are generally easily identified as non-resuscitatable and nothing can or could have been done. They are generally under-developed, deformed, or show signs of necrosis. Some are born at full-term and appear to be recently deceased but have obvious outward signs of defects making it evident that long-term survival would be a challenge.

Most stillborns are fully developed normal pups who should have been born alive. Either the pup was delayed in its travel from the uterine attachment to outside the fetal membranes, or the efforts to resuscitate the pup were not timely or aggressive enough. Many bitches can whelp and resuscitate their pups without human intervention. But this is not always the case. With an appropriate degree of human intervention to aid the bitch in delivery, removing fetal membranes and clearing the airways, the pups should thrive. If there is prolonged labor, assistance in whelping or C-section should be offered. Some pups that are born alive but have had prolonged deliveries may survive only a few hours to a few days. In retrospect, a C-section might have improved neonatal survival rates.

Some clients would rather lose a few puppies than to subject the bitch to a C-section. Some clients expect the highest puppy survival rate they can achieve; in most cases, this can be provided by offering a C-section before there is fetal and bitch distress. Pro-active or elective C-sections have been shown in studies to allow for the highest puppy survival rates at birth, 2 hours and 7 days post-whelping. However, to maximize Caesarean success, advance planning and staff training are mandatory.

Managing a dystocia

Dystocia means abnormal or difficult birth. It can include maternal and fetal causes, and failure for labor to start (Figure 6-5).

Maternal dystocias

Maternal causes account for approximately 75% of dystocias. Maternal dystocia includes either an obstruction of the birth canal or uterine inertia. There are several types of obstruction; these include

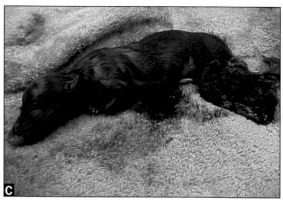
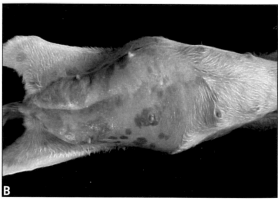
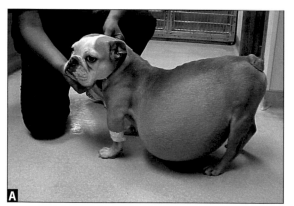

Figure 6-5.
A. A bitch with a high risk pregnancy. *B.* Dystocia pup sideways. *C.* Dystocia pup from previous photograph. Born dead from prolonged labor.

a narrow pelvic canal; vaginal stricture, septa or other restriction; uterine torsion; uterine rupture; scarring, tumors, vaginal hyperplasia, or other malformations.

Some causes of dystocia can be determined at C-section and some remain mysteries. Most causes are not believed to be inherited. Because there are so many causes including fetal and unusual causes that are unlikely to recur, it is not possible to say with certainty that a bitch who needs a C-section should not be allowed to breed again. It may be possible for a bitch who has had a C-section to have a vaginal birth at a subsequent pregnancy.

Primary uterine inertia is failure of the uterus to contract adequately to expel the fetuses. This is not fully understood in the dog and is considered rare. Secondary uterine inertia is the inability to progress from stage I to stage II labor, and is common. Some breeds are predisposed to primary uterine inertia; other causes include overstretching of the uterus with very large litters or oversized pups; insufficient hormones to initiate labor in very small litters; uterine torsion; hypocalcemia; obesity; and when fetal obstruction due to oversized or malpositioned pups causes exhaustion of the uterus and failed delivery (Figure 6-6). Torsion See Chapter 9.

Fetal dystocias

Fetal causes account for approximately 25% of dystocias. The causes include mal-presentation (fetal position that is not linear with the birth canal) and fetuses that are too large relative to the size of the birth canal. There are multiple positions that cause fetal dystocia. Puppies may present sideways, neck first, head flexed back, breech, head in one horn and torso in the opposite horn, or in pairs. Puppies that are too large relative to the size of the birth canal include those that are simply too large and puppies that have deformities that prevent normal delivery. There are many breeds that are predisposed to fetal oversize. Some, such as the brachycephalic breeds, have high rates of dystocia because the head of the puppy is oversized relative to the size of the mother's pelvis. For these breeds, a scheduled C-section is a good option.

Most causes of dystocia will require medical or surgical intervention. Some causes of dystocia, such as relative oversize, cannot be resolved by medical therapy. When medical therapy fails, or is destined to fail, proceeding to C-section may save the bitch and the pups.

Breech delivery

With a breech delivery the pup is born tail, not rear feet first. It is considered normal for approximately 40% of puppies to be born in posterior presentation, this means the back

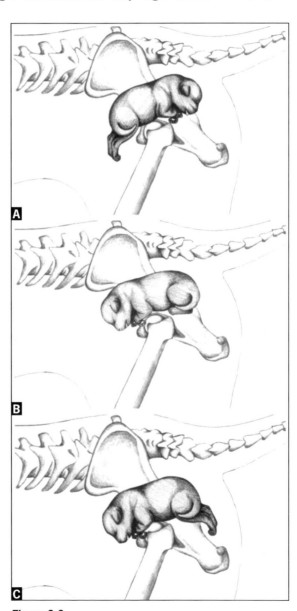

Figure 6-6.
A. Normal birth position shown with the pelvis cut away (60%).
B. Breech presentation. C. Posterior presentation (40%).

feet are presented first. This alone is not a cause of dystocia; it is only a dystocia if there are other causes such as relative oversize. A puppy positioned with its back feet first is not a breech birth. A breech birth is when the pup is presented with its tail first and back feet forward. This can cause dystocia and make it difficult to manipulate the pup.

Tocodynamometry

Tocodynamometry is a computer-based method of uterine contraction monitoring. There is currently only one service available for animals – WhelpWise™. This service is particularly valuable for the bitch in premature labor, the bitch with a history of dystocia, the owner with little experience, or for the bitch in a breed or line of dogs with a predisposition to dystocia. Since the availability of the equipment is limited, reservations must be made upon confirmation of the pregnancy.

The service includes 2 pieces of equipment: tocodynamometer and fetal Doppler and the associated interpretation of the data. The tocodynamometer is used to assess uterine contractions and the fetal Doppler is used to assess trends in fetal heart rates. In routine cases, data is collected by applying a transducer to the clipped abdomen for one hour twice daily. This can be done from home or the veterinary hospital. The data is downloaded from the transducer through a modem to a 24 hour service, located in Colorado. A phone call is made to the breeder and/or attending veterinarian with an interpretation of the data. This data includes information about the onset of labor; timing and strength of uterine contractions; efficacy of medical intervention; and objective data on whether medical or surgical intervention is indicated. High risk cases or bitches in active labor will have more frequent monitoring periods. Medical and surgical therapy is recommended based on these results, combining data pertaining to the uterine contractions and fetal viability.

All medical therapy is based on the objective data collected and the attending veterinarian's treatment plan.

A study involving Guide Dogs showed a reduction of fetal death from 9% to 2% when using Whelpwise™ (Figure 6-7).

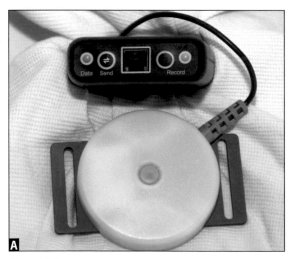
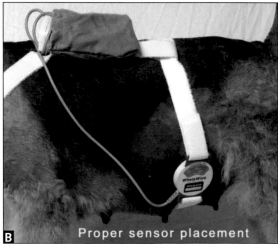

Figure 6-7.
*A. Whelpwise equipment – a uterine contraction monitor used for tocodynometry during labor. **B.** Whelpwise equipment shown showing correct sensor position on the bitch's abdomen.*

Managing the C-section
Procedure
In this section, we will lay out one suggested set-up and sequence of events. In the beginning, your staff will find this guideline will make their job in a busy practice faster and less stressful. After you become more experienced in this process, you and your staff will likely have modifications which will make this protocol suit your hospital.

Prior to induction for the surgical procedure, the doctors and staff should briefly discuss their plan for managing the puppies and bitch to be certain they are familiar with equipment location, have adequate drugs and supplies, and all staff is familiar with their duties to maximize efficiency.

C-section set up
(Appendix A-5)
Paperwork
- Patient Record, including breeding dates and ovulation timing and medical history
- Surgery consent form – signed by the owner, after informed consent is given.
- Anesthesia form (Appendix D-8)
- C-section surgical report (Appendix D-9)
- C-section discharge sheet (Appendix C-12)
- Patient ID band

Induction/IV setup
- Mouth Gag
- Endotracheal tube
- Ties for Endotracheal tube
- Laryngoscope
- Bland eye ointment
- IV Catheter
- IV injection port
- 1" white tape for IV catheter
- Saline flush for IV flush
- Sterile skin prep for catheter placement

Surgery room set-up
- Lactated Ringer or fluid of the doctor's choice, kept warm for abdominal flush
- Colloids – hetastarch if necessary
- Surgery table
- V-tray or surgery table with V capability
- Heating source for bitch – be careful to avoid anything that could cause thermal burns
- Towels ready to support rear of bitch if needed
- Sterile Lap towels – 2 large and 4 small
- Surgery gown – 1 per person scrubbing in
- Surgery caps and masks for all in the surgical suite
- Scalpel blade
- Suture for closing the uterus, abdominal wall, subcutaneous tissue and skin
- Surgery pack, large – with a system for an instrument and gauze count
     Suggested surgical pack with accurate instrument count
     4 to 8 towel clamps
     1 Metzenbaum scissors
     1 Mayo scissors
     1 thumb forceps

1 scalpel handle
2 straight carmalts
2 curved carmalts
5 curved Kelly forceps
3 curved mosquito forceps
1 needle holder
Serrated straight Mayo scissors for episiotomy
Surgery gloves – 2 pair for each person scrubbing in
Duct tape to keep long coated hair away from the incision site
Puppy ID towels – 1 set of each colored sterilized/non-sterilized

Drugs to set-up for the bitch
- Atropine injectable
- Butorphanol injectable
- Buprinex injectable
- Calcium for SQ injection
- Famotidine
- Lidocaine or bupivicaine
- Metoclopramide injectable (Reglan®)
- Oxytocin from refrigerator
- Post-op pain medication injectable as preferred by attending veterinarian
- Propofol injectable
- Solu-Medrol 1 to 24 hours pre-op

Drugs to set-up for the neonate
- Caffeine*
- Ceftiofur – keep in freezer reconstituted until use*
- Dexamethasone
- Dextrose
- Dopram – 0.01 cc per pup
- Epinephrine diluted 1:10*
- Lasix injectable
- Vitamin K injectable

*Pre-dilute just prior to anesthetic induction

Puppy set-up
- Non-sterilized set of colored towels matching sterilized set in the surgery suite
- Heating pads
- Puppy scale (weight in kilograms preferred)
- Stethoscopes
- Laryngoscope to aid in neonatal intubation
- Otoscope with large tip to aid in neonatal intubation
- Sterile umbilical pack (needle holder and hemostat)
- Suture for umbilical cords
- Laundry baskets or large styrofoam boxes for pups
- Bulb syringes
- DeLee mucous traps
- Endotracheal tubes suitable for puppies – Cole tube, tom cat catheters, red rubber feeding tubes cut and end smoothed to allow for ventilation or large bore IV catheters (prepare these in advance, clean and can be reused)
- Stylet for endotracheal tube
- Face masks, small fitted with diaphragm for neonatal ventilation

- Tincture of iodine, in contained to dispense to client – to dip cords in, disposable
- AmbuBag, pediatric
- End to adapt endotracheal tube to fit Oxygen hoses or Ambu bag
- O2, with regulator turned on
- Fish tank or O2 chamber/incubator
- Hair blow-dryer to aid in drying off wet neonates
- Dog dish, disinfected, for warm water bath to use to warm neonates

Additional set-up to keep work area clean and safe:
- Place non-slip mat in under surgery table
- Place towels in work area and around surgery table

Sequence of events
(Appendix A-5)
- Confirm the bitch's due date prior to proceeding to C-section and that there are pups present
- Arrival of the bitch with possible or confirmed dystocia
- Exam room with blanket for bitch to nest on during evaluation
- Palpation/vaginal digital exam
- Episiotomy if indicated (pup trapped in vagina by stricture) should be done ASAP
- Technician to take history and assist with examination
- Assess the bitch
    PE/TPR/Blood pressure of bitch
    Preparation for possible radiograph
    Radiograph and or ultrasound as indicated
- Examination glove and lubricant (KY jelly®, Nolvalube®, or J-lube®)
- Incubator or basket with heat source for pups
- Towels
- Supplies and drugs as listed for neonatal resuscitation
- Owner signs consent form to allow anesthesia and surgical procedure after informed consent with doctor, discussing options and risks
- Pre-surgical blood panel with protime if available/progesterone if available
- +/– Doppler or abdominal ultrasound to assess pups heart rates if available
- Place IV catheter and start fluids – stabilize before proceeding if indicated
- Administer drugs to the bitch:
    - small animal atropine injectable (1 cc per 20 pounds SC or 0.02 to 0.04 mg/kg (0.01 to 0.02 mg/lb) IV, IM, SC, using atropine 0.54 mg/ml),
    - Metoclopramide injectable at 0.3 cc per 10 pounds SC, (dosed at 0.2 to 0.4 mg/kg, using metoclopramide 5 mg/ml),
    - 10% calcium at 0.5 ml per 10 pounds SC and
    - Solu-Medrol® SLOWLY IV (at 1 mg/lb based on the bitch's body weight, using 125 mg/2 ml). Give Solu-Medrol® first to provide maximal time from administration to induction.
- Start oxygen by face mask or other administration if tolerated by bitch.
- Administer antibiotics only if indicated by condition of bitch and pups
- Shave abdomen before anesthesia
- STOP! LOOK AROUND TO BE SURE ALL SUPPLIES AND STAFF ARE IN PLACE AND READY TO MOVE QUICKLY
- GO!
- Move bitch to surgery room
- Induce anesthesia with Propofol® at 1 cc/5 pounds (start with 1/2 to 2/3 and give as needed)
- Bland eye ointment apply to protect her eyes
- Mouth gag
- Intubate and inflate cuff/secure tube with tie
- Place bitch on surgery table with left side slightly rolled down
- Attach anesthetic machine and monitors

- Continue IV fluids at rate on chart per hour (see chart in appendix)
- Scrub the site with Nolvasan® and alcohol alternating preps or routine surgical prep per your hospital protocol while the doctor is scrubbing in
- Roll her onto back and secure in final position as doctor prefers – be sure she is in a comfortable position with her head, neck, and back level, avoid tipping head down (avoid gastric reflux which can cause irreparable damage to esophagus)
- Prep again in case final positioning contaminated surgical field
- Open supplies – gown/gloves/surgery pack/blade/towel clamps/drape/suture/lap towels/ puppy towels (Table 6-2). Preform instument count prior to making incision.

Table 6-2 Caesarean section procedure	
Bitch	Pups
Increase gas anesthestic if light or titrate with Propofol	Clear membranes off the face ASAP, keeping pup tilted head down and face out of pooled fluids. Hand to waiting tech in sterile colored towel to start rubbing.
Metacam® (at 0.18 ml/10#sq) or Rimadyl® (at 4.4 mg/kg sq) after last pup is out	Suction with bulb syringe and/or DeLee mucus trap
Suture uterus	Monitor/assist with respirations
Oxytocin p r n	Stethoscope and Doppler to check for heart beat if not obvious
Belly flush and eliminate soiled lap towels	Oxygen as needed – face mask or chamber
Re-glove	Acupuncture if needed 25 g needle in upper lip
Closure of abdominal wall, sq and skin	Dopram® and/or Caffeine to stimulate respirations (controversial). Dopram® must not be given unless the airway is open, oxygen is being administered and the pup is at least 10 minutes old if needed
Wash disinfectant off skin with saline along mammary chain so pups can nurse without ingesting Nolvasan®	Use "accordion" technique if still not breathing
Assist pups in nursing	Intubate trachea if needed, or use face mask ventilation, begin ventilations with O2
Apply DAP collar	Check for cleft palates and other defects/treat
Prepare discharge instructions	Ligate umbilical cord/treat with tincture of iodine
Make up meds for owner to take home – Metacam®/ Reglan®/ Nolvasan®/ Nemex®/ +/– Antibiotics	Mark pups with corresponding color to map of uterine location
Remove IV catheter AFTER entire dose of IV fluids have been administered and OK with attending veterinarian	Weigh pups and placentas, record Record APGAR scores @ 1 and 5 minutes
	Photographs of pups
	Assist pups in nursing
Discharge the bitch and pups, being sure you have shown the owner how to tube feed and care for the pups, and all instructions and supplies are sent home with the breeder	Reweigh pups after nursing
	Blot or dab pups with reserved amniotic fluid to increase bitch's acceptance of pups
	Administer plasma to ineffective nursers or all pups if colostrum is not available
	Place in oxygen/incubator or warmed basket
	Prepare warmed transport container for travel home
	Discharge pups and bitch to owner

When a C-section is the best choice

The decision to proceed with a C-section or allow a bitch to attempt to whelp is usually difficult. This section will attempt to make the process less emotionally and mentally challenging. It is not uncommon to reflect upon the C-section you did and wonder if you acted too impulsively, that she could have done it; and for every one of those decisions, you will have an equal opportunity to look back on a whelping gone wrong and wish you had reacted more aggressively.

Many factors are involved in the decision to perform, or not to perform a C-section. It is not uncommon to have a client break down in tears at the mention of a caesarian, usually because they or a friend have a bitch and/or puppies that had an unfortunate outcome. This is most commonly due to a delay in the decision to go to surgery which led to a higher than necessary puppy mortality.

To reduce your angst when the inevitable phone calls come, here are some guidelines.

A well executed C-section statistically will produce a higher percentage of live pups than vaginal delivery. It is, however, obvious that not every litter should or could be delivered surgically. The current trend in human medicine is toward ever increasing caesarians, with predictions that it may soon approach 50% of U.S. births. Many reasons are listed, but the primary goal we consider justifiable in veterinary medicine is to increase puppy survival rates.

In a study published by Paula Moon, et. al. while an anesthesiology resident at Cornell, she compiled data from 807 Caesarian derived litters in 109 practices across Canada and the United States totaling 3,908 pups. The purpose of her study was to evaluate peri-operative risk factors affecting neonatal survival after canine C-section in a clinical population once the decision was made to undergo the surgical procedure. She did not dictate any anesthetic or treatment protocols, but collected and analyzed for survival immediately, at 2 hours and 7 days after delivery as summarized and adapted below (Table 6-3).

Of the 757 dams for which information was available, maternal mortality at seven days was 1.2%. Emergency surgery accounted for 58% (n=453 of 776) of the cases for which information was available. For both elective and emergency surgeries, the bulldog was the most frequently represented breed (17%; n=138). The following factors increased the likelihood of all puppies being alive: the surgery was not an emergency; the dam was not brachycephalic; there were four puppies or less in the litter; there were no naturally delivered or deformed puppies; all puppies breathed spontaneously at birth; at least one puppy vocalized spontaneously at birth; and neither methoxyflurane nor xylazine was used in the anesthetic protocol. Isoflurane and propofol were associated unconditionally with a positive effect on neonatal survival at seven days.

The value of her study is two-fold. One, it aids us in anesthetic selection. Two, it aids both breeders and veterinarians in making well-informed decisions, with the knowledge that well-executed C-sections have the potential to maximize puppy survival. Clearly, our patient selection is limited in that we cannot select away from the brachycephalic patient. However, it does allow us to minimize some of the risk factors known to increase maternal and fetal morbidity and mortality.

Table 6-3 Puppy survival rates		
Time after delivery	Puppy survival by C-section birth	Puppy survival by vaginal birth
0 hours	92%	86%
2 hours	87%	83%
7 days	80%	75%

Moon et. al.

A scheduled C-section is a better choice for:
1. High Risk breeds such as Bulldogs.
2. Bitches with diagnosed pelvic fractures or vaginal strictures.
3. Bitches with illness diagnosed during pregnancy predicted to cause dystocia such as diabetes mellitus or intervertebral disc disease.
4. Bitches with previous primary uterine inertia (75% of C-sections are due to maternal causes).
5. Large litters (more than 9 pups).
6. Small litters (1 to 2 pups).
7. Highly valuable puppies such as litters conceived from frozen surgical inseminations.
8. Bitches predicted to develop dystocia based on radiographs taken pre-partum – films which show malpresentations, log-jams, or oversized pups.
9. When the client is unable to manage a whelping.

Timing is critical for puppy survival, as a few hours too early or too late will lead to significant puppy mortality. The ideal planned C- section is scheduled based on ovulation timing. Normal pregnancy in the bitch is 63 days from ovulation, plus or minus 24 hours. The dates in the literature that state pregnancy can last 58 to 67 days are based on dates from breeding, not ovulation. Progesterone timing has revolutionized several aspects of canine reproduction and is very valuable in this setting. (See chapter 3.)

We can calculate that the bitch is anticipated to go into labor 63 days from ovulation plus or minus 24 hours using a progesterone level of 5 ng/dl (from many referral labs) or the progesterone level that your referral lab indicates signal ovulation. Typically, we schedule our bitches for C-section 62 days **from ovulation providing colostrum or milk is present in the mammary glands** and there are no contraindications for anesthesia and surgery. Bulldog and other bulldog type breeds are scheduled for C-section 61 days from ovulation. The bitch and pups MUST be ready for the C-section for it to be safe. Bitches with larger litters tend to have a slightly shorter pregnancy (0.25 day per puppy shorter) and bitches with one to two puppy litters tend to have a slightly longer pregnancy. Convenience should not override good sense and patience. Lactation represents more than nutrition for the pups; it represents a physiological and psychological preparedness for the bitch to feed and mother her pups and a physiological and psychological preparedness of the pups to nurse strongly and manage themselves in the whelping box.

Why and when to be aggressive in early dystocia intervention

Puppy survival can be maximized by early intervention. The longer a bitch labors or the longer over day 63 (based on ovulation date) her pregnancy extends, the greater the chance that puppies will be born dead. This is a result of poor placental blood flow associated with placental separation due to prolonged labor or placental aging.

We cannot overemphasize the need for a rapid decision making strategy and response. At the first inkling of a possible dystocia, the staff must initiate decisions regarding the care of the pregnant bitch. They must advise the owner of how and when to proceed, alert the doctor of the potential crisis, and be prepared for care of the bitch and neonates by the time the client arrives at the hospital.

Most unsuccessful neonatal outcomes are the result of taking a wait-and-see approach. None of us would tell a client with a dog showing evidence of any other life-threatening condition to stay home and wait it out. But many veterinarians make this recommendation to clients with bitches in whelp. In this situation, you are not only putting the bitch at risk but you may be making life and death decisions for up to 15 patients.

If you have a client on the telephone that is concerned about how the bitch's labor is progressing, and they either have no experience in whelping and need trained assistance, or they know they have a litter in trouble and are prepared to travel to your hospital for assistance, HAVE THEM PACK THEIR SUPPLIES AND START DRIVING. If they are well equipped for the trip (**See Appendix C-3**) and have someone to drive, the worst thing that can happen is that they will call and tell you the bitch started whelping in the car en route. The opposite scenario occurs when you advise the client that it is better to wait while the fetal survival rate plummets on the basis of your conservative advice.

How to determine if a bitch has a dystocia

Guidelines for clients and staff are imperative for rapid assessment of a potential dystocia and loss of puppy vigor. Providing clients and staff with a list of questions for evaluation of the bitch and your instruction that they are to immediately notify the staff doctor on duty of findings and concerns can rapidly and effectively improve communication and is critical in preventing possible bitch and fetal mortality.

Questions for the veterinary staff to evaluate the bitch at home or at the hospital indicating the probable need for an EMERGENCY C-section: (Appendix B-4)

1. Has the bitch been in hard labor (abdominal pushing) over 2 hours on the first or 1 hour on subsequent pups?
2. Did the bitch initially show good abdominal contractions and stop without producing a puppy?
3. Is there is green vaginal discharge PRIOR to the delivery of the first puppy?
4. Does the bitch seem distressed? Frantic? Sick? Weak or unable to stand? Tremoring? Repeated vomiting?
5. Is this labor pattern different than her previous ones?
6. Has the bitch been unwilling or unable to eat and/or drink for over 12 hours?
7. Has WhelpWise™ indicated there is a problem with fetal heart rates (<160 BPM) or uterine contraction patterns?
8. Have any pups been born dead?
9. Did a previous radiograph or ultrasound suggest there could be a problem? (low heart rates on ultrasound or pups without visible heartbeats?) (Malpresented or very large pups)
10. Is a pup palpated on vaginal examination and in an unusual position or not progressing through the birth canal?
11. Did her temperature drop to 98 degrees and rise to normal (over 101.0) and stay there more than 4 hours?
12. Has her pregnancy exceeded 63 days?
13. Does she appear to have a very large or very small litter?
14. Does she have a previous history of dystocia?
15. Is she a breed at risk for maternal or fetal causes of dystocia?
16. Does she have unexplained or unusual discharge from her eyes?
17. Is she having weak or non-productive contractions with multiple puppies left?
18. If oxytocin has been used, has there been a minimal or no response?
19. Are any puppies weak, crying excessively, or do they have any obvious physical abnormalities?
20. Does the breeder or veterinary staff member have a feeling that something is going wrong? Trust their intuition.

If the answer to any of these questions is yes, you may need to assess the bitch as soon as possible and advise your client that the bitch should proceed to emergency surgery unless you can immediately correct any cause for dystocia.

How to minimize the risks of C-sections

Benefits and risks

When assessing the risks and benefits of caesarian, as in any invasive procedure, a balance must be achieved. The primary difference with this procedure is that the stakes are higher – your decision must weigh the lives of many. Most breeders may have already indicated that the bitch is their top priority; that if they must decide between puppies and the bitch, they will always opt to do what is best for the bitch. Fortunately, it is unusual to have to make a decision between the two.

Benefits for the bitch: The most obvious benefit is for the bitch who simply cannot deliver a litter. Both primary and secondary uterine inertia can occur, as can physical inability to deliver. In these cases, the obvious benefit is that the bitch will likely survive if veterinary intervention is provided.

She will not exhaust herself in the process of parturition only to need surgical intervention when she is a higher risk candidate, she will not labor so hard as to rupture her uterus or cause other damage associated with parturition, and she will not need to go to surgery later for a deceased retained pup when she is ill.

Risks for the bitch: There are risks associated with anesthesia including respiratory and/or cardiac arrest and death. Surgical complications may include hemorrhage, hypovolemic shock, infection of the abdominal incision, peritonitis, dehiscence of the uterine or abdominal incision, adhesions, and esophagitis as well as others. These are reported in 1.2% of the bitches in the study done by Moon et al in the U.S. and Canada.

Benefits for the puppies: Statistically, puppies have a 4 to 6% higher survival rate when born by C-section. Risk of premature placental separation and prolonged delivery causing weak or deceased pups is prevented by a rapid and successful surgical delivery. Even if a pup is born alive, a stressful and prolonged delivery can result in the pup or pups dying the first several days after birth. This is generally the strongest motivation for a client to proceed with a scheduled caesarian.

Risks for the puppies: Although more pups are born alive by C-section, it can be more difficult to initiate nursing and maternal instincts. Btches who have C-sections are more likely than bitches who have vaginal births to initially be unwilling and unable to allow pups to nurse. In these cases, the bitch may need close supervision, pharmaceutical assistance in lactation and developing maternal skills, and the pups may require supplemental feeding and/or plasma.

Benefits for the owners: The owner can plan for a specific time of day and arrange their personal and work schedule around the delivery. The owner can arrive at the veterinary hospital and return home organized, well-rested and better able to manage the demands of caring for their bitch and her puppies. Few would consider this a primary reason for surgical intervention.

Risks for the owners: The only risk we experience is the cost. However, in the long run, the client will often come out ahead financially with the increased puppy survival offsetting the cost to deliver the pups.

Benefits for the veterinary staff: The primary benefit to the veterinarians and staff is the opportunity to schedule procedures, reducing after hours care and scheduling conflicts during routine office hours. For veterinary hospitals covering their own emergencies, advance planning and appropriate scheduling can reduce stress.

Planning protocols
(Appendix A-7)

1. **Keep a calendar** showing predicted whelping dates of all known breedings. This can be done in a software program like Repro Manager®, or by having your receptionist keep a handwritten calendar. A staff member can check the calendar daily and contact the bitch owner that is due that day. By doing so, you can reduce the "hour of guilt" phone calls that come as you are closing or going to bed. This allows you to intervene at home or have the bitch visit your hospital for evaluation before too much time has elapsed to ensure a good outcome.

2. **Great staff-to-staff and staff-to-client communication** will allow your staff to take a complete history, do an initial assessment on the bitch and puppies, and minimize lag time in doctor intervention.

3. **Practice procedures** so that your staff and doctors are experienced in handling neonatal and bitch emergency care. Learning how to place an endotracheal tube in a neonate is a task most certified veterinary technicians can learn to perform, but the time to learn is not under fire.

4. **Have adequate numbers of trained assistants** to properly monitor the bitch and resuscitate puppies. It is ideal to have 1 staff member for every 1 to 2 puppies anticipated. This is in addition to the veterinarian doing the procedure and a technician monitoring the patient during anesthesia. Hospital policies regarding owner participation in the resuscitation of puppies should be established in advance if the hospital staff is insufficient after-hours.

5. **Develop a protocol or apply the one supplied** in this book. By doing so, everyone on the veterinary team knows what the anesthetic protocols, neonatal resuscitation techniques, and sequence of events should be. Assigning specific tasks to individuals will minimize confusion during induction and neonatal resuscitation.

6. **Organizing your supplies and equipment** will allow rapid and efficient setup. Having drugs, supplies, equipment and instruments designated for this purpose and stored together significantly reduces set-up time. Clients and staff alike will appreciate the reduced stress of searching for an essential drug or equipment during an emergent situation.

7. **Establish a protocol for after hours care in advance.** With the increase in available 24 hour emergency care in many municipalities, your hospital may opt to send clients to a referral facility. If that is your policy, let your clients know in advance that you will not be available and that they may be asked to make difficult decisions without your familiar guidance. Counsel them in advance about decision making on how to decide if a caesarian is indicated, if they are told their bitch needs an emergency hysterectomy, and what level of supportive care they may chose for possible critically ill neonates.

8. **Always use IV fluids** prior to and continuously during the procedure for the bitch undergoing C-section.

9. **Do not wait too long to intervene surgically.** If medical management is not successful in producing effective uterine contractions and delivery of live pups, discuss the advantages of a caesarian or referral to a veterinarian experienced in this procedure. You are not a hero by avoiding a caesarian. Your client will measure your success by the number of live pups they have at the time of weaning, not by the caesarians you avoided.

10. **Determine in advance if your clients are allowed into the treatment and surgery areas of the hospital.** Many breeders prefer to be involved and your staff should know how you want them to handle these requests.

11. **A well-coached client** will know if they have a dystocia, have supplies ready in advance, and will have superior husbandry skills. Many breeder clients will come to you with excellent skills but it is still essential that your staff spend time at discharge to be certain all aspects of post surgical and neonatal care have been covered.

12. **Great written discharge instructions** are essential to client education and to legally document your post partum instructions. (See Appendix)

13. **Establish a fee schedule** that includes fees to support an appropriate number of staff members, supplies, equipment, drugs and time to provide excellent medical care to the bitch and pups and to educate and support the owner.

Now that we have this ammunition for ourselves and to bolster our clients knowledge base and emotions, we can determine if we should plan a C-section for high risk patients or reserve the decision for a time if a problem develops during whelping.

Your staff – The key element to success

Staff plays two key roles in managing a well run reproduction service. The first is in communication prior to, during, and after the appointment. The second involves techniques and procedures related to the pre-breeding evaluation, at the time of the breeding and at the time of the C-section. While you may designate 1 or 2 key staff members to handle most communication and procedures of pre-breeding and breeding, you many need all "hands on deck" when the first call regarding a possible dystocia comes in and when the bitch arrives for a C-section.

Excellent staff training and utilization are essential to maximizing bitch and puppy survival rates. Communication starts prior to the breeding, at the time of the client's first contact with the hospital. Well trained staff will be able to explain the services your hospital provides. They will also be able to educate clients regarding the importance to maximal bitch fertility of pre-breeding examinations and the value of progesterone testing. They can provide client education relating to neonatal and post-partum care to improve the success of your C-section.

C-sections need a team approach to patient care. While the veterinarian and one veterinary technician concentrate on the bitch's surgery and anesthesia, an entire team of highly trained staff (and in the right circumstances client participation) is imperative to achieve maximal neonatal resuscitation and survival. Be certain you have spent the time in advance of an emergency rehearsing how the staff should handle neonatal care.

Techniques for success

This section will cover the process from arrival at the hospital through discharge of the bitch and litter to the care of the owner. A step-by-step checklist follows for staff and doctors which will help with rapid and efficient patient care **(See Appendix A-5)**.

Telephone assessment of the bitch in labor or with suspected dystocia

Doctor, staff and client have agreed that the bitch's labor is not proceeding normally. On this basis, she is being transported to the hospital.

Preparation for the arrival of the pregnant bitch

Prior to arrival of the bitch and any pups she may have already delivered, you have an examination room ready as follows.

Clients like to have a large blanket on the floor as many bitches prefer to nest or lie down on the blanket while in labor. We find it preferable to sitting on our exam room furniture. For larger bitches, the examination can be done on this area of the floor. For smaller bitches, a towel or mat can be placed on the examination table to allow for better footing for the bitch during the doctor's examination.

A laundry basket lined with towels and a heating pad set on low or other safe heat source should be available and ready should she arrive with newborns or a pup is delivered shortly after her arrival to the hospital.

Towels, bulb syringes, DeLee mucus traps, gauze squares, Dopram®, and any other drugs and supplies you anticipate will be needed quickly should be in the room or readily available from the workstation you plan to use to resuscitate the pups.

The patient record, history from telephone calls if not in the file, and consent forms should be available.

Radiology should be prepared in advance if necessary.

For the examination, a rectal thermometer, stethoscope, examination gloves, lubricant, and blood pressure monitor should be readily accessible.

Arrival of the pregnant bitch and client

Upon arrival, a technician or assistant should be ready to assist the owner into the hospital. The technician should walk behind the bitch to be sure she does not deposit a puppy in your parking lot unnoticed (this happens), and should bring in the supplies necessary to transport the puppies home.

A technician or assistant should be either in the examination room with the client and bitch at all times or readily available should it appear a pup is about to be delivered. This is particularly important if the owner is inexperienced; you do NOT want them to have to come looking for your help.

A complete and comprehensive physical examination should be done on the bitch on arrival. Start your examination by checking for any pup in the birth canal. You will likely need restraint assistance from a staff member as many bitches are not cooperative at this point. Once it is determined that there is no pup in eminent danger from incomplete delivery, the physical examination should be as complete as that for any pre-surgical patient. It should include checking the general status of the patient, mucus membrane color and refill, hydration, ausculting the thorax, palpation of the abdomen, palpation of lymph nodes, assessment of the mammary system, and any abnormalities brought to your attention by the client or staff. The routine T/P/R or temperature, pulse rate and respiratory rate should be assessed. Blood pressure evaluation is also valuable if available.

If a pup is lodged in the birth canal and it appears that an episiotomy will be needed, it be should be peformed immediately.

Radiographic and ultrasonographic assessment

Radiographic and ultrasonographic assessment of the litter should be your next step in most cases. NEVER take a bitch to surgery without verifying that she has one or more retained fetuses. A uterus that is irritated by abdominal palpation or oxytocin can feel large and firm enough to be mistaken for a retained fetus. If you cannot be absolutely certain that what you are palpating is 1 or more fetuses, take the time to ultrasound or radiograph the bitch.

Ultrasound can be helpful in quickly assessing fetal viability. It is also a great tool for assessing fetal heart rates. You cannot guarantee a client that a pup with a heartbeat on the ultrasound can be resuscitated. However, it is a valuable tool for assessing the general condition. Because deceased pups are frequently the cause of dystocia, if one or more pups without heartbeats are seen on ultrasound, the client should be advised of this prior to caesarian. It is probable that a caesarian will be needed If there are pups with low heart rates. IV fluids and atropine should be administered, and the patient should be taken to surgery as quickly as possible. (The definition bradycardia in a fetus is somewhat controversial. General consensus suggests that 180 to 220 is normal, less than 120 is a sign of fetal distress, and 140 to 160 is open for interpretation.

Fetal Doppler monitoring, can be a valuable tool in assessing fetal distress. These units are available for sale and some clients may already own one.

Radiographs can be valuable in determining whether the bitch is a surgical candidate or can be managed with conservative medical therapy. (see chapter 5). If there is evidence of emphysema (air pockets) surrounding the fetus, peritonitis, significant loss of detail, 1 or 2 fetuses as the total in the litter, oversized or malpresenting fetuses, brachycephalic pups, fetuses outside the uterus, over 10 fetuses, pelvic fractures or a disproportionately small pelvis, C-section should be recommended.

Preparation for surgery
IV catheter placement and IV fluids
Fluids should be started immediately. Continuous IV fluids are imperative for any patient undergoing C-section. Because of the puppy volume compressing the abdominal veins, there will be a sudden drop in pressure as those veins fill when you lift the uterus.

Surgical consent forms
The completed forms should be presented to the client for discussion and their signature. The doctor should explain the benefits and risks of surgery and anesthesia to the client (some states require the veterinarian to do this, not delegate it to staff), and be certain the history is complete. This discussion should include any known anesthetic complications, drug allergies, when and what she ate last, medications , if she has vomited or had any recent symptoms of illness not explained by a healthy pregnancy, previous surgical procedures paying particular attention to abdominal procedures including gastropexies, and other history the client or doctor may deem pertinent.

Pre-surgical lab work
If available on a stat basis, lab work should be drawn and run. If possible, a CBC with platelet count, chemistry panel and protime be completed. If this is a scheduled C-section, the lab work can be done the day prior to the surgery.

Pre-surgical EKG
This is advised if available on a stat or in-house basis.

Atropine
This drug is routinely administered at many hospitals for most C-sections. It should be avoided in cases where atropine is contraindicated such as narrow angle glaucoma. Dose atropine is preferred at 1 cc per 20 pounds of pregnant body weight using the small animal product (0.54 mg per ml). We prefer atropine to glycopyrrolate because it will cross the placentas and aid in maintaining fetal heart rates. (There is some controversy surrounding the use of atropine.)

Buprenorphine or Butorphanol
Either drug may be useful for pre-emptive pain management. However, these drugs may be contraindicated because they can cause an altered mental state in the post-op period, putting the pup's well-being at risk. For post-op pain management, buprenorphine can be dosed at 20 to 30 ug/kg IM (mcg/kg – dose carefully) just prior to induction. Administering buprenorphine at induction provides post-op analegesia but because it takes 45 minutes to take effect, the effects on the neonates are minimized. By starting buprenorphine prior to anesthetic induction, wind-up post-op pain can be reduced. Butorphanol will aid in analgesia as well as sedation if this outcome is desired.

Metoclopramide
This drug is routinely administered subcutaneously (0.3 mg/kg sq or 0.6 cc per 20 pounds pregnant body weight) pre-op unless it was given orally prior to admission or if she has sufficient milk. Metoclopramide has been shown to improve lactation in approximately 75% of bitches by its prolactin secretion stimulation effects. It may protect the bitch from gastroesophageal reflux during the C-section. Metoclopramide should be avoided in bitches with known hypersensitivity to the drug.

"Metoclopramide is excreted into milk and may concentrate at about twice the plasma level, but there does not appear to be significant risk to nursing offspring" (Plumb). Bitches who have had

C-sections tend to exhibit agalactia more frequently than bitches who have experienced vaginal births. In cases where the C-section was scheduled, she may not have entered the phase where her glands were fully developed for milk production. Passage of feti through the cervix stimulates prolactin secretion – a stimulus lacking if all pups are delivered by C-section, unless the surgeon performed digital stimulation of the cervix prior to closing the uterus.

Famotidine can also be useful for reducing gastric reflux and post-op esophageal strictures but should not be given within 2 hours of administering metoclopramide.

Calcium
Calcium is anecdotally reported to improve maternal skills. It also aids in uterine contractility, reducing post-op hemorrhage. It can be given subcutaneously (be sure the product you have is labeled for this use because some products can cause skin sloughs) in 2 separate sites prior to induction.

Steroids
When C-sections are scheduled, rather than when the bitch goes into labor, short-acting cortico-steroids appear to be beneficial. Steroids are theorized to decrease progesterone, prevent shock, and improve the production of surfactant in the neonatal lung; all beneficial to the pups and bitch.

Ideally, steroids are given 8 to 24 hours in advance of a planned C-section. However, there is anecdotal evidence that even when administered 1 hour prior to C-section, the pups seem to be more vigorous and more able to breathe with less technical intervention. Both Solu-Medrol® and Solu-Delta-Cortef® have published doses for this use. The prednisolone sodium succinate (Solu-Medrol®) dose is 1 mg/pound of body weight administered slowly IV. Vials are reconstituted at 125 mg/2 ml and once reconstituted, are discarded if not used within 48 hours. (Lopate, Cheryl. SFT list, 15 April 2007.) The improvement in puppy survival is worth the small additional cost.

Caution should be used in administration of steroids if there is any sign that the bitch or pups have an underlying infection.

Surgical preparatory shaving
This should be completed prior to anesthesia if tolerated by the bitch. DO NOT place patients directly on their backs for shaving because it will compromise the movement of the diaphragm and compress the aorta; instead move her side to side gently to complete the prep. Be certain to have the hair shaved from the vulva to cranial to the xyphoid process and laterally past the nipples. Many bitches will experience post-partum effluvium ("blow their coat" to dog owners) so authorize your staff to prep a large enough area to assure that the field will be adequate to extend the incision if necessary.

Stabilize the bitch
Prior to C-section she should be stabilized if it appears that she is not a surgical candidate on admission. This decision must be balanced by the owner's instructions regarding the value of the pups.

Antibiotics
These are seldom indicated for routine C-sections. When the cervix is closed, uterine contents are nearly always sterile. If there has been excessive vaginal manipulation or you have other concerns regarding bacterial contamination, cefazolin or amoxicillin with sulbactam (Unasyn®) may be given intravenously (assuming that there is no known hypersensitivity to this drug or other beta lactams). Administration after the pups have been delivered is preferred as it will cross the placenta. Ceftiofur or amoxicillin with clavulanic acid should be administered and dispensed for all pups born with meconium in their fetal membranes or that appear to be compromised (See Chapter 8).

Dog appeasing pheromone collar

This is an analog that mimics the pheromone naturally found in the amniotic fluid of dogs and the mammary glands of lactating bitches. Its function is to reassure and calm puppies, and aid in bonding between the bitch to her pups. Its effects last into adulthood and it can also be used to reduce anxiety in many settings. Since the bitch who has had a C-section is not exposed to the pheromone in the amniotic fluids, maternal skills take longer to develop (up to 72 hours). Maternal skills can be hastened by the use of the Adaptil™ collar. Although Adaptil™ comes in collar, room diffuser and spray forms, the collar works more quickly. The collar can be used on the bitch for several days prior to her planned whelping or C-section or can be applied at the C-section. The collar will last for up to 4 weeks, carrying you easily through the development of good mothering skills. The collar is not a substitute for careful observation to assure that she is not threatening to harm her pups.

Anesthesia

(Appendix D-8)

Prior to anesthesia, it should be determined where induction will be done. We prefer **the surgical suite** (remember, the surgical shaving is already done) to reduce the time from induction to delivery of the pups and to reduce the manipulation of the bitch. Walk her to the side of the surgery table, use supplemental oxygen (avoid stressing the bitch with forceful use of a face mask) and induce by Propofol injection. Many of these bitches are large breed dogs and the additional weight and girth of a pregnancy makes moving her under anesthesia both hard on her and the staff.

Pre-oxgenation of the bitch

This is frequently recommended and in theory is a great idea. Often, the bitch has respiratory compromise due to the pressure of the expanded uterus on the diaphragm and many are also brachycephalic. However, there are some patients who will fight the face mask and make the effort counter-productive, i.e. she uses up more oxygen fighting you than she takes in. Techniques employing blow-by oxygen can be useful but only if they do not create excessive delays or stress to the patient. In this situation, or if there is a need for speedy induction, this step can be omitted. Rapid induction with injectable propofol and intubation to control the airway may be appropriate.

Propofol® induction

Administer propofol® through an IV catheter followed with isoflurane or sevoflurane maintenance via endotracheal tube. This has proven to be a highly successful technique for both the bitch and pup recovery. Propofol is dosed at 4 to 6 mg/kg, IV, to effect over 30 to 90 seconds. This dose should be reduced to 1 to 4 mg/kg IV if the patient is depressed or sedated. (At 10 mg/ml, this is approximately 1 cc per 5 pounds body weight.) (source: http://www.vasg.org/induction_protocols.htm). An easy dosage regimen is to prepare 1 cc per 5 pounds of body weight plus 2 to 10 extra ccs, in a syringe, and give to effect. Approximately 1/3 to 2/3 can be given slowly to induce, the remainder to effect as necessary to allow intubation and transition to inhalant anesthesia. Some bitches will need the additional Propofol® IV to attain a plane of general anesthesia. Propofol® does cross the placenta but rapidly crosses back and what remains on the puppy side is metabolized quickly by the pups.

Recently, the price of Propofol® has decreased. Additionally, clinical experience has made this induction technique preferred. If your practice does not stock or use Propofol®, you may consider including it in your inventory and use it several times on "routine" surgical patients so you are familiar with the nuances of this protocol prior to anesthetizing a pregnant bitch.

Gas anesthetic induction: With the advent of Propofol®, induction by face mask using any gas anesthetic agents **is no longer the preferred approach**. The inevitable excitement phase all dogs go through during face mask induction reduces blood flow to the placenta, obviously jeopardizing the fetuses. Many patients who require caesareans are brachycephalic breeds and ventilate much better when rapid anesthetic induction allows for immediate intubation and oxygen support. In addition, pressure from the uterus increases the risk of regurgitation and aspiration, meaning managing the airway of any caesarian patient is in everyone's best interest.

Anesthetic maintenance
Most practices use either isoflurane or sevoflurane to maintain the bitch in a plane of surgical anesthesia for the remainder of the procedure. The MAC decreases by as much as 40% during pregnancy. This must be accounted for when maintaining with gas anesthesia.

It is possible to maintain the bitch quite successfully on propofol® if isoflurane or sevoflurane anesthesia is unavailable. In this situation, a syringe may be used intermittently to infuse propofol® as necessary to maintain a good plane of anesthesia.

Even if inhalant gas anesthesia is not used, it is essential that an endotracheal tube be placed to maintain an airway with oxygen and good ventilatory support.

Spinal anesthesia: This technique can be used by those skilled in its application but should never be used alone, or for the first time when performing a C-section. Without some form of sedation, which will affects the pups, control with local anesthesia is rarely attainable. Most veterinarians will find it safer and faster to proceed with general anesthesia than to rely on local anesthetics for a C-section. Epidural anesthetic administration is beyond the scope of this book. If used, ensure the use of an epidural product that does not contain preservatives.

A local lidocaine block can be useful to reduce the induction agent dose needed and to assist in managing post-op pain but should never be used alone. Lidocaine without epinephrine (0.5 to 1.0%) diluted with sterile water should be injected along the incision line. The dose must not exceed 10 mg/kg body weight.

Remember, (how could you forget – the client is there reminding you) you are not just anesthetizing one patient, you are anesthetizing the entire litter too. You must attempt to minimize stress to the mother, keep her in an ideal plane of anesthesia, and minimize anesthetic effects on the puppies. Any stress will reduce blood flow through the uterus. Avoid keeping the anesthesia too "light" as pain will result in sympathetic stimulation, reducing blood flow to the uterus. Too deep a plain of anesthesia will also reduce uterine circulation secondary to hypotension and will result in excessive anesthetic effect on the pups. Careful titration of anesthesia and utilizing a technician skilled at anticipating the ups and downs of anesthetic monitoring will allow you to achieve a successful anesthetic procedure.

Contraindicated anesthetic agents
Many anesthetic agents used in routine veterinary surgical procedures are contraindicated for C-sections. Many of these agents reduce uterine blood flow. These drugs include xylazine (Rompun®), diazepam (Valium®), ketamine (Ketaset®), Domitor® and methoxyflurane.

Isoflurane and propofol are unconditionally associated with a positive effect on neonatal survival at seven days. If no propofol is available, thiopental IV or isoflurane induction are preferable to the contraindicated injectable anesthetics listed above.

Monitoring parameters during anesthesia
Anesthetic monitoring during caesarean is critical and demands the full attention of a dedicated and trained staff member to oversee the respiratory and hemodynamic changes that occur during anesthesia. The parameters monitored include: 1. spO_2 2. heart rate 3. respiratory rate and 4. blood pressure. Also helpful are 1. EKG 2. CO_2 monitoring and 3. temperature. The guidelines established for these parameters should be the same as for any patient. Prior to exteriorizing the uterus, the patient may require ventilatory support in the form of "bagging" with O_2 (not too much inhalant gas –

keep her anesthetized but not too deep) or a mechanical ventilatory system may be employed if you are so equipped and experienced in its use. Her SpO_2 should be over 95%, heart rate over 100, and respiratory rate over 12. When the uterus is removed from the abdomen, weight is removed from the vena cava and may cause blood pressure to drop precipitously. This should be monitored and anticipated – be sure IV fluids are running at an appropriate rate and colloids are available.

Surgery – The C-section and delivery of the pups
Making the final decision
The attainment of a high puppy survival rate requires a combination of early intervention, and rapid induction, incision and removal of pups from the uterus. The C-section should not be performed if it is contraindicated for a sound medical reason.

If the patient is a poor surgical risk, the owner should be advised of their options and a decision made that is in the best interest of the bitch. If it is apparent that both the mother and pups cannot be saved, it will be necessary to determine which to try to save. The literature reports a 1% mortality rate in bitches undergoing C-section in the United States. (Moon supra)

Reducing the surgical risks
Many bitches undergoing anesthesia for C-section may be oxygen deprived secondary to exertion, stress and pressure on the diaphragm from the gravid uterus. They are often dehydrated, although neither parameter is evident clinically. Most bitches have not eaten for several to 24 hours, are not interested in drinking, some have vomited, they have been straining and stressed in labor, and have thoracic compression because of expanded uterine volume. Some are also hypoglycemic and hypocalcemic.

We stress them further by presenting them to the veterinary clinic, no dog's favorite place to visit. We manhandle her during examination, radiography, and ultrasonography and proceed to place a catheter, and prep her for surgery.

We must attempt to do all we can to minimize the stress to the bitch and the pups by keeping everyone calm (dog and owner), starting IV fluids, managing the bitch's pain and anxiety, doing an efficient anesthesia and surgical procedure, and providing oxygen if accepted by the bitch.

The last steps before induction and surgery – Communication and organization
It is now time to move quickly. Minimizing the time from induction to delivery of the pups strongly correlates with maximizing neonatal survival rates. And minimizing surgical time minimizes bitch morbidity. Speed is of the essence!

Before the bitch is induced and the surgery begins, it is beneficial to stop briefly and review the surgical and treatment areas to be certain all necessary equipment, supplies and drugs are readily available. Taking time to allow the doctors and staff to review their step-by-step plan and familiarize themselves with their roles and the location of supplies and equipment will definitely save time and lives. It also reduces stress on the staff and inspires greater confidence in a distressed owner when they see the staff working as a team, making every move effective.

It is time to start the surgical procedure. The physical examination, EKG and blood work are completed, the IV catheter has been placed, the indicated medications and fluids have been administered, she is prepped for the surgical procedure as much as possible without undue stress, and has been pre-oxygenated if appropriate.

Each staff member has been assigned specific duties for monitoring, setting up the anesthetic monitor, the surgical scrub, and handling surgical packs, gowns and gloves. Puppy resuscitation duties should also be pre-assigned.

Induction of anesthesia and monitoring

In many hospitals, induction is done in the surgical suite. This minimizes the time from induction to delivery of the puppies.

The bitch is induced with propofol to effect, the endotracheal tube is immediately placed and secured, the cuff inflated. She is maintained on either Isoflurane or Sevoflurane.

Methoxyflurane, ketamine, diazepam, xylazine, and thiamylal are contraindicated because they adversely affect puppy survival rates. Face mask induction with anesthetic gas increases the bitch's oxygen needs due to anxiety and the struggle at induction, causing reduced blood flow to the uterus and oxygen depletion to the fetuses. It is also putting your staff at risk by increasing the anesthetic gas in the environment and injury while handling an unruly bitch. Therefore, induction with Propofol followed by immediately securing the bitch's airway and anesthetic maintenance with isoflurane or sevoflurane is the currently preferred anesthetic protocol.

Additional Propofol® should be readily available in case the bitch's anesthetic plane is inadequate while she is transitioning to the inhalant anesthetic.

IV fluids are started, and monitoring sPO_2, CO_2, blood pressure, EKG, heart rate and respiratory rates is initiated.

Depth of anesthesia must be managed carefully, even more so than in other abdominal procedures. If the plane of anesthesia is too deep, the bitch will become hypovolemic and blood flow to the puppies will be compromised. If too light, pain will result in sympathetic stimulation, reducing blood flow to the uterus.

The surgical prep

Place the patient on her back rolled slightly to the left (left side down) and secured in preparation for the surgeon. Positioning with the left side tilted downward minimizes the weight of the gravid uterus on the aorta, allowing better blood flow to the uterus, and instead the spleen is compressed (arguably not much with small puppies and small litters). The table should NOT be tilted with her head down as gastric reflux with esophageal scarring and constriction are potential sequella.

If there is adequate staff, the surgeon should begin the surgical scrubbing at the start of induction. If staff is short, the surgeon should be certain the patient is in a stable plane of anesthesia prior to scrubbing in (Appendix A-5).

Cap and mask for all in the surgical suite, routine scrubbing, gowning and gloving of the surgeon should be initiated.

When the surgeon is ready to drape the bitch, she should be rolled into the final position and the final surgical scrub applied. The surgeon should routinely drape the patient, being certain to use plenty of lap towels. Ideally, there should be a pre-counted pack of instruments and gauze, and the lap towels identified with a radio-opaque system (i.e. safety pin).

The surgical approach

Speed and efficiency are of the essence. With great planning and staff assistance, the first pup can be delivered less than 10 minutes after induction, with an average of 1 pup per minute thereafter (Figure 6-8).

The gloved and gowned surgeon should make a routine ventral midline celiotomy from caudal to the umbilicus caudally as far as necessary to easily exteriorize the uterus. The incision can be extended cranially and caudally as indicated. Here, the linea can be much thinner than the surgeon may be

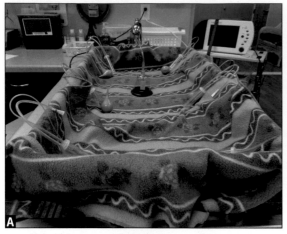

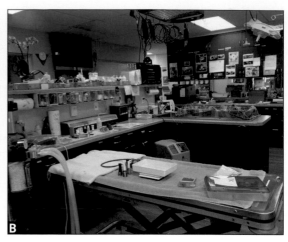

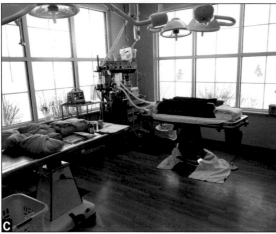

Figure 6-8.
A. Puppy Resuscitation Center – Plastic tray lined with heating pads and a blanket. Oxygen mask. DeLee Mucus traps ready for each assistant to use to suction pups. **B.** Puppy Care Setup – 2 workstations for puppy resuscitation, puppy weighing, identification, and umbilical cord care. **C.** Surgical Suite Setup – ready for the bitch, with padded, heated v-tray, towels on the floor for staff safety, surgical packs and sterile towels.

accustomed to and the uterus and/or bladder distended. Other organs may be displaced so that they are dangerously close to the incision and care is required. An incision is made with a scalpel through the skin to the subcutaneous tissue. Using a pair of Metzenbaum scissors sharply dissect through the subcutaneous tissue approximately 1 cm on each side of the incision to facilitate closure of the linea. With a pair of thumb forceps, lift the linea and make a nick through it with the scalpel, blade directed up. A full-length incision is made in the elevated linea with a pair of Metzenbaum scissors.

Once the incision appears to be long enough, the surgeon can identify the uterus and assess its position. The uterus should NOT be incised without exteriorization and packing off at least a portion with lap sponges. The uterus can be carefully exteriorized by locating a puppy in mid-horn position (they are the most accessible and mobile) and lifting by holding the puppy and uterus in the same hand. It can also be helpful to have an assistant, not scrubbed in, apply gentle pressure to the lateral abdomen on the side the puppy is on, below the drape to avoid contaminating the sterile surgical field, to facilitate exteriorizing the first puppy. Care should be taken in manipulation of the uterus, as it is easy to tear or puncture the uterus during this process. If the incision is too small, it should be extended either cranially taking care not to extend it so cranial as to reach the xyphoid process or caudally as far as the pubic bone, to prevent undue trauma to the pup or uterus. The incision often seems to need to be unduly large, but remember it must be large enough in cases of multiple pups in a horn to allow 2 pups folded in a V to be exteriorized simultaneously. Place lap sponges along the abdominal incision. The towels can be moistened if there is time, but the uterine contents will do this nicely within a few minutes (Figure 6-9).

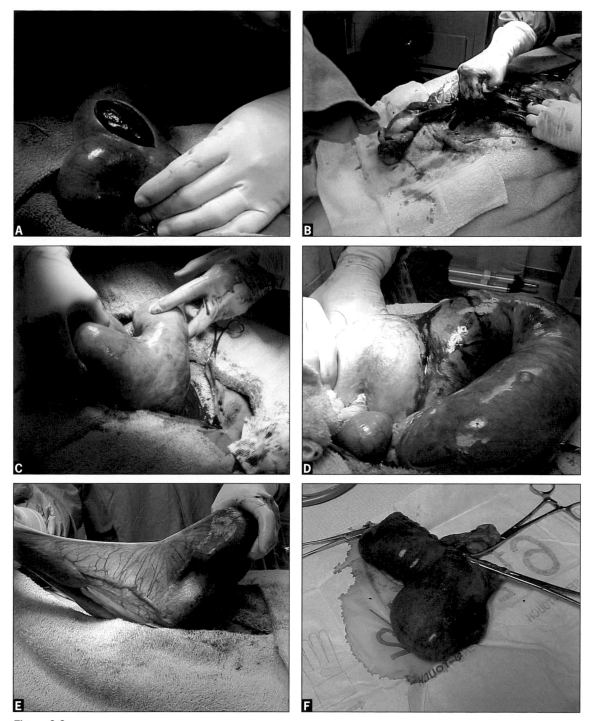

Figure 6-9.
A. C-section incision in the uterine horn, near the uterine body, on the dorsal aspect of the horn. **B.** C-section with pup delivered, head below pup's hips to allow fluid to drain while placenta is removed from the uterine wall. Note there is no fluid near the pup's face so no fluid will be aspirated. **C.** Pup in a transverse presentation. The head of the pup is in one horn with the rump of the pup in the opposite horn. **D.** The green area shows where a previous C-section incision was made and healed. **E.** Segmental aplasia. One uterine horn is normal, the other uterine horn did not have a lumen that connected to the uterine body. There was purulent material trapped in the horn, a pyometra unilaterally. **F.** Segmental aplasia with horn removed from the dog in the preceding photograph. The opposite uterine horn was left in situ, and this bitch went on to have a litter of 4 pups on her next breeding. Her daughter had a normal uterus and normal fertility.

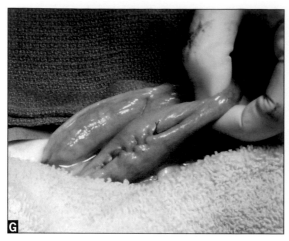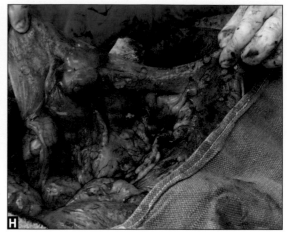

Figure 6-9. (continued)
G. Routine uterine closure after a C-section using a Utrecht Suture pattern, absorbable suture, not penetrating into the lumen.
H. Uterine horn with a narrowing, causing dystocia. Note the serosal cysts are an incidental finding and not a cause of infertility or other disease.

Depending on the size of the bitch and the litter, several or all of the pups inside the uterine horns can be exteriorized. If the litter or pup size is very large, do not exteriorize the entire uterus at one time or it is likely to tear from shear weight alone.

If possible, locate the uterine body by following a horn caudally and exteriorize this portion. Place lap sponges strategically to minimize abdominal contamination by uterine contents.

There is currently discussion over whether it is appropriate to ovariohysterectomize the bitch at C-section. The current recommendation by many veterinarians heavily involved in canine reproduction is NOT to remove the uterus at the time of C-section. This is a relatively recent change of philosophy. Although the ovaries are not necessary for lactation, removal of the uterus can cause tremendous blood loss, induce DIC, and cause other physiological changes that can greatly increase surgical risk for the patient.

Even use of the laser will not make ovariohysterectomy safe at C-section. The blood loss is primarily from blood contained in the uterus, not from the incision sites. We do not recommend ovariohysterectomy unless the uterus is surgically irreparable or the bitch is at risk of serious complications by leaving a toxic uterus in situ. This situation is very rare.

The pups should be removed from the uterus. If there is any hope of survival, the uterus should NEVER be removed with the pups in situ. They need to be removed swiftly and individually while the uterine and ovarian arteries are still supplying blood and oxygen to the fetuses.

Delivery of the puppies
It is useful to develop a system for labeling puppies rapidly at removal to allow for "mapping" their location in the uterus and to facilitate tracking resuscitation, if any, of individual puppies. Several systems are often used. The surgeon can have a sterilized set of colored hand towels for the assistants to receive the puppies into, with a matching non-sterile set available for the corresponding puppy once it is breathing well and is dry. Alternatively, color banded mosquito hemostats can be applied to the umbilical cord either by the surgeon or the assistant. An effective tracking system will later prove to be valuable for entering data in the patient record (Figure 6-11).

Most surgeons prefer to lift the uterus and retract it caudally, exposing the dorsal surface. Make 1 longitudinal incision into the uterus on the dorsal side of the uterus near the uterine body between placentas and remove as many pups as possible. The surgeon should make a light-handed full thickness lengthwise incision with a scalpel over one end of a puppy or between puppies in a healthy area of the uterine body or horn approximately 1/2 to 2/3 the length of the puppy. If this is impractical for any reason, another area of the uterine horn may be incised in a healthy area lengthwise on the anti-mesenteric border as just described. Avoid incising the uterus and puppy concurrently with the linea.

The first visible puppy is exposed, the face quickly cleared by the surgeon by tearing full thickness through the membranes with a gauze square, while holding the puppy head down. (it is not necessary to use scissors to do this.) This can be done while the placenta is still attached to the uterus so the pup is still receiving oxygen through the placenta as it takes its first breath of air. After the membranes are removed from the pup's nose, the pup can be laid down briefly on the lap towel so the placenta can be detached from the uterine wall using both hands. Watch to be sure the pup's nose is not submerged in blood and fetal fluids that pool on the drapes and lap towels. In litters born at term, the placenta is usually easily freed from the uterine wall by finding the edge of the attachment and hooking an index finger from one hand between the placenta and uterine wall, and lifting the placenta away while the thumb of the other hand helps separate the placenta and is stabilizing the uterus, taking care not to damage the uterine lining or tearing the uterine wall. If the placental attachments are very secure, or the umbilical cord tears, the pup can have its face cleared, umbilical cord clamped 1 inch from the pup's abdominal wall with a hemostat by the surgeon to detach the pup from the placenta. The retained placentas can be removed after delivery.

With or without the placenta attached, the pup is handed to a waiting assistant holding a sterile color-coded hand towel. By using sterile hand towels placed fully open by the surgeon in to the hands of assistants, the surgeon can maintain a sterile field without chancing that a pup will be dropped in the handoff to the assistant. Our technicians prefer to have the pup handed to them with the pup's face toward their fingertips, and the pup's rump toward their elbows, allowing them to tilt the pup's head downward for fluid drainage and easier access for suctioning fluids with the DeLee mucus trap as they are walking from surgery to the treatment area to continue resuscitation of the pup. This process is then repeated until all pups are delivered.

If the pups are high risk or trouble is suspected prior to C-section, interventional resuscitation at removal from the uterus may be useful. An assistant can scrub in, aid in exteriorizing the uterus, supporting the uterus to prevent tearing, and begin to resuscitate pups as their heads are exposed from the uterus. The assistant can use a sterile DeLee mucus trap (straight out of the original sterile packaging) and begin to rub the pups and suction the secretions as the surgeon delivers the pup and separates the placenta from the uterus. Although each placenta does not need to be delivered with each pup (it can be left in situ and the umbilical cord can be clamped off at delivery), the placenta will be in the surgeon's way as the next pups are delivered. This pre-emptive resuscitation may improve puppy survival rates.

Frequently, the next pup in line will slide into the uterine incision. The pups should be removed from the uterus in the order that makes delivery of each most efficient. The remainder of the pups should be removed from the uterus as previously described. When the uterine incision can be well planned, the surgeon can usually remove all of the pups through one uterine incision. This is preferred because the uterine closure will be faster, minimizing surgery time and the uterus will heal with less scarring, improving the bitch's chances to have another successful breeding.

A second, or rarely third uterine incision may be required. If it is obvious that the delivery will be prolonged by fighting to move the pups down to the incision, an additional incision is indicated. In some cases, the uterus is so long and the pups so numerous that it is impractical to quickly remove all pups through one incision. Oxygen deprivation by prolonging the delivery is counter-productive. In some cases, there is a bifurcation of the uterine body (the intercornual septum) that will interfere with delivering pups from 1 horn through an incision on the other side. In these cases, an additional incision must be made.

In some cases, the uterus is friable and heavy and the uterine horn may tear. If this occurs in a location that would serve for delivery, the incision can be thoughtfully extended lengthwise to avoid further tearing. If the uterus is going to tear, it is likely to tear circumferentially, not longitudinally – this is undesirable. Do not to exteriorize the uterus too aggressively or so far that the weight causes it to tear.

Once all the pups have been delivered, the uterus should be carefully examined. BE ABSOLUTELY CERTAIN THAT ALL PUPPIES HAVE BEEN DELIVERED – the uterus should be examined from ovary to vagina on both sides. Be sure there is not a fetus left in the pelvic canal where it cannot be visualized. If there was a uterine rupture, the abdominal cavity should be explored for fetuses and other uterine contents. If there are placentas in the uterine lumen, they should be manually removed only if this can be done without causing trauma or hemorrhage. Large blood clots should also be gently removed. IF there is any fetal material, purulent material, or mucoid material that suggest fetal resorption sites, this should be removed or lavaged from the uterus. The uterine lavage can be done with either a large syringe attached to a red rubber feeding or comparable tube or a bag of warmed IV fluids via a venoset. All equipment and supplies must be sterile.

Closure of the incisions
Prior to closing, cultures, placentas and uterine biopsies for pathology may be collected if indicated. Additionally, brief digital manipulation of the cervix may be performed; this is reported to simulate vaginal delivery of pups and improve maternal acceptance of her newborns.

The uterus should be thoroughly examined on the serosal surfaces to assess for small tears through the serosa or broad ligament. If any are located, they should be repaired with a 2-0 or 3-0 absorbable suture, taper needle. Serosal or muscularis tears must be repaired to create a seal. Tears in the broad ligament should be sutured to prevent other abdominal organs from slipping into the rent but close carefully to avoid compromising uterine circulation.

The uterine incision(s) should be closed, carefully creating a seal of serosa to serosa contact. There are several techniques. The author prefers a Utrecht pattern with 2-0 or 3-0 absorbable suture (usually polyglycolic acid) with a taper needle. The suture should be meticulously placed so as not to penetrate the mucosal surface. Avoid suturing the remaining placentas into the incision as this will increase the risk of developing metritis (Figure 6-10).

When the uterus is closed, the incision line should have a good seal with only the knots peeking through on the exposed end. This will permit excellent healing with minimal adhesions or damage, inside or outside the uterus. In most cases, the uterine incision will heal well enough to allow a return to normal fertility, allowing the bitch to conceive, carry and whelp another litter(s).

Prior to closing the abdomen, perform an instrument and gauze count – this is the type of surgery that can lead to an overlooked gauze sponge or instrument.

The uterus and abdominal cavity should be examined for uterine content contamination and lavaged thoroughly. Soiled lap sponges should be replaced with fresh sterile towels, and the assistant can aid in the lavage directly or via the use of a sterile system. Either sterile warmed (99-101° F) Lactated Ringers or Normal Saline should be used. Routine generous lavage with 1 to 2 liters of fluids will reduce abdominal contamination of the abdomen with blood clots and fetal fluids. The surgeon should attempt to remove as much material as possible from the omentum, but if contaminated by placental material it can be difficult to fully cleanse. The uterine contents should be sterile, so bacterial contamination from this source is probably not great. The major volume of fluid used to lavage should be sponged or suctioned from the abdomen although it is not harmful to leave some fluid.

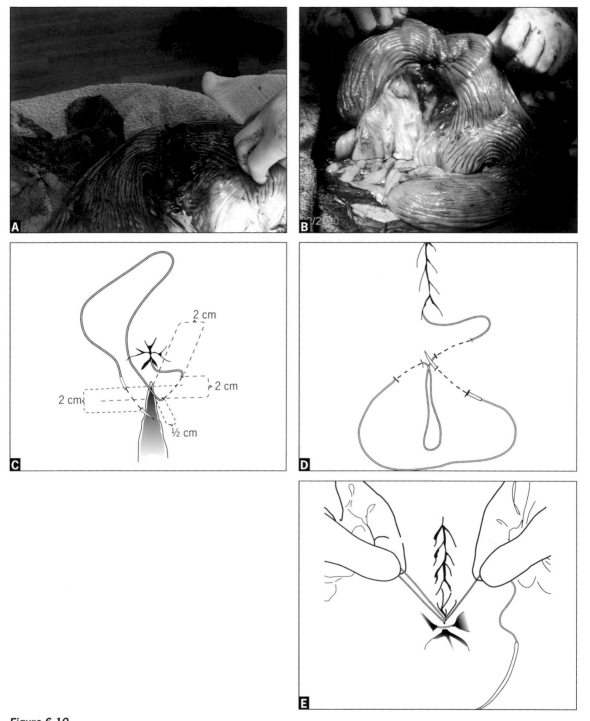

Figure 6-10.
A. Uterine tear at C-section. This can be repaired by careful suturing. **B.** Uterine tear at C-section repaired with a Utrecht suture pattern and absorbable sutures. This will not impair fertility at the next breeding. **C.** Utrecht suture pattern to close the uterus at C-section showing placement and proportions. **D.** Utrecht suture to close uterus at C-section. **E.** Utrecht suture pattern to close the uterus at C-section showing the final tie. With permission from the Drost project.

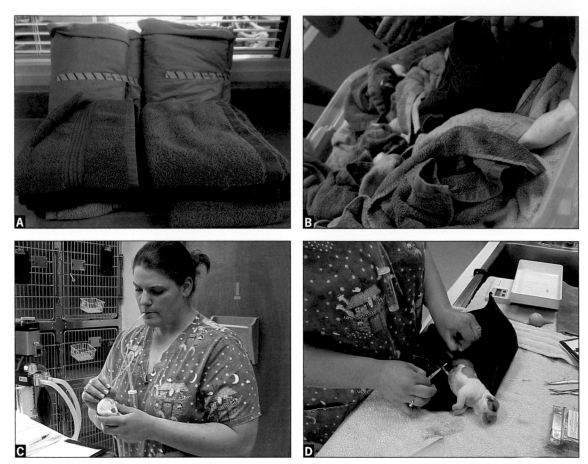

Figure 6-11.
*A. Puppy Towels – matching set of non-sterile and autoclaved towels, allows color coding pups for tracking neonatal resuscitation and uterine location. **B.** 16 pups wrapped in their colored towels for identification. **C.** DeLee Mucus trap used to aid in clearing fluids from the airways of the pups. **D.** Technician tying off the umbilical cord with suture after the C-section.*

The surgeon should remove soiled lap towels and reglove.

There are individual preferences for abdominal closure. One option is to use 2-0 polyglycolic acid absorbable suture material in a simple interrupted pattern in the linea. Size 0 absorbable or non-absorbable suture may be considered an alternative in giant bitches or where wound healing may be compromised. Continuous suture patterns can be risky in the abdominal wall where there is a large incision with a great deal of activity and edema. Many of these patients will have a following procedure, whether a routine ovariohysterectomy, a surgical breeding, or a subsequent C-section, and non-absorbable sutures may cause complications during future surgical procedures. For the subcutaneous, subcuticular and skin closures, avoiding placing suture in the mammary tissues, the pattern can be done at the surgeon's preference. For speed, a Ford Interlocking suture pattern with a non-absorbable material may be used in the skin. This is well tolerated by the bitch and puppies. Some surgeons close with the subcuticular layer as their final pattern. Surgical staples may not be suitable for skin closure because they do not lay as flat to the skin and can interfere with the puppies when they are nursing. An occasional bitch may feel the need to remove her own sutures.

Now you can give her drugs
After all the pups have been delivered and the uterus closed, the use of Oxytocin can be very helpful. Administered slowly IV or directly into the uterine muscle (myometrium), Oxytocin rapidly causes uterine contractions, reducing the size of the uterus and minimizing ongoing hemorrhage from

placental attachment sites. The dosage varies widely (1 to 20 U/dog) and should be based on the needs of the patient. There is often a transient reduction in the bitch's heart rate, but this will resolve spontaneously.

All of the concerns we have about the use of Oxytocin prior to delivery of the puppies, such as restricting uterine blood flow or causing uterine rupture are clearly no longer an issue.

A non-steroidal anti-inflammatory may also be appropriate. The decision to use or not use a non-steroidal anti-inflammatory must be based on the overall health of the bitch – her blood pressure during the procedure, renal and liver function, and her tolerance of NSAIDs. There is no product currently labeled for this use and it is unlikely the pharmaceutical industry will apply to the FDA for a label claim for this application. However, the author has used injectable Metacam® for over 10 years with no known ill effects. Others have used Rimadyl® with success. The human literature, which is the only source of data available, suggests that little passes into the milk and is safe for the mother as well as nursing offspring.

The first dose is administered by injection and followed by oral medication for 3 to 5 days post-op. Buprenorphine can be used to manage pain until the Metacam® takes effect. Others prefer tramadol for pain management. There are other medications commonly prescribed for post-op pain management, but care must be taken to select one which will not pass in large quantities through the milk and will not cause the bitch such a change in attitude or mental capabilities that she could inadvertently or deliberately cause harm to the puppies.

There is no comprehensive study to support the use of more than one dose of pain medications in the post-op C-section bitch. It is easy to extrapolate from the human that there is post-op incisional pain. Because the incision for the C-section is one of the largest abdominal incisions routinely made in the dog, it stands to reason that pain management should be considered essential. Add to that the edema in the region associated with lactation and the activity of the newborns along the incision line, and failure to prescribe some form of post-op pain medication represents a serious lapse in judgment. It is finally recognized in veterinary medicine that pain management is essential to the practice of quality medicine. Anecdotally and logically, bitches who have their pain adequately managed seem to make better mothers. They feel better, eat and drink better, consequently lactate better, can move around more comfortably, and are better able to care for their newborns. Not only is it more medically appropriate to administer pain medications, it is more ethically appropriate to provide pain relief to a post-surgical patient.

Resuscitation of the neonate at vaginal birth or Birth by C-section
Airway and breathing, including ventilatory and pharmaceutical support if needed
This is the recommended sequence of events for resuscitation whether the pups are born by C-section or vaginal birth (See Table 6-2).

Many newborns show no or poor respirations at birth due to hypoxia and hypotension during delivery, inadequate surfactant, excessive fluids in the airways, or aspiration of meconium (Figure 6-12).

All equipment should be laid out and organized in advance so it is readily available as needed. The pups which are usually born vigorous and vocalizing and need little assistance. If the bitch or pups are distressed, promptly applied resuscitation techniques are the difference between sending home a happy client with a basket full of healthy newborns and a disappointed client with little to show for their efforts (Figure 6-14).

It is ideal to have 1 assistant for every 1 to 2 pups. Initial resuscitation should consist of assuring that the mouth and nose are free of fetal membranes and the free fluid in the oral cavity is suctioned

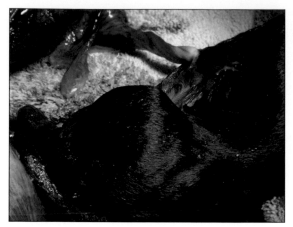

Figure 6-12.
Meconium on pup indicating fetal distress prior to birth. Antibiotics are indicated for this pup.

out with a soft-tipped bulb syringe. At the same time, the assistant should vigorously rub the pup with the towel, tip the pup head down to allow fluids to drain from the airway, check the umbilicus for excessive hemorrhage and to be certain the abdominal wall is complete (no exposed intestines). The pup should be placed on a heated surface or a heating pad should be folded taco-style with the pup and towel in the fold. Swinging the pups is not recommended as this can cause excessive intracranial pressure, sub-dural hemorrhage and forces stomach contents into the airway.

With rubbing, the pup should be vocalizing and breathing spontaneously. If this is not the case, suctioning with a bulb syringe and De Lee mucus trap should be started. A bulb syringe is most effective in removing thick mucus, and can be alternated with a De Lee which is better for thin watery fluid. The DeLee mucus trap can also be used to remove excess fluid from the stomach if it is distended and interfering with respiration. Gently shaking the pup by the scruff of the neck can also aid in stimulating respirations. If there is excess fluid in the lungs, the assist can lay a pup on a board or other surface, tilting the head downward at a 45 degree angle. This can be done while also supplying oxygen and supplemental heat (Figure 6-13).

If the pup is still non-responsive, it should be evaluated for obvious physical defects, such as a cleft palate or other deformity, that would make ongoing attempts to resuscitate futile.

If the pup appears normal but is not breathing, the thorax should be auscultated for a heartbeat. If the pup has a curled tongue and/or a heartbeat, efforts to revive the pup should be continued.

If the pup is breathing, but not well, face mask oxygen should be supplied. If there are a number of pups who need oxygen, they can be lined up in a glass aquarium on its side or other chamber with plastic wrap across the front so the oxygen level is high and the assistants can monitor the pups as they receive oxygen.

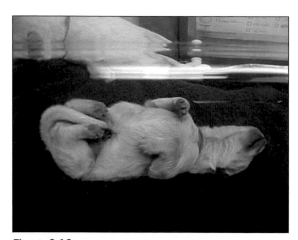

Figure 6-13.
Head down position of pup after delivery to aid in fluid fluid drainage draining from the respiratory tract.

If the pup is not breathing, this may be stimulated by use of GV26, the acupuncture point. To do this, a 25 gauge needle is inserted into the upper lip until bone is hit, then it is turned. This is the respiratory stimulation point.

The airways should again be cleared, and the pup rubbed.

If no spontaneous respirations have started by 10 minutes after delivery, an injection of doxapram (Dopram®) may be administered. This product can be administered as 1 or possibly 2 doses, of 1 to 2.5 mg per puppy each, injected into the umbilical vein, followed by a saline flush to deliver the Dopram® to the circulation. As an alternative, 0.01 ml Dopram® can be administered into the caudal thigh muscle or 0.1 ml dropped under the tongue, and the pup can be monitored for a response, seen as a red flush to the mucus membranes. It can be repeated if necessary. Injection into the tongue may lead to pain and reluctance to nurse. It is essential that the airway be clear prior to this injection as damage will be done to the pup if it attempts to inhale against a closed airway or aspirates fluid deeper into the airways. Dopram is controversial in humans as it can cause brain damage by increasing the brain's demand for oxygen. However, we believe from clinical experience that there are pups who have survived with normal skills that may have died without this intervention.

Atropine is contraindicated in the neonate.

If any drugs requiring reversal were used, the reversal agents should be administered. Naloxone can be administered via the endotracheal tube at two times the injectable dose, but is only effective if opioids were used. Dexamethasone Sodium Phosphate or Solu-Medrol® (0.1 to 1 mg) may aid surfactant production and help respiration.

For respiratory support, endotracheal intubation is favored, but it requires special equipment, highly trained staff, and can be difficult to perform, particularly if there are several pups in trouble simultaneously. For these reasons, doxapram and face mask ventilation is a useful alternative.

Endotracheal intubation should be performed if the neonate is not breathing. (It is a very good idea to practice this in advance.) Tubes that can be used include the Cole tube, a red rubber feeding tube with the end cut off and flamed smooth, tom cat or large bore IV catheters. The Cole tube provides the best seal. The pup should be positioned sternally. The intubation can usually be done by one person. For a right-handed person, the tongue can be held out of the mouth with a gauze square in the left hand, with the thumb of the left (same) hand on top of the tongue, and the fingers of the left hand curled under the jaw. The left hand will also support the head with the lower jaw horizontal to the table and the upper jaw vertical to the table. In the palm of the left hand, the same hand holding the tongue, the technician can hold a laryngoscope or otoscope with a large tip. This instrument will illuminate the airway and simultaneously hold the tongue downward so the arytenoids can be visualized. The handle of the otoscope/laryngoscope can be supported by the technician holding it against his or her own trunk. The right hand of the technician will be used to clear fluid from the airway with cotton swabs, a bulb syringe, or a DeLee mucus trap. As soon as the tracheal opening is visible, an appropriately sized endotracheal tube can be passed.

An alternative way to illuminate the larynx for intubation is for an assistant to the technician to place the tip of a transilluminator against the neck adjacent to the larynx. This will light the area without the blade of the laryngoscope interfering with the placement of the endotracheal tube.

Once the tube is verified to be in place, the tube should be secured with a strip of tape around the tube and around the back of the pup's skull. Initiate ventilation. The first breath is the most difficult and requires the most force – it is the one that will open the alveoli and spread the surfactant over the alveolar surface.

The first ventilation can be administered by use of 1 ml of air in a syringe. Care should be taken to avoid overexpansion of the lungs as this may cause pneumothorax. Ventilations should not exceed 15 to 25 bpm. A pediatric Ambu bag or rebreathing bag with only oxygen flowing through an anesthetic machine can be used to deliver oxygen to the lungs. Use of a manometer will assure that the lungs are not overinflated. If PEEP (Positive End-Expiratory Pressure) is available, it should be used. This will prevent the alveoli from collapsing. The maximum PEEP value should not exceed 5.

If intubation is not an option, a face mask with a tightly fitted diaphragm attached to an Ambu bag or anesthetic machine can be placed over the nose and mouth of the pup and used to inflate the lungs.

Efforts to resuscitate a puppy should be continued for up to 20 minutes, with owner consent, if the pup is grossly normal in appearance and has a heart beat. It is possible for the pup to have normal vision and cognitive skills even with prolonged apnea.

If no heartbeat is ausculted, cardiac compressions should be started immediately. This should be done by placing the thumb on 1 side of the thorax and the forefingers on the opposite side. Compressions should be given at 100 to 120 per minute, alternating with ventilations through an endotracheal tube. Epinephrine should be given initially at 0.01 mg/kg (10 mcg/kg) for the first dose (into the umbilical vein or at two times the injectable dose into the endotracheal tube) followed by 0.1 mg/kg for subsequent doses.

Once the pup is breathing spontaneously, oxygen should be administered by face mask or in an oxygen chamber. This should be continued until the tongue stays pink without supplemental oxygen. Eventually, the pup can be moved from the oxygen source and evaluated for cyanosis. A pulse oximeter can also be used to monitor spO_2. Arterial blood gases are not practical to monitor the newborn.

If the number of pups needing oxygen support is large, an incubator or an aquarium or translucent storage box on its side with heating pads under it and clear plastic wrap across the front can be used as an oxygen chamber. Nasal oxygen delivery can be designed by suturing a small red rubber feeding tube near or in one nostril of the pup and continuous oxygen flow hooked up. Many owners are willing to assist technical staff by monitoring the stable pups thereby freeing veterinary staff to care for the pups needing additional resuscitation.

It is common for newborns to breath irregularly at first. If they are pink, breathing, have a heartbeat, and are crying, they are probably OK.

The "accordion squeeze" technique can also be used to stimulate breathing and remove excess fluid. To use the accordion squeeze, the head and shoulder of the pup are held firmly in one hand while the pelvis and rear legs are held firmly in the other hand. With the head held downward (no swinging), the pup is folded and extended alternately in the abdomen region, this pressure is thought to draw air into the lungs while stimulating cardiac activity. Other methods can be interspersed at the same time – CPR, dopram, oxygenation, and suctioning.

Don't give up if there is a curl to the tongue and a heartbeat you can hear with a stethoscope.

It is important for the veterinary staff to practice neonatal resuscitation protocols in advance of the C-section. In most cases, the veterinarian and one staff member will be concentrating their efforts on the anesthetic and surgical care of the bitch and will need additional skilled staff to handle the newborns.

The veterinary staff should also be trained to assess each pup for vitality. There is no standardized method in veterinary medicine, but use of an APGAR-type method will help to produce consistent record-keeping and improve the doctor's ability to assess which pups need more careful post-partum monitoring and care (Table 6-5) (Appendix A-1).

Umbilical care
Once the pups are stable, and no longer in need of oxygen or other support (other than thermal support), the umbilical cords can be tied off from the placentas. A sterile hemostat should be positioned approximately 1 inch (2 cm) from the pup's abdominal wall, and used to clamp the umbilical cord. The hemostat is removed and sterile suture used to ligate the umbilical cord in the crushed site of the umbilical cord. After the umbilical cord is ligated and transected, the umbilicus should then be dipped in tincture of iodine solution (in the container to be dispensed with the client) to minimize bacterial contamination of the cord. This infection, omphalitis, can lead to secondary

Table 6-5 Proposed APGAR for puppies			
Parameter	0 pts	1 pt	2 pts
Activity, muscle tone	Flaccid	Some tone in extremities	Active movements
Pulse, heart rate	Absent – < than 110 bpm	110 – 220 bpm	> 220 bpm
Reflexes when stressed	Absent	Some movement	Crying out
Mucous membrane color	Pale or cyanotic	Slightly cyanotic	Pink
Respiratory rate	Absent	Weak, irregular	> 15/min, rhythmic

Interpretation:

Total points	Vitality
0-3	Weak
4-6	Moderate
7-10	Normal

bacterial infection, peritonitis, sepsis, pneumonia and rapid death. The placentas can be discarded unless needed for histology and culture.

Fluids and nutritional support

Some pups that are distressed due to prolonged labor and delivery will be dehydrated and hypoglycemic and will benefit from supportive care. Oral or parenteral dextrose and fluid administration can be very successful. As soon as the pups appear to be warm and unlikely to aspirate, they may be fed warmed formula diluted 50% with normal saline. This should be dosed at 0.5 to 1 ml per ounce of body weight, administered by feeding tube every 2 to 3 hours. This should be continued, gradually increasing to full strength formula, until the pups can nurse independently.

If the pups and bitch are willing and able, the pups can be allowed to nurse prior to discharge from the veterinary hospital. Prior to introducing the pups to the bitch, her mammary chain should be wiped with sterile saline to remove the residue of surgical scrub, minimizing the pup's oral exposure of the product used as this tastes bad and deters the pups from nursing. Once this is completed, the puppies can be allowed to begin nursing with close supervision by the veterinary staff. In large litters, the pups can be rotated. An attempt should be made to feed all pups with the bitch's colostrum prior to discharge to the owner's care. (Figure 6-14).

The pups should be weighed before and after their first nursing to assess if they were effective nursers. Thawed fresh frozen plasma can be administered SC or orally to the pups if the bitch has scant colostrum or the pups do not appear to be nursing. (See chapter 8). Antibiotics should be administered and dispensed to the pups if they had meconium in their fetal membranes or appear to be otherwise compromised.

Discharge of the bitch and her litter
(See Appendix C-12)

A typical C-section takes 45 to 60 minutes from induction to closure. The owner/breeder client will often want to remain at the hospital during delivery, either to observe or participate in neonatal care. Hospital policy should be established in advance which areas of the

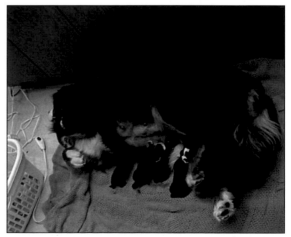

Figure 6-14 .
Post C-section bitch nursing before she goes home.

hospital clients are to have access to and whether photographs or videotaping will be permitted.

Medications and supplies dispensed should be prepared. During the recovery which is usually under 1 hour, the bitch owner should be instructed on post-op care including incision care, pain medications, dewormers, care of the newborns including daily examinations, nursing instructions, umbilicus care, weigh-ins, and tube feeding techniques.

Unless there are complications, the bitch and puppies can be discharged as soon as the pups have nursed and the bitch can ambulate. Round-the-clock care by experienced breeders is often better given in the home setting than in the veterinary hospital, particularly in hospitals without 24 hour care. Most veterinary hospitals are not set up with enclosures that are large enough for the bitch to be with her pups, and often these enclosures have small gaps newborns can slip through and become separated from the bitch and litter. They would require constant monitoring. Most breeders have a whelping box that is secure enough to contain the puppies and allows them to be monitored carefully in their own home setting.

Encourage your clients to ask for help, in advance, from friends, family, and other breeders to assure they remain well-rested enough to provide good post partum care and decision making for the pups and bitch (Appendix C-9).

CHAPTER 7
Managing the Immediate Postpartum Period in the Bitch

Health care

Prior to whelping, the bitch should be eating a quality commercially manufactured performance, puppy, or pregnancy diet. Approximately 1 week prior to the delivery, she should be radiographed to assess the number of pups due. Most bitches whelp at home without veterinary intervention.

If the bitch has not been radiographed prior to whelping, or if she does not deliver the expected number of pups, she should be scheduled for an appointment as soon as possible. Ideally, she should be seen immediately, upon completion of whelping, but no longer than 24 hours of whelping. The longer the delay from whelping to the appointment, the greater the risk to the bitch and the retained pup(s).

The minimum examination of the bitch should be a physical examination including hydration, mucus membrane color and refill, rectal temperature, abdominal palpation for retained fetuses, character of vaginal discharge, and evaluation of the mammary glands for character and quantity of colostrum/milk. If there is any question regarding uterine palpation, for instance if the bitch is thick-bodied or the contracting uterus cannot be distinguished from retained pup(s), a lateral abdominal radiograph should be taken to confirm that the bitch has completed her delivery.

Many veterinarians and breeders are familiar with an injection of oxytocin following the delivery of the last pup. In the lingo of breeding, this is called a "clean-out shot." It is surrounded by some controversy. Purists may state that oxytocin is not necessary if all pups and placentas are accounted for. Others feel it can aid in expelling any retained placenta or fetuses, to hasten uterine involution, decrease postpartum hemorrhage and aid in milk let-down. Subjectively, intramuscular oxytocin at 5 to 20 units or 2 units/kg, up to 20 units, has not been harmful.

In general, this oxytocin injection is unlikely to cause harm, although the bitch may experience transient cramping. On the other hand, it is an opportunity to schedule a post-partum evaluation for the bitch and pups. You may discover a retained pup, another health concern with the bitch, or a pup whelped at home with a cleft palate or other defect. Early intervention is good medicine for the bitch or pup and it allows for more efficient scheduling at the veterinary hospital. Most veterinarians would rather see a patient and have the opportunity to intervene early than have to deal with a serious problem after hours.

All pups should be examined within 24 to 72 hours of birth. This examination should include body weight, temperature, examination of the mucus membranes, examination of the oral cavity for cleft palates and other defects, palpation of the skull for open fontanelles, auscultation of the thorax for murmurs, examination of the ventral abdomen for hernias and umbilical infections, evaluation of the limbs, examination of the rectum for patency (feces present) and evaluation of the presence and color of urine on a cotton ball swabbed across the urethral opening.

At this visit or within 5 days of birth when the pups are deemed strong enough, dewclaws and tails can be removed as appropriate for the breed.

Unless the bitch was on the 4 week fenbendazole protocol, at 2 weeks of age, the bitch and pups should be wormed with oral pyrantel pamoate (Nemex®). This should be repeated at 4 and 6 weeks. Heartworm preventive can be given to the bitch throughout lactation. Heartworm preventive can be started for the pups at 6 weeks.

Vaccines can be administered to the bitch at the time the pups receive their first dose – at 6 to 8 weeks of age as indicated by risk factors and colostrum ingestion (Appendix C-11).

Nutrition and exercise

The feeding location and type of food and water dishes chosen for the post-partum bitch must be based on where she will be willing to eat/drink and where the pups will be safe. Care must be taken so that pups cannot fall into the water and food dishes. Some bitches become protective of their food, even to the point of becoming aggressive toward their own newborns.

Many bitches will not eat very well for the first few days. It may be necessary to tempt her with canned or home-cooked food to keep her eating, hydrated, and to control diarrhea.

New mothers often develop a ravenous appetite within a few days. By the 3rd week of lactation, many will require 2 to 4 times their maintenance caloric needs to lactate adequately without losing body condition. They will need to be fed a high quality commercially prepared performance or puppy diet. Calcium supplements or food high in calcium such as cottage cheese may be fed post-partum – these should not be fed pre-partum because calcium supplementation will predispose the pregnant bitch to eclampsia.

After weaning, most bitches will continue to eat more than a maintenance diet for a few weeks. Care should be taken to avoid obesity.

Excessive hair loss, known as post-partum effluvium, is normal and will resolve on its own. It can make the bitch look unkempt at the time puppy buyers are arriving to visit.

The bitch should be exercised in moderation. Many bitches will not leave their pups during the first days to weeks except for a quick trip outside. As the pups become more independent, the mother will be more willing to leave and normal activities can be resumed. Care should be taken to protect the mammary glands from trauma. Swimming can be resumed once the vaginal discharge is minimal, presuming the cervix is closed.

Post partum bitches should not be taken to areas such as dog parks and dog-related activities to avoid exposure to infectious diseases that could be transmitted to the pups.

Anthelmenthics
Post-natal preventive anthelmintic treatment

These protocols, both prenatal/postnatal for the bitch and early treatment protocols for the puppies are safe and effective. Nevertheless, many breeders may be resistant to their use. The breeder and veterinarian share in the responsibility of protecting puppy buyers and their families and friends from exposure to zoonotic diseases which have the potential to cause serious health threats in humans.

If the pregnant bitch did not receive an entire round of prophylactic anthelmintic treatment with fenbendazole, ivermectin, or selamectin, the puppies must be treated with anthelmintics early and frequently to prevent patent infections.

Pyrantel pamoate is the drug of choice for very young kittens and puppies, and is appropriate for their lactating mothers as well. Puppies should have treatment starting at 2, 4, 6, 8, 12, 16, 20 and 24 weeks of age, with their mothers being dosed at the same time. The bitches and queens should be treated concurrently with their puppies and kittens because they frequently ingest the neonate's feces. This protocol will reduce roundworms and hookworms in the pups. Kittens do not have transplacental transmission of parasites, only transmammary. Kittens should be treated at 3, 5, 7, and 9 weeks of age. Pyrantel pamoate is considered safe for lactating bitches and queens.

Puppies, kittens, and their mothers need anthelmintic treatment prior to the typical first wellness visit at 6 to 8 weeks of age. Send the worming medications home with the client at an earlier visit, such as the breeding appointment, the prenatal appointment for ultrasound or radiographs, or the post-partum check-up. The breeder is much more likely to treat the puppies if they already have the wormer at home for both the pups and bitch.

Puppies from bitches treated prenatally with anthelmintics or pups treated starting at 2 weeks of age are thriftier, gain weight faster, utilize their food better, and have less diarrhea. These pups are easier to raise because they tend to be sick less often and are easier to keep clean. Pups with early intestinal parasite infections can have hookworm anemia, vomiting, diarrhea, dehydration, poor weight gain, and in some cases die prior to their 6 week veterinary visit. This can easily be prevented by early worming.

Common disorders of the immediate post-partum period: Diagnosis and treatment

Mastitis

(Appendix B-6)

Mastitis is a bacterial infection of 1 or more mammary glands. Mastitis is the most common cause of fever and lethargy in the post-partum or post-C-section bitch. Initially, when the client reports that the bitch is vaguely ill, she may be febrile but the gland and milk may appear normal. In this early stage, careful gross and microscopic examination of the milk expressed from each gland may be required for a diagnosis. Cytology on a drop of milk from each gland may aid in diagnosing subclinical or early mastitis. The milk and gland may look grossly normal. Normal milk contains a few neutrophils, macrophages, and lymphocytes. Milk from an infected gland will contain many degenerative neutrophils and bacteria, either cocci or rods. Oxytocin may be helpful in collecting the milk sample – pain associated with mastitis may deter the bitch from letting down her milk. Total cell counts have not been correlated to severity of mastitis or neonatal illness, and are not helpful diagnostically.

The bitch usually presents with signs of illness. In some cases the infection may be subclinical or so early that changes in the mammary gland are subtle. The 2 routes of infection are through the teat ducts (trauma from the pups or contamination from vaginal secretions or fetal stools) or through a hematogenous spread (from the uterus or other sites of bacterial infection). The bacteria most commonly found include Staph spp., Strep spp, E. coli, Klebsiella, Proteus, and Pasteurella.

Staphylococcus aureus is the most common cause. The patient will have a fever; lose interest in food and water, and be lethargic. There will be marked swelling, redness and inflammation of one or more glands associated with abnormal milk production. The involved gland will sometimes develop a necrotic area which can abscess through the skin surface.

Within a few hours of developing malaise, one or more glands will be red, swollen and hot. The milk may be obviously different in appearance from normal milk. On CBC, the white blood cell count will probably be elevated with a left shift. Chemistries will probably be normal, unless the bitch is septic. If septic, she may have a decreased glucose and albumin, and elevated liver enzymes.

If mastitis is suspected, but is not clinically apparent, ultrasound of the glands can help pinpoint a diagnosis. A normal mammary gland on ultrasound should have organized layers of medium echogenicity and an overall coarse granular structure. The mastitic gland will lose its organized layers; instead the tissue will be randomly organized with reduced echogenicity. Most veterinarians do not routinely scan the normal mammary gland with ultrasound so it is useful to scan all of the glands for comparison. Only 1 or 2 glands are typically infected, so there are usually others on the same bitch that can be used for comparison.

Cytology, culture and sensitivity will be useful in developing a treatment plan. Note if rods or cocci are seen. The sample for culture and sensitivity should be collected aseptically. Clip the hair, clean the skin with 70% rubbing alcohol and allow it to dry. Wearing gloves, express milk from the teat. Discard the first drop and collect the next drop(s) on the sterile swab, taking care to avoid touching the skin.

An appropriate antibiotic is the treatment of choice and is best based on a drug shown to be safe during lactation and sensitivity testing. However, treatment must be initiated prior to the availability of sensitivity results. The best choices for safety and efficacy are amoxicillin, amoxicillin with clavulanic acid (if cocci are seen), or trimethoprim-sulfa if the bitch cannot tolerate the penicillins. Enrofloxacins (if rods are seen) should be used with care but are probably safe for ingestion by the pups in the milk if they are under 2 weeks of age. Because of the inflammatory changes in the mammary gland, nearly any antibiotic will cross the blood-mammary barrier. Antibiotic treatment should be at label doses for 3 to 4 weeks.

Warm compresses are also helpful. IV or SQ fluids and non-steroidal anti-inflammatories may be indicated. Pups should be allowed to nurse unless there is a necrotic gland or they are old enough and eating independently enough to wean. If there is open necrotic tissue, this should be covered with light tape to keep the pups away from the lesion. In most cases, antibiotics, warm compresses and time to heal will adequately treat open abscesses. In rare cases, the necrotic tissue may need to be surgically debrided and drains placed.

If the bitch is toxic or is developing gangrenous mastitis and a sloughing gland, it may be necessary to remove the pups and hospitalize the mother. She may require IV fluids and IV antibiotics. IV glucose is indicated if she is hypoglycemic from septicemia. Non-steroid anti-inflammatories will reduce the fever and inflammation, and speed her recovery.

Cabergoline administered for 2 to 3 days (5 mcg/kg once daily) will reduce lactation if indicated. This can be reversed by withdrawing the drug and instituting metoclopramide or domperidone. The pups will require supplemental feeding unless they are old enough to wean. (See chapter 8).

If early weaning is necessary, but the breeder would like to leave the bitch with the pups, she can be placed in an appropriately sized t-shirt or one-piece bathing suit so that the social interactions that will benefit the pups can continue without allowing them to nurse.

The prognosis is very good and recurrence at subsequent breeding is unlikely.

Metritis and retained placentae

Metritis is a post-partum infection of the uterus. Retained placentas are placentas that did not pass at whelping or were not removed at C-section. Although retained placentas are the most common cause of metritis, retained placentas in the dog rarely cause metritis (Figure 7-1).

Metritis is a far less common cause than mastitis of fever and malaise in the immediate post-partum bitch. Metritis is typically noted in the first 3 to 5 days after whelping; mastitis can occur at this time, but is more common several weeks after whelping. The cause is bacterial colonization of the uterus, with or without retained placentae and without the hormonal influences that cause pyometra.

The bitch may run a fever, be lethargic, be anorexic like with mastitis; but will have a foul-smelling thick red to brown cloudy vaginal discharge. The pups may also show signs of illness. Diagnosis is based on ruling out mastitis, post-op wound infection if a C-section was performed, or other causes of illness and the atypical fetid odor to the discharge. Confirmation is based on cytology and culture of the uterine discharge; cytology will show toxic neutrophils with intracellular bacteria. Ultrasound may show retained fetal or placental tissues. This is not the same disorder as pyometra.

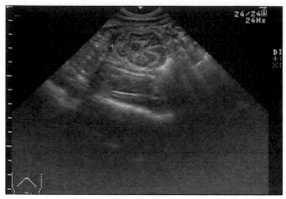

Figure 7-1.
Retained placenta seen on ultrasound post partum.

Treatment consists of appropriate antibiotic therapy (amoxicillin, amoxicillin with clavulanic acid, or trimethoprim-sulfa for bitches that cannot tolerate the penicillins). Prostaglandin F2 alpha (Lutalyse) and its analogues (Cloprostenol) may help evacuate the retained tissues and fluids from the uterus. Oxytocin is of little value – by this time post-partum, the uterus responds poorly to oxytocin. IV or SQ fluids and anti-inflammatories may be indicated. On rare occasion, ovariohysterectomy may be necessary. If the bitch is too ill to care for the pups, a surrogate mother or supplemental feeding may be necessary.

If the infection can be managed medically, the prognosis for return to fertility is very good. Recurrence at subsequent breeding is unlikely.

Retained pups

This is an unfortunate and preventable cause of illness in the bitch. By simply presenting the bitch for post-partum abdominal palpation, or radiographs post-partum, this will never have to happen. Even better than postpartum evaluation is a pre-partum puppy count on radiograph to allow accurate prediction of the number of pups expected.

ALL bitches, regardless of their owner's experience, should have veterinary care at the time of whelping (either pre-partum with an accurate puppy count or post-partum for a follow-up radiograph, or both in the case of a large litter difficult to count on pre-partum radiographs) to assess for complete delivery of all pups. The attending veterinarian should NEVER feel the need to apologize to the client for taking a post-partum radiograph that shows there are no pups left: this is great news for the client and it is practicing good medicine within the standard of care.

If there is a retained puppy, the bitch will either be normal or as time elapses, sick, febrile, painful, depressed, dehydrated, and in need of immediate medical attention. The mother has a litter of pups depending on her at a time when she is too sick to care for them. You not only have a sick mother to treat and income loss from the loss of the retained pups, you also need to manage the care of the remaining pups.

Conservative treatment is infrequently appropriate. If there is a retained dead pup (based on ultrasound), and the bitch is not febrile or ill; initially, she may be treated with vaginal lavage of warm saline. She can be sent home for the client to monitor for 24 hours. If the pup is not passed within 24 hours, surgery will probably be necessary to prevent metritis.

Treatment is usually surgical. The uterus is likely to be non-responsive to oxytocin when it is no longer "estrogen primed". It is likely to be friable and at risk of rupture if made to contract by aggressive use of pharmaceuticals (prostaglandins) in an attempt to expel the retained pup(s). The risk is that the uterus will contract around the pup(s), decreasing the likelihood that they will pass, or it will rupture, creating a life-threatening peritonitis.

If surgery is indicated and if the patient is not febrile or ill, she can be treated as a routine surgical patient. She should have pre-op laboratory work, IV fluids, an appropriate anesthetic protocol, and hospital care. Antibiotics should be administered because the risk of post-op metritis is high.

If febrile and ill, she should be stabilized pre-op. The owner should be advised that she could die. Treatment should include: IV fluids, hetastarch as indicated by lab values, antibiotics, and other care as indicated. Once stable, her abdomen should be explored. If the uterus is in good condition, remove the retained pup(s) from the exteriorized uterus, lavage the uterus while packed off from the abdomen, close the uterus, lavage and routinely close the abdomen. If the uterus is in poor condition AND the owner has given consent, an ovariohysterectomy may be performed. Adhesions are possible. Prior to closure, if there is evidence of uterine rupture, the abdomen should be explored for uterine contents, lavaged, and an appropriate abdominal wall closure for potential peritonitis performed. Post-op antibiotics, IV fluids, and pain management are indicated. In extreme cases, adhesions and peritonitis may require referral to a board-certified surgeon or 24 hour facility for nursing care.

Post partum hemorrhage

Hemorrhage or shock post-whelping to a degree requiring treatment is rare. Post-op hypovolemic shock is more common after Caesarean section than whelping and can be prevented by adequate fluid therapy during the procedure. NO bitch should have a Caesarean section without IV fluids. Clinical judgment dictates the need for colloids, plasma, or blood transfusion. Ovariohysterectomy at her C-section is a serious decision because it can lead to blood loss, shock and/or the development of DIC.

Poor appetite

Many bitches do not eat or drink well in the immediate post-partum period. This may be related to exhaustion, not feeling well, ingestion of all placentas, illness, or such total devotion to the pups that she will refuse to leave them to eat, drink, or eliminate.

Clinical judgment and client impression are important tools. If the bitch is seen in the immediate post-partum period and it is determined by radiograph that all pups have been delivered, a conservative approach may be warranted. If the uterus is empty, the patient is not febrile, not vomiting, and the client feels she is in good spirits, she is probably OK to treat at home.

If she has not had pre or post-partum radiographs, or if she is vomiting, running a fever over 103° F, or the owner sees or suspects something serious, she should be seen as soon as possible. You are not just treating her; the entire litter is at risk and may become your patients if she is not able to care for them.

If it is determined that she is not ill , she can be encouraged to eat by adding warm canned dog food or table food such as meat or cottage cheese to her meal. Mildly salting the diet may be helpful and improve her lactation. Sometimes the location of feeding must be changed, or hand-feeding can be used to jump start her appetite. Her appetite should improve by the time the pups are 2 to 3 days old. If this is not the case, she runs a fever or develops other symptoms, veterinary intervention is required.

If it is determined that she is ill, mastitis, metritis, retained placentas and retained pups are the first differentials to rule out. The post-partum bitch, however, can have nearly any other canine disorder, and a complete diagnostic work-up is in order if she does not have a postpartum issue or fails to respond to conservative therapy.

Diarrhea

Most bitches, whether they ingest placentas or not, seem to develop diarrhea shortly after delivery. Adequate hydration and dietary manipulation to minimize diarrhea (rice, bland diet, canned pumpkin, yogurt or a commercially formulated intestinal dog food) and Kao-Pectate® (real kaolin-pectin, not Bismuth Subsalicylate) are important. If drug therapy is indicated, consult veterinary resources to assess safety during lactation. Fluid therapy may be indicated to maintain lactation. Many breeders can use SQ fluids at home.

Unless fenbendazole was administered in the pre-partum period, by 2 weeks post-partum, the bitch and all her pups should receive their first dose of worming medication – pyrantel pamoate is the drug of choice. This should be repeated at 4, 6, and 8 weeks, according to the Companion Animal Parasite Council. These guidelines are available at www.capcvet.org.

Fenbendazole is used in late pregnancy and early lactation to reduce transplacental and transmammary transmission of T. canis and A. caninum. Fenbendazole (Panacur) is dosed at 50 mg/kg PO once daily from the 40th day of gestation to the 14th day of lactation.

Agalactia

Agalactia is the inadequate availability of milk while lactation should be occurring. This can be due to inadequate milk production or poor release of milk from the mammary gland. Too high an environmental temperature, too little food and water intake, too many previous litters, a C-section done too early, or any systemic illness can lead to agalactia. Some bitches seem to produce milk poorly with each litter. A complete history and physical examination may reveal the underlying cause.

The bitch should be assessed for illness including mastitis. If no underlying cause is found that merits treatment, the following therapy can be instituted.

1. **Increase fluid intake** by adding water to canned or dry dog food, offering broth or ice cream to drink, adding moderate amounts of salt or salty food to the diet, and/or giving SQ fluids. Many breeders have fluids on hand and are capable of handling this at home.
2. **Increase food intake.** Increase the total caloric intake.
3. **Metoclopramide therapy** (Reglan®) – can be given by SQ injection or orally in liquid or tablet form. It is useful when there is no apparent milk in the glands, based on the palpation of non-distended mammary glands (different from milk being present but not being released.) This is an important side effect of the drug that many veterinarians are unaware of (but lots of breeders are – thanks to the internet).
   In the CNS, metoclopramide appears to antagonize dopamine at the receptor sites, which stimulates prolactin release. Metoclopramide is excreted into milk and may concentrate at about twice the plasma level, but there does not appear to be a significant risk to nursing offspring. It is widely used with few limiting side effects.
   Metoclopramide is prescribed at the same dose as for gastrointestinal use: 0.2 to 0.4 mg/kg TID PO or SQ. It may be discontinued after 24 hours or can be continued after effective lactation occurs. It can be restarted if necessary. Some bitches may develop CNS signs ranging from drowsiness to restlessness and tremors. The drug should be discontinued if these symptoms occur.
4. **Domperidone** blocks the action of dopamine (dopamine inhibits the release of prolactin), allowing the release of prolactin. It is dosed at 0.05 to 0.1 mg/kg PO BID to improve lactation. It's use should be avoided in Collies and Collie-related breeds with the MDR-1 mutation. Both metoclopramide and domperidone are commonly used to increase lactation. Neither drug stimulates let-down, only increased production (Figure 7-2).
5. **Oxytocin** – can be given to aid in milk let-down, when milk is apparently present in the mammary glands but the bitch is unable to lactate effectively. It must be administered by injection; there is no oral form. Oxytocin may be given subcutaneously at 0.25 to 1 u total dose SQ every 2 hours to augment lactation.
   Oxytocin appears to work best if the pups are removed from the bitch, the oxytocin is given, the bitch has warm compresses applied to her mammary glands for 15 to 20 minutes, and then the pups are returned to her for nursing.
   Whelpwise™ recommends the following oxytocin protocol to improve lactation:
   1/2 unit SQ q 2 hours X 4 doses, then
   1 unit /SQ q 2 hours X 4 doses, then

2 units SQ q 2 hours X 4 doses, then
3 units SQ q 2 hours, then increase time between injections to 4, then 6 then 8 hours, then
discontinue when lactating well.
6. **Acupuncture or acupressure** are reported to improve lactation.

Domperidone Dosing in ml at 30 mg/ml:
For agalactia – 2.2 mg/kg of pound weight, po BID for 4 to 6 days, or longer if needed. May be started prior to whelping.

Dog by weight in pounds	ml of medication	Dog by weight in pounds	ml of medication
7.5 pounds	0.25 ml	15 pounds	0.50 ml
25 pounds	0.83 ml	30 pounds	1.0 ml
45 pounds	1.5 ml	50 pounds	1.67 ml
69 pounds	2.0 ml	70 pounds	2.33 ml
75 pounds	2.5 ml	90 pounds	3.00 ml
100 pounds	3.33 ml	110 pounds	3.67 ml
125 pounds	4.17 ml	150 pounds	5.0 ml

Figure 7-2.
Domperidone dosage chart.

Aggression toward the puppies

Some bitches may be aggressive toward their pups after vaginal or Caesarean delivery. This may last from 24 to 72 hours and is more common in first-time mothers. Within 72 hours, most bitches have settled into motherhood and tolerate the pups well but a few are never tolerant of the pups. Bitches should have human supervision, particularly if they are recovering from anesthesia, until the breeder is certain that they will accept the pups. Postoperatively, good pain management with drugs that are not likely to cause dysphoria is recommended. Buprenorphine, tramadol, Rimadyl® and Metacam® are good choices.

Some bitches will not tolerate any contact, even nursing; some will tolerate nursing but no movement around the head and shoulders. Most if they are aggressive will growl and sneer at the pups; of course this communication is of no value to the pups as they can neither hear nor see. Rarely, the mother will ravage the litter; this is devastating. If pups are disappearing, an abdominal radiograph will confirm or disaffirm that the bitch has ingested them.

There are several proposed causes for maternal aggression. Some suggest that it is genetic, but it is not always a trait seen in mother and daughters. Stress, underfeeding, overcrowding, and deafness have all been proposed as possible causes. A low stress environment means a quiet room with no other dogs or unfamiliar people in the same area or within sight or hearing range.

Anecdotal reports suggest that hypocalcemia may play a role in maternal aggression, particularly in bull terriers. There is no study currently available to show that low measured ionized calcium levels have been correlated with this behavior. In addition to maternal aggression, there are strange behaviors including hiding, staring at the pups, and having a glazed over look. Rarely, the bitch exhibits aggression toward humans. There seems to be a positive correlation between the need for calcium to stimulate oxytocin uptake and the need for oxytocin to achieve normal mothering skills. Treatment consists of SQ calcium supplementation, followed by oral calcium supplements for several days. The immediate improvement in maternal skills upon calcium supplementation supports the correlation between low ionized calcium levels (not total calcium) and maternal aggression.

Dog Appeasing Pheromone (DAP) can be used to minimize aggression and anxiety. This is an analog that mimics the pheromone naturally found in the amniotic fluid of dogs and the mammary glands of lactating bitches. Its function is to reassure and calm puppies, and aid in bonding between the bitch and her pups. Since its effects last into adulthood, it can also be used to reduce anxiety in many settings. The bitch who has had a C-section is not exposed to the pheromone in the amniotic fluids so maternal skills take longer to develop (up to 72 hours). Development of maternal skills can be hastened by the use of the Adaptil™ collar. Although DAP comes in collar, room diffuser and spray form, the collar works more quickly than the other forms. The collar can be used on the bitch for several days prior to her planned whelping or C-section or can be applied at the C-section. The collar will last for up to 4 weeks, carrying you easily through the development of good mothering skills. The collar is not a substitute for careful observation to assure that she is not threatening to harm her pups.

If there is a stressful environment, such as multiple other pets in a small area, changing the environment is indicated. If there is no response to calcium supplementation, the DAP collar, or the environment is not stressful, keeping the bitch muzzled while with the pups and not leaving her with the pups unsupervised may be the only option to completely removing the pups from their mother. In most cases, patience with the bitch, crating her next to the whelping box, and only allowing (or forcing in some cases) her to be in contact with the pups to nurse every 2 to 3 hours may be required. It is beneficial to the pups to have several days of colostrum and milk from their own mother prior to changing to hand-raising or placing them with a surrogate bitch.

Eclampsia, Post-parturient hypocalcemia, or Milk fever

Eclampsia is a condition caused by low ionized calcium in the extracellular fluid. In dogs, the initial symptoms are neglect of the pups; scratching at the face; restlessness and nervousness; stiff goose-stepping type gait and muscle tremors; panting; dialated pupils; hypoglycemia; and hyperthermia. This can progress rapidly if unnoticed or undiagnosed to lateral recumbency; rigid muscles; seizure activity; and death (Figure 7-3). In cattle, more commonly affected by hypocalcemia, the opposite presentation occurs; the clinical signs are weakness and flaccid muscles seen as "down cow" syndrome.

A presumptive diagnosis is made on clinical signs, history, and is confirmed by laboratory tests showing low calcium. The typical patient is a small-breed dog with a large litter of puppies at peak lactation – between 1 and 4 weeks post partum. They are frequently on an unbalanced diet or were supplemented with calcium during pregnancy.

Laboratory tests show a total serum calcium of 7.0 mg/dl or less. Differentials include hypoglycemia, epilepsy, toxicity, metoclopramide overdose, and other neurologic diseases. However, on physical examination, a bitch with seizures and mammary development should be presumed to have hypocalcemia until proven otherwise.

Slow intravenous calcium supplementation should begin immediately, while carefully monitoring the heart rate with a stethoscope, or preferably with an EKG. Administration must be discontinued if bradycardia, tachycardia, arrhythmia, or vomiting occurs. Administer calcium gluconate 10%, warmed to body temperature, at a rate of 50 to 150 mg/kg or 0.5 to 1.5 ml/kg over 20 to 30 minutes. An alternative IV treatment is 1% calcium glycerophosphate plus calcium lactate (Calphosan solution 1%) administered at 2.5 to 7.5 ml/kg, over 20 to 30 minutes, stopping if the heart rate changes.

Additional calcium can be administered SQ or IM, but the product must be labeled for this route. Calcium chloride CANNOT be given IM or SQ as it will result in tissue sloughs. If 10% calcium gluconate solution is available, it can be diluted 50% with normal saline and administered SQ every 8 hours until the oral calcium takes effect. Oral calcium treatment in tablet form (gluconate or carbonate) is available for dogs and humans over-the-counter. It should be dosed at 500 mg TID per 20 lbs and continued throughout lactation. An oral calcium gel is also available and but is very bitter and administration can

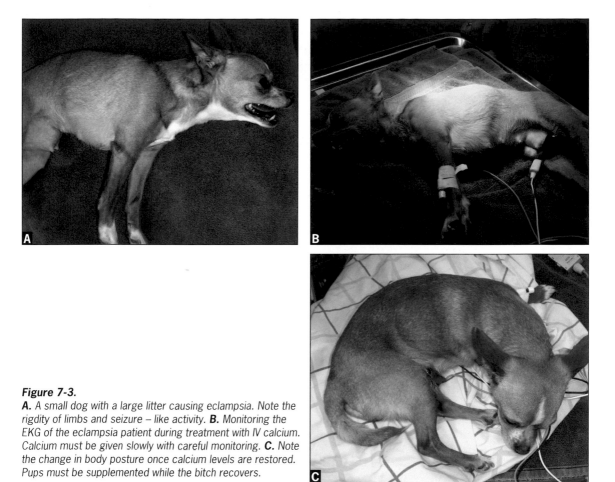

Figure 7-3.
A. A small dog with a large litter causing eclampsia. Note the rigdity of limbs and seizure – like activity. **B.** Monitoring the EKG of the eclampsia patient during treatment with IV calcium. Calcium must be given slowly with careful monitoring. **C.** Note the change in body posture once calcium levels are restored. Pups must be supplemented while the bitch recovers.

be difficult. Tums® contain 500 mg calcium carbonate which supplies 200 mg calcium.

Some bitches need additional treatment if the symptoms are severe. This may include glucose supplementation if she is also hypoglycemic; IV fluids for hyperthermia and dehydration; cooling with water to control hyperthermia; and diazepam (1 to 5 mg IV) or barbiturates if seizure-type activity persists.

To prevent recurrence, puppies should be removed for weaning or removed temporarily and hand-fed until the bitch can care for them. Additionally, oral calcium may be administered during lactation, but not during pregnancy.

Uterine prolapse

Uterine prolapse is rare in dogs. It can occur following whelping while the cervix is still open. This emergency requires repositioning the uterus as soon as possible. To do so, the dog should be anesthetized, the uterus lubricated with sterile lubricant, flushed with sterile saline, and repositioned. After replacement, oxytocin should be administered (5 to 10 IU IM) to aid in uterine involution. If it cannot be reduced, hypertonic saline or 50% dextrose can be used to reduce uterine edema. If the uterus cannot be reduced by external manipulation, a midline abdominal incision should be made and the uterus reduced by internal manipulation. If the uterus is necrotic or cannot be repositioned, an ovariohysterectomy may be performed.

SIPS

Subinvolution of placental sites or SIPS is failure of the placental attachment sites to heal completely. This is a common disorder. It is most frequently noted in bitches after their first litter. The only symptoms are an ongoing vaginal discharge with blood for more than 3 weeks and up to 4 months post-partum. The bitch and pups do not show signs of illness; the vaginal discharge contains bright red blood or mucoid blood but does not look cloudy or have an odor; and the delivery was typically normal. There is anecdotal evidence that SIPS is less common in bitches treated with oxytocin post-whelping. (Hutchison, VIN online communication 18 July 2008.)

Diagnosis is usually based on history, lack of other findings in physical examination, and vaginal cytology. Cytology will show red blood cells, with only a few normal white blood cells and a few bacteria. A CBC may assure the veterinarian and owner that she is neither anemic, thrombocytopenic, nor suffering from metritis. A protime to assure that clotting time is normal is recommended if the blood loss seems excessive or there is possible exposure to rodenticides or other causes of coagulopathy.

There is generally no indication for treatment, medical or surgical – this is a self-limiting disease and it will resolve spontaneously and probably not recur at future whelpings. Bitches may be left intact, bred again, and usually do not have a recurrence of the condition. Lutalyse® can be used if the discharge is severe or if the client is concerned. If the disorder becomes problematic, prostaglandin F2 alpha (Lutalyse®) may be used at 50 mcg/kg subcutaneously twice daily until the red blood cells disappear on vaginal cytology. If the bitch is ovariohysterectomized for another reason near this time, bands of green tissue identified as healing placental sites may be noted in the uterine lining.

If the client or the veterinarian elect to have the bitch with suspected SIPS examined, it is best done by the veterinarian going out to the car to do an examination and vaginal cytology. This will minimize the bitch's exposure to contagious diseases that may be present in the veterinary clinic.

If an underlying coagulopathy is found as the cause of the long-standing or severe vaginal blood loss, the underlying cause should be treated (See Chapter 9).

CHAPTER 8
Neonatal and Pediatric Care

Introduction

Breeders and veterinarians share 2 great fears: the first and most devastating is the loss of a bitch "in whelp". The second is the loss of a litter or an overwhelming number of pups.

A 10% to 40% loss of pups is reported to be a "normal loss". This remarkably high figure is difficult to substantiate and sources do not always indicate if it includes loss from conception to 12 weeks of age or from birth to 12 weeks of age. This is a staggering figure. In general, any time losses exceed 10%, veterinary investigation is warranted. If an underlying cause can be determined, the remaining pups in that litter as well as pups in subsequent litters can be protected. History, physical examination, and diagnostics will be described in this chapter.

Good breeding and husbandry practices and high quality veterinary care can minimize losses. But even under the best circumstances, we must recognize that there will be unavoidable losses. Neonates are fragile; disorders that are mild in an adult or slight alterations in environment often have much more severe consequences in the neonate.

The following information is meant to equip you and your staff to provide the highest quality care possible. The first step is to assist in selecting top quality stock. The second step is to assist in achieving a successful pregnancy. Third is to minimize fetal distress at delivery. The final step is to work cooperatively with your clients to raise every pup.

Teamwork with the breeder-client is essential. Most pups are born at home and are not frequently examined by a veterinarian. Those born vaginally or by C-section at the veterinary hospital will be raised at home after they are discharged. The breeder who either intuitively recognizes a sick pup or through objective evaluation (numerical assessments based on body weight/gain, rectal temperature, and urine color) is usually the person who recognizes the need for veterinary intervention. Veterinarians and their staff may also detect health problems when the pups are delivered, at office visits to remove dewclaws and tails, or at routine scheduled visits.

To develop the client-staff team, you can:
1. Teach your client how to monitor the whelping and pups in the early post-partum period. Objective measurements including rectal temperature, urine color, and weight gain are easily quantified and trends can alert you early on if there is a problem.
2. Train your staff to ask the "right" questions on the phone. Combined, the client and staff will learn to recognize early signs of disease. (Appendix B-2)

The normal neonate
(Table 8-1)
The first week of life

The normal newborn sleeps and nurses approximately 90% of their time. They should cry very little and be able to find a nipple without assistance most of the time. They should form a tight seal on the nipple and nurse for several minutes before dropping off or falling asleep. Pups often twitch and move intermittently when sleeping. They should be near their littermates, but should not stack on top of each other. Their only interaction with the mother is nursing. Their only interaction with littermates is competition during nursing, snuggling when resting, and occasional nursing on one another. They are born with their eyes and ears sealed closed. They need to be stimulated to urinate and defecate by their mother licking their perineum.

When held, a healthy puppy has a good "feel" to its body – it feels well filled out, with good firm body tone. Flexor dominance is present at birth, which means extending their neck causes flexion of all 4 limbs for up to the first 4 days. They should be able to right themselves, suckle and root for a nipple spontaneously. Although they can feel, there is no strong withdrawal reflex until day 7.

Table 8-1 Normal puppy development from birth to 6 weeks of age				
What is normal?	Week 1	Week 2	Weeks 3-4	Weeks 5-6
Temperature, rectal	96 - 98° F	96-99° F	100° F	100 - 101° F
Ambient temperature	75 to 80°F	70 to 80° F	70 to 75° F	65 to 75°F
Heart rate & blood Pressure	200 to 240 beats per min; Blood pressure 61	200 to 240 beats per min, sinus rhythm	160 to 200 beats per min, sinus rhythm; blood pressure 139	Varies with breed
Respiratory rate	15 to 35 per min	15 to 35 per min	15 to 25 per min	15 to 25 per min
Mucus membranes Color/ CRT	Pink to hyperemic if recently nursed	Pink/1 second	Pink/1 second	Pink/1 second
Urine color	Very pale yellow, <1.020	Very pale yellow, <1.020	Pale yellow	Pale to moderate yellow
Weight	May lose up to 10% in the first 3 days. Birth weight: Toys 100-200 gms; Large 400-500 gms; Giant 700 gms	Gaining 5 to 10% daily, many double birth weight by day 10. Calculate weight gain of 2-4 gm/day/kg anticipated adult weight.	Calculate weight gain of 2 -4 gm/day/kg antici-pated adult weight.	Calculate weight gain of 1 -4 gm/day/kg anticipated adult weight. Giant and large breeds gain at faster rate than small breeds.
Activity	Sleeps & eats 90% of time, twitch while sleeping	Sleeps & eats 90% of time, twitch while sleeping	Beginning to crawl, then stand and walk by day 21. Start to play when eyes open. Can sit.	Walking, climbing, play-ing, may bark, begin to explore environment, mouthing. Normal postural reflexes.
Attitude	Quiet, cry infrequently.	Quiet	Quiet, more active	Start to develop "person-alities",
Body tone and reflexes	Flexor dominance for 1st 4 days, then extensor. Righting, rooting, weak withdrawal.	Extensor dominance, righting, rooting, crossed extensor. With-drawal developing.	Approaching normal for adult. Suckling reflex & crossed extensor disap-pears.	Normal adult
Vision and hearing	No vision but blink with bright light. Limited hearing.	None to limited vision and hearing, menace present but slow initially. Limited hearing, waxy discharge.	Vision blurry, Pupillary light reflex present within 24 hours of eye-lids opening, respond to sound. Startle reflex develops.	Approaching full vision and hearing
Teeth	None	None	Deciduous incisors & canine erupt	Deciduous premolars erupt
Breeder's interaction	Assure pups are nursing, supplement if necessary. Daily temp, weight, urine & stool character. Start Early Neurologic Stimulation day 3-16	Assure pups are nurs-ing, supplement if necessary. Daily temp, weight, urine & stool character. Continue Early Neurologic Stimulation day 3-16	Continue to assure pups are thriving, begin to enrich environment by variation of toys, surfaces.	Continue to assure pups are thriving, continue to enrich environment. Lots of human interac-tion for socialization
Veterinary care	Assess & treat if not thriving, taildocks and dewclaws prior to 5th day	Assess & treat if not thriving. Dispense pyran-tel pamoate to use on day 14 after birth.	Assess & treat if not thriving. Dispense pyran-tel pamoate to use on day 28 after birth.	Veterinary wellness visit – assess pups for any ab-normalities for breeder to sell pup with full disclosure. First vaccina-tions (DAPPv). Dispense pyrantel pamoate to use on day 42 after birth.
Food and water	Nursing only. If supplementing, 60 ml/lb/24 hours divided by 12, fed every 2 hours.	Nursing only. If supplementing, 70 ml/lb/24 hours divided by 8, fed every 3 hours.	Offer water, then gruel to start weaning. If supplementing, 90 ml/lb/24 hours divided by 6, fed every 4 hours.	Teething. Many pups weaned, on full food and water, some still nurse for social interaction.

Small Animal Pediatric Medicine Tufts Animal Expo 2002 Johnny D. Hoskins, DVM, Ph.D. DocuTech Services, Inc. Baton Rouge, Louisiana, USA

Early neurological stimulation should start on day 3 and be completed on day 16. These simple manipulations will improve an individual dog's ability to tolerate stress (Figure 8-1).

The rectal temperature of a normal newborn should start at 96° F and goes up 1 degree per week, while the ambient temperature at the pup's contact surface should start at 90 to 95° F and be lowered 5° F per week. If the contact surface is warm, the ambient air temperature can be between 70 and 75° F. Incorrect environmental temperatures, both too hot and too cold, are common causes of a pup's failure to thrive.

Normal vital signs are a body temperature of 96° F, heart rate of 200 to 240, no murmur, and irregular respirations at a rate of 15 to 35 respirations per minute with no pause between inspiration and expiration. They have bright pink gums, a PCV equal to their mother's, total protein of 5 to 6, BUN of 7 to 10 and glucose of 40 to 60. The urine color should be very pale yellow on a cotton ball and <1.020 specific gravity.

Normal birth weight should be 100 to 200 gms (4 to 7 oz) for toy breeds, 200 to 400 gms (7 to 16 oz) for medium breeds, 400 to 500 gms (16 oz) for large breeds and 700 gms (24 oz) for giant breeds.

Many pups lose weight in the first 24 hours – but this should not exceed 10% of their total body weight. After the initial loss, weight gain should be 5 to 10% of their birth weight daily. Another way to calculate weight gain is to use this formula: Pups should gain 2 to 4 g/day/kg of anticipated adult weight. Many breeders want the birth weight to double in the first 7 to 10 days. Most pups should be receiving all of their fluid and nutritional needs by nursing. Careful monitoring of rectal temperature, weight gain, urine color, and overall well-being will indicate if some or all the pups require supplemental feeding.

The second week of life

The pups still sleep and nurse aggressively most of the time, twitch while sleeping, and should cry little. They may move more frequently but should still cluster together when not nursing. They do not interact with any thing in the environment because their eyes and ears are still closed – they move around the whelping box like bumper cars. They only interact with the bitch to nurse and with littermates when competing for a nipple (many show a preference for a favorite spot on the bitch), when suckling on each other, or to snuggle when asleep. They still depend on the bitch to stimulate them to urinate and defecate. At sometime in the first 2 weeks, extensor dominance replaces flexor dominance – they should extend their limbs when their neck is extended. They should be able to right themselves, suckle and root for a nipple spontaneously. They should be able to support themselves on the front legs.

The temperature of the contact surface should be 85 to 90° F and the ambient temperature of the room should be 70 to 75° F. Normal vital signs are a body temperature of 96 to 98° F, heart rate of 200 to 240 with a sinus rhythm, no murmur, and more regular respirations at a rate of 15 to 35 breaths per minute. Urine color should remain very pale yellow on a cotton ball with <1.020 specific gravity.

Weight gain should be at 2 to 4 g/day/kg of anticipated adult weight. They should receive all of their fluid and nutritional needs by nursing. The first dose of wormer, pyrantel pamoate, should be given at the end of the second week.

Abnormal findings in the first 2 weeks

Despite the varied disorders in newborns, their clinical signs may be so similar that they don't help distinguish the cause. The most obvious complaint is incessant crying or mewing. This grabs the

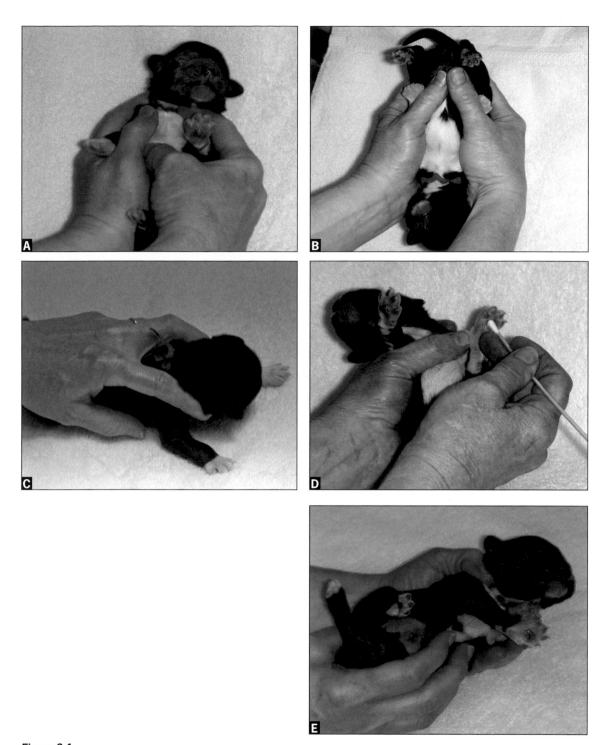

Figure 8-1.
*There are 5 steps of early neurologic stimulation, each performed for 5 seconds from day 3 to day 16 of age. **A.** Step 1. Hold the pup head up for 5 seconds. **B.** Step 2. Hold the pup head down for 5 seconds. **C.** Step 3. Hold the pup on a cool towel for 5 seconds. **D.** Step 4. Rub the bottom of one foot of the pup for 5 seconds. **E.** Step 5. Hold the pup on its back for 5 seconds. These can be done in any order.*

attention of even the most inattentive owner and bitch, but may not identify the sickest pups. Sick puppies move very little, and make no or weak efforts to nurse. They do not twitch while sleeping. Sick pups are often separated in the whelping box from littermates, not cuddled in the group. They are not gaining weight or worse, are losing. Body temperature is below 94° F (this is a chilled pup who should not be fed milk until warmed to 96° F) or above 98° F (this is a fever in a neonate). If the rectal temperature of all pups is high, this may either indicate all the pups are sick or that the environmental temperature is too high. Urine color on a dry cotton ball is an obvious color of yellow. Milk may flow from the nostrils of pups with cleft palates or other swallowing defects.

Sick pups have a look and "feel" that can be difficult to describe. The general appearance is unthrifty and either overly active or overly still. When picked up, they feel limp and scrawny. Frequently, there is a history of prolonged labor. If a breeder says there is something wrong, but they can't describe it fully, believe them. These are pups that require medical attention.

Diarrhea, nasal discharge, inflammation of the umbilicus, and/or sloughing of the toes and/or tail tips are early symptoms of illness in newborns.

If a pup seems to be sick or abnormal, take a rectal temperature. If below 96° F, warm the pup inside the breeder's shirt or carefully with an external heat source. A heating pad covered with a towel, hot water bottle, or sock filled with heated white rice can be used, but care must be taken to avoid burning, overheating or warming too quickly.

Once warmed, assist the pup in nursing or tube feed. There are many reasons a pup may be under nourished and dehydrated. The underlying problem needs to be addressed (sick mother, sick puppy, too large a litter), but the first thing to do is warm and supplement the pup. Feeding a pup with a rectal temperature below 96° F will result in ileus and fermentation of the milk in the gut. This leads to aspiration and perpetuates the pup's distress. Tube feeding is recommended over bottle feeding. Most breeders can be quickly trained to tube feed (see tube feeding in Appendix C-16 for client handout material). Done correctly, it is a safe, fast, and effective method.

Low birth weight and failure to ingest colostrum has a strong correlation with failure to thrive. Pups that are 25% below the weight of the average pup in the litter are at increased risk of hypothermia, hypoglycemia, hypoxia, and septicemia. Pups that lose more than 10% of their birth weight in the first 24 hours are sick enough to seek veterinary attention. Treatment including supplemental feeding, fluid therapy, supplemental heat, antibiotics, as well as plasma infusion, and oxygen therapy should be initiated. Diagnostics may also be indicated.

Some pups requiring supplemental feeding have serious medical or genetic disorders. More, however, are just off to a rough start. The least we can do is support them with the warmth and nutritional care they require. Most pups who start off poorly begin to thrive with a few feedings a day and a little extra TLC. Clients who are willing to invest the extra effort should be encouraged and educated to promote this. **More pups are lost to starvation than to any other problem in the immediate post-partum period.** Make it your goal to do all you can to prevent your patients from starving to death. Fear of tube feeding should not be an excuse.

If warming and feeding do not return the pup to normal, veterinary diagnostics and care should be initiated.

The third and fourth weeks of life
By now, the pups are not so fragile and everyone feels a sense of relief. It is easier to detect problems and the pups are more resilient when faced with an illness or disorder.

The pups are up on all 4 legs and moving, but at first cannot see where they are going. By the end of the second week and beginning of the third, the ears and then eyes open. Pupillary light reflexes and corneal reflexes are present within 24 hours of the eyelids opening. However, the corneas are cloudy and gray and the pup's vision is probably blurry for the first few days. Tear production should begin. There will be some waxy debris in the ear canals as they open, but it should clear on its own. It is a good idea to have the lights and noises softened as the pups adjust to a world of vision and hearing. Early neurologic stimulation should be discontinued by day 16.

They try to play with each other and with toys, but are awkward and fall down often.

The body temperature should be 99 to 100° F and the ambient room temperature should be in the 70 to 75° F range.

Most pups are still very dependent on the bitch for fluid and nutritional needs but weaning can start. By the third week, a dish or water bottle (Figure 8-2) can be offered (take care to avoid drowning), and by the third to fourth week, gruel can be offered. Introducing gruel and water should be done gradually so all pups are skilled at eating and drinking before the bitch is no longer accessible. Gruel can be made of puppy food soaked and ground up with warm water or a combination of chicken baby food, yogurt and baby rice cereal. Royal canin makes a product to aid in weaning called starter mousse, which eases the transition from nursing to eating solid food. The gruel can be placed in a shallow dish or on the edge of the palm of your hand for introduction to the pups. When they are ready to wean, they will quickly learn to eat from a dish. The breeder should monitor this closely

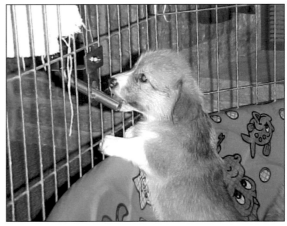

Figure 8-2.
Pups can easily be taught to lick water from a water bottle by applying a tasty paste such as peanut butter. Use of a water bottle assures a clean safe water source that pups can't fall into or soil.

as some pups in the litter may eat aggressively and some may be more reluctant to try. In large litters or when there are some pups who are significantly more aggressive than others, the pups may benefit from being fed in small groups or separately. Shallow heavy dishes should be used – there are commercially available pans. The gruel should be very thin, and thickened gradually.

In all but the toy breeds, the deciduous incisor teeth are beginning to erupt. They can now defecate and urinate without stimulation; a litter tray for elimination can be introduced into the whelping box (Figure 8-3).

Administer a second dose of wormer, pyrantel pamoate, at the end of the fourth week.

The fifth and sixth weeks of life
The pups are a lot more fun and a lot more work. Personalities, which have been developing all along, are easier to describe. They seem more independent, but socially still need to be with their mother and littermates – they are not ready to be moved into new owner's homes. The pups can remain in the whelping box, if it is large enough,

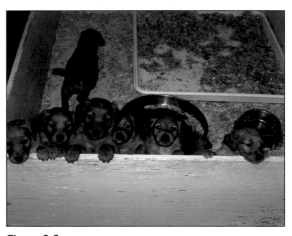

Figure 8-3.
Use of a custom built box with a litter tray for pups to eliminate in and food and water dishes.

or be moved into a pen that is safe for small puppies. A "litter box" can be used to start housetraining and in some climates at some times of the year, they can be outside for parts of the day.

This is a good time to move the pups to a less isolated part of the breeder's home – they should have an opportunity to see and begin to interact with other dogs with supervision, to hear normal house sounds (TV, telephones, and kitchen noises) and to explore new environments. Environmental enrichment can begin – this can be accomplished by adding and removing toys and obstacles from the pen. At night, the pups can begin to sleep in crates in close proximity to one another. This step will make the transition to a crate in the new owner's home much easier.

The body temperature should be approaching that of a normal adult – 99 to 100° F. The pups can now regulate their own temperature and no longer need supplemental heat. Room temperature should be maintained at 65 to 75° F.

Teething is progressing – toy breeds will have deciduous incisors erupting and most other breeds will have premolars erupting. Weaning should be progressing, and may be complete for many puppies. Water should be available at all times, in a shallow dish or drinking bottle – if using a drinking bottle, be certain all the pups can reach it and know how to use it. The pups should be fed 3 to 5 times a day, using a gruel of quality commercially available puppy food. Softened food should be used because pups of this age can easily choke on dry food. They should be monitored to assure that they are not being over or underfed. No nutritional supplements, no meat, no cottage cheese, and no raw meat diets should be fed – the pet food manufacturers have formulated excellent puppy foods for small, medium and large breed puppies. These diets cannot be improved upon by supplemental feeding.

The pup's vision and hearing should be normal. Neurologically, the pups should be normal.

Administer the third dose of wormer, pyrantel pamoate, orally at the end of the 6th week. The first set of canine vaccinations can be administered at the end of the 7th week. Vaccines and vaccination protocols change rapidly. It is advisable to review the current literature, products available, the environment of the pups, and the area of the country in which you practice to develop an appropriate vaccination protocol (Appendix C-11).

Advanced in-home care – The breeder as the health care provider
Breeder skills and supplies
Most breeder clients are exceptionally successful at raising puppies. They are highly skilled and intuitive, experienced, hard working, and they put their hearts and souls into the process. Many have husbandry skills that outshine anything we can hope to achieve as veterinarians. Some count on it for income or to support their dog-habit, some do it as a labor of love, and many do it for both.

A well-educated breeder paired with a well-educated veterinary staff and a veterinarian willing to learn from their breeder-clients make a formidable team. Veterinarians and veterinary staff can learn as much from their breeder-clients as they can learn from us.

There are a few things that set a great breeder apart from a good breeder. They are time, great husbandry skills, exemplary record keeping, secure whelping and nursery area, and basic equipment.

Time
There is very little that can replace the time a breeder spends with the pups. They know their bitch and what normal parturition looks like. They recognize signs of dystocia early and are quick to intervene with veterinary assistance. They see subtle changes in the pups early. They provide basic needs and medical care to the bitch and pups immediately. They provide essential social interaction for the pups.

They take the time to carefully consider who should be bred and why. They monitor the pups and reflect on their successes and failures.

Great husbandry skills

These clients keep their dogs and their environment meticulously clean. Parasite and disease control is optimal. The dogs are impeccably groomed. They often spend more time and effort preparing food for the dogs and ensuring that they have a comfortable home than they spend on themselves.

They are also "intuitive." They have things so well in order that they can notice the early changes – the first time the dog urinates inappropriately, the first abnormal stool, the first picked-at meal, the first hair out of place, the tiniest lump.

They see subtle changes with clarity. Unfortunately for us, some of them find changes we have difficulty diagnosing because they are so early and so subtle. The important thing is to never doubt them. They are almost always right. The challenge is to identify the changes they notice and try to predict with accuracy if the changes they have identified are serious, may become serious, or are minor or self-resolving conditions. We are there to put their concerns in perspective, diagnose and treat what we can, and come to terms with what we cannot control. Our role is to always take them seriously and provide the service we can to help them meet their goals.

Clients who report health changes early allow us the opportunity to diagnose and treat disorders and conditions early, enabling us to provide them with the best possible outcome.

Exemplary record keeping

(Appendix C-6)

The most essential step in good record keeping is to be able to definitively identify each individual in a litter. This is useful for several reasons, including tracking health, weight gain, monitoring medical care, and identifying the purchaser. In large kennels, this also applies to adults (Figure 8-4).

For pups born at the veterinary hospital: There are several techniques that can be used for tracking individuals in the litter. With one system, sterile colored hand-towels are used to receive the neonates during C-section. This allows birth order and each pup's immediate neonatal care to be more easily recorded following resuscitation. The towel color is translated into permanent marker or nail polish and the information is mapped onto a uterine diagram with one copy maintained in the hospital record and one copy provided to the owner. (Appendix D-9).

For pups born at home: If the pup has distinctive markings or colors, they can be sketched or photographed with a digital camera and included in the record. If the pups are similar, markings of different colored permanent marker, non-toxic fabric paint or fingernail polish, or notch marks can be clipped into the coat in different locations. Although many breeders use a variety of different materials for neck bands to identify pups, there is a risk associated with anything restrictive placed around the neck.

Ideally, a tracking system should be planned prior to the birth of the pups. This prevents trying to backtrack and recall what occurred during middle-of-the-night whelpings or rapid fire delivery at C-section. Beginning record-keeping at vaginal births or C-sections allows the breeder and veterinarian to track birth order, location in the uterus (when delivered by C-section), time of birth and length of time between births, identify pups adjacent to abnormal pups, and medical care given to each pup. Once a system is developed, it should be maintained. Markings change in many breeds, colors need to be reapplied, and clipped areas need to be re-shaved.

This information may become vital in monitoring an at-risk pup more carefully or establishing a diagnosis of illness in a newborn (Figure 8-5).

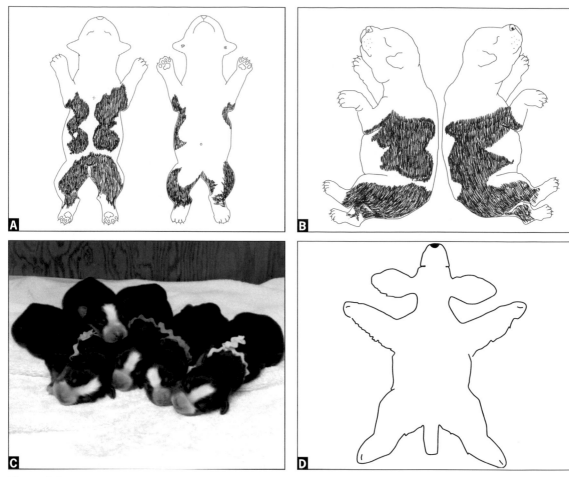

Figure 8-4.
A. Outlines of pups with markings added by hand for individual puppy identification. *B.* Lateral outlines of pups with markings added by hand for puppy identification. *C.* Puppy identification using colored rickrack for neckbands. This is not recommended. *D.* Outline of puppy used for identification.

Once the pups are identified, a tracking record must be started for each pup. Tracking each pup's progress is essential to assure that no pup is overlooked in a litter. There are many different types and each breeder can easily develop their own or purchase or borrow a format from another breeder (See Appendix C-6 and C-8).

The most commonly and objectively tracked parameters are:
1. **Weight at birth** and at least twice daily; (Appendix C6 and C8)
2. **Temperature** at least twice daily;
3. **Heart rate and respiratory rate** at least once daily
4. **Mucus membrane color** at least once daily
5. **Urine color** at least daily – should be almost clear color on a dry cotton ball used to stimulate the pup by rubbing the perineum;
6. **Stool character** at least daily;
7. **Medications administered**, if any;
8. **Intervention at birth to resuscitate** – drugs, techniques, and oxygen – if any;
9. **Early Neurologic Stimulation maneuvers completed** – 1 time a day from day 3 to 16;
10. **Volume of formula fed**, if any;
11. **Owner concerns or observations**;
12. **Any other findings noted**, if anything out of the ordinary.

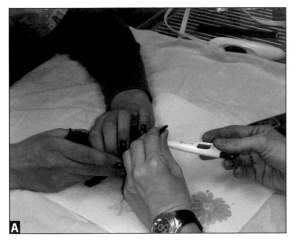
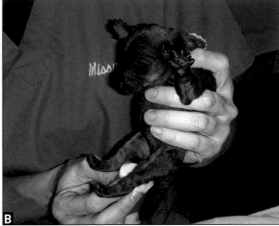
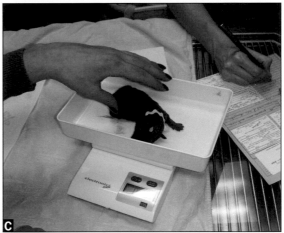

Figure 8-5.
A. *Use a rectal thermometer to check on newborn pups. Pups can accommodate the size of the thermometer tip if petroleum jelly is applied first.* **B.** *Check urine color on a newborn pup with a dry cotton ball rubbed gently on the perineum of the pup. The urine color should be pale yellow if the pup is well fed and well hydrated.* **C.** *Use a digital food scale to weigh pups. They can be weighed in grams or ounces.*

If the breeder objectively (based on body weight, urine color and body temperature) or subjectively indicates that there is a concern with one or more of the pups, this data is invaluable at the veterinary phone call or office visit. Not only can the breeder clearly identify their concerns, but the veterinarian can also make clinical judgments and adjustments in the care provided by the breeder.

Secure whelping and nursery area
The importance of a clean, secure, warm, easily-accessible, safe, easy-to-clean area to whelp and raise the pups in cannot be overemphasized. This does not need to be expensive or elaborate. A quiet, small, warm room that can be equipped with a child's wading pool, and the following supplies is all that is needed.

Basic equipment to have at home
(Figure 8-6) (See Appendix C-6)
- Record keeping system.
- Method to re-mark puppy's identification.
- Room thermometer to track temperature at the puppy's surface.
- Rectal thermometer, digital is ideal, to monitor the bitch's and pup's temperatures.
- Scale to weigh pups, easiest with a bowl type platform. A kitchen scale is ideal. This should weigh in ounces or grams.
- Cotton balls to check urine color of pups.
- Feeding tube and appropriate syringes if supplementation is necessary.
- Formula to feed, if supplementation is necessary.

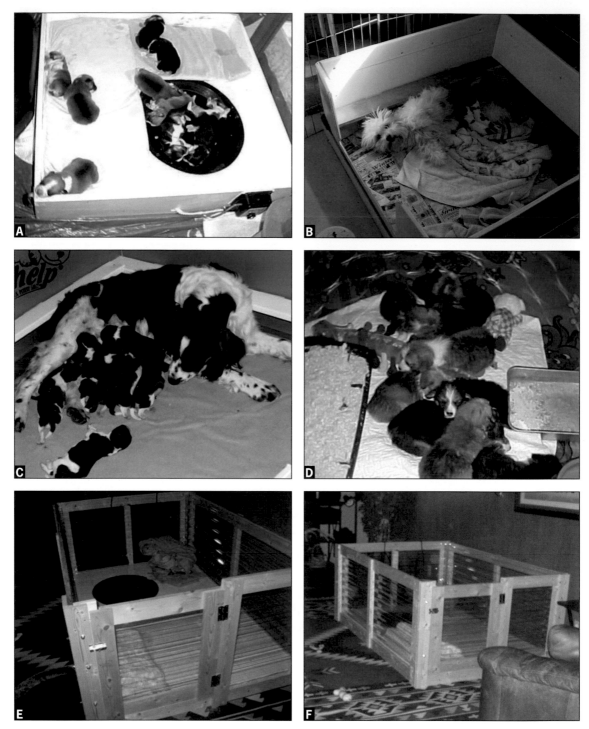

Figure 8-6.
A. A custom built box with a heated T. E. Scott whelping nest installed. **B.** An unheated whelping nest with rails to keep the mother from lying on the pups. This is more important for heavier bitches. **C.** A Durawhelp pre-made whelping box with rails to protect the puppies. **D.** A whelping box with litter. **E.** A clear sided whelping box, with heated T. E. Scott whelping nest. The clear sides are plastic for easy cleaning, high enough to contain a large bitch, and clear so that the pups can be observed from across the room. **F.** The finished whelping box.

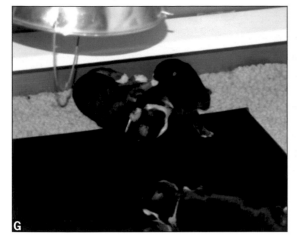

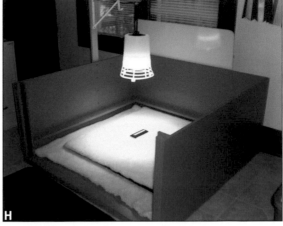

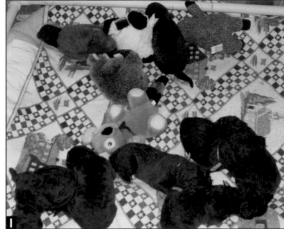

Figure 8-6. *continued*
G. *Dangerous use of a heat lamp. It is too close to the pups and flammable surfaces. Not recommended.* **H.** *A home-built whelping box with rails, fleece beds and a lamp overhead.* **I.** *A home-built whelping box with PVC rails, bedding, and varied toys for environmental stimulation.*

- Tincture of iodine - to dip the umbilicus in at birth, 2 and 8 hours post partum.
- Chlorhexidine disinfectant solution – to disinfect surfaces in the whelping and nursery areas – available through your veterinary suppliers or local farm stores.
- Bulb syringe or DeLee Mucus Trap.
- Laundry basket or ice chest (do not seal with the lid and monitor temperature to prevent overheating or chilling) to keep pups in during daily evaluation – makes sorting who is done and who isn't easier and faster. This can also be used to hold the bigger pups outside of the whelping box temporarily to allow the smaller ones less competition nursing.
- Heating pads, rice bags, or Snuggle Safe® – to keep pups warm during sorting – heating pads often have safety shut-offs so are difficult to keep warm. Rice bags are stockinette or socks filled with long-grain white cooking rice microwaved to warm pups. After microwaving, roll the rice around to avoid a hot area that could burn. Snuggle Safe® – a microwaveable disc made to warm puppies, available on line.
- Towels, blankets, tarps and flannel-backed vinyl table cloths to keep the pups and room sanitary.

Each item on the list should cost less than $20.00. Great husbandry isn't expensive, but it is time-consuming and a lot of hard work.

Many puppies will be evaluated and be treated at the veterinary hospital but most will not remain in the hospital overnight. Most clinics are not staffed overnight and puppies usually benefit from being at home with their dam and littermates. In addition to tube feeding, many breeders already can, or can be taught to give injections, administer SQ fluids, manage catheters, and monitor vital signs. Many prefer having the pups at home, at least for overnight care and will return the pup to the hospital for care during the day, particularly if they will be at work. This combination of care allows for constant monitoring, frequent feedings, and medicating on schedule.

Causes of neonatal mortality
(Appendix B-2)

Early recognition and effective medical care can significantly reduce neonatal illness and death. This can be divided by age range into three time periods. First are problems that occurred in utero or during whelping (from pre-birth to two weeks of age); second are problems that occur early in the post partum period (from 2 to 5 weeks of age); and third are those in the post-weaning period (from 5 to 12 weeks of age). Common causes of neonatal illnesses include: dystocia, physiologic or nutritional causes, environmental causes including poor husbandry, genetic and congenital causes, trauma, teratogens and toxins, and infectious diseases.

There is no specific disorder known as "fading puppy syndrome". However, this term is thrown about as a catch-all phrase for any pup with an undiagnosed illness, failure to thrive or unexplained death. Simple diagnostics and supportive care can often turn these pups around, and they will begin to thrive. While a diagnosis is pending, or if no diagnosis can be made, survival of these pups is dependent on promptly providing the basic supportive care needed to prevent sepsis, maintain body temperature, blood glucose, blood volume, and adequate oxygenation.

Remember, puppies can have most of the same diagnostics used on adults – blood chemistries, CBC's, ultrasound and radiographic imaging. Different normal values must be applied, and diagnostics and treatments must be modified, but they are just small dogs in many respects and their small size and immaturity should not put off the veterinarian as the diagnostic plan is developed. Many of the in-house veterinary chemistry and blood count analyzers now use such a small blood volume that nearly any size patient can be evaluated safely.

Dystocia and prolonged labor – Occurs in the immediate post partum period
Early intervention with veterinary assistance including C-section at the first sign of maternal or fetal distress can prevent neonatal illness and loss.

Fetal stress/distress with oxygen deprivation during birth is a common cause of neonatal illness and early death, usually in the first hours to days after birth. This may not be apparent until the pup is 2 to 3 days of age and begins to "fade". Pups that were distressed at birth or that were noted to have a prolonged delivery should be watched carefully. Injectable ceftiofur or unasyn, or oral clavamox can prevent the development of septicemia. Should they begin to drop behind in weight gain or seem to be weak, supportive care should be initiated.

One study showed a higher percentage of neonatal death in pups born to an older dam. This reinforces the importance of careful monitoring of the bitch in whelp and the need for early intervention during delivery if pups are in distress.

Physiological causes – Occurs in the immediate post partum period
The pups are totally dependent on the bitch and breeder for care. Frequently, first time mothers will need assistance determining how and where to lay down so that the pups can nurse. Some bitches attempt to leave the designated whelping area with or without their pups and require confinement so that the pups are all together and secure. Some bitches do not have enough milk initially so supplementation is necessary. Some need help in learning to lick the pups so that they urinate and defecate. With patience, an Adaptil collar, and on occasion calcium supplementation of the bitch, this will be resolved within the first 72 hours. Ongoing problems will require assessment by the veterinarian to see if there is a physical problem including mastitis or a retained pup. The household needs to be arranged so that there is a private area where other dogs and non-essential humans are denied access until the bitch is comfortable.

Nutritional causes in the neonate – Occurs any time prior to completing weaning

It is common for a bitch to require several days to lactate sufficiently to support a litter without assistance. This is most common in those with very small litters (1 to 2 pups), very large litters (10 or more), bitches who have been ill during pregnancy, who have not been fed appropriately or were unwilling to eat during pregnancy, who deliver pups prior to the whelping date, or have undergone a C-section. Some bitches are reluctant to allow the pups to nurse and some pups are too weak or sick to nurse.

The bitch may be allowed to eat food that is not ordinarily part of her normal diet. This can include meat that is not too fatty or spicy, ice cream, scrambled eggs, or commercial diets meant for nutritional support such as Iams Maximum Calorie® Diet, Hill's Prescription A/D® or Royal Canin Recovery RS® Diet. Other foods including human food may be used if appropriate for her individual needs. Bratwurst sausages and oatmeal may be helpful in improving lactation. After the first few days of lactation, most bitches will begin to eat well on their own, in spite of "spoiling" them.

Fluid therapy can be useful in improving lactation. Subcutaneous fluids can be administered, often by the clients at home, after all other causes of agalactia have been addressed.

Oxytocin can aid in milk letdown **(See Chapter 7)**. By contrast, metoclopramide or Domperidone can help increase lactation in approximately 75% of bitches. It affects the CNS and appears to antagonize dopamine at the receptor sites. This action is thought to be related to prolactin secretion stimulation effects. Metoclopramide is excreted into milk and may concentrate at about twice the plasma level, but there does not appear to be significant risk to nursing offspring. Oxytocin and metoclopramide may be used simultaneously.

The metoclopramide dosage is similar to that for GI use: 0.2 to 0.4 mg/kg subcutaneously or by mouth (tablets or syrup) three times a day as indicated. Continue for 3 to 5 days, but the use can be prolonged if needed. The maximum dose should not exceed 1 mg/Kg daily. Monitor and discontinue if extrapyramidal signs (movement disorders) are detected. Metoclopramide is contraindicated in any bitch with GI hemorrhage, GI obstruction or perforation, a hypersensitivity to the drug, or a seizure disorder.

If the pups are undernourished, it may be necessary to supplement their diet while waiting for fluid therapy, oxytocin, metoclopramide therapy, and the bitch's improved appetite to kick in.

The neonatal diet can be supplemented in several ways. If the client has another litter of comparable age, and the other bitch is not overwhelmed with her own litter, she will often accept the new pups. Some clients will seek out a "wet nurse", a lactating bitch from another breeder and move the pups to that location. This can be risky. The surrogate bitch may refuse the pups, or the facility may have infectious or husbandry problems that could lead to puppy illness or loss. This approach can also create liability issues.

Tube feeding is the most reliable supplemental puppy feeding technique. It ensures that the required volume is delivered efficiently, even to a pup too sick to nurse **(See Appendix C-16)**. Many breeders and some veterinary staff fear tube feeding. When done correctly the technique is highly successful.

Bottle feeding is a commonly used technique. This can work well if the correct bottle and nipple can be found, and the pup(s) is strong enough to suckle on a bottle. If the pup is too weak or unwilling to take a bottle, or if the opening in the nipple is too large, the pup may aspirate formula and develop aspiration pneumonia and/or death.

Supplemental feeding with an eyedropper is dangerous and not recommended. The administration rate is often too fast and the pup cannot control the flow rate.

Parenteral supplementation will not deliver adequate nutrition and should not be considered a substitute for using the GI tract.

IT IS CRITICAL THAT YOU NOT ALLOW ANY PATIENT TO STARVE TO DEATH, ADULT OR PUPPY. Standard of care dictates that your client should be informed of their options. Nutritional support via oral-esophageal tube feeding should be included in the list of options they are offered.

Environmental causes – Housing and husbandry

Disorders related to housing and husbandry can occur at any time. Access to good food, clean water and safe shelter are the backbone of basic needs in any species (Figure 8-7).

Prior to whelping, a member of the veterinary staff should discuss basic husbandry with the breeder. Enough time needs to be invested to assure that the breeder has the facility and equipment necessary for a successful whelping and to raise the pups to adoption age. Even breeders with a great deal of experience will benefit from a review and assurance that they have all supplies and equipment in order.

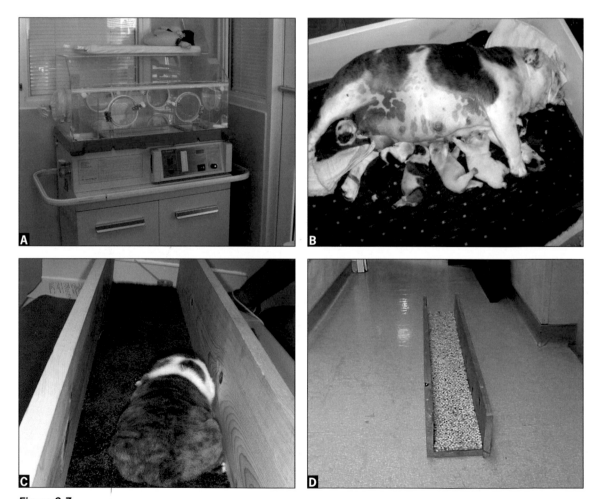

Figure 8-7.
A. Infant incubators modified for use for neonatal pups. They are used for warming pups as well as oxygen administration if indicated. B. Note the pups with extremely straight hocks and stifles, and feet rotated into an atypical position. Most will return to a more normal conformation within a few weeks. C. A custom built "trough U" to support pups with difficulty learning to walk. D. A custom built U trough to support pups with difficulty learning to walk.

The whelping room/puppy raising facility must be easy to clean and well-ventilated. The bitch will be less stressed if isolated from other dogs in the household. A small room, if available, is ideal. If this is not a viable option, a partition can be placed in a larger room. Even the most even-tempered bitch can become aggressive if she feels her pups are threatened.

The ideal flooring should be impervious to fluids, easy to clean, and not too slippery. If the room selected does not have this kind of flooring, plastic sheets/tarps can be used as a base with washable rugs or bedding placed on top with a heat source. A wading pool or whelping box can be a very convenient area in which to confine the bitch and her puppies. Some small breed dogs can be housed in a plastic dog crate that is opened, so that only the bottom half is used. An exercise pen surrounding the wading pool can be used to insure that the bitch and her pups stay in the area that the breeder has made safe for them. Prebuilt whelping boxes can be purchased commercially.

The whelping area should be scrupulously clean. Several times daily, waste should be removed and the whelping box should be cleaned with an appropriate disinfectant such as diluted bleach or Chlorhexidine. Take care to allow for adequate ventilation to prevent airway irritation from the disinfectants. Dry the surface prior to placing the pups back in the box to avoid skin irritation. Washable absorbent bedding should be used to keep the pups clean and dry and to provide good footing. For the first 2 to 3 weeks, little urine or stool will be in the bedding because the bitch will usually clean up after the pups. Bedding must be washed frequently with an appropriate laundry detergent (detergents for baby laundry work very well) and diluted bleach. Nursing home pads for incontinence work very well, are absorbant and launder well.

As the pups approach 3 to 4 weeks of age, a shallow tray of pine shavings or shredded newspaper (avoid pelleted newspaper as some pups will eat it) can be placed in 1 corner of the whelping box. Over time, the pups will begin to housebreak because they are naturally drawn to that area to eliminate. The bitch will stimulate the puppies less and the volume of waste in the tray will increase.

Water should be offered in a shallow dish or drinking bottle at about 3 weeks. Take care to make the dish shallow enough so that a pup will not fall or walk in and be unable to get out. Food, in gruel form, can be offered at 3 to 4 weeks, shortly after drinking is learned. Special "flying saucer" dishes can be used, but any heavy shallow dish that allows enough room around the circumference for all the pups to eat at once will do nicely. Food and water dishes should be washed and bleached regularly because some pups will walk through, defecate in or lay down in the dishes. Royal Canin Starter mousse is an easy diet to use when transitioning from nursing to solid food (Figure 8-2 and 8-3).

Genetic and congenital disorders
These may be noted at any time. Congenital defect are disorders present at birth. Many are genetic, that is inherited, but there are other causes such as infections, hypoxia, trauma, toxins and teratogens as well. Genetic defects may include physical malformations, inborn errors of metabolism, and increased susceptibility to disease. In many cases, these disorders overlap.

Physical defects grossly visible
Congenital defects may present as an **anatomic defect**, some visible on examination, some internal and not recognizable without diagnostic testing; but some are **disorders of metabolism**, immunity, or microanatomy and are more difficult to identify and treat. Up to 20% of neonatal pups may have one or more congenital defects.

Inborn errors of metabolism
Metabolic diseases, also called inborn errors of metabolism, are genetic disorders which represent a defect in the biochemistry of the protein molecule. The protein defect is either in the structure or function of a protein molecule.

While many congenital defects are lethal, some can be diagnosed and managed successfully.

Congenital defects often account for pups that are stillborn, weak, or fail to thrive. If there is an obvious anatomic defect, the diagnosis is straightforward. However, many are internal (inborn errors of metabolism, immune system deficiencies, or microanatomic), and can be very difficult to diagnose in time to manage. Some congenital defects appear at birth or early in life, others may not become apparent until later in life.

Differentiating the pup with a serious or terminal congenital defect from a normal pup that merely needs supportive care is challenging. The decision must often be made to provide general supportive care instead of a diagnostic work-up or while diagnostics are pending. Puppies do not have the physiologic resources that adult dogs have and may not be able to tolerate a complete diagnostic evaluation prior to initiating treatment. The pup can be assessed for improvement or progressive deterioration after supportive care is initiated, and the treatment plan adjusted as indicated (Table 8-2).

Table 8-2 Congenital defects of dogs					
Age of Diagnosis	At Birth	Neonatal and Pediatric	Early Adulthood	Middle Age	Advanced Age
Anatomic	Cleft palate, spina bifida, umbilical hernia and other midline defects, limb anomalies, agenesis of portions of GI tract, pectus excavatum	Patent Ductus Arteriosis, Portal systemic shunts, Hydrocephalus, Persistent right aortic arch, heart valve disorders.	Hydro-cephalus, OCD, Atlanto-occipital instability, megaesophagus, pyloric stenosis, prognathism, brachygnathism, patellar luxation, cataracts. Congenital portal hypoplasia.	Elbow dysplasia, spinal stenosis.	Hip dysplasia
Micro-anatomic			Renal dysplasia		
Immune system		Thymic disorders, severe combined immunodeficiency.	Cyclic haematopoiesis	Immune mediated lymphocytic thyroiditis, hypoa-drenocorticism.	Degenerative Myelopathy
Metabolic		Congenital Diabetes Mellitus, growth hormone deficiency. (Pituitary dwarf-ism) Centronuclear myopathy (CNM).	Amyloidosis, Copper toxicosis, MPS disorders, hy-pothyroidism, von Willebrand disease. Exercise induced collapse (EIC).	Uric acid deposi-tion, Cystinuria	Dialated cardiomyopathy

Failure of passive immunity

Puppies may have inadequate passive immunity, immunity acquired from their mother, for 3 reasons. 1. The bitch was not immunized. 2. The bitch, although immunized, was a low-responder or no-responder to the vaccine and this failure to mount an antibody response was not detected by blood titers. 3. The pup was colostrum deprived, either because of inability to nurse or lack of opportunity to nurse in the first 24 hours.

These puppies are vulnerable to diseases normally protected against by routine immunization protocols. Ninety-five percent of passive immunity is acquired through colostrum within 24 hours of birth, only 5% is transferred transplacentally.

If the bitch was not immunized prior to breeding,or if she is a no or low responder, she should not be vaccinated during pregnancy (Canine herpesvirus is the only unique exception to this rule). In these cases, Fresh frozen plasma should be administered to the pups, who should be isolated from potential sources of infection until after their second vaccination. Vaccines should be administered starting at 4 weeks instead of 8 weeks.

All pups should be closely observed to determine if they have been adequately nursed in the first 24 hours. This is essential not only for nutrition and fluid intake, but also to transfer passive immunity. If the bitch does not have enough milk, is unavailable, or if the pup(s) are not able to nurse, supplementation of milk or milk replacer, fluids, and plasma or serum should be instituted. There is no diagnostic test for failure of transfer of passive immunity in the dog – monitoring for adequate nursing includes observation for effective nursing, increase in body weight, and dilute urine color, using hydration status as an indicator of nursing ability.

Teratogenic effects and toxins during pregnancy

The first trimester of pregnancy (3 weeks in dogs and cats) is when the developing fetus is most susceptible to teratogens and toxins.

Halothane anesthetic gas, glucocorticoids, phenobarbital, ketoconazole, chemotherapeutic agents, griseofulvin, environmental pollutants and some, plants, vitamins, hormones, and radiation therapy all have teratogenic effects in dogs. Pregnant dogs should have limited exposure to clients who are undergoing radiation therapy (including prostate brachytherapy) as the research here is not conclusive. This list is not all inclusive and new drugs as well as newly reported drug adverse effects are introduced frequently. To assure accuracy, each drug should be researched prior to initiating treatment. Drug package inserts, veterinary drug formularies, and human drug formularies are excellent resources.

In general, pregnancy should be as drug-free as possible. Most commonly prescribed products for heartworm, intestinal parasites, flea, and tick control are safe during all stages of pregnancy. The first trimester (the first 3 weeks in the dog) is the time during which the fetus is most vulnerable to the teratogenic effects of drugs. For planned breedings, these medications can be administered just prior to breeding, and will not need to be administered for another 4 weeks.

Some drugs are so necessary during pregnancy that they must be administered regardless of the risks. Alternative drugs are sometimes available. The veterinarian should discuss balancing the risks versus the benefits of the drug with the breeder so that a mutual decision can be made.

Infectious diseases

Infectious diseases are a significant cause of death in the post-weaning period.

Neonates and adults are susceptible to most of the same organisms. Neonates are especially vulnerable to bacteria, viruses, and parasites to which the adults are immune or more resistant. Therefore, sanitation and parasite control are of utmost importance to the well-being of the neonate.

The neonate is more vulnerable to these diseases for several reasons. They are fragile – have little body fat, scant glycogen reserves, dehydrate easily, cannot thermoregulate, have no protective intestinal flora, do not have a fully developed immune system, and have not developed immunity to many of the organisms they are exposed to. They may have one or more congenital defects, be inadequately nourished, chilled, and be affected by multiple infectious diseases simultaneously. Neonates need careful monitoring and protection.

Bacterial diseases and sepsis

Bacterial diseases commonly seen in the neonate include Staphylococcus, Streptococcus, Pasteurella, Esherichia, Enterobacter, Enterococcus, Klebsiella, Pseudomonas, Clostridium, and

Salmonella species. Brucella, though uncommon, should not be overlooked. The bacterial organisms may invade through the skin, the umbilicus, the oral cavity and GI tract, the respiratory tract, the eye, or the urinary tract. Some of these organisms are normal flora of the bitch (and neonate as they mature), some are the result of environmental exposure, and some are the result of a pathologic condition in the bitch or other dogs in the household. Pups can be septic at birth.

Regardless of the route of exposure, the neonate may quickly become bacteremic/septicemic and critically ill. They have limited resources with which to ward off infections and must be treated quickly and aggressively.

Supportive care and antibiotic therapy must be initiated immediately. Samples should be collected for culture and sensitivity testing, but an initial antibiotic must be chosen while culture and sensitivity results are pending. Cytology can be useful in empirical antibiotic selection.

Sudden death, or sloughing of the extremities are symptoms of severe septicemia. Symptoms also include fussiness and crying, hypothermia, poor weight gain, diarrhea, weakness, either restlessness or profound inactivity and weakness, respiratory distress, abdominal distension, abdominal wall discoloration (blue coloration) hypoglycemia, and hematuria.

Toxic milk or Toxic metritis
Both mastitis and metritis may be associated with sick and dying neonates.

A bitch with toxic metritis may initially present with sick and dying pups, and no symptoms. This typically occurs when the pups are 1 to 5 days old. Symptoms include fever with a foul smelling vaginal discharge. This is a true emergency. The bitch and her pups should be present at the veterinary visit. The mother needs treatment with antibiotics, fluids, and possibly Lutalyse®. She should be evaluated to confirm that there are no retained pups. The owner should be taught to tube feed the pups until mom is better (See Chapter 7).

She should be examined for coexisting illness because she may also be sick from any number of causes unrelated to toxic metritis. Particular attention should be paid to the uterus, mammary glands, and C-section incision site/abdomen.

Viral diseases
Maternal antibodies, naturally acquired and as a result of vaccination, play an important role in protecting the neonate from viral diseases. It is important that the bitch be appropriately vaccinated well before her planned breeding date, as vaccinations are not recommended during estrous and pregnancy. Even when the bitch is vaccinated, there can be failure of passive immunity. She may not have responded to the vaccinations; the pups may have failed to take adequate colostrum during the critical period for absorption; or the pups may be exposed to a virus for which there is no vaccine commercially available. Additionally, the bitch and/or pups could be exposed to a virus the bitch has no natural immunity to.

Canine Herpesvirus (CHV) is a common cause of neonatal death, from the pre-partum period up to 6 weeks of age. In the older pup and adult dog, CHV looks like an upper respiratory infection or kennel cough. If Herpes is acquired by the bitch during pregnancy, she may resorb the pups which can masquerade as failure to conceive; or develop fetal mummification, abortion, premature labor; and/or the birth of small pups who fail to survive (Figure 8-8).

The pups can be exposed to CHV during the birth process, if fresh vesicles are present on the mucosal surface of the vulva. If these are present prior to delivery, C-section delivery of the pups may be recommended to reduce exposure of the neonate to the virus. If the pups are a few days to a few weeks of age at the time of exposure, they may be mildly ill or die. Pups are most vulnerable

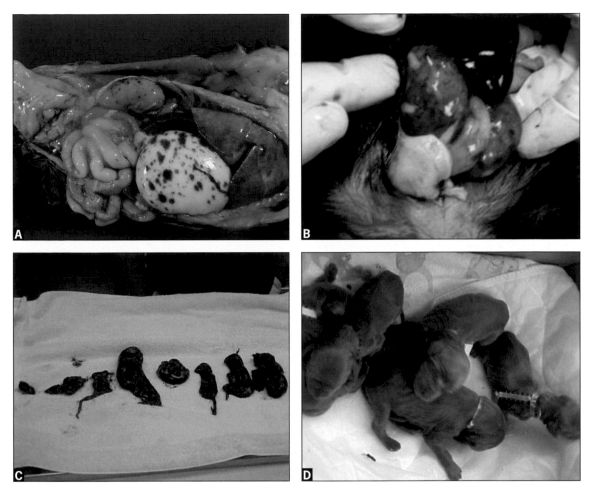

Figure 8-8.
A. A 1 week old puppy that died acutely of Canine Herpesvirus. Post mortem findings. *B.* A 1 week old pup that died of herpesvirus. Note the characteristic petechial hemorrhages on the liver and kidneys. *C.* A litter of pups whose dam contracted Canine Herpesvirus during pregnancy. Note the difference in size of the pups, demonstrating the various neonatal ages when the pups succumbed. Some pups were carried to term and survived. *D.* Littermates to the pups shown above. These five pups survived but were small at birth.

from 9 to 14 days of age. Symptoms range from sudden onset of persistent crying (mewing), respiratory distress, abdominal pain and bloating, hypothermia, depression, anorexia and weakness. This often quickly progresses to death within 4 to 24 hours.

Treatment is largely supportive including oxygen, fluids, hyperimmunized plasma, supplemental feeding, and antibiotics to manage any secondary bacterial infection. There is one report of successful treatment with Acyclovir dosed at 10 mg/kg as a suspension PO q 6 hours until 3 weeks of age.

Canine Herpesvirus (CHV), as with herpesviruses in other species, lives preferentially on the mucus membranes of the extremities where the temperature is slightly below body temperature. It is believed that this is the main reason the neonate suffers from a more serious syndrome when affected by Canine Herpesvirus than a mature animal with a body temperature over 100° F. For this reason, increasing the ambient temperature may aid in preventing and/or treating affected or exposed neonates. Care should be taken that the increased ambient temperature does not lead to dehydration.

Diagnosis is confirmed at post-mortem, based on observation of classic spotted lesions in the liver and kidneys, pneumonia, and by histology or PCR testing.

It was thought that once a bitch was exposed to CHV, her subsequent litters would be protected. Newer research contradicts this indicating that each litter a previously exposed bitch produces can be vulnerable to CHV due to the short life of protective antibodies. However, a bitch that has had CHV affected puppies can go on to have a normal litter.

In Europe, a commercial vaccine is available for use in pregnant bitches. The manufacturer has demonstrated that bitches immunized produced increased litter size, higher birth weights, and lower neonatal death rates. Two doses of the vaccine are given during pregnancy, and need to be repeated during each pregnancy. It appears unlikely that this vaccine will be approved for use in the United States.

Canine Parvovirus 1 or the Minutevirus is another significant cause of conception failure, birth defects, and early neonatal death. Symptoms of Parvovirus 1 are vomiting, diarrhea, respiratory distress, constant crying, and sudden death, clinically indistinguishable from Canine Herpesvirus. Supportive care is the only treatment, but is often unsuccessful. Diagnosis is confirmed at post-mortem.

Canine Parvovirus 2 is a common cause of death in the unvaccinated pup from 6 weeks to 6 months of age, with 10 to 12 weeks of age the time of greatest risk. Puppies can also contract this disease if maternal antibodies wane between protective vaccinations. Death from severe enteritis, dehydration, shock, septicemia, bone marrow suppression, and cardiac involvement is common. Treatment consists of supportive care, including use of hyperimmunized plasma given IV at 5 to 10 ml per pound of body weight IV slowly over a period of 2 to 4 hours. There are reports of response to Tamiflu®.

Many other viruses, even those that cause mild disease in the adult, can cause fatal disease in the neonate (Figure 8-9).

Parasitic diseases
Both internal and external parasites can lead to illness and death of the neonatal puppy.

Intestinal parasites such as roundworms (Toxocara) and hookworms (Ancylostoma) can create such heavy burdens that pups can be lost. Antihelmintic medications, wormers such as pyrantel pamoate, should be administered to all the pups and the bitch every 2 weeks starting at 2 weeks of age. These should be administered even if no parasite ova are seen on fecal flotation, because the prepatent period lasts for at least the first 3 weeks of the pup's life.

Roundworms and hookworms can cause significant diarrhea and nutrient depletion in neonates. Intestinal intussusceptions and rectal prolapses are also sequella of worm infections. Hookworms can cause significant anemia in the neonate. Zoonotic infections of the breeder, their family, the veterinary staff, and puppy buyers pose liability issues for the breeder and veterinarian. Guidelines published by the Companion Animal Parasite Council are available on line at www.capcvet.org.

There are three treatment protocols that can be used during pregnancy to minimize the carrier state of the bitch that had parasites as a puppy. These are the first protocols that have prevented the transmission of parasites across the placental membrane and through the milk to the pups. Both require administration during pregnancy but are safe and effective. Routine worming of the bitch will not prevent this route of transmission.

Fenbendazole dosed at 50 mg/kg PO once daily from day 40 of gestation through day 14 of lactation (the last 14 days of pregnancy through day 14 after delivery) will minimize transmission of roundworms and hookworms through the placenta and the milk.

Ivermectin can be administered once weekly at 200 µg/kg from 3 weeks before to 3 weeks after whelping to reduce roundworm and hookworm infections in neonates. Dogs who carry the MDR-1

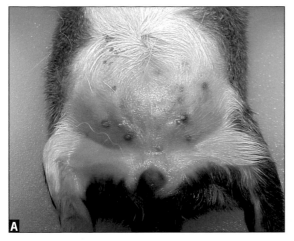

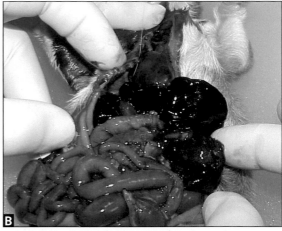

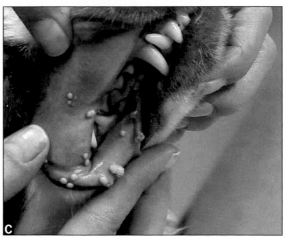

Figure 8-9.
A. *Deceased neonatal pup with skin lesions. Post mortem showed death was caused by an adenovirus.* **B.** *Adenovirus post mortem.* **C.** *Warts on the mucus membranes of a young pup, a non-fatal disorder.*

gene should not be treated with this protocol. Selamectin applied topically to the bitch at 6 mg/kg 6 and 2 weeks before whelping and 2 and 6 weeks after whelping, reduced roundworm burdens in puppies by 98%, and reduced egg shedding by 99.7% in the dams.

Both the fenbendazole and ivermectin regimens have been documented to reduce roundworm infections (T. canis and A. caninum) in puppies up to 98 to 100%. This not only reduces worm burdens and the commonly associated diarrhea in pups but also reduces exposure to these zoonotic parasites for anyone handling the pups.

External parasites, in low numbers such as fleas and lice, can be controlled by managing the environment. Baths using non-insecticidal shampoo and flea combs can be used to remove fleas. Vinegar rinses are helpful in dislodging louse eggs (nits) from the coat. Fipronil (Frontline®), nitenpyram (Capstar®), and selamectin (Revolution®) are all labeled as safe for use during pregnancy. Organophosphates and pyrethroids/ permethrins should not be used during pregnancy or the early neonatal period. Fleas and other external parasites can cause significant blood loss and anemia in the neonate.

Heartworm microfilaria can cross the placenta and enter the circulation of the fetus if there are micro-hemorrhages during pregnancy. These microfilaria cannot cause disease in the affected pup without transmission through a mosquito, but the pup can serve as a source of infection for other dogs. Ivermectin, selamectin, and milbemycin are labeled as safe during pregnancy. As a precaution, the administration of the medications can be timed so that they are not given during the first 3 weeks of pregnancy.

Behavioral problems

Several behavioral problems exhibited by the bitch can create health concerns for the neonates (Figure 8-10).

The bitch may have poor maternal skills. Bitches can be reluctant to give up their position with their owners and spend adequate time with their puppies. Bitches can be aggressive toward other canine members of the household, and fail to adequately concentrate on caring for their pups. After vaginal or Caesarean delivery, bitches can be in pain and can be reluctant to allow pups to approach them for nursing – improved pain management may help alleviate this problem. Use of a Dog Appeasement Pheromone collar, prior to or at the time aggression is noted, can help calm the bitch **(See Chapter 6**).

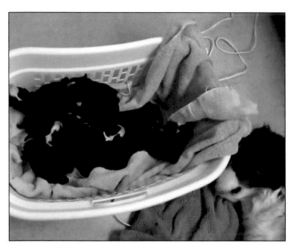

Figure 8-10.
Preparing the new mother and her thirteen pups for the ride home after a C-section.

Hypocalcemia may lead to maternal aggression. The theory is that calcium is needed for oxytocin uptake, the key hormone in maternal recognition of her pups. Although the total calcium is normal, the ionized calcium may be low. The clinical picture described is that the bitch becomes glassy eyed, stares, growls at her pups, and may become aggressive toward the owner, the pups, or other dogs in the household. Calcium (Calphosan® SQ) is reported to lead to resolution of symptoms within 30 to 45 minutes of administration.

All bitches, particularly post C-section first time mothers, should be monitored very carefully for the first 72 hours after delivery. Some will growl and snarl at their pups as the pups crawl away from the mammary glands and past the shoulder approaching the head. Even ordinarily trustworthy bitches can become aggressive. Commonly, 72 hours after delivery, a switch flips and the bitch changes from aggressive to maternal. During the first 3 days, or any time a bitch may be aggressive, she should not be left alone with her pups. Either an adult person should be present at all times in the room, or she should be moved from the whelping box to a crate when she is unsupervised. Use of a Dog Appeasement Pheromone collar may shorten the time until she accepts the puppies.

Cannibalism is an extreme form of maternal aggression. An entire litter can be destroyed in a few minutes so caution should be taken with any new mother and her pups.

Breeders frequently report that they have lost a pup or puppies as a result of the bitch lying on the pup. It is possible in many of these cases that the pup was sick or otherwise debilitated, which predisposed it to death in this manner.

Trauma

With careful housing and supervision, trauma should not occur. The dam should not be left unattended with her pups until she has been observed to be trustworthy, especially if she is recovering from anesthesia from a C-section. Other dogs and puppies in the household should not be left alone with the pups until the pups are substantial in size and able to fend for themselves (Figure 8-11).

Collars, flea collars, or other neck bands should not be used on the pups. The room where the pups are housed should be safe and secure in a location where no where the pups can fall, become stuck,

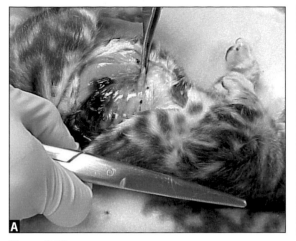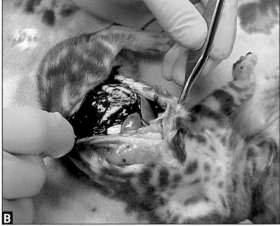

Figure 8-11.
A. A kitten at post mortem that died of splenic hemorrhage caused by the mother biting the kitten through the abdominal wall. **B.** The kitten in **A** at post mortem, showing free blood in abdomen.

become burned, chew on electric cords, choke on foreign bodies, fall into water dishes, or knock heavy objects onto themselves.

If a pup presents with signs of trauma – bite wounds, fractures, electrocution, or burns – they should be treated in the same way that an adult would be treated.

Anesthesia can be induced with propofol and maintained with isoflurane or sevoflurane if surgery is warranted.

Maternal nutrition

Excellent maternal nutrition is essential to support pregnancy and lactation. A high quality commercial dog food – pregnancy, puppy and performance diets are currently recommended. She should be at an ideal body condition prior to pregnancy. During the first 4 weeks of pregnancy, no diet changes or increase in quantity is indicated. During the last 5 weeks of pregnancy, she will benefit from an increase of 20% to 50%, depending on the size of litter she is expected to have. No nutritional supplements are necessary if she is fed a commercially available diet for puppies, performance or pregnancy.

Uncooked diets put the pups at risk of developing bacterial and parasitic conditions.

Low birth weight

Low birth weight is a strong predictor of neonatal illness.

Thymic disorders

Thymic disorders are typically undiagnosed except at post mortem. The thymus should be present until puberty. It may atrophy prematurely due to viral diseases (canine distemper, canine parvovirus) or may be hypoplastic and the cause of death due to immunosuppression.

The thymus should be identified and submitted at any complete post-mortem examination.

Diagnostics for the sick neonate
Neonatal examination, supportive care, symptoms, and diagnostic work-up
The importance of an office visit – Assistance when they need it most
Veterinary intervention can be the difference between life and death for the neonate. This needs to be offered on an emergency basis because sick pups can deteriorate quickly when they become ill.

Use of a telephone triage form **(See Appendix B-6)** will allow your staff to efficiently collect data from the client. Neonatal examination, history, supportive care, diagnostics, and specific treatment are similar to that offered adult and pediatric patients.

Handling the newborn at the veterinary hospital should be done with great care. Two disinfected laundry baskets with a heat source and towel should be ready prior to the arrival of the client. The pups can be moved from one basket to the next as they are handled to prevent confusion regarding which pup has been examined and treated.

All staff should wash their hands thoroughly and wear examination gloves prior to touching the pups. The examination room should not have recently been used by a patient with a potentially contagious disease. A circulating water blanket or heating pad should be placed under a clean towel as an examination surface. Although the bitch should be present for an examination (to evaluate for a retained pup or placenta, metritis, mastitis, or other illness), she may be more comfortable in the car or another room during examination and treatment of the pups.

The entire litter should be presented for examination so sick pups not identified at home may be diagnosed and so healthy pups can be compared with sick pups diagnostically. The physical exam should be similar to that of any patient. Vital signs including rectal temperature, heart rate, respiratory rate, and mucus membrane color/capillary refill time should be taken. Urine color (including urine specific gravity) and stool character should be evaluated. Precise weights should be taken and compared to those in the breeder's records and at the C-section if the information is available. All of this data can be recorded by a veterinary technician or assistant. (Appendix D-4).

Supportive care or "Treat for the Treatable"
Neonatal and pediatric patients can be treated with the following protocol (unless there is a contra-indication) until they return to a clinically normal state or a diagnosis can be confirmed, allowing for a specific protocol. These patients are fragile and deteriorate so quickly when ill that treatment should be initiated while diagnostics are pending. Sick neonates symptoms include respiratory distress, constant crying, weakness, abdominal distention or pain, anorexia, poor weight gain, poor nursing, restlessness, and isolation. None of these symptoms are pathognomonic for the underlying cause.

In many cases, a "shotgun" or multi-pronged approach is taken. Treatments are listed in the order indicated based on need; 1. Oxygen therapy; 2. Thermal support; 3. Nutritional support; 4. Fluid therapy; 5. Antibiotics; 6. Passive immunity with plasma or serum infusions; 7. Transfusions; 8. Vitamin K injections; and 9. Basic hygiene and assistance with eliminations. Assume the sick neonate has a treatable disease and initiate care until proven otherwise (Table 8-3).

Oxygen
Hypoxia is common in the newborn. Oxygen therapy can be used in obvious cases of hypoxia (cyanotic mucus membranes) and dyspnea, but can also improve the status of any sick puppy. Many sick pups vocalize continuously so are less distressed in an oxygen enriched environment. Pups born prematurely, that aspirate amniotic fluid or meconium, that are traumatized or oxygen-deprived at birth, will benefit from supplemental oxygen therapy (Figure 8-12).

Table 8-3 Summary of empirical treatment of the sick neonatal puppy
Identify the sick individual(s) The entire litter should be present for examination
Oxygen
Warm the hypothermic pups slowly until rectal temperature reaches 96° F
Provide nutritional support in the form of tube feeding formula or IV/PO/IO glucose
Fluid therapy PO/IO/SQ
Antibiotic therapy and topical treatment of the umbilicus
Plasma or serum administration
Transfuse
Vitamin K
Hygiene and elimination
Initiate diagnostics – blood work, urine testing, radiographs, ultrasound
Reintroduce normal diet – nursing, tube feeding, puppy food
Continue to carefully monitor with temp/weight/urine color twice daily
Consider hand-raising the pup(s) and using empirical antibiotics and supportive care on the entire litter if no source of infection can be found.

The decision to use oxygen is generally based on clinical judgment since arterial blood gases are not practical and often unavailable. There are no reports of oxygen causing vision deficits after use in neonates and it does not appear to be contraindicated.

Intubation and ventilation may be necessary immediately following birth **(See Chapter 6)**.

Supplemental oxygen can be administered by nasal cannula or placement of an IV catheter in the trachea, if only 1 pup is affected. It can also be administered to 1 or more pups by use of an oxygen chamber, either at the veterinary hospital or at home. There are many techniques for constructing an oxygen chamber. An empty aquarium or clear plastic storage box can be

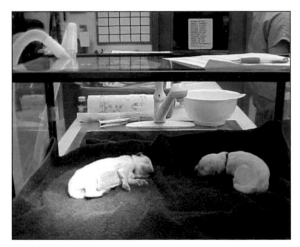

Figure 8-12.
Oxygen administration to newborn pups using an aquarium on its side.

used with the oxygen tubing inserted through a hole in a plastic lid or plastic wrap. Oxygen tanks or concentrators can be used to deliver a continuous supply of oxygen.

The greatest limitation to oxygen use is restriction of the treatment group of pups from association with their dam and littermates. The benefits versus limitations must be considered.

IMPORTANT

Thermal support
Hypothermia: Normal body temperature for newborns is 96 to 98° F, rising 1 degree a week until 4 weeks of age, when they can maintain their own body temperature. Thermal support is frequently necessary. Great care is needed at the hospital, during transport, and at home to prevent chilling or overheating.

It is essential to avoid overheating puppies that are in a confined space with no ability to move away from the heat source. A range of temperatures and space should be provided which allows the pups to move closer to or away from the heat source. If overheated and dehydrated, young pups can die in a short time, therefore careful monitoring is essential.

Heat sources include heating pads, heat lamps, heated microwave pads, heated rice bags, incubators, and hot water bottles. Enclosed housing and transport devices include crates, x-pens, whelping boxes, laundry baskets, and ice chests. The right combination of warmth and ventilation is essential.

The ideal ambient temperature for a litter and the bitch is 70° F with a relative humidity of 55 to 65%. Ambient temperatures of 85 to 90° F are only necessary for orphaned or sick pups or those removed from the care of the bitch. The temperature of the contact surface should be 70 to 95° F dependent upon the age and health of the puppies.

Achieving the correct ambient temperature for a litter can be difficult. Pups can easily be too warm or too cold. A room thermometer should be placed at the surface the pups are housed on to monitor the ambient temperature. A rectal thermometer must be available for monitoring the pups. Digital thermometers register fast and are easy to read.

Newborn pups cannot maintain their own body temperature without adequate thermal support along with the bitch and littermates. A healthy newborn can only maintain a body temperature of 12° F above the ambient temperature. A sick newborn is even more vulnerable to hypothermia. The newborn's inability to shiver and lack of peripheral vasoconstriction leave them dependent on an external heat source for maintenance of a safe core temperature. This situation is exacerbated by their lack of body fat and a relatively large surface area allowing for heat loss. Poor mothering skills, such as moving the pups out of the warm whelping area, pushing a sick pup aside, or excessive licking of the pups is a common cause of chilling, which leads to illness.

Low body temperature (less than 96° F) is a very common and often life-threatening problem in the neonate. It should be suspected in any sick pup or pup that is unusually quiet or still. Bradycardia is often secondary to hypothermia, dropping the heart rate from 200 bpm to the 100 to 150 bpm range.

If pups are too warm, they are usually fussing/crying or overly active. They fail to thrive and gain weight although the bitch is healthy and lactating well. To distinguish between the ambient temperature being too warm and a fever, all pup's temperatures should be taken rectally. If the ambient temperature is too high, all of the pups will usually have a rectal temperature over 100° F. If only a portion of the pups have rectal temperatures over 100° F, it is more likely that the hyperthermic pups are febrile and ill.

If some or all of the pups are hypothermic, with rectal temperatures of 96° F or below, they should be carefully and slowly warmed over 30 to 180 minutes. Care must be taken to prevent thermal burns from direct contact with a heated surface or being too close to a heat lamp. (Heat lamps are not recommended.) The patient should be moved every 20 to 30 minutes to prevent burns and allow for uniform heating. Their temperature should be taken hourly until it reaches 99 to 100° F. If a rectal thermometer is unavailable, a wired indoor/outdoor thermometer can be used. The sensor can be used as a rectal probe when encased in a plastic sleeve. As the pup warms, heart and respiratory rates increase, nursing attempts return, the gut begins to move and the glucose level rises. Feeding should not be attempted, by nursing, bottle or tubing, until the rectal temperature can be maintained at 96° F.

Human electric heating pads can pose a risk of thermal burn or electrocution if the dam or pups chew through the cord. Many of the newer pads have an automatic shut-off. They do not maintain consistent heat but can reduce the chance of overheating.

There are several safer alternatives to the use of a heat lamp. Human or veterinary neonatal incubators or whelping nests with an electric heat source are safe and very effective. Circulating hot water blankets are also a safe and can be wrapped around the pups. Commercially-produced forced air patient warming systems are another safe and effective method of warming.

RICA surgical produces a countertop incubator/fluid warmer that can be used with oxygen. It is small enough and affordable enough for clients to purchase.

Hot water bottles, SnuggleSafe®, or bags filled with rice or oats that can be heated in the microwave will temporarily warm the pups, but must be frequently reheated. Water bottles that cool will actually draw heat from the puppies so must be monitored frequently. Any of these can be set up with 1 heat source in each of the 4 corners of a box with the pups in the center. Effective heating will provide a 1 degree rise in body temperature every 10 to 30 minutes.

A pup that becomes chilled rapidly WILL develop a life-threatening condition. A chilled pup does not nurse effectively. When the rectal temperature drops below 94° F, peristalsis slows. The pup is at risk of vomiting or backflow followed by aspiration pneumonia. When the rectal temperature plummets below 85° F, bacterial overgrowth occurs in the gut, often followed by sepsis, and the pup becomes hypoglycemic. If allowed to progress, the pup's rectal temperature will approach room temperature; the pup will not move, breathing becomes almost indistinguishable, the heart rate slows and cannot be palpated, and the pup appears dead.

Nutritional support including tube feeding

Symptoms of inadequate nutrition and hypoglycemia include crying, weakness and inability to nurse effectively. Supplemental feeding can be done in several ways. The most reliable technique is tube feeding. It assures that the volume necessary is delivered efficiently, even if the pup is too sick to nurse. It is, however, feared by many breeders and some veterinary staff. When done correctly, the technique is highly successful.

Prior to initiating nutritional support, it is important that the rectal temperature of the pup is 96° F or slightly higher and that it is well-hydrated. Gentle and slow warming of the pup should be initiated prior to feeding to prevent ileus. Most sick neonates are also hypoglycemic. Nutritional support early in the course of treatment is critical.

If the pups have diarrhea, the milk replacer can be diluted 50/50 with equal parts of Ringer's and 5% dextrose. As the diarrhea resolves, the milk replacer can slowly be returned to the exclusive diet.

Tube feeding is usually initiated by the veterinary staff, but can easily be continued at home. With appropriate training and equipment, nearly every client can be taught to safely tube feed a puppy.

The most effective way to tube feed a neonate is to pass a soft silicone feeding tube through the oral cavity into the stomach at each feeding. An NE tube can be placed and sutured into position for long-term nutritional support. Surgical placement of a pharyngostomy or esophagostomy may also be indicated for long term feeding. This can be done with a brief anesthetic period using gas induction and/or propofol induction and maintenance. Despite the tendency of some pups to gag on the tube when fed past the second week of life, as they mature, many pups see the feeding tube and become very excited and cooperative as the tube is passed making surgical placement unnecessary.

Tube feeding can be used as the sole means of nutrition for orphaned pups or those with congenital abnormalities such as cleft palate which precludes nursing. It can also be used as a supplemental feeding technique when the bitch cannot adequately meet the needs of the neonate. It can easily serve as a bridge from the time the pups fail to receive adequate nutrition until they are strong enough or mature enough to eat semi-solid food without assistance.

Some breeders and veterinarians are reluctant to tube feed for fear of harming the puppy. The pups are generally at greater risk of starving than they are to developing a tube feeding complication. Complications include passing the tube into the airway, feeding too large a quantity causing aspiration, and puncturing the esophagus or stomach. All of these are possible and serious, but less likely to occur than death by starvation in cases where the puppy cannot or will not nurse or the bitch cannot adequately feed the puppy.

Some clients and veterinarians fear that by supplementing, the pups will have no drive to nurse, the bitch will not have enough milk, or that they are keeping a puppy alive that nature would select out. Tube feeding will NOT reduce the pup's drive to suckle and stimulate the bitch to lactate. The pup that gets off to a rough start and needs nutritional support often turns out to be a truly outstanding specimen. At birth or the first few days that follow, it is not possible to tell how the pup will develop. We should be very careful not to "discard" a pup for lack of nutritional support.

Puppies require 22 to 26 kcal per 100 gm of body weight for the first 12 weeks. This translates into 13 ml of formula per 100 grams of body weight per day per pup for the first 7 days. This increases to 17 ml/100 gm for week 2, 10 ml/100 gm body weight for week 3, and 22 ml/100 gm body weight for week 4. This should be divided into a minimum of 4 feedings per day.

Another easy to remember formula is based on the stomach capacity of the newborn, rather than a caloric intake. A neonate stomach can accommodate 1 ml = (1 cc) of formula per 1 oz of body weight. This calculation is much easier for clients with a pound scale when they are trying to do calculations under duress. However, the first several feedings should be approximately 30% lower than the calculated formula to allow for the stomach capacity to accommodate this volume. A smaller quantity should also be fed if the pup appears to have nursed. The stomach can be gently palpated prior to feeding to estimate fullness. If the pup is found to be over-fed after being tubed (overdistended and crying), the tube can be passed again with an empty syringe attached and the excess volume removed by gentle suction.

Pups should gain 1 to 2 gm per day per pound of anticipated adult body weight. This equals 5 to 10% of their birth weight daily. Most breeders expect their pups to double their birth weight by 7 to 10 days of age.

Tube feeding equipment should be washed out with hot soapy water and allowed to dry between uses. It is not necessary to boil the equipment between uses. The feeding tube and syringes should be replaced frequently and between litters to keep the tube flexible and the syringe plunger moving freely. Feeding tubes come in a variety of sizes and materials; neither feeding tubes nor syringes are expensive. Equipment that works well makes tube feeding less stressful.

Feeding with a bottle works if the pup has a strong suckle reflex and normal oral anatomy. Pups that are too weak to take a bottle, who refuse the nipple, or have oral defects (cleft palate or lip, mismatches of upper to lower jaw, oral trauma, or other oral pathology) will need nutritional support via feeding tube until they recover or the defect can be corrected. Clients frequently prefer bottle feeding. If the correct bottle and nipple can be found, and the pup(s) is strong enough to suckle on a bottle, this can be an effective method. If the pup is too weak or is unwilling to take a bottle, or if the opening in the nipple is too large, it is common for the pup to aspirate the formula and develop aspiration pneumonia.

Supplemental feeding with an eyedropper is dangerous and not recommended. Aspiration is all too common because the flow rate is often too fast and cannot be controlled by the pup.

Total parenteral nutritional support, i.e. feeding intravenously only, is impractical in most cases due to the small size and unique nutritional needs of the patient.

IT IS CRITICAL THAT YOU DO NOT ALLOW ANY PATIENT TO STARVE TO DEATH, ADULT OR PUPPY. Standard of care dictates that your client should be informed of their options. Nutritional support via oral-esophageal tube feeding should be included in the list of options the client is offered.

Puppy milk replacer formulas can be purchased commercially, made at home with a recipe, or goat's milk can be used. The commercially available formulas are preferred as their amino acid and fat/protein ratios most closely match bitch's milk. Pups fed home-made diets or goats milk often develop nutritional cataracts.

Pups require a relatively dense caloric intake (energy requirement is 2 to 3 times that of an adult) to support their basic maintenance needs and to allow for rapid growth. Additionally, they do not have adequate stores of protein and glycogen and have decreased or poorly developed gluconeogenic enzymes, so hypoglycemia can develop easily, particularly in small breed pups.

Normal blood glucose should exceed 70 mg/dl (goal 80 to 150 mg/dl). Symptoms include episodes of weakness, tremors, stupor, coma and seizures. This is frequently associated with anorexia, vomiting, diarrhea, sepsis, or a low birth weight. Congenital glycogen storage diseases are rare, but should be considered in the differential. Although the immediate episode must be treated with oral and/or injectable glucose, long term management includes correcting the underlying cause and feeding a diet high in protein, fat, and complex carbohydrates in multiple (every 2 to 3 hours) small meals per day. Continued use of oral glucose-containing products will cause wide fluctuations in blood glucose levels.

If a puppy is presented in a hypoglycemic crisis, an IV catheter should be placed in the jugular vein if possible (use the largest vein possible or the Intraosseous (IO) route to reduce the likelihood of phlebitis). Then 1 to 2 ml/kg of 5% to 20% dextrose should be administered slowly IV. IF an IV or IO catheter cannot be placed, 50% dextrose, honey or corn syrup can be rubbed onto the gums and/or administered by stomach tube when the pup is warm enough (over 96° F). Alternatively, 2.5% Dextrose and 0.45% NaCl can be given subcutaneously if the IV or IO route is unavailable. For patients that present in a coma or in shock, 20% dextrose administered IV or IO should be used, but with care.

Care must be taken to avoid creating a hypertonic or hyperglycemic state. Hyperglycemia can lead to hyperosmolarity and death. Blood glucose levels should be monitored intermittently to assess that the patient is remaining euglycemic.

Food should be offered as soon as the pup is alert enough to eat. 5% dextrose can be continued IV. Prior to discharge from the hospital, the pup must be weaned off the dextrose and must be eating an appropriate diet to prevent relapse of the hypoglycemic episode.

Fluid support and methods of administration – IM, IO, IP, IV, PO, PR, and SQ
Dehydration may occur because of inadequate nursing or secondary to diarrhea, fever and/or other illnesses. Neonates are more susceptible to dehydration because of a higher ratio of surface area to body mass and the inability of their kidneys to concentrate urine.

Hydration status can be assessed on tacky mucus membranes, history of loss and/or inadequate intake, urine with a specific gravity exceeding 1.020 or that is dark yellow in color. Hydration status of the newborn and neonate cannot be assessed by skin turgor due to a lack of subcutaneous fat. Nearly all sick pups will benefit from fluid replacement therapy. Care should be taken to avoid overhydration.

There are multiple routes of fluid administration in the neonate and pediatric patient. The route selected will be based on many factors including the ability of the gut to effectively absorb fluids, the severity of the illness, preference of the client, associated costs, size of the patient, and skill level of the veterinary staff.

The fluids given by any of these routes should be warmed to body temperature (95° to 99° F or 35° to 37° C) before being administered. Neonatal fluid maintenance is 60 to 180 ml/kg of body weight per 24 hours. This needs to be reduced according to fluids taken in by nursing and supplemental feeding or increased for ongoing fluid loss (vomiting, diarrhea), fever, dehydration, and sepsis.

If indicated, fluid loading can be initiated by using warmed fluids at a rate of 1 cc per 30 gm of body weight over 5 to 10 minutes, continuing until the patient shows improved mucous membrane color. The fluid maintenance rate can then be increased to 30 to 50 cc/lb/24 hour period (60 to 100 cc/kg/24 hour period) based on deficit and ongoing loss. Potassium chloride can be supplemented via the fluids or orally (using KCL elixir) if the potassium is below 2.5 meq per L.

The IV and IO (intraosseous) routes are most effective for debilitated patients but are more costly, require hospitalization and separation from the dam and littermates and increased levels of veterinary skills.

IV fluids
The jugular vein is the largest, most accessible vein in the neonatal and pediatric patient. An IV catheter (20 g to 24 g, up to 1 inch in length) can be placed, with or without a cutdown, and sutured into place with a tape butterfly. If the skin is difficult to pierce without damaging the catheter, a 20 g needle can be used to nick the overlying skin allowing easier introduction of the catheter. The catheter can be supported with a light tape bandage, taking care to protect the patency of the catheter and the comfort of the puppy. A bandage that is too heavy and restrictive can be detrimental to the pup. In larger pups, other peripheral veins can be accessed. If the catheter is expected to be indwelling for over 12 hours, a sterile skin prep (Betadine®, or Nolvasan®) should be applied to minimize complications. To minimize clotting of the catheter if it is used intermittently, 0.5 cc of 50% dextrose can be injected into the catheter at the end of each injection cycle. Heparin should be avoided.

Fluids that can be administered via the IV route include 2.5% dextrose and 0.45% NaCl, Ringers, normal saline, dextrose 5%, hypertonic fluids such as 50% dextrose and 7% saline, hetastarch, other colloidals, blood and blood products as well as drugs labeled for IV administration. Lactate cannot be metabolized by the neonate. It is better avoided if there is an alternative fluid source, but can be used if LRS is the only fluid option available.

If IV fluid administration is desired but a vein cannot be catheterized, either intermittent IV injection or intraosseous fluid administration may be substituted.

IO fluids
The intraosseous route (IO) allows rapid absorption of fluids or blood/blood products by administration directly into the vascular space. It is easier to place an IO needle than it is to cannulate a small vein on a neonatal patient. Equipment needs are simple – either a 22 gauge spinal needle or a hypodermic needle, size 20 to 25 gauge, materials for a sterile prep, bandaging materials, and a routine IV administration setup with an extension set. The sites most commonly used are the trochanteric fossa of the femur, the tibial tuberosity, and the trochanteric fossa of the proximal humerus, taking care to avoid injuring the growth plates (Table 8-4).

This route of fluid administration should be limited to patients that are depressed or unconscious because of the associated discomfort and for a maximum of 24 hours at any one site.

IO Needle placement technique
Palpation of the various sites is done to determine the location best suited for this patient. The site should be 1 cm distal to the trochanteric fossa of the femur or humerus, or 1 cm distal to the tibial tuberosity. The site is clipped and a sterile prep is applied, taking care to avoid overuse of fluids

Table 8-4 Intraosseous catheter placement-set up
Needle – 20 gauge usually. Spinal needle with stylet is preferred if available.
Stylet – from IV catheter or smaller needle to clear lumen of needle if plugged.
Gauze squares
1 inch white tape
Saline flush
Sterile gloves – depends on doctors size
Nolvasan® surgical scrub
Antibiotic or Betadine® ointment
Injection port

which may cause chilling of the patient. A small bleb of lidocaine or bupivicaine can be administered if indicated by the patient's condition, taking care to use a minimal dose as neonates have a reduced tolerance for these drugs. A small nick is made in the skin with a scalpel blade. The limb should be stabilized with the free hand cupping the stifle or other joint distal to the insertion site, and the middle finger parallel to the long bone to aid in directing the needle into the lumen. A 22 g spinal needle or a hypodermic needle is selected to suit the size of the patient's intramedullary space. The needle is inserted by attaching an injection port to the hub to maintain sterility, then twisting the needle as it is advanced. If a hypodermic needle is used and the lumen is plugged at insertion, the first needle should be removed and a second smaller needle or IV stylet should be placed through the needle to dislodge the obstruction. The needle should feel securely seated in the bone when correctly placed.

Tape the needle into place with a figure 8 strip of 1 inch white tape around the hub of the needle, around the limb on each side, and crossing over near the distal joint. Place an antibiotic cream around the opening in the skin. Position folded gauze squares around the hub of the needle to support the needle and administration set. Tape the needle and administration set securely to the patient to avoid dislodging the needle or discomfort to the patient. Complications from IO administration are rare. This technique does require removal of the pup from the other healthy littermates and dam.

Fluids that can be administered via the IO route include Ringers, normal saline, 5% dextrose, hypertonic fluids such as 50% dextrose and 7% saline, hetastarch, other colloidals, blood and blood products and drugs labeled for IV administration.

SQ fluids
Subcutaneous fluid administration is a very simple method of rehydrating a neonatal patient. The patient must be warm and have adequate peripheral circulation to pick up the fluids. This can often be done by the client at home. This route has the advantage of keeping the affected neonates with their littermates and dam. It is also more affordable for the client.

Not all fluids can be administered via the SQ route. Lactated Ringers, normal saline, 2.5% Dextrose with 0.45% NaCl, serum and plasma and drugs labeled for subcutaneous administration can be given via this route. 5% dextrose is not recommended for administration subcutaneously.

Warm the fluids to body temperature and inject them into 1 or 2 sites in the interscapular space. Injection with a 22 gauge needle and appropriate sized syringe is easier than use of a bag of fluids with a venoset. The typical dose is approximately 1 cc per 1 oz of body weight per time of administration.

Overhydration can be a serious complication. Rapid or labored respirations are a symptom of overhydration and indicate that fluid therapy rates must be adjusted.

PO fluids

Fluids can be administered by mouth or by feeding tube, if the gut is working. This means that the rectal temperature of the pup must be over 96° F, the gut is patent (stools have been passed) and there is no ongoing vomiting.

If the pup is strong and has an adequate suckling response, a small "preemie" nipple and bottle or a small bottle (15 ml) designed to administer oral medication to infants can be used. Many pet nursers and human baby bottles are not well suited to this because the pups do not take the nipple well and the bottle is so large it is difficult to assess how much fluid the pup has taken.

Initially, a sick pup can be fed electrolytes (warmed Lactated Ringers) or a 50:50 mix of milk replacer and LRS, mother's milk extracted from the bitch, or goat's milk combined with warmed Lactated Ringers or other appropriate oral electrolyte solution. This can be administered by bottle or by feeding tube, but never by eyedropper as this is too likely to lead to aspiration. Alternatively, a 5% to 10% dextrose solution can be given by feeding tube at 0.25 ml per oz of body weight. There is a small but serious risk of aspiration or perforation of the gut when a tube is used for oral supplementation, but when done correctly, the risk is very small and the benefits are great.

Antibodies can be absorbed through the gut only during the first 24 hours of life. These antibodies can be in the form of canine colostrum, serum, or plasma. If the pups are premature, sick, or weak, or the bitch does not appear to be producing adequate amounts of colostrum, plasma or serum can be administered by stomach tube within 24 hours of birth. This product can be purchased commercially (HemoPet, Appendix A-4) or collected from the bitch or other dog in the breeder's kennel, processed in the veterinary hospital's lab and administered by feeding tube. Testing for failure of transfer of passive immunity is impractical due to associated cost and turn-around time. If the pups are suspected of having inadequate colostrum intake, plasma or serum should be administered immediately.

Commercially available canned milk replacers may state they contain colostrum on the label. However, they contain heat processed bovine colostrum that has no protective immunity to the newborn puppy.

Antibiotics
Treating the puppy

Antibiotics should be considered a first line of defense and started immediately for any sick or debilitated pup. This includes pups born distressed, with diarrhea, with meconium in the fetal fluids, or born after a protracted labor. They should be started at the first sign of illness or preventively. The decision to treat the affected pup only or the entire litter is a clinical decision and will vary from case to case.

Antibiotics can be administered to neonates through the same routes that are labeled for an adult dog. Orally, or through a feeding tube, is a reliable route if the gut is working. The intraosseous route, which may be preferred if IV administration is not possible, can be substituted for any antibiotic labeled for IV administration. IV injection into the umbilical vein can be useful if the use is indicated at birth. Subcutaneous injection can be used when the pup has adequate peripheral circulation. IM administration should be used with caution due to the small size and limited circulation of the target site. The intraperitoneal route is no longer considered appropriate for antibiotic administration.

Bacterial infections, as a primary cause of disease, as a secondary invader, and as sepsis are common in the neonate. A minor health concern in a more mature dog can be very serious in a neonate. Maternal antibodies are not protective against many bacterial infections.

Many of these bacteria in pups are are relatively antibiotic sensitive. This, and the immature metabolism of a neonate, make penicillin, amoxicillin, amoxicillin with clavulanic acid and cephalexin antibiotics of first choice. These can be given through the feeding tube if the gut is working and at home. Injectable penicillin can be administered subcutaneously by a client if the patients have adequate peripheral circulation. Ampicillin/sulbactam (Unasyn®) can be used via the IV or IO route. The Unasyn® dose for neonatal sepsis is 50 mg/kg IV or IO every 4 to 6 hours as long as necessary.

Amoxicillin can be dosed at 25 mg/kg IV or IO (preferred), IM, SQ or PO. After 2 to 3 days, the dose may be reduced to 10 mg/kg if there has been a good clinical response.

Ceftiofur can be used as an injectable for newborns that have had meconium in their fetal membranes. Knowing which pups need antibiotics is a very important reason to track individual pups born vaginally or by C-section – so they can be identified and treated as indicated. Naxcel® or ceftiofur is dosed at 2.5mg/kg SQ q 12hrs 5 days maximum.

Potentiated sulfonamides must be used with caution and only in the well-hydrated newborn patient. This is an appropriate drug choice in a lactating bitch with metritis, mastitis, or other bacterial infections. Aminoglycosides are rarely indicated and should only be used based on culture and sensitivity results.

The fluoroquinolones are reported to cause defects in the formation of articular cartilage and they are contraindicated from 8 weeks to beyond 8 months of age, depending on the length of the growth phase in different breeds. Drugs in this class can probably be safely used up to 4 weeks, and to 8 weeks of age if absolutely necessary, but only if based on culture and sensitivity results and if there is an adequate risk-benefit ratio (when articular cartilage damage is a better outcome than a fatal disease.) This drug class can also be used in the lactating bitch with pups under 4 weeks of age, but only if necessary because there are other preferred antibiotics for this application.

Articular cartilage damage has been reported due to use of fluoroquinolones. Small breed puppies are at lowest risk, minimizing activity by crating large breed puppies minimizes but does not eliminate damage.

The tetracyclines should not be used in pups prior to eruption of all adult dentition due to alteration of the enamel color.

The umbilicus should be closely evaluated and treated by continued dipping with tincture of iodine. The umbilicus is a common source of infection in the neonate, causing fatal peritonitis.

Treating the bitch
The carbapenems (amoxicillin, penicillin, amoxicillin with clavulanic acid and cephalexin), macrolides (erythromycin and azithromycin) potentiated sulfonamides and lincosamines (lincomycin, clindamycin) are generally safe choices for use in the lactating bitch, if she is not sensitive to the products. Most of these antibiotics will be distributed in the milk, in varying percentages. Although clindamycin may cause nursing puppies to develop diarrhea, the American Academy of Pediatrics considers clindamycin compatible with breastfeeding.

Although many drugs cross into the milk, in no case should this be considered an adequate route of administration for antibiotics (or any drug) to the neonate.

Passive immunity – Plasma or Serum
Newborn pups are dependent on ingestion of colostrum in their first 24 hours of life to develop adequate passive immunity to carry them through their first few months of life. The passive immunity transmitted transplacentally in the dog (and cat) is insufficient protection.

If the pups are premature, sick, or weak at birth, or if the dam does not appear to be producing adequate amounts of colostrum, or for any reason the pups will not be able to nurse adequately, plasma or serum can be administered by oral, subcutaneous or intraosseous injection.

Fresh frozen plasma is available commercially (HemoPet Appendix A-4). It is practical to have this product on hand, frozen, in practices with a large breeder client base or if a current client is expecting a high-risk litter. It has a one year shelf life if kept in a chest freezer and can also be used for other applications in the pediatric and adult patient. Overnight shipping is also available for unexpected needs.

Alternatively, blood can be collected (then harvest plasma or serum) from the dam or another dog from the same kennel. The commercially available product is harvested from health-screened dogs. Although there are reports that suggest using non-commercial colostrum, serum, or plasma harvested from facilities other than the breeder's kennel, this risks introducing non-endemic diseases. The product from the individual breeder's kennel has the advantage of offering passive protection to the newborns to diseases they will be exposed to in their own environment.

The dam can be used if she is physically able to withstand the associated blood loss. This is not recommended if she has just undergone a C-section or is otherwise debilitated. The candidate should be a resident of the breeder's kennel, have not previously had a blood transfusion or a pregnancy, be young and in peak health. A larger dog should be selected because she will be able to tolerate having a larger volume of blood withdrawn. The average puppy will require 45 to 60 ml of whole blood (that translates into (16 cc of plasma or serum) after centrifugation).

Collection of the plasma or serum
Prep the donor dog aseptically over the vessel selected. Collection and harvesting of the blood must also be handled aseptically. In most cases, jugular venipuncture with physical restraint will provide adequate volume.

A healthy 60 to 70 pound (30 kg) dog can donate up to 500 cc (1 unit) of blood if IV fluids are administered concurrently. This can be repeated every 4 to 6 weeks.

Either plasma or serum can be harvested and administered. Serum is the non-cellular fluid from clotted blood; plasma is the non-cellular fluid from unclotted blood. Studies indicating the efficacy of passive immunity transfer were done with serum; no comparable studies were done on plasma. It may be assumed, however, that the two blood products are interchangeable. The advantage of plasma over serum is that it contains clotting factors. The advantage of serum over plasma is that it is easier to harvest in a clinical setting.

To harvest plasma, the blood can be drawn into a syringe with ACD anticoagulant and transferred into the tubes, or directly into an ACD blood collection bottle or bag. If using tubes to collect and harvest serum, the blood should be collected into sterile non-barrier red top tubes that have had the tops wiped with alcohol (and allowed to dry) or chlorhexidine to prevent introduction of bacteria. The blood should be allowed to clot at room temperature for 20 minutes, then centrifuged. If collecting as plasma, the blood can be spun in a centrifuge. The plasma or serum must be removed from the cells aseptically with a sterile needle and syringe, taking care to avoid including red blood cells in the harvest. The serum or plasma can be frozen for later use; it should be kept refrigerated only if it is to be used immediately. It is most practical to store the plasma or serum frozen in 5 ml aliquots. The desired IgG is stable for up to 1 year if frozen properly. Thaw in slightly lower than body temperature water (lower than 100° F or 36° C), never warmer, and never microwaved as the protective antibody proteins will be inactivated.

Administration of the plasma or serum

IgG antibodies are well absorbed when administered subcutaneously. They can also be given IO but this route is more complicated and cannot be done by the breeder for the second and third doses at home. IP administration poses significant risk and does not offer any benefits over SQ administration. PO administration is inferior to SQ when comparing absorption rates of antibodies. PO administration has been suggested to provide local immunity in the gut.

Plasma is often used in place of serum, but there is no documentation of the absorption in the neonate by any route. If used, it should be citrated (ACD) plasma, not heparinized plasma. ACD Plasma does have the advantage of providing the neonate with coagulation factors. This can be valuable in the premature neonate with coagulopathy (Table 8-5).

The published dose for a puppy is 16 cc of plasma administered SQ aseptically in divided doses over 24 hours.

Kittens require smaller doses, 5 cc SQ 3 times in 12 hours, and show high levels of circulating antibodies within 12 hours of administration.

Most breeders can be taught to administer SQ fluids including plasma at home **(See Appendix C-13)**.

Table 8-5 Fresh frozen plasma for neonatal puppies
Keep all plasma frozen until use.
To thaw, carefully warm the plasma to body temperature. Only warm the tubes you will be using at each administration – keep the remaining tubes in the freezer. Thawing is best done by placing tube against your body or in a pocket for warming. Do NOT heat in warm water or microwave as this will denature/damage the proteins and render the product ineffective. Gently rock the tube during thawing; do not shake.
The dose is 5.4 cc per puppy 3 times over a 24 hour period, totaling 16.2 cc per puppy. If this can be administered in the first 24 hours after birth, it can be given orally with a feeding tube. After the pups are over 24 hours old, it must be given by SQ or IO injection to be effective systemincally.
Draw 5.4 cc of warmed plasma into a 6 cc syringe. Using a feeding tube (only if the pups are less than 24 hours old) or a 20 or 22 gauge needle (for pups over 24 hours old), inject the warmed plasma. If given SQ, hold the skin pinched to prevent outflow from the injection site. If given by feeding tube, carefully follow instructions for feeding tube administration.
Repeat 2 more times in the next 24 hours. Change to SQ injection if the pups have exceeded 24 hours of age before the doses are administered.

Transfusion

Anemia severe enough to merit a transfusion is rare in the puppy. Neonatal Isoerythrolysis, seen in some breeds of kittens, is not a condition seen in the puppy.

Puppies are born with a normal hematocrit, which declines from approximately 42% to 24% by the 8th week of age. From this point on, the hematocrit should rebound to that of a normal adult by 5 months of age.

A pup with severe anemia or a hematocrit of less than 15%, and associated symptoms, may require a whole blood transfusion. Blood is administered at a rate of 10 ml/lb of body weight over 2 hours IV or IO. The whole blood should be collected with a citrated anticoagulant and administered with a standard Millipore blood filter. Administration of blood IP should be done as a last resort only.

Vitamin K injection

Any neonatal pup under 4 days of age showing symptoms of hemorrhage (internally or externally) should have an injection of Vitamin K1 administered at the rate of 0.25 to 2.5 mg SQ or IM once. Neonates are deficient in thrombin and may show signs of hemorrhage associated with sepsis, trauma, or other illness.

Basic hygiene and assistance with eliminations

Pups up to 4 weeks of age lack the ability to urinate or defecate without assistance. Every 4 hours, or after each feeding, the abdomen and rectal region of each pup should be wiped in a circular motion with warm wet cotton balls to stimulate elimination.

If the pups appear soiled with feces or look greasy, they should be carefully washed to reduce contamination without chilling the pups.

In some cases, the pups will have a gas accumulation in the stomach and/or intestinal tract. Gas in the stomach can be relieved by passing a feeding tube and allowing the gas to escape. This type of tube can also be passed rectally if there is gas in the colon or if an enema would benefit the pup. If there is a frothy gas in the stomach or the gas is lower in the intestines, simethicone can be administered orally. A pediatric formulation is easily found over the counter in most stores.

The literature suggests the use of a trocar to relieve gas. Because of the risk of peritonitis, other better options should be considered.

Adjusting drug doses for the neonate

The dosage of most drugs needs to be adjusted for the neonate. There is no published information for most drugs and there are many physiologic differences between the neonate and the adult patient. The neonate has a relatively lower body fat and higher water content than the adult; the neonatal blood-brain-barrier is more highly permeable to drugs; the neonate has reduced albumin so has a lower protein binding of drugs; the neonate has reduced renal clearance of drugs; and the neonate has lower hepatic clearance and altered metabolism of drugs due to an immaturity of enzyme function. Even the site and type of administration in the neonate has an altered absorption rate compared to the adult; drugs administered by IM injection have a lower absorption rate and drugs administered by SQ injection and PO routes have an increased rate of absorption compared to adults. Routes of administration such as intraosseous (IO) not used in adults are options in the neonate.

Critically ill or septic pups should have antibiotics administered by injection, not by PO route.

Selected drugs, particularly antibiotics used for sepsis, should be administered by injection (IO, SC, IM), for more reliable drug absorption. Although the beta lactam antibiotics are considered safer for neonates (cephalosporins and penicillins), they only offer protection against gram positive bacteria. Neonates, commonly stricken by septicemia caused by gram negatives, may need the more broad spectrum antibiotics in other drug classes such as ceftiofur and potentiated sulfonamides or fluoro-quinolones. Because the bacterial flora of the gut is altered by antibiotic administration, probiotics should be included with an antibiotic regimen.

In general, drugs that are water-soluble should have the dose increased to compensate for the higher percentage of body water in the neonate. Drugs that are fat-soluble should have the dose decreased (up to 30% to 50%) to compensate for decreased clearance.

Each drug dosage should be researched and calculated based on the case. Many antibiotics have a wide margin of safety, and this needs to be considered when drugs are selected. The benefit-risk ratio of each drug should be carefully assessed and the breeder/owner should be included in this discussion. The Johns Hopkins formulary in *The Harriet Lane Handbook: A Manual for Pediatric House Officers* book is very useful and available used for a very affordable price. This focuses on drugs used in human pregnancy; the data can be extrapolated to veterinary use if necessary.

> **Prior to administering any drug to any patient, particularly a neonate, the following thought process is useful:**
> 1. Is there a better alternative treatment? Do we need a drug at all? Do we need this drug?
> 2. Are the risks of treatments balanced by the benefits?
> 3. What do we know about this drug in this type of patient considering the physiology of the neonate?
> 4. Is there data we can use to compensate for lack of knowledge about this drug in this type of patient?
> 5. Do we have informed consent of the owner?
> 6. What parameters will we use to assess treatment success? Toxicity?
> 7. Should littermates also be treated?

Although many drugs cross into the milk, in no case should this be substituted as an adequate route of administration to the neonate. Many drugs, however, will be found in the milk and may affect the pups, and this needs to be considered in drug selection. In most cases, with precautions, pups can continue to nurse. In the rare circumstances where the bitch's milk may cause harm to the pups, they should be hand-fed but left with the bitch so she can mother them. Use of a garment (human swimsuit or dog body suit similar to that found http://www.retrieverworld.com/lycra_full_bodysuit. htm) will interfere with the pup's ability to nurse but will allow her to spend time with them without causing harm (Tables 8-6 and 8-7).

S.O.A.P. (Subjective/Objective/Analysis/Plan)
(Appendix D-5)
A complete and systematic history and physical examination, like that for adults should be done on neonates.

Symptoms
The breeder usually notes symptoms such as puppies that are sick, crying inconsolably, vomiting, coughing, losing weight, dehydrated, have diarrhea or dying. Sometimes, they know something is wrong with 1 or more pups, but can't quite describe it. In either instance, this is an emergency and the bitch and entire litter should be scheduled for an appointment the same day. Sick neonates deteriorate quickly.

> **For the appointment, the client should be instructed to bring:**
> 1. The entire litter.
> 2. The mother of the litter.
> 3. A way to keep the pups warm and safe in transit. To keep the live pups or kittens warm in transit the breeder can use a heating pad, an ice chest lined and covered with a towel to prop the lid open. A thermometer to monitor temperature to prevent chilling or overheating is essential.
> 4. The recorded notes and charts the breeder has kept of data on puppies or kittens weights, temperatures, vaccinations, worming, medications, urine color, stool character and diet fed.
> 5. ALWAYS BRING ALL THE DEAD PUPS (OR KITTENS) THEY HAVE FOR EXAMINATION AND POSSIBLE TESTING.
> 6. A fresh fecal sample from the pups.

Knowing if some or all of the pups are sick can help determine the urgency and start preparation of a differential diagnosis list. The earlier the pups are evaluated, the sooner appropriate therapy can be instituted.

Table 8-6 Key drugs, dosages and indications for Pediatric Patients

Key Drug	Indication	Dose Range (dose adjusted for neonates and pediatric patients)	Frequency	Route	Precautions	Reference	Margin of Safety
Acyclovir	Herpes virus infection	10 mg per kg as suspension	Every 6 hours until 3 weeks of age.	PO	Anecdotal only.	Kampschmidt and others. Unpublished observation	Narrow
Amikacin	Gram Negative Septicemia	Up to 20 to 25 mg per kg (with caution)	Every 36 to 48 hours if under 6 weeks.	IV	May cause renal and ototoxicity. Reserve for suspected severe life-threatening gram negative infections. Monitor blood levels.	Plumb	Narrow
Amoxicillin	Infection	10 to 22 mg per kg	Every 12 hours	PO		Various	Wide
Amoxicillin/ Clavulanic Acid	Infection	12.5 to 25 mg per kg	Every 12 hours	PO		Lee	Wide
Ampicillin	Infection	22 mg per kg	Every 8 hours	IV		Lee	Wide
Cefazolin	Infection	10 to 30 mg per kg	Every 8 hours	SC or IO	Decrease dose if diminished renal function.	Root Kustritz	Wide
Cefotaxime	Infection	25 to 50 mg per kg	Every 8 hours	SC or IO		Root Kustritz	Wide
Cephalexin	Infection	10 to 30 mg per kg	Every 8 to 12 hours	PO		Various	Wide
Chloramphenicol	Mycoplasma Infection	22 mg per kg (Puppies only)	Every 8 hours (up to 7 days total)	PO	Reserve for CNS disease or cases where bacteria are resistant to other antibiotics. Use minimized due to human health risk when handled.	Poffenberger	Narrow
Fenbendazole	Anthelminthic	50 mg per kg	Every 24 hours for 3 days	PO	5 days if treating for Giardia.	Various	Wide

Drug	Indication	Dose	Frequency	Route	Comments	Reference	Spectrum
Fluoroquinolones	Infection	5 to 20 mg per kg per day PO 5 to 20 mg per kg every 12 hours IV for sepsis	5 to 20 mg per kg per day PO. 5 to 20 mg per kg every 12 hours IV for sepsis.		To protect against cartilage damage, avoid use from 8 weeks to 8 months of age.	Various	Narrow
Metronidazole	Giardia or anaerobic infection	10 to 25 mg per kg in pups at least 2 weeks of age	Every 24 hours for 5 to 10 days	PO	Neurotoxicity or "intoxication"	Plumb	Narrow
Pyrantel Pamoate	Parasites	5 to 10 mg per kg	Every 14 days starting at 14 days of age	PO		Various	Wide
Sulfadimethoxine	Coccidiosis (not labeled for this use)	50 mg per kg first dose, then 25 mg/kg	Every 24 hours for 5 to 10 days	PO	Avoid if under 4 to 5 weeks of age. Can cause renal precipitate if patient is not well hydrated. May cause KCS or thrombocytopenia.	Plumb	Narrow
Trimethoprim-sulfadiazine or Trimethoprim-Sulfamethoxazole	Infection	30 mg per kg	Every 24 hours	PO	Same as for sulfadimethoxine	Various	Narrow
Vitamin K 1	Neonatal hemorrhage	0.25 to 2.5 mg total dose SQ or IM once.	Once	SQ, IM	Use small gauge needle. May cause anaphylaxis by injection. PO is better absorbed.	Various	Narrow

Table 8-7 Drugs to avoid in neonates and pediatric patients	
Drug name:	Reason to avoid:
Doxycycline and tetracyclines	Discoloration of teeth and alteration in bone development
Fluoroquinolones	Damage to cartilage in pups over 8 weeks and under 8 months.
Griseofulvin	Liver damage – diminished liver clearance
Ivermectin	When neonates, blood-brain barrier too permeable
Metronidazole	When neonates, blood-brain barrier too permeable
NSAIDS	In the neonate, renal function may be damaged
Long acting corticosteroids	

Gelens, Hans. "Drug Therapy in Pediatric Practice." Western Veterinary Conference, Las Vegas, 2003.)

Diagnostic workup
History
A thorough history is essential, and should be taken by a technician or assistant. The SOAP form is useful to ensure that the unique information required for a complete history of the neonates is not overlooked.

Physical exam step by step
(See Appendix D-4 & D-5)
A complete physical examination should be performed on each pup. If only 1 pup is ill, it is helpful if the breeder brings other "normal" puppies for comparison. If there is any question, all the pups as well as the bitch should be brought. The bitch's examination often provides clues regarding the source of the illness. You may also find early signs of illness in seemingly normal littermates that reduce morbidity and mortality.

A towel placed over a heating pad makes a suitable location for the examination. It is ideal to have 2 laundry baskets with a heat source lined with towels ready when the pups arrive. The use of 2 laundry baskets, each with a heat source and lined with towels helps to sort pups, to keep track of which pups have been examined, treated or are still in line for evaluation and treatment.

The bitch should be thoroughly examined first, paying particular attention to her abdominal palpation (to assess for retained pups or C-section incision), vaginal discharge, and mammary glands. If she is ill, it is most likely related to the pregnancy, but don't forget to include any other canine disorder in your differential.

She should be separated from the pups for treatment, diagnostics, and holding so that handling the pups does not upset her.

A SOAP form is useful when examining the neonate. A pediatric, neonatal, or electronic stethoscope should be used because the smaller size of the neonate makes finding murmurs more difficult with a larger stethoscope head.

Almost any physical abnormality that is noted in adults can be seen in neonates. There are a few unique findings worth noting.

Vital signs are moderately different in the newborn as compared with the adult and gradually shift to adult normals as the pup matures. The mucus membranes should be pink, but may be hyperemic if the pup has just nursed or has been vocalizing. By 8 weeks of age, its mucus membranes become more pale, then gradually return to pink. Heart rates are higher, respiratory rates and blood pressures are lower as neonates, then gradually normalize.

Assessment should include body tone, body condition, and hydration. Reflexes start as flexor dominant, but become extensor dominant by 5 days of age.

Eyes and ears are closed until approximately 10 to 14 days of age. Swelling behind the eyelids prior to opening is clinically related to neonatal opthalmia and should be addressed immediately. (See section in this chapter for treatment.) The eyes (corneas) are cloudy for the first few days after the eyelids open. Distichia and entropion are common causes of eye discharge, redness, and corneal ulcer (Figure 8-13). Sloughing of the ear tips is clinically related to septicemia.

Any cleft in the upper lip, nostrils, or palate (look carefully at the soft palate with good lighting) is important and needs to be discussed with the breeder at once (Figure 8-14A-C).

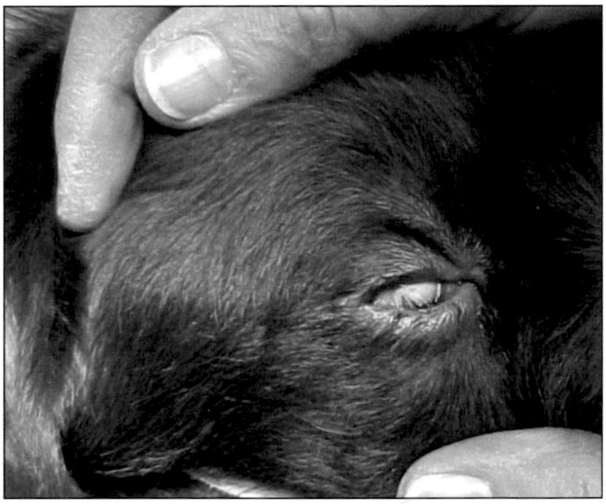

It is normal for the lower jaw to look disproportionately long at birth as this aids in nursing. This normalizes as the pup approaches weaning age. Malocclusion and retained deciduous teeth are common and may require correction to prevent pain and improve dental alignment with maturity but are seldom a cause of acute illness. Discomfort upon eruption of adult dentition is also a rare cause of clinical disease (Figure 8-14D).

Many puppies, particularly toy breeds, have an open fontanelle at birth. This should close as the pup matures. If it is excessive in size or

Figure 8-13.
A 9 week old pup with lower eyelid entropion.

length of time open, this may predict potential neurologic disease. This can present in the form of developmental delays or seizures. Particular care should be taken when handling this pup to prevent inadvertent damage to the unprotected brain.

The nares should be wide enough to allow for ease in inspiration. Stenotic nares are common in the brachycephalic dogs and may require surgical intervention to prevent a lifetime of respiratory distress. Elongated soft palates, everted laryngeal saccules, and disproportionately narrow tracheas or overly stretched tracheal membranes are also often seen in the toy and brachycephalic breeds and should be noted.

Even in the newborn pup, heart murmurs are abnormal. Any murmur may be clinically significant. Innocent murmurs are common and typically can no longer be ausculted by 12 weeks of age. These innocent or functional murmurs are usually soft, no louder than a grade II on a scale of VI, are loudest at the left base, and change with the position of the patient. In most cases, this pup is one of the larger and more active in the litter. The functional murmur is often associated with fever, anemia, or other illness. A murmur that is severe, III or greater on a scale of VI, often with a precordial thrill, in an unusually small or weak pup, and that persists past 12 weeks is significant. A pup with this finding should not be sold as normal; a referral for a complete workup with a cardiologist should be offered.

Neonates have a higher heart rate, lower blood pressure, and a sinus rhythm.

Lung sounds should be similar to that of an adult.

The abdominal wall should be complete. The umbilicus should be small and the umbilical cord should have dried up and fallen off in 3 to 4 days. Inflammation of the umbilical region is significant. Examine for umbilical and/or inguinal hernias. These are common and in rare instances can allow for strangulation of abdominal contents. Abdominal wall defects can allow intestines and other

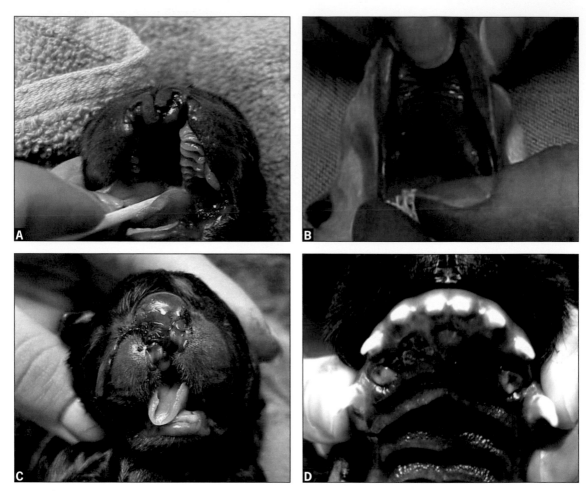

Figure 8-14.
*A. A newborn pup with severe cleft palate and lip. **B.** A newborn pup with cleft palate. **C.** A newborn pup with cleft lip. **D.** A narrow lower jaw with lower canine teeth causing trauma to palate.*

abdominal contents to be exposed at birth. In some cases, these can be surgically corrected at birth. Umbilical hernias or hernias of the midline cranial to the umbilicus can suggest the presence of a diaphragmatic or peritoneo-pericardial diaphragmatic. Patent urachus is rare in dogs.

It should be possible to see urine and stool on all normal pups. The absence of urine suggests dehydration, anuria, or urinary obstruction. Gently palpate the abdomen for the presence of an overly full bladder or free fluid. If feces are absent, diarrhea, constipation, or ani atresia should be considered. Normal bowel sounds should be present. The stool character should be noted.

Evaluate the vulva for evidence of abnormal structures suggesting intersex. Sticky or purulent vaginal discharge is common in the young female pup and rarely associated with clinical disease (Figure 8-15).

If a male pup is not urinating, evaluate the tip of the penis for calculi. If the bladder is distended and the pup is distressed, evaluate for urethral calculi. Both testes should be palpable in the scrotum by 3 weeks, but may still "normally" descend up to 14 weeks of age. Acute abdominal pain in a male pup without both testes palpable in the scrotum should be evaluated for testicular torsion.

Blood work
Blood work can be very useful in making a diagnosis in the neonate. The newer lab equipment available

in many veterinary hospitals can provide results with microsamples and rapid turn-around times. The smallest possible sample should be taken and should not exceed 1.5 ml. Normals for neonatal-pediatric patients are shown in Tables 8-8 and 8-9.

Titers

Titers show 1 of 2 aspects of a patient's ability to mount an immune response against a disease. One mechanism is cellular and the other is antibody production. This antibody test is called a titer. If a titer is high enough, it is said to be protective. The level determined to be protective varies from one infectious agent to the next. Passive immunity is from antibodies transferred from mother to neonate via the colostrum; active immunity are antibodies developed in the pup.

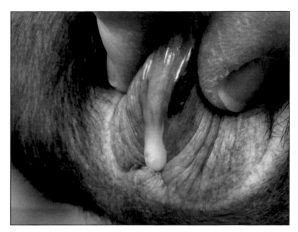

Figure 8-15.
Puppy vaginitis, common finding.

Exposure to disease and immunizations will cause an antibody response. Titers are used in clinical practice to either diagnose a disease or to evaluate the efficacy of a vaccination program. Most veterinarians and breeders use titers to determine if the dog needs to be revaccinated according to a pre-set schedule. However, titers can be even more valuable to determine if a patient has responded well enough to a vaccination to develop protection. Surprisingly, up to 15% of all dogs fail to respond adequately to routine vaccinations. Up to 5% of all dogs fail to mount any immune response to immunization (called no-responders) and 10% fail to mount a high enough response to be fully protective to either parvovirus or distemper virus (called low-responders).

Upon completion of the puppy vaccination series is the best time to determine if a patient is a low-responder or a no-responder. Ideally, a titer should be done at approximately 18 to 20 weeks. If the dog is a low or no-responder, an additional vaccination is recommended, followed by another titer. If the second titer still shows a poor response, a booster with a vaccine produced by a different manufacturer is recommended. If the dog still fails to respond, the recommendation is to limit the dogs exposure to situations that may allow disease transmission. If this patient is the mother of a litter of pups, the pups should be treated as pups with a failure of passive immunity. The use of immune plasma in the neonate and early vaccinations of the pups can help protect them from disease. The heritability of this failure to respond is unknown, the pups of this bitch should be titered at 18 weeks of age, with the same protocol followed for them if they show limited response to vaccine.

Table 8-8 CBC (Table of normals for the neonate)		
Parameter	Range	Age
PCV/Hct	42 to 48%	Birth
PCV/Hct	30%	21 days
PCV/Hct	26%	28 days
PCV/Hct	24%	8 weeks
PCV/Hct	Increasing	9 weeks
PCV/Hct	Adult range	20 weeks
WBC	Adult range including differential but poor bone marrow reserve	

Table 8-9 Chemistry panel (Table of normals for the neonate)		
Parameter	Normal range	Reason
ALP	Increased up to 4000 IU/L	Bone growth
ALT	Normal	
BUN	Increased 1st 7 days, then declines to low end of adult normal	Immaturity
Glucose	80 to 150	
Total Protein and Albumin	TP 4.1	
Albumin	Low	
Specific Gravity	1.006 to 1.017	immaturity
Urine protein	Mild proteinuria normal up to 6 weeks of age	
Urine glucose	Mild glucosuria normal up to 6 weeks of age	
Electrolytes	Normal	

Urinalysis

Urine specific gravity can be used to estimate the hydration status of a puppy. Remember, skin turgor is not an accurate estimation because there is too little body fat in the neonate.

Urine can be collected by rubbing the perineum with a dry cotton ball and collecting the urine in a tube or directly onto the refractometer's screen. In the neonate under 8 weeks of age, the specific gravity should be between 1.006 and 1.017. Urine in this range is typically very pale yellow. If the urine is dark enough to look yellow, the puppy is dehydrated and needs additional fluid supplementation – increased time nursing, more tube feeding, or more IV/SQ/IO fluids. This is a good skill to teach the breeder. A skilled breeder can supplement fluids prior to the appointment.

Dipstick

Very little urine is required for testing on a urine dipstick. In the very young, when urine quantity is limited, the sticks can be cut in half the long way. It is considered normal for puppies under 6 weeks to have mild amounts of glucose and protein in the urine.

Organic acids

There are many biochemical pathway errors in mammals; they are commonly enzyme deficiencies. These pathway errors lead to illness and death. Because they are not readily apparent on physical examination, but cause significant clinical signs, early detection is vital.

Inborn metabolic pathway errors are diagnosed by testing for amino acids, organic acids, and carbohydrates. These are more readily detected in the urine compared to the blood.

Symptoms include early neonatal death, unthriftiness, slow development, cloudy corneas, anorexia, chronic vomiting and/or diarrhea, skeletal defects, and enlarged livers and/or spleens. Urine testing for these metabolites can be useful in making a diagnosis on pups exhibiting symptoms for which no physical exam findings or other diagnostic testing can reveal a cause.

The Metabolic Screening Laboratory, section of Medical Genetics of the Veterinary Hospital of the University of Pennsylvania provides these tests. Sample requirements, fees, and submission information can be found on their website by searching for penngen.

Cultures – Samples and techniques
Viral cultures
Viral cultures are usually taken for electron microscopic analysis. These are samples of feces, corneal scrapings and other tissues that may be found to contain the virus.

Newer tests, PCRs, are replacing electron microscopy in many cases. Prior to sampling, check the submission information at your reference lab for a list of the most recent and accurate tests, how to sample, and how to submit a sample.

Bacterial cultures
Bacterial samples need to be collected carefully to avoid outside contamination and maximize accuracy. Each area to be sampled has particular requirements. The person taking the sample should wear gloves to avoid contamination of the sample by contact with their skin. Sterile intruments and collection devices should be used.

Samples for culture should be taken prior to collection of samples for histology or PCR for example, to minimize contamination. For instance, on a post mortem exam, samples for culture of the solid organs should be collected prior to opening the intestinal tract. Specialized swabs with media to support bacterial growth should be used. For blood cultures, vacuum tubes are available and should be stocked. Solid tissues can be placed inside sterile bags or tubes for transport. If bacterial cultures are not to be performed at the clinic, refrigerate them and send to a reference laboratory as soon as possible.

EKG lead II
Although cardiac disease is rare in pups, it can occur. A lead II electrocardiogram is a fast, non-invasive and easy screening test available in many veterinary facilities. It can be used to detect both primary cardiac arrhythmias as well as electrolyte disorders with secondary cardiac changes.

Cardiac disease with auscultable murmurs is a more common cardiac manifestation in the young pup. Although cardiac chamber enlargement can be detected on EKG's, interpretation can be more challenging. Consultation with a cardiologist may be necessary. EKGs and auscultation are not diagnostic of the underlying cardiac pathology.

Many pups, under 12 weeks of age, may present with soft systolic murmurs. Some may be innocent the pups will outgrow them. For pups with loud or persistent murmurs, or who are small and tire easily, cardiology referral is recommended. Prior to sale, referral to a cardiologist or internist with an interest in cardiology for evaluation, including an echocardiogram may be useful in diagnosing the specific cardiac disease and developing a prognosis and treatment protocol.

Radiographs
Radiography in the young can be challenging but still provide important information. Many disorders can be diagnosed radiographically, even in the very young. Restraint can be difficult. Sedation and the use of tape and other devices such as sandbags can be of great assistance in positioning the patient well (Figure 8-16).

The young pup has a lack of detail on abdominal films due to lack of abdominal fat. Non-screen cassettes or special screens (such as mammogram cassettes) can be used to improve detail.

Radiography is sometimes bypassed because of concern that interpretation of normal is difficult in a neonate. If this is a concern, radiographing a littermate can be a useful "control." Ask the client if they are willing to allow a radiograph – don't assume that they will decline just because the patient is so small.

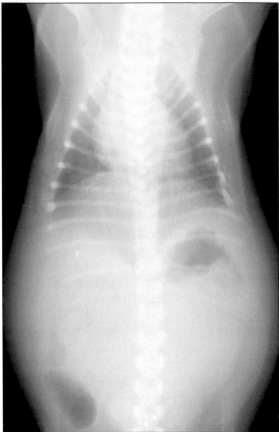

Figure 8-16.
A radiograph of a newborn pup.

Thoracic radiographs can be more enlightening than abdominal radiographs. These can be used to evaluate for pneumonia, rib fractures, hemorrhage, an enlarged heart, and a incomplete diaphragm. Relative to adults, the lungs will be more opaque and the heart larger. Gas in the GI tract is readily apparent. Some foreign bodies can be easily seen. Bones will have a mysterious array of growth plates and very little mineralized structure if the pup is very young.

Ultrasound

Ultrasonography can be very useful in the neonate and pediatric patient. The lack of abdominal fat, and thus detail on a radiograph, is not an issue with ultrasound. However, the neonate does not have the same relative organ sizes as an adult and the ultrasonogram should be interpreted carefully. Nearly any ultrasonic study that can be done on an adult can also be done on a neonate.

Ultrasound is a very useful tool for collecting urine by cystocentesis. It can also be helpful when assessing for and collecting free fluid in the abdomen and thorax.

Many cardiologists use echocardiograms to assess for cardiac disease. Puppies under 10 weeks of age are generally not candidates for echocardiography.

Function testing
Gastrointestinal function testing

TLI (Trypsin-Like Immunoreactivity): The TLI test is not considered to be a classic function test. It assesses normal exocrine pancreatic function to check for the ability to secrete normal digestive enzymes. This problem is most common in adolescent German Shepherds, but other breeds are also affected.

Following a comprehensive physical examination, evaluation for intestinal parasites and appropriate use of a broad spectrum wormer, a TLI test should be a routine part of any work-up for canine small bowel diarrhea. It is available at Texas A and M University and can be ordered alone or in combination with cobalamin and folate. The patient must fast for 12 hours for these tests to be accurate. (See:http://www.cvm.tamu.edu/gilab/)

Hepatic function tests
Bile acids

This test assesses liver function. In the pediatric patient, it is used to detect a suspected porto-systemic shunt. These are most commonly run in pairs, fasting or pre-prandial and after a meal, or post-prandial. However, a single bile acid that is significantly elevated is often considered diagnostic. Some pathologists prefer using the blood ammonia test to diagnose a portosystemic shunt, but there are logistic problems with this test – it must be kept anaerobic until run, on ice, and a control from a normal patient is often required with each sample submitted. For these reasons, the bile acid test is often preferred.

Renal function

Iohexol clearance test

Diagnosing renal disease is a challenge. The tests we rely on – the BUN and Creatinine tests – do not become elevated until the patient has suffered damage or loss of over 75% of the renal tissue. In dogs and cats, we sometimes rely on urine specific gravity to detect renal disease, but it does not drop into the isothenuric range (1.008 to 1.012) until 66% of the renal tissue is damaged.

It is obvious that a more sensitive test is needed for earlier diagnosis of kidney damage. The iohexol clearance test is valuable for this application, but seldom used in private practice.

Although this is not a difficult test to perform, it does require attention to detail and advance planning. Its value is that it specifically measures the glomerular filtration rate (GFR), which is directly related to the functional renal mass.

Iohexol is used as a radiographic contrast medium for myelograms and IVPs. It works because it is not protein bound and its elimination by the kidney tracks the GFR. The test is sensitive, accurate and linear.

Prior to testing, contact the reference laboratory you intend to use to be certain that the protocol has not been updated. The test is currently run on serum. A 300 mg iodine/kg bolus is injected as a one-time injection IV with a catheter. The precise time of the injection must be recorded. At 2, 3 and 4 hours after administration, additional samples should be drawn. The sample size should be sufficient to harvest at least 1.2 ml of serum from each of the 3 samples. All samples should be allowed to clot in serum clot tubes, and centrifuged. Label each sample with the owner's name, the patient's ID, and the time the sample was drawn, to the closest one minute. Transfer the blood into plastic transport vials with the above identifying information on them and submit by shipping overnight to the reference lab in an insulated container (Figure 8-17).

Urine Protein Creatinine Ratio (UPCR)

A urine protein creatinine ratio (UPCR) is useful in determining if there is evidence of protein loss in the urine. There are multiple causes of proteinuria, including pre-renal, renal, or post-renal. This is a simple test requiring a small volume of urine. Any value greater than 1 is considered abnormal. Interpretation complex and is beyond the scope of this book.

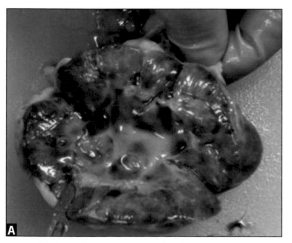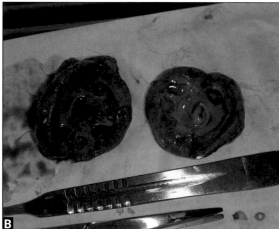

Figure 8-17.
A. Congenital renal disease. **B.** Renal dysplasia in a pup.

Post mortem exam

A post mortem examination is recommended whenever a pup dies. It is rare in companion animal practice to sacrifice a sick pup for the benefits of post mortem examination. The information gained from post mortem examination can be invaluable. With prompt results and institution of appropriate therapy, other pups in the litter may be saved.

In house

The gross post mortem can be done in the veterinary clinic, taking care to note and record any physical abnormalities. Tissues and other samples should be collected for histopathology, culture, DNA, organic acids in the urine, and toxicology. Digital photographs are useful. The particular differences to note between the neonate and adult are the relative difference in organ size, and the presence of the thymus in neonates and pediatric patients. A systemic approach to the post mortem and record keeping will prove useful for both this client and future clients.

Reference laboratory

The body may also be refrigerated, not frozen, and submitted it in its entirety with gel packs to a reference lab. Prior to shipment, develop a relationship with a lab and pathologist that will accept intact neonates and is interested in diagnosing causes of neonatal death. Diagnostics include gross findings, histology, PCR, toxicology, urine organic acids, and microbiological findings (bacteria, viruses, and parasites).

If the lab prefers a complete post mortem on fresh tissues, the body should be wrapped in plastic, boxed with frozen gel packs and enough packing material to absorb any liquid that may be present, and shipped overnight or by lab courier. If the lab personnel prefer fixed tissues, both body cavities and the skull should be opened and the body submerged in formalin at a 10 to 1 ratio of formalin to pup. Prior to fixation, fresh tissues for PCR, DNA and culture should be harvested. After 24 hours, drain the excess formalin and ship the body with just enough formalin to keep the tissues moist.

Be certain all paperwork is complete including a clinical history and the veterinarian's signature if required (Figure 8-18).

Managing the neonate in the hospital

It is difficult to manage patients overnight in hospitals without 24 hour staffing. This is especially true for the neonatal patient due to the need for frequent feedings and the potential for frequent changes in treatment protocols. This often necessitates separating the sick pup(s) from their dam

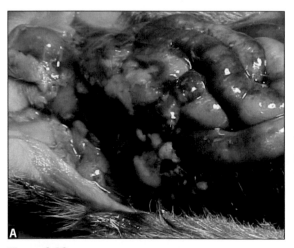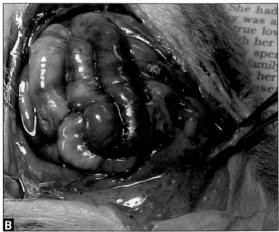

Figure 8-18.
Post mortem evaluation of a neonatal pup. The pup died of peritonitis secondary to omphalitis, an infected umbilicus.

and littermates, causing additional stress and nutritional deficits.

Breeders frequently prefer outpatient management, or daytime hospitalization alternating with nighttime care at home. Many injections can be administered by the breeder.

This approach should be discussed with the breeder in advance. Overnight care can also be arranged at a 24 hour emergency clinic.

Illness syndromes in the neonate

This discussion, covers common disorders by symptom rather than by etiology. It is not intended to be all-inclusive.

"Fading puppy syndrome"

There is no specific disorder known as "fading puppy syndrome". This is a catch-all phrase for any undiagnosed illness, failure to thrive or death. While diagnostics are pending, or if no diagnosis can be made, survival of these pups is dependent on basic supportive care to maintain body temperature, blood glucose, blood volume, prevent sepsis, and adequate oxygenation. Keep the patient warm; provide plasma and/or fluids; supplement oxygen, food and antibiotics. This is often all that is needed.

Poor weight gain

Poor weight gain has a strong correlation with pups that fade and die. This can involve either individual pups who are unable to compete for food or the bitch's inability to produce enough milk for the entire litter.

Evaluate the bitch for disorders that reduce lactation. These include mastitis, metritis, inadequate post-Caesarean pain management, diarrhea, and any other illness that reduces food and fluid intake. Correct the underlying disorder, hydrate the bitch and administer metoclopramide and oxytocin to the bitch by injection or orally.

Administer plasma SQ to the pups and start supplemental feeding. Heat, oxygen, antibiotics, and other supportive care may be required. Continue supplemental feeding until they reach their ideal weight, then drop 1 feeding per day if they continue to gain weight as anticipated.

Diarrhea

Almost every litter has one or more pups that are affected with diarrhea. The prognosis and treatment are determined by the age and size of the pups, severity of the diarrhea, and presence of other symptoms such as vomiting. Symptoms include crying, failure to nurse, bloating, dehydration and depression. The diarrhea may not be obvious because the mother has licked away all traces.

All pups over 2 weeks old should be wormed every 2 weeks unless the bitch was on the 4 week fenbendazole protocol while pregnant and in early lactation. If they have diarrhea and are not vomiting or too sick to worm, and have not been wormed in the past 2 weeks, worming should be done at once. Owners should be advised to practice good hygiene and cautioned about the zoonotic potential of intestinal parasites.

The bitch should accompany her pups to the clinic for evaluation. If she is not ill, it may be advisable to examine her in the car to prevent exposure to diseases in the clinic. Check her for mastitis and metritis.

Diagnostics should include fecal flotation and fecal centrifugation. Evaluate a fecal smear stained with Dif-Quick® for the type of bacteria present. Rods should predominate. If all the rods look the same, if there is an abundance of cocci, or if Clostridium is noted, administer an appropriate antibiotic. Bacterial cultures can be set up at the clinic or submitted to a reference lab. In house tests are now available for Parvovirus and Giardia, providing results in 20 minutes. Parvovirus is of greatest concern in unvaccinated pups over 10 weeks of age or in vaccinated pups 10 to 14 weeks old.

Determining and treating the underlying cause of diarrhea should be the goal. Adding baby rice cereal and probiotics or live or active culture yogurt to the diet can be very useful. This can be syringe fed. If the pups are on solid food, they can be fed a commercially available diet to control diarrhea. Kaolin/Pectin suspension can also be used.

Constipation
Constipation is less common than diarrhea, but some owners will see pups straining to defecate. This can progress to vomiting. It can be related to inadequate water or food consumption.

It is important to distinguish between constipation and urinary obstruction with inability to urinate.

Sometimes, a well-lubricated thermometer can stimulate defecation. If not, and a patent rectum has been confirmed by finding feces previously, treatment should consist of SQ fluids, oral Karo syrup, glycerin suppositories, and/or gentle soap suds enemas with warm water administered with a soft red rubber feeding tube. Do not overcorrect the problem. Constipation is a common sequella to overcorrecting diarrhea and it is easy to swing back and forth between the 2 conditions.

Fussy
A fussy puppy can be suffering from anything imaginable. Attentive owners can usually assess and correct the situation. The most common causes are environmental temperatures that are too high or low, hunger, thirst, being dirty or wet. If the problem cannot be resolved by phone, the pups should be examined for signs of illness.

Pneumonia
Pneumonia is common secondary to aspiration of food, fluids, or medications. It may also result from exposure to infectious diseases such as Herpesvirus.

Prevention is the most effective way to deal with pneumonia. Neonates should not be allowed to nurse or be tube fed if their body temperature is less than 96° F. Avoid feeding by bottle or with a syringe or eye dropper because it can lead to aspiration of formula.

Radiographs can be used to diagnose pneumonia, even in the very young. To aid in radiographic interpretation, an unaffected littermate can also be radiographed for comparison.

Treatment consists of:
1. Antibiotic therapy for primary bacterial disease, treatment of aspiration, or to treat secondary invaders following viral infection.
2. Fluid therapy to keep secretions loose and for general supportive care.
3. Oxygen, by tank or oxygen concentrator. +/– nebulizer
4. Hyperimmunized plasma to aid in infectious disease management.
5. Nutritional support.
6. Warmth if Canine Herpesvirus is suspected.

Refusal to nurse
Pups often refuse to nurse if they are too cold. When warmed and returned to the bitch, most will regain the drive to suckle. Other causes are cleft palates (usually limited to 1 pup in the litter), poor maternal skills, inadequate lactation, or a sick bitch or pup.

Regurgitation

First, distinguish regurgitation from vomiting. This is usually done by asking the client questions or by describing the difference and giving the client symptoms to watch for. On occasion, the pup may be observed in the act at the hospital.

Regurgitation is often noted at the time of weaning, when solid food is introduced. If only one episode is noted, overeating is the probable cause. If one or more pups are regurgitating after each solid meal, losing weight, and/or have aspiration pneumonia, they need to be evaluated. Radiography, including barium swallows, can be done in most practices. Referral for functional imaging should be considered if barium swallow and observation are inconclusive. Differentials include megaesophagus, vascular ring anomalies, cricopharyngeal achalasia, esophageal foreign bodies, esophageal strictures and fistulas, and other more unusual disorders.

Megaesophagus

Supportive care can be rewarding because many but not all, pups will either "outgrow" or improve with age. Predicting which pups will improve is difficult. The breeder should consider keeping the affected pups, sometimes for months, until radiography shows that the disorder is resolved.

Owners must monitor for early signs of aspiration. Appropriate antibiotic therapy based on culture and sensitivity may be indicated from time to time. Frequent small meals from an elevated position are recommended. "Bailey chairs" may be built or purchased to keep pups elevated during and after meals. The front end of the pet should be supported for a short time after each meal. Different food textures ranging from solid to liquid diets can be tried to determine which kind each patient tolerates best. Gastrotomy tubes can be placed surgically if required.

Drinking bottles mounted above the pup's head also allow gravity to improve swallowing. Over-the-counter products that thicken drinking water (developed for use in nursing homes for human patients) are useful.

Sucralfate suspension is recommended for all patients with megaesophagus. (*Gaynor et al.,* 1997) Medicate affected animals with oral sucralfate suspensions (1 g tid for large dogs and 0.5 g tid for smaller dogs. Bethanechol may improve esophageal contractility in some patients but should be used with caution. Bethanechol can be dosed at 5 to 15 mg/dog p/o TID or 0.5 to 1.0 mg/kg PO TID.

Megaesophagus does not lend itself to surgical correction. Gastro-esophageal intussusception is rare. The incidence is highest in male German Shepherd pups. The stomach, and occasionally other organs including the pancreas, spleen, duodenum, and omentum ascend into the esophagus. Emergency surgical or endoscopic intervention is required.

Vascular ring anomalies

Vascular ring anomalies can mimic esophageal foreign bodies, esophageal strictures, megaesophagus, and other swallowing defects. Presenting signs are a thin, underweight puppy that was gaining and growing well while nursing, but fails to thrive and begins to regurgitate when solid food is introduced. Pups with vascular ring anomalies must be distinguished from those with a cleft palate. Pups with a cleft palate will show milk in the nostrils after nursing and fail to thrive from birth; pups with other swallowing defects become clinically affected at the time of weaning.

Although vascular ring anomalies are always included on the comprehensive differential list, they are far less common than primary megaesophagus. Several different vascular ring anomalies, involving different blood vessels, with and without a patent ductus areteriosium, have been described. Persistent right aortic arch is the most common, with aberrant subclavian arteries second. It is thought to be hereditary.

A vascular ring anomaly is a congenital defect caused by an abnormal location of the great vessels cranial to the heart, leading to entrapment of the esophagus. This anatomic defect interferes with the passage of solid food through the thoracic esophagus. It results in regurgitation. Regurgitation can be clinically distinguished from vomiting by the lack of retching and the tubular shape of the food. A previously well-conditioned pup with a vascular ring anomaly will begin to drop behind its littermates in size at the introduction of solid food, become thin, and may show signs of fever and lung congestion associated with aspiration pneumonia. The breeder may present the pup before it aspirates and has evidence on radiography of pneumonia. Although a dialated esophagus can be seen on survey radiographs, a carefully performed barium swallow is useful in distinguishing megaesophagus from a vascular ring anomaly. Because these conditions differ in treatment and prognosis, the barium swallow should be offered to the client.

Diagnosis is made by clinical suspicion and a barium swallow (esophagram). Take a non-barium survey radiograph to assess the lungs and radiographic technique. Carefully feed a small amount of barium (1 to 5 ml), alone or mixed with meat baby food just prior to the radiographic exposure. Do not use a feeding tube, because it will bypass the portion of the esophagus to be evaluated. The affected pup will have a pouch of barium and food in the esophagus just cranial to the heart. This is distinguished from a normal esophagus (no collection of barium, just slender stripes) or from a megaesophagus (where the barium accumulates in the esophagus but does not end abruptly at the base of the heart).

Fluoroscopy, endoscopy, and angiography may also be indicated in rare cases. There are no specific changes noted on blood tests. The pup may have an elevated white blood cell count with a left shift if aspiration pneumonia is present.

Treatment is surgical, by thoracotomy. There is often poor esophageal motility following surgery, and the prognosis for full recovery is guarded. Bethanachol may improve esophageal motility.

Swallowing defects (Dysphagia)
This is a group of disorders where the dog has difficulty prehending and/or swallowing food. These can include foreign bodies, anatomic defects and neurologic deficits. Observation of the dog attempting to eat is helpful in determining if there is a swallowing defect. Visually inspect for a string under the tongue. If no obvious cause is found referral, for videofluoroscopy and endoscopy, is indicated for a definitive diagnosis.

Sepsis
Sepsis is a common cause of illness or acute death in neonates, and they must be monitored closely. Symptoms can include crying (mewing in puppies), lethargy and weakness or restlessness, a distended belly with a blue hue to the skin, hypothermia, petechial hemorrhages, and discoloration and sloughing of the distal extremities (toe tips, ear and tail tips) or sudden death.

Affected pups may have an increased white blood cell count with a left shift, or a profoundly low white blood cell count due to consumption of the cells. There is often a low blood glucose and low platelet count.

Septicemia should be treated on an emergency basis. Begin supportive care including correction for low body temperature, hypoxia, low blood glucose, and dehydration. Begin antibiotics after collecting appropriate samples for culture. IV or IO antibiotic administration is more reliable when the pups are debilitated. Ceftiofur or amoxicillin/clavulanate potassium are the drugs of choice until culture and sensitivity results are available. Hyperimmunized plasma may also be administered.

Sepsis occurs easily in neonates due to chilling, inadequate colostrum ingestion, hypoglycemia, secondary to viral infection or parasitism, or metritis or mastitis in the dam. Bacteria may enter through the umbilical cord (remember to treat the cord with tincture of iodine solution 3 times in the first 8 hours after birth), gastrointestinal tract, respiratory tract, or skin. A post mortem with bacterial cultures should be performed as soon after death as possible. The information yielded regarding the source of infection might save the remaining littermates.

Herpes
Canine Herpesvirus (CHV) can cause fetal death or early neonatal illness and death. (See previous section in this chapter).

Husbandry problems
Husbandry problems can involve inadequate maternal skills, inadequate food and water, and unsanitary, cold, poorly ventilated, or otherwise unsafe environments. The veterinarian should visit the facility if husbandry problems are suspected. Direct observation of the dogs and their environment is an invaluable tool in resolving these issues.

If this is impractical, photographs, video along with a complete history and physical examinations of the dam and pups can be very useful.

Dermatitis
Infected umbilicus or Omphalitis: A moist, inflamed umbilicus can lead to peritonitis and rapid death. Prevention consists of dipping the cord up to the abdominal wall in tincture of iodine (not Betadine) at birth, 2 hours and 8 hours post-partum until the umbilical cord drops off. The cord typically dries and falls off after 3 days. Diagnosis is made by observation of redness, swelling, and discharge in a sick puppy. Treatment, if diagnosed in time, consists of topical cleansing of the umbilicus and systemic antibiotics. It can be diagnosed post-mortem by the presence of localized or generalized peritonitis or abscesses in the liver and lungs.

Impetigo: Is a common bacterial skin disease in puppies. It is seldom serious. The symptoms include multiple pustules on the unhaired ventral abdomen, near the genitals. Once the pustules rupture, they leave a yellow crusty debris in the area, and may be followed by dark pigment that soon resolves. Treatment may only require antibacterial shampoos such as chlorhexidine or benzoyl peroxide. Systemic antibiotics are a last choice and seldom necessary. This form of staph pyoderma is not indicative of poor health or predictive of long-term skin disease.

Puppy strangles or Juvenile cellulitis
Although this is uncommon in puppies, it is dramatic in its severity and response to treatment. Presenting signs are acute onset of large submandibular lymph nodes (thus the name strangles), deep pyoderma, weeping skin lesions on the lips, around the eyes, and inside the ear flaps and canals, depression, fever, and loss of appetite. Frequently, several to all pups in a litter are affected. Rarely, there is joint involvement with joint swelling and lameness. The drama is in the rapid onset, the number of pups affected, and the poor response to antibiotic therapy (Figure 8-19).

Cytology of the pustules is needed prior to treatment to confirm the presence of cocci and white blood cells. To confirm the diagnosis, skin scrapings and fungal cultures can be collected to rule out other disorders. Additional studies such as skin biopsies are seldom indicated and may delay treatment.

Although this is considered by most to be a bacterial disease, it's failure to respond to antibiotics suggests that there is an associated immune component. It is possible that this is a staphylococcal hypersensitivity. Concurrent therapy with corticosteroids and topical Dome-boro® can lead to rapid and complete resolution. Failure to quickly initiate a combination of antibiotic and corticosteroid therapy can lead to a long course of disease, permanent scarring of the affected areas on the face, and possible death. Appropriate therapy involves the use of a cephalosporin or amoxicillin-clavulanic acid combination at label doses, prednisolone or prednisone at 2.2 mg/kg daily for 14 days with a

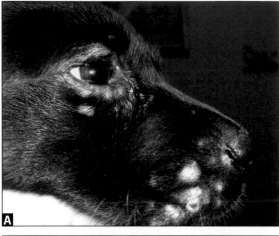

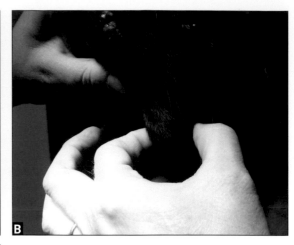

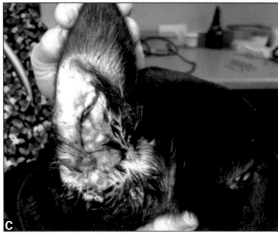

Figure 8-19.
A. Skin lesions on the face of a Labrador Retriever pup with Puppy Strangles or juvenile cellulitis. **B.** Lymphadenopathy caused by puppy strangles or juvenile cellulitis. **C.** Puppy strangles or juvenile cellulitis with exudative lesions inside the pinnae.

slow tapering, and careful application of Dome-boro® solution on cotton pledgets with no rubbing or abrasion. The importance of corticosteroid use cannot be overemphasized.

Pups affected by juvenile cellulitis are often between the ages of 4 weeks and 6 months. The breeds commonly affected are Golden Retrievers and Golden Retriever mixes. This suggests a genetic component.

Demodecosis
Demodex mites are a relatively common cause of hair loss. Dogs with demodex can present at any age, with hair loss in patches on the face, trunk, feet, ears, or generalized hair loss. If more than 6 lesions are identified, it is considered generalized. Approximately 10% of dogs with demodex develop generalized disease.

It can occur in dogs under 1 year of age, and in older dogs with immunosuppressive disorders. It is considered to be a genetic disorder, probably autosomal recessive, caused by abnormalities of both the humoral (antibiodies) and cellular (T cells) immune systems. Demodex in the pediatric patient is not considered predictive for long-term immune system dysfunction. All dogs are considered to be exposed to demodex mites shortly after birth, but only dogs with this specific immune deficiency develop the disease. It is not considered contagious. Dogs with this disorder should be removed from the gene pool.

Dogs with demodex are usually not itchy. They may present with one patch of hair loss, several patches of hair loss with no associated inflammation, lesions on the feet, otitis with no other symptoms, or generalized hair loss that usually starts on the face or feet. It may also present as a pustular dermatitis. In generalized cases, the dog may present ill, with a fever and generalized lymphadenopathy.

The pattern of hair loss is suggestive of demodex but should be confirmed by identifying demodex mites on deep skin scrapings. Areas of suspected demodex should be scraped with a slightly dull scalpel blade, while squeezing the skin, until blood shows. The material should be placed in oil on a glass microscope slide with a coverslip, and examined at 40x. Rarely, skin biopsies are needed to make the diagnosis.

Until recently, generalized demodex was sometimes fatal. The development of new parasiticides has made it highly treatable.

Treatment of demodex
Goodwinol ointment (rotenone) has been used for decades to treat individual lesions. If demodex becomes generalized following treatment with Goodwinol, it is not a treatment failure.

Patients with associated pyodermas should be treated with antibacterial shampoos and systemic antibiotics prior to the use of topical miticides.

Amitraz as a dip is the only FDA approved product for the treatment of generalized canine demodex. The label directions are complete. In some states, only personnel with pesticide training are permitted to apply the product. Prior to treatment, the patient should have the hair clipped with a 40 blade. The pet should be bathed with benzoyl peroxide shampoo the day before dipping. The applier should wear gloves and protective eyewear. The dip should be diluted according to label directions, with a fresh dilution for each treatment. Apply it to the entire body for 15 minutes, with the feet covered by dip, and allowed to air dry (no toweling or blow-drying). The dips should be applied every 2 weeks for at least 3 treatments, and 1 month beyond 2 consecutive negative skin scrapes at 1 month intervals. Many dogs are lethargic for 24 hours after treatment. Some also develop itching and redness of the skin, diarrhea, and low body temperature. Toy breed pups should be closely observed after treatment and may require supportive care.

Up to 40% of dogs will not resolve completely with amitraz treatment. Some will need intermittent treatment throughout their lifetimes, while in others, the disease resolves after they mature. Extralabel use of amitraz at higher doses and higher frequency may be required.

Other treatment options include ivermectin, milbemycin, and an amitraz-metaflumizone combination product. Some dogs are highly sensitive to these products and they should be used carefully. It is advisable to use the MDR1 test to evaluate the patient's tolerance for these drugs prior to initiating treatment.

Neonatal ophthalmia
This is a true emergency in the neonate that has not yet opened its eyes. It is obvious clinically. The diagnosis is made on the observation of a swelling behind the eyelid(s) and/or purulent drainage from the inner corner of the eye.

All breeder clients should be educated to monitor their pups for this. If it is suspected or observed, the affected pups should be seen by the veterinarian immediately. The treatment consists of gently opening the eyelids. Soften the lid margins with baby shampoo and a warm compress. The lids can be manipulated open by using dry gauze on the fingers for traction. If this is unsuccessful, a curved mosquito forceps can be carefully used to open the seal between the eyelids. Collect a sample of the purulent discharge for culture and sensitivity testing. Staphylococcus is the most common organism cultured. All affected pups should be treated with an antibiotic ophthalmic ointment preparation.

All affected eyelids should be opened. In some cases, opening the eyelids on all the puppies in the litter is indicated. Frequently, purulent material is found behind eyelids not yet showing distention. Opening the lids prematurely will not cause damage to the pup's vision. Failure to treat this condition promptly may lead to permanent eye damage.

The condition has been attributed to pups raised in unsanitary surroundings. However, experience shows this has not been the case – in fact, this is seen in households where the pups are kept fastidiously clean. Be cautious in communicating to clients that they may not be raising pups in sanitary conditions (Figure 8-20).

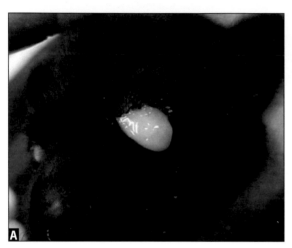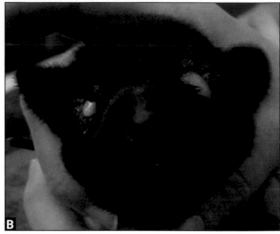

Figure 8-20.
A & B. A 1 week old pup with a purulent ocular discharge. This condition, known as neonatal ophthalmia requires opening the eyelids and treating promptly to prevent permanent damage to the eyes.

Birth defects
Birth defects are defined as abnormalities of structure, function, or body metabolism that are present at birth. Over 4,000 are known in humans. It is not possible to make a comprehensive list.

The most common structural defects in neonates include the cleft palate, heart defects, umbilical hernia, gastroschisis and omphalocele (open abdominal wall), spina bifida, underweight neonate, swimmer puppy, and abnormal rear legs. The following defects should be recognized early and are often treatable.

Cleft palete
This defect is visible with a good oral examination and good lighting. All veterinary staff should be trained to evaluate pups for this at assisted births or when a pup is presented for failure to thrive. Clients can be instructed to look for this at the time of the pup's birth. Often, the shape of the head is different in the affected pup; experienced staff will frequently detect this at delivery.

Although this is surgically correctable in some cases, management until surgery is taxing on the owner. Tube feeding is recommended until the pup is old and large enough for surgical intervention. Allowing the pup to nurse or eat and drink from a dish can lead to aspiration pneumonia in many cases. Some pups have multiple other defects, making correction of the palate defect impractical. After surgery, some pups will require a soft diet for the rest of their lives to prevent perforation of the unsupported soft tissue by dry dog kibble, hard treats and chew toys. Some clients find managing these pups to be rewarding. Most clients opt for euthanasia when the defect is discovered or if the management becomes too difficult.

Heart defects
All pups should be ausculted for murmurs within a few hours to days of birth. They should have a complete physical examination including careful thoracic auscultation, in a quiet setting prior to placement in their adoptive homes. Most murmurs are audible by 6 weeks, but some will not be noted until the dog is an adult.

Many murmurs that are audible in the very young are innocent and will disappear as the pup matures. All murmurs should be noted and the breeder should consider advanced evaluation of the pup's cardiac function prior to placement in homes if the murmur persists beyond 8 weeks.

Some murmurs are benign and others result in a very short life expectancy. Some can be surgically corrected and some can be managed medically. The cause of most murmurs cannot be definitively identified with auscultation, so any murmur that persists or any pup with clinical signs associated with the murmur (such as a small pup that tires easily) should be referred to a cardiologist prior to sale or if kept by the breeder.

Umbilical hernia
Keep the umbilicus clean and disinfected until the cord dries and falls off. Very large or vulnerable hernias should be corrected prior to the sale of the pup. Smaller stable hernias can be corrected by the new owner, often at the time of the spay or neuter. Nearly all umbilical hernias are inherited (they are not usually caused by trauma to the umbilicus at birth), they are not serious and are easily corrected. Many breeders will use the affected dogs for breeding. Compared to other more serious defects that are life-threatening, using these dogs for breeding is not the sign of an irresponsible breeder.

Gastroschisis and omphalocele
These are relatively common defects in the newborn human and puppy. Gastroschisis is a defect in the abdominal wall, not at the umbilicus, but usually just right of it, allowing intestines and other abdominal contents to be exposed. The exposed abdominal contents are not covered by peritoneum. It is a genuine emergency requiring immediate surgical correction. It is not usually associated with other defects and the pup often will do well if the surgery is prompt and goes well, and antibiotics are used. Omphalocele is an opening around the umbilicus, where gut is exposed but covered by peritoneum, and requires requires prompt attention. A primary difference between gastroschisis and omphalocele is that an omphalocele is caused by failure of the 3 portions of the embryonic gut to form correctly. Because of this embryonic error, a portion of the gut may be incomplete and difficult to detect in neonates. In humans, both of these defects are detected by ultrasound, allowing Caesarean intervention and immediate care. In pups, they are usually born with no advance awareness. Usually only a single pup is affected in the litter and heritability in the dog is unknown. It is not thought to be heritable in humans where it is most common in mothers under 30 that are smokers.

Whether born by vaginal birth or C-section, the umbilicus should be closely examined at birth. If any defect is noted, the area should be covered with a moist sterile dressing and the pup immediately transported for surgery. Some pups with gastroschisis (over 75% in the author's experience) can be saved by rapid intervention if the intestines are not compromised. Many of these dogs enjoy normal lives with no other associated defects.

Correction of an abdominal wall defect is best achieved by immediate surgery. Anesthetize the pup by face mask gas anesthesia (intubation is often difficult due to the small size of the patient). Prep the area with a disinfectant that will not harm exposed tissues. Use sterile gloves and a sterile pack. A stomach tube may be passed to relieve gas, making it easier to return the gut to the abdominal cavity. The defect in the abdominal wall may need to be enlarged to allow the exposed contents to be repositioned without force. A 2 layer closure is sufficient. The first layer, the linea, should be closed with a simple interrupted pattern of 3-0 or 4-0 absorbable suture. The subcutaneous layer is not visible in most newborns. The second layer, the skin, can be closed with the same suture or a non-absorbable suture. The umbilical cord should remain exposed, and may need to be ligated to prevent hemorrhage. The pup can be discharged to the owner with its littermates. The incision should be kept clean with tamed iodine or chlorhexidine. Administer systemic antibiotics, usually amoxicillin-clavulanic acid drops or injectable ceftiofur, to prevent peritonitis. Pups with gastroschisis can usually be saved, while those with omphaloceles do not have as high a rate of survival rate due to associated multiple gastrointestinal and thoracic wall defects (Figure 8-21E and F).

Spina bifida
This is another midline defect, like umbilical hernias and cleft palates, but much more rare. There is little information regarding treatment. Some pups will survive without intervention if the defect is mild (Figure 8-21A).

Underweight newborn
Often this pup is normal other than its small stature. Commonly, the pup was crowded or had poor placental blood flow. With supportive nutritional care, those with no associated defects will often thrive (Figure 8-22A).

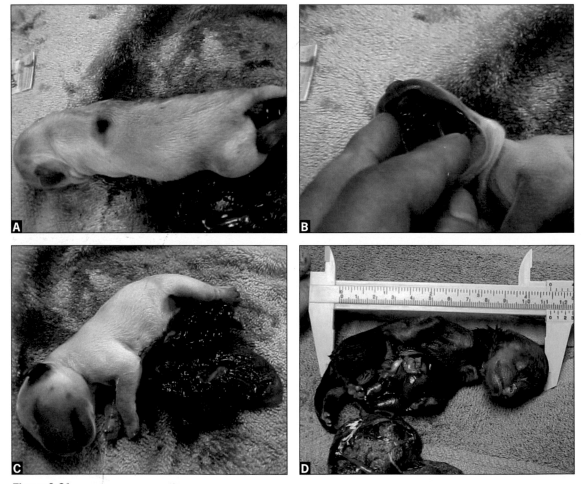

Figure 8-21.
A-C. Newborn pup with 3 midline defects: cleft palate, spina bifida and open abdominal wall. **D.** Neonatal pup born with open abdominal wall and open eyelids.

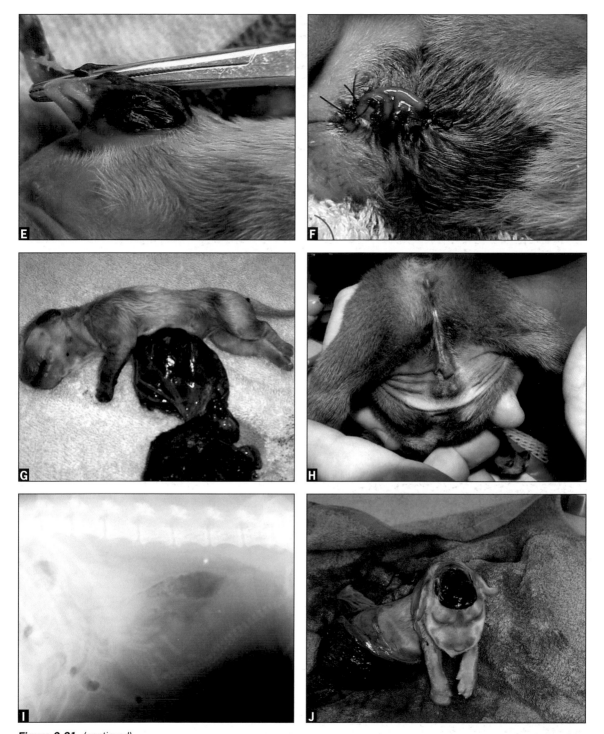

Figure 8-21. (continued)

E. *Neonatal pup born with gastroschisis.* ***F.*** *Neonatal pup born with gastroschisis with a successful repair of the defect done immediately after birth.* ***G.*** *Neonatal pup born with open thoracic wall. This pup did not survive.* ***H.*** *A newborn pup with hypospadias, a failure of the midline to close. This pup survived* ***I.*** *A radiograph of a bitch with distocia. The pup was known to have anencephaly prior to delivery by C-section.* ***J.*** *A neonatal pup born with anencephaly.*

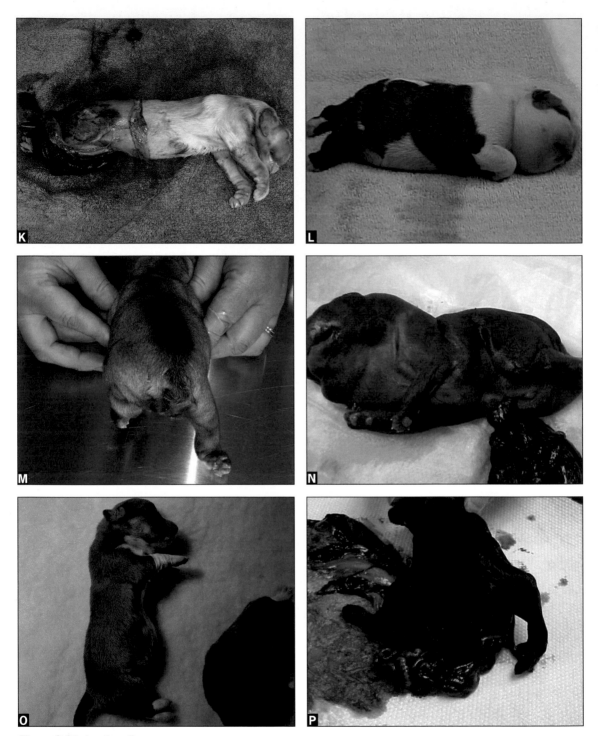

Figure 8-21. *(continued)*
K. *A neonatal pup born with anencephaly. The pup did not survive.* ***L.*** *Severe anasarca or walrus puppy. This puppy could not breath and did not survive.* ***M.*** *A neonatal English Bulldog pup born with the feet rotated. Within a few days, this will self – correct.* ***N.*** *A neonatal pup born with multiple defects. This pup did not survive.* ***O.*** *A Pembroke Welsh Corgi pup with a thoracic wall defect which developed 3 days after birth. In mild cases, some of these pups survive.* ***P.*** *Neonatal pup born with schistosomus reflexus. This pup did not survive.*

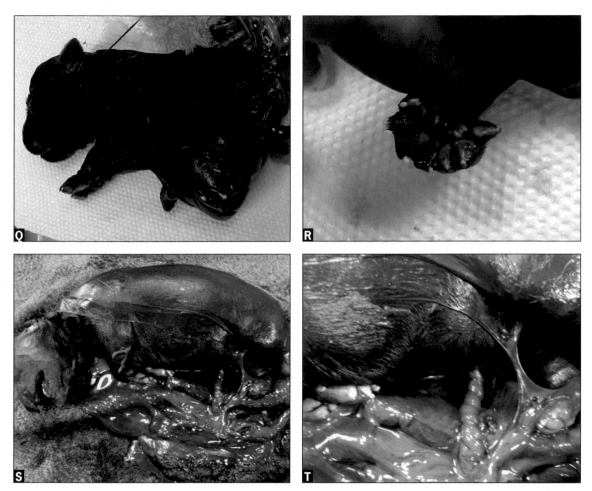

Figure 8-21. (continued)
*Q. Neonatal pup born with schistosomus reflexus. This pup did not survive. **R.** Neonatal pup born with Schistosomas Reflexus and a paw with extra toes. This pup did not survive. **S.** Pup stillborn at C-section, appears to have died several days prior to birth due to inadequate blood flow to the pup through the twisted umbilical cord. **T.** Close up of the twisted umbilical cord in the previous illustration.*

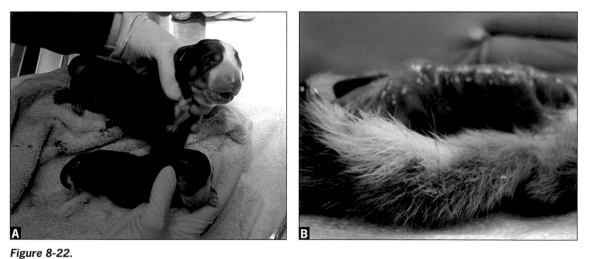

Figure 8-22.
*A. Littermate neonatal pups with size disparity due to placental dysfunction. **B.** Pembroke Welsh Corgi pup with ribcage defect seen at post mortem demonstrating extreme deviation of shape of thorax. This developed at the 3rd day of life, was not present at delivery by C-section.*

Swimmer puppies

Swimmer pups have a flattened chest wall and difficulty supporting their weight on their legs. This "diagnosis" is based on the appearance of the pup. Swimmers need to be distinguished from a more severe form of thoracic wall defect, pectus excavatum, which has a poor prognosis.

They are usually normal in appearance at birth, but change quickly by several days to weeks of age. Some are very heavy relative to their littermates. Providing better footing on an egg-crate mattress will prevent them from laying flat on a hard flat surface. Some breeders hobble the legs together, but this must be done carefully to prevent compromising blood flow to the lower limbs. As they begin to walk, some breeders place them for several short sessions a day in a U-shaped narrow carpeted trough with high sides to help support their weight. With supportive care, many will improve (Figures 8-22B and 8-7C and D).

Abnormal rear legs

Some pups, particularly English Bulldogs, are born with the lower portion of their rear legs twisted. The hocks are often rotated laterally and the paws are rotated upward. Euthanasia at birth is not advised. The legs often roll into a normal position by 4 to 7 days of age and have "normal" ambulation as they mature Figures 8-7B-D and 8-21M).

Seizures

Seizures occur in patients of all ages. Determining if the patient had a seizure or other type of episode can be difficult. Other syndromes that can mimic seizures include: cardiac episodes, pain, intense itching, or other behaviors.

Seizures may be divided into 2 categories: intracranial and extracranial. Intracranial causes include epilepsy, trauma, inflammatory lesions, and hydrocephalus. Extracranial causes include metabolic diseases such as hypoglycemia, portosystemic shunts and toxicity. Inborn errors of metabolism are a rare cause of seizures in the dog, but can be intracranial or extracranial.

Evaluate extracranial causes first. Hypoglycemia (glucose < 40 mg/dl) is easily determined. If suspected, a blood should be drawn before treatment is initiated.

If the glucose is normal without supplementation, evaluate for a portosystemic shunt with bile acid or blood ammonia testing. Treat the patient symptomatically based on a presumption of a shunt while diagnostics are pending.

Often, the dog suspected of a portosystemic shunt is a small pup who does not keep up mentally and physically with its littermates. Some may seize and show other neurologic signs of circling, ataxia and disorientation; some are very quiet; and some may just have unusual behavior, particularly after high protein meals. Some dogs are not diagnosed until they are older and other symptoms develop such as bile-containing bladder stones. (See section Nutritional Support earlier in this chapter.)

In some cases, the presence of a shunt can be confirmed by abdominal ultrasound. There are 2 general types of shunts – intra-hepatic and extra-hepatic. Surgical correction of the intra-hepatic shunt is very difficult and often cannot be accomplished. An extra-hepatic shunt is somewhat easier to access, but requires a skilled surgeon. Some surgeons ligate this abnormal vasculature while others use an embolization coil to correct this vascular flow defect. The patient will require careful pre-op and post-op management with medications to reduce the likelihood of seizures and other complications.

> **Managing theportosystemic shunt patient medically prior to surgery to minimize symptoms. Management includes the use of:**
> 1. **Metronidazole** to reduce the ammonia levels produced by anaerobic bacteria.
> 2. **Lactulose** to decrease GI transit time and minimize ammonia absorption from the gut.
> 3. **Medications** such as propofol, sodium and potassium bromide, and levetiracetam to manage seizures and reduce the probability of post-op seizure complications.
> 4. **Low protein diet.**
> 5. **Proton pump** of H-2 blockers if indicated for GI bleeding.
> 6. **Manitol, furosemide and mild hypothermia** to manage elevated intracranial pressure.

Inflammation in the CNS is a documented cause of seizure in the dog. Although rare in most regions, canine distemper virus remains a cause of acute encephalitis in young dogs with inadequate immunity. Seizures caused by canine distemper are difficult to manage with medications. Other causes include bacterial disease in the brain, Cryptococcus, Toxoplasmosis, Ehrlichiosis, and steroid-responsive meningoencephalomyelitis.

Trauma may lead to seizures within a few days of the event. The seizures may be progressive.

Toxins are a common cause of seizures, particularly in the pediatric patient with a tendency to ingest inappropriate products. The list of toxins is long. Diagnosis and treatment depend on the agent involved. Consultation with the ASPCA's National Animal Poison Control Center at 1-800-548-2423 should be recommended to the client if a toxin is suspected.

Intracranial causes of seizures include trauma, hydrocephalus, inborn errors of metabolism, hypoxia at birth, inflammation, infection, parasitism, and idiopathic epilepsy. Specific diagnostics include: ultrasound of the brain to assess the size of the ventricles of the brain if the fontanelle is open; CSF tap; EEG; and MRI or CT scan. In many cases, advanced diagnostics are not an option or may be delayed by the need for referral. Presumptive treatment may need to be initiated (Figure 8-23).

Hydrocephalus may be suspected based on a dome-shape skull (can use littermates for comparison) and an open fontanelle. Breeds at increased risk include Boston terriers, Chihuahuas, Pomeranians, Pugs and Toy Poodles. Pups with hydrocephalus may be disoriented, slower to learn than littermates, and seize. Confirm the diagnosis by ultrasound of the brain if there is access through the open fontanelle to assess the size of the ventricles, MRI, CT, and EEG. Presumptive treatment should

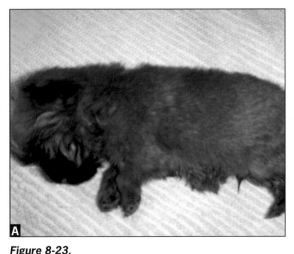 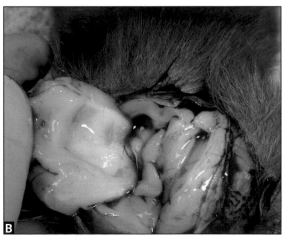

Figure 8-23.
A. Terrier pup with hydrocephalus at euthanasia. *B.* Same pup with skull opened at post mortem showing ventricles of the brain with thinned walls due to fluid accumulation.

include prednisone (0.25 mg/kg to 0.5 mg/kg once daily to BID) and furosemide (0.5 mg/kg to 2.0 mg/kg once daily to BID) to reduce CSF accumulation. Some patients are candidates for shunt placement for better long-term management, but these are not without complications. The long-term prognosis is guarded.

Seizures caused by hypoxia prior to and at birth may be seen in very young neonates. You may only be able to offer supportive care and patience while the brain is allowed to heal.

If idiopathic epilepsy is suspected, based on age, breed, and elimination of other possible causes, and the seizures are progressively worsening, treatment may be necessary.

Breeds commonly affected by idiopathic epilepsy include: Beagles, Belgian Tervurens, Boxers, Cocker Spaniels, Collies, Dachshunds, Dalmatians, German Shepherds, Golden Retrievers, Irish Setters, Irish Wolfhounds, Keeshonden, Labrador Retrievers, Pointers, Poodles (all varieties), Saint Bernards, Schnauzers (miniature and standard), Siberian Huskies, Vizslas, Welsh Springer Spaniels, and Wire Haired Fox Terriers. The most common age range is 4 months to 5 years. It appears to be heritable, so affected dogs should not be included in the breeding program.

Treatment for suspected or diagnosed idiopathic epilepsy is initiated when justified by the frequency or severity of the seizures. Emergency management using injectable diazepam, barbiturates and sodium bromide may be indicated. Long-term treatment with oral phenobarbital and/or potassium bromide may be useful. These drugs can be used in puppies as young as 12 weeks, and even younger if necessary. Use lower doses in younger pups. Serum levels can be used to fine-tune the dosages. If the seizures are well controlled, slow withdrawal of medications may be indicated after 6 months of therapy.

Anasarca or "Walrus" or "Water" puppy
Anasarca pups, also known as walrus or water puppies, are pups born with excessive fluid accumulation in their subcutaneous tissues. It is most commonly seen in English bulldogs, but has been recognized in many other unrelated breeds. The cause is not understood. It usually affects one puppy in a litter, although entire litters have been affected.

These pups are profoundly abnormal in gross appearance at birth. They are very heavy and the skin is distended with subcutaneous fluid. Some appear to respond to treatment.

Assure that the airway is open and the pup is breathing. If the breathing is spontaneous, administer face mask oxygen. Tracheal intubation may be indicated but is often very difficult as the edema makes visualizing the tracheal opening nearly impossible. Retrograde intubation may be attempted. If intubation and ventilation is possible, initiate it at once to a non-breathing pup with a pulse. If there is no pulse, further resuscitation efforts may not be indicated.

Once the pup is breathing or is being ventilated, administer furosemide by injection. There is controversy regarding the success and specifics of therapy. Because furosemide is not contraindicated and the cost is reasonable, the effort is probably worthwhile. The prognosis is highly variable and some pups survive if mildly affected. The cause is unknown, but a heritable component is suspected.

There is a protocol widely circulated on the internet that may be requested by clients. Accurate application of the protocol is difficult and it is likely to result in overhydration as the excessive fluid from the subcutaneous tissues enters the circulation. Treatment failures occur if the airway is obstructed by excess fluid or if pleural effusion is so severe that the lungs cannot inflate. Diuretic use is reasonable, but Potassium must be supplemented to prevent excessive loss on day 2 of treatment.

Theoretically, the pregnant bitch could be monitored for excessive weight gain and if noted, that she be treated with a diuretic. However, assessing what her exact weight gain should be is difficult if only one affected pup is present.

The following protocol is presented by Dr. Hoskins:
1. Provide an open airway and keep the pup in a warm location with its littermates.
2. Weigh the pup and record the weight in grams or ounces.
3. Administer a dose of 0.2 ml furosemide IM.
4. Weigh a "normal" sized littermate for comparison.
5. Determine the difference in weight between the normal and affected pup and record this.
6. Move the affected pup frequently and stimulate urination.
8. Reweigh and record the affected pup's weight every 3 hours. Keep the pup warm.
9. Repeat the furosemide injection every 3 hours until the affected pup weighs no more than 45 grams or 1.5 ounces more than a normal littermate. Discontinue the furosemide when the pup has been reduced in size to within 45 grams of a normal littermate.
10. Every 3 hours, administer 1 meq of potassium chloride for every 30 gms or 1 ounce of weight lost. The potassium chloride can be administered orally. A 10% potassium chloride solution contains 1 meq in 1 ml (1 ml = 20 drops). Discontinue the potassium chloride when the furosemide is discontinued.

Feeding in the critical period (Recipes)
Tube feeding directions (See Appendix C-15)

Materials:
1. Goat's milk, (pasteurized is preferred), or commercial milk replacer
2. Feeding tube, silicon or red rubber feeding tube 5 to 14 French
3. Permanent magic marker
4. Syringe of appropriate size
5. Puppy scale
6. Rectal thermometer

Steps:
1. Establish a well-lit warm location where you can hold the pup comfortably and all materials are within reach. Be attentive and do not rush.
2. Take the puppy's temperature rectally - do NOT feed unless the rectal temperature is between 96° F and 99° F. If the temperature is below 96° F, gently warm the pup before feeding.
3. On a safe surface, hold the pup with the neck extended. Hold the tapered end of the feeding tube even with the last rib of the largest pup to be fed. Lay the tube along the side of the pup, mark the tube even with the tip of the pup's nose. The tube should be marked (Figure 8-24).
4. Fill the syringe with the calculated amount of formula or milk (20 cc/16 oz body weight or approximately 1 cc per ounce of body weight) plus 1 cc of air. Pre-warm the formula to body temperature in a warm water bath – avoid microwaving. Feedings should be administered every 3 to 6 hours as indicated by weight gain and hydration status (Figure 8-25).
5. Attach the syringe to the feeding tube.
6. With the pup fully awake, warm (over 96° F rectal temp) lying horizontally on the chest, gently pass the tube over the center of the pups tongue, applying gentle pressure to slide the tube up to the mark. Keep the pup's chin below its ears and pass the tube along the left side of the throat to reduce the chance of mistakenly introducing the tube into the trachea instead of the esophagus. If resistance is met, remove the tube and start over.
7. If you are right handed, cup your left hand around the back of the pups head and hold the tube between your index and middle finger of the left hand to prevent it from moving out of the correct position while feeding. Reverse this if you are left handed (Figure 8-26).

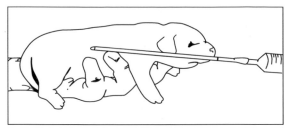

Figure 8-24.
Hold the pup with the neck extended. Hold tapered end of the feeding tube even with the last rib of the largest pup to be fed. Lay the tube along the side of the pup and mark the tube even with the tip of the pup's nose.

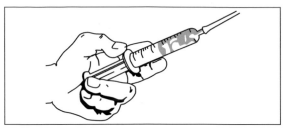

Figure 8-25.
Fill the syringe with the calculated amount of formula or milk (20 cc/16 oz body weight) plus 1 cc of air and attach the syringe to the feeding tube.

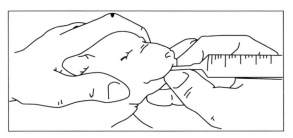

Figure 8-26.
With your left hand if you are right handed, cup your left hand around the back of the pups' head. Hold the tube between your index and middle finger of your left hand to prevent it from moving out of the correct position while feeding.

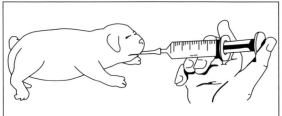

Figure 8-27.
Depress the plunger on the syringe, not too quickly, delivering the calculated amount of formula or milk.

8. BEFORE FEEDING, firmly pinch the pup on the foot or tail. If the pup vocalizes, the tube placement is correct and you can proceed with feeding. If the tube is mistakenly in the trachea, the pup will struggle but will not be able to make any sound – STOP IMMEDIATELY, REMOVE THE TUBE AND START THE PROCESS OVER.

9. With your right hand, depress the plunger on the syringe, NOT too quickly, delivering the calculated amount of formula followed by the 1 cc of air, stopping sooner should milk reflux out of the mouth or nose (Figure 8-27).

10. Flex the tube on itself to prevent milk from being aspirated in to the pup's airway. Repeat for each pup.

11. Wash syringe and tube with hot soapy water and allow to air dry until next feeding.

12. Stimulate the external anal and urinary orifices with a warm moistened cotton ball or washcloth to effect defecation and urination.

Remember the 5 P's of safe tube feeding:
1. Premeasure the tube
2. Pass with the chin down
3. Pass along the left side
4. Pinch to assure the pup can vocalize before feeding
5. Prewarm the pup and formula before feeding

Hand-rearing the orphaned, sick, cleft palate, or abandoned pup
Hand-raising may be necessary if the mother dies or is too ill to care for the pups. It may be required if the bitch refuses to care for one or more pups or if she fails to lactate. It may be indicated if the pup is too sick to nurse on its own or if a cleft palate prevents the pup from nursing without aspirating the milk. Only a few feedings may be needed until the pups become competitive with littermates.

Pups raised without their mothers must be kept warm – at 90° F to 95° F. They must also be stimulated to urinate and defecate at each feeding and wiped with a damp towel at least once a day.

In any of these circumstances, tube or bottle feeding must be used. Some pups, if healthy enough not to aspirate, may take a bottle. Most pups will require a feeding tube. Multiple tube feedings are possible each day for most pups and for most breeders.

If long-term nutritional support is needed, a naso-esophageal tube may be placed and sutured in place. If the pup can be anesthetized, or is so sick that anesthesia is not necessary, an esophagostomy feeding tube may be placed.

If the pup is totally dependent upon this form of feeding, feed at a rate of 1 cc per 1 oz of body weight. Initially feedings may be needed every 2 to 3 hours around the clock. Feedings can be further apart as the pups gain strength. Skipping the middle of the night feeding first is a practical way to begin adjusting the schedule.

Dish feeding can start for hand-raised pups at 2 weeks of age, gruel at 3 to 4 weeks, and puppy food at 5 to 6 weeks if they are able to eat and swallow normally.

Raising the "Singleton" puppy

Sometimes, only one pup is born or survives. Appropriate calorie intake is a primary concern; some bitches over-lactate and some have scant milk production The bitch may require medications (metoclopramide or domperidone) to lactate. If the pup is being hand-raised, frequent feedings and an adequate formula are needed to assure good growth with minimal diarrhea. IF the pup never received colostrum, hyperimmunized plasma should be administered by oral or subcutaneous route. (See section on Passive Immunity earlier in this chapter). If the pup is overeating, the time allowed to nurse may need to be restricted.

Appropriate stimulation is also a concern. These pups are frequently spoiled by their dam and owners. They never have the normal frustration or tactile stimulation that pups raised with littermates experience. Unless these experiences are provided by their owners, many of these pups will grow up with unusual and sometimes dangerous personalities.

Dr. Patricia McConnell (personal consultation) recommends that the pup be handled several times daily from day 1 on. Several times a day, it should be pushed off the nipple while nursing by a human holding a stuffed animal to simulate competition at the nipple (frustration) and touch (tactile stimulation). Once the pup is larger and can begin to interact, it should be exposed to age and size appropriate puppies to enhance social skill development. If the bitch is not available, supervised exposure to an appropriate adult dog may also enhance the development of social skills. Frequent human interaction in a typical household (not isolated kennel) setting is also important to allow the pup to integrate into a human family. The first critical social period for pups ends at 12 to 16 weeks, so appropriate social interaction must be started by 8 weeks of age or younger to prevent the development of fearful or aggressive behavior.

In special circumstances, a surrogate mother and/or littermates may be a solution. There is a potential liability to both the owner of the bitch (that the pups may expose her bitch and pups to disease) and to the owner of the pups (that the bitch and other pups may expose the pups to disease and that the bitch and/or pups may cause trauma to the newly-introduced pups).

Taildocking and dewclaw removal

Removal of dewclaws and taildocking are often requested by breeders. Both procedures are under consideration for change in the United States. The surgery is usually done when the pups are 3 to 5 days old, during their first veterinary visit.

Vital signs and a thorough history are needed on all the pups prior to surgery. Vital signs include temperature, weight, weight gain since birth, urine color on a cotton ball, heart and respiratory rates. If the pups are not identified by the breeder, they can be marked with colored markers. As part of the examination, auscultate the chest and check the mouth of every pup for cleft palate.

If the pups are vigorous, the dewclaws can be removed at their dam's C-section. Taildocks should not be done at C-section. The change in relative size of the pup to its own tail by 3 to 5 days is surprising; taildocks should be done at this age to improve the accuracy of tail length. Additionally, taildocking is more stressful so is better done once the pups are gaining weight.

Local anesthesia may be used. Use the appropriate doses of lidocaine in the neonate, to avoid toxicity. General anesthesia is not routinely used for these procedures at this early age.

Dewclaw removal

Prep the pup for surgery. The veterinary assistant should hold the pup in lateral recumbency parallel to the table, with 1 hand supporting the head and shoulders and the other hand supporting the rump. All the feet should be pointed toward the veterinarian, with the dorsum of the pup toward the assistant. The hand supporting the head and shoulders can also be used to extend and restrain the most ventral forelimb.With the index finger of the assistant cranial to the elbow and the 3rd finger of the assistant caudal and proximal to the elbow, the limb can be held in abduction. This allows the veterinarian to manipulate the foot without having to pull. Prep the dewclaw with 1 or more scrubs of Nolvasan® or Betadine®. The veterinarian gently holds the foot closest to the table with pressure on the carpal pad. Using a curved iris scissor, make an incision in 1 cut in the area where the skin reflects along the dewclaw. The scissors should be parallel to the long axis of the leg, at approximately a 45° angle from caudal to cranial. Carefully remove the pad associated with the dewclaw. Make a second incision with the tip of the iris scissor to remove the remaining bone fragment of the dewclaw. Without removing pressure from the carpal pad, to maintain hemostasis, place a drop of surgical glue around the rim of skin and slide the skin into apposition. If necessary, styptic powder and/or direct pressure can be used to control hemostasis. A hemostat is often used to crush or pull the dewclaw off, but this does not leave as pleasing a cosmetic result. The objective is to leave a clean looking leg with no bump, pad, and scar at the surgical site. Silver nitrate sticks are often used for hemostasis, but they burn the pups, causing increased discomfort. **ALWAYS** check for dewclaws on both rear legs because they are variably present in some pups within the same litter (Figure 8-28A-E).

Taildocking

Tail length is the most important concern. The best way to assure the correct length is to request that the breeder mark the tail at the preferred length.

There is great variation in preferred tail length, even within the same breed or litter. Charts are available with specific measurements in fractions of inches or millimeters, calculations based on the percentage to take or leave, where the tail meets the tip of the vulva, how many vertebrae to leave, where the tail changes width, which coin (nickel, quarter, etc.) to use under the tail to measure, and so on. The question of whether to measure from the top of the tail or under the tail at the rectum remains. Variation can be dependent on the size and age of the pup. If the breeder leaves the decision of length up to the veterinarian, it is recommended to use a table with published standard lengths. The veterinarian will be relieved of fault if they follow the breeder's preferences (Figure 8-28F-K).

The sterile surgical pack for taildocks includes: 1 Serrated Straight Mayo Scissors, 1 pair of Needle Holders, 1 pair of thumb Forceps, 1 Mosquito Hemostat, 1 pair of curved Iris Scissors and sterile gauze squares.

Clip the hair from the tail, before or after the length is marked by the breeder using a permanent black

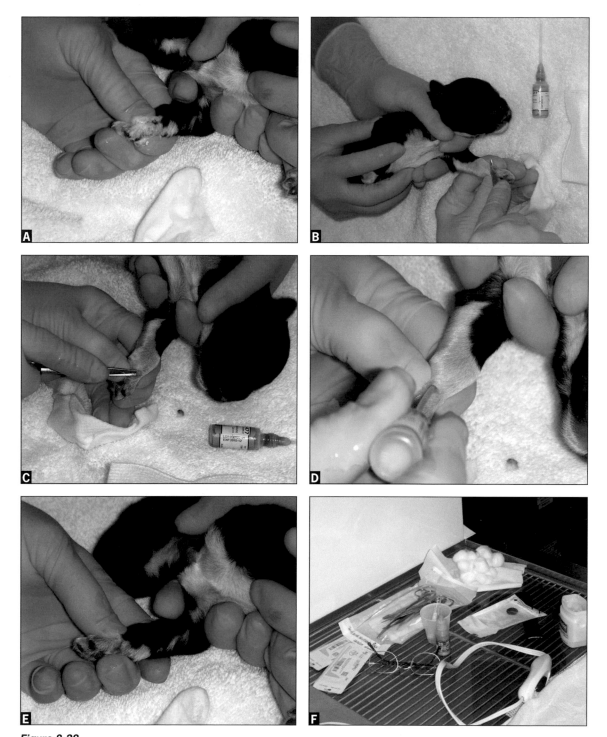

Figure 8-28.
A. Surgical preparation of the dewclaw for excision. **B.** Making the first incision to remove the dewclaw. **C.** Making the second incision to remove the remaining portion of bone from the declaw excision. **D.** Closing the dewclaw excision site with surgical glue. **E.** Dewclaw excision completed and closed. **F.** Surgical instruments and supplies ready for taildock procedure.

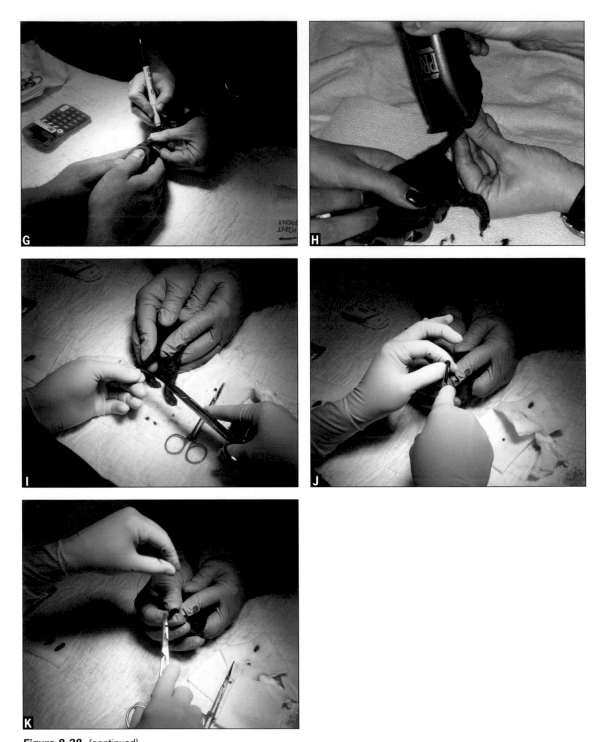

Figure 8-28. (continued)
G. Marking the tail length with a permanent marker and ruler prior to docking the tail. The client's input is invaluable in this decision. **H.** Shaving the tail in preparation for docking. **I.** Making the horizontal incision to dock the tail. The scissors are best held horizontally for a long taildock and vertically when the tail is to be shorter, near the rectum. **J.** After the tail is docked, use the iris scissors to remove the remaining portion of the transected vertebrae, allowing the skin to be pulled over the tip of the tail to minimize tension on the sutures and scarring. **K.** Closing the taildock site with sutures.

marker or tissue pen. Use a sterile pack, and prep with Nolvasan® or Betadine. Stimulate the pups to defecate prior to the procedure.

The assistant holds the head at a 45° angle down, with the legs directed ventrally. The assistant can use both hands to support the pup and restrain the legs. The assistant must be careful not to restrict the pup's breathing.

If the tail is to be docked level to the rectum, leaving no vertebrae or only 1 vertebra, the scissor is held perpendicular to the table and angled 45° cranially. Carefully avoid catching the rectal mucosa in the scissors. In 1 firm cut, the entire tail should be transected from ventral to dorsal, using a serrated Mayo scissor. Use the tip of the iris scissors to remove the remaining bone fragment. Close the wound using 4-0 Vicryl® in a continuous suture pattern.

The procedure is done differently If the tail is to be docked leaving several vertebrae. The scissors are held parallel to the table going from right to left (left to right if left-handed). Two techniques may be used for the incision. One is to make the cut in 1 incision straight across the tail, but with the upper blade of the scissors angled more caudally than the lower blade. This creates a flap of skin longer dorsally than ventrally, allowing the skin to be sutured on the underside of the tail. This creates less scarring.

The alternative is to make 2 cuts from proximal to distal, meeting in a V pattern in the center of the tail. This also allows a flap to form, reducing scarring.

With either technique, the extra piece of vertebrae is removed with iris scissors and 1 or more interrupted sutures of 4-0 Vicryl® are placed in the skin. The sutures can be removed 24 to 48 hours after placement to reduce scarring which is particularly noticeable in some short-coated breeds. Styptic powder can be applied along with direct pressure if necessary to achieve hemostasis. Consistency in the order of removal reduces the likelihood that the surgeon will overlook removing some of the dewclaws, particularly when the pup has dewclaws on the rear legs.

Feeding and housing at weaning
The veterinarian should understand basic husbandry to serve as a resource for the client.

Pups can be weaned between 3 and 6 weeks of age. Some bitches will wean the pups on their own, while others need to be separated from the pups. Many breeders use a plastic child's swimming pool (without the molded slide) to house the pups. It can be encircled by an exercise pen (X pen) to minimize escapes. To prevent slipping, bedding can be provided. Shallow food and water dishes should be used. A drinking bottle is an easy way to keep the pups dry and provide a constant source of clean drinking water. Pups quickly learn to use this drinking bottle if baby food is applied to the tip to draw their attention. Be certain all of them are using it effectively before it is used as their only source of drinking water.

Many pups will begin to housebreak if given the opportunity. Some breeders allow the pups to follow their mother outdoors to eliminate. Alternatively, a shallow plastic tray (like a litter box) filled with pine shavings or shredded newspaper can be provided. Many pups will use the tray. Avoid the use of cedar shavings because they are too aromatic. At adoption, send some of the litter material with the puppy to help them identify an appropriate location to eliminate. This works best on shorter-coated dogs.

By 6 weeks, the pups can be placed in individual crates in a communal area during the night. This simple step will make the transition to a new home much easier.

No pup should be placed in a new home until they are at least 7 weeks of age. Pups placed earlier will not have the necessary social interactions with littermates and dam. Pups placed when they are too young tend not to eat and sleep well and are fussy. Many breeders who raise dogs for competition will keep their pups until 10 weeks and up. This allows them to better assess the litter and determine which pups are best suited for which homes. These pups are usually immunized and wormed several times and transition into new homes more easily (Figure 8-29).

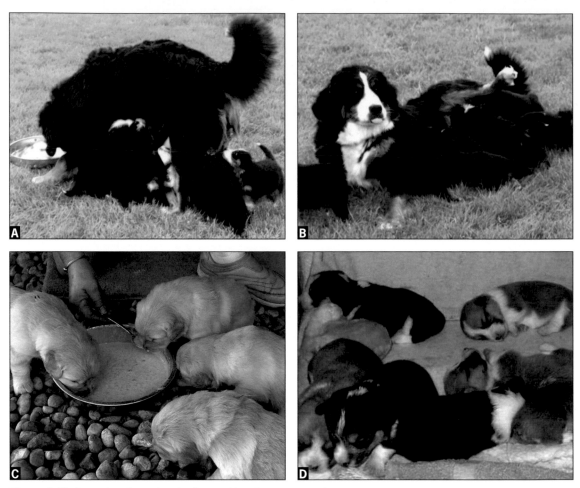

Figure 8-29. *Examples of weaning, feeding, and housing young puppies.*

Preparing the puppies to leave for a new home
Physical examination
(Appendix D-4 and Chapter 2 The Veterinary Examination)
Prior to placement, each pup should receive a comprehensive physical examination by a veterinarian. Some states require a certificate of veterinary inspection prior to sale and/or transport.

Vaccinations
(Appendix C-11)
Each veterinarian has preferred vaccination protocols. These change as new diseases, vaccine technology, and information on response to vaccines becomes available.

Breeders have long been skeptical about veterinary recommendations. The attached protocol may be modified according to each breeder's needs (Table 8-10).

Deworming
Recommendations by the Center for Disease Control (CDC) and Companion Animal Parasite Council (CAPC) have updated worming protocols. The CAPC website, www.capcvet.org may be reviewed by

Age/Date Next Visit	Examination	Vaccinations	Heartworm Test and Other Lab Tests	Medications	Other
			Table 8-10 Recommended canine vaccine and care protocol		
2 and 4 Weeks	As needed	–	–	Pyrantel Pamoate	–
6 to 8 Weeks	Veterinary Puppy Visit #1	DAPP(No Lepto)	Fecal No Heartworm test due	Heartworm preventive with pyrantel q 4 weeks, with pyrantel 2 weeks later Flea/ Tick Control*	
9 to 11 Weeks Due	Veterinary Puppy Visit #2	DAPP (No Lepto) Bordetella	Fecal No Heartworm test due	Heartworm preventive with pyrantel q 4 weeks, with pyrantel 2 weeks later Flea/ Tick Control*	Obedience Class
12 to 16 Weeks due	Veterinary Puppy Visit #3	DAPP/Lepto 4 way* Lyme* Rabies Canine influenza vaccination*	Fecal No Heartworm test due	Heartworm preventive wormer Flea/Tick Control* Pyrantel pamoate fenbendazole	Vaccinations may be divided so fewer are administered at each visit Large Breed: X-ray hips for laxity
16 to 20 Weeks due	Comprehensive	DAPP/Lepto 4 way* Lyme* Canine influenza vaccination*	Fecal No Heartworm test due	Heartworm preventive Flea/Tick Control*	
2 weeks after last vaccination	Distemper/Parvo Titer Blood test		Titer for Distemper and Parvovirus	Recommended to assess response to vaccination	Repeat boosters if low or no response to previous vaccinations
6 Months or older	Presurgical	Complete series if not yet done	Presurgical blood test, Heartworm test if not on preventive	Heartworm preventive Flea/Tick Control*	Spay/Neuter – if appropriated medically or dependent on owner's plans. Microchip
15 Months due	Comprehensive	DAPP/Lepto* Rabies Bordetella Lyme* Canine Influenza*	Heartworm test	Heartworm preventive Flea/Tick Control*	

* Varies with region of the country

the veterinarian and pet owner for most current recommendations.

Pups and their dams should receive their first worming when the pups are 2 weeks of age. Repeat at 4, 6, and 8 weeks, then place on monthly broad-spectrum heartworm anthelmintics that are effective against parasites with zoonotic potential.

Fecal examinations should be performed 2 to 4 times during the first year and repeated 1 to 2 times a year for adult pets. Use of fenbendazole during pregnancy will minimize transmission of roundworms and hookworms through the placenta and the milk. (See section on Antiparasiticides during pregnancy in chapter 5).

Nutrition

A high quality manufactured puppy food, appropriate for the breed is recommended. Start at weaning by softening the food with warm water. No other food or nutritional supplements are necessary. Many pet owners opt to supplement their pet's diet but this should be discouraged. Feed the pup every 3 to 4 hours, gradually reducing the number of meals to 3 per day until the pup is 6 months old.

Puppy shopping list

To have prior to bringing your new puppy home

1. Crate, exercise (x) pen or playpen
2. Washable bedding
3. Ceramic or stainless steel food and water dishes
4. Puppy food appropriate for the breed
5. Appropriate chew toys
6. Kong toy and food to stuff
7. Leash and collar
8. Long line to allow puppy to run safely
9. Dog shampoo
10. Towel or blanket from puppy's mom
11. Treats for housebreaking
12. An empty bottle to take water home from the breeder's water source for the first few days in the new home.

To do upon purchase

Schedule an appointment for a wellness veterinary examination

Vaccination schedule

DAPPv at 6 to 9 weeks of age
DALPPv at 12 and 16 weeks
Rabies, based on local legislation
Bordetella if in classes, boarding, grooming, daycare
Lyme if at risk
NO Lepto before 12 weeks
Worming schedule
Heartworm preventive and flea/tick control based on region of the country
Spay/neuter schedule

Appointment for puppy grooming
Visit a boarding kennel
Sign up for puppy socialization class

Placing the puppies

The responsible breeder will have had the pups examined by a veterinarian, vaccinated at least once, and wormed several times. If the pup is over 8 weeks old, it should also be on a monthly broad-spectrum anthelmentic. Some breeders will use topical external parasite control.

The pups are often microchipped. Many breeders will have the buyer sign a contract. If the pup is purebred and eligible for registration with a purebred registry, paperwork for this may accompany or follow the pup once it is received by the breeder. Receipt of registration paperwork is often delayed, particularly when litters are produced using shipped or frozen semen.

Some pups will be crate-trained and on their way to being housebroken.

Zoonotic diseases

There is increasing pressure on veterinarians and breeders to provide parasite-free pups as pets for the protection of the buyers. For this reason, multiple wormings and negative fecal examinations should be completed prior to sale. The pup should also be bathed just prior to or after sale to reduce the number of parasite eggs in the coat. This is particularly important if the pup is to be placed in a household with immunocompromised individuals including children or those who are mentally disabled.

Registering litters

Litters produced using fresh chilled or frozen semen, multiple sires, or with co-owners in different households cannot be registered on-line; the paperwork requires more time to file and receive from the purebred registries.

The American Kennel Club (AKC) allows breeders to sell pups to buyers on a limited registration. This means that the pup is registered but cannot have his or her pups registered. This is done because the breeder does not consider the pup to be of "breeding quality." A pup sold on full registration and without restrictions in the contract of sale may have pups registered with the AKC.

CHAPTER 9
Infertility and Reproductive Problems in the Valuable Bitch

The "Normal" estrous cycle

The "normal" estrous cycle is considered to occur every 6 months, commonly in the spring and fall. *Estrous* is the entire cycle, *estrus* is the fertile period within the estrous cycle.

The bitch is in proestrus for 9 to 12 days (range 3 to 17 days); during this time she has a firmly swollen vulva, a bloody vaginal discharge, and is not receptive to the male dog. During proestrus, most male dogs are attracted to the bitch, but most experienced males are only moderately interested. Vaginal cytology shows non-cornified epithelial cells; large lightly stained cells, rounded and containing nuclei, and many red blood cells in the background. A large number of bacteria of many sizes, rods and cocci, may be present. Few white blood cells should be seen. Vaginoscopy shows large, edematous, pink, moist folds, making the lumen difficult to follow. Progesterone levels, usually started approximately 6 days after the onset of bloody vaginal discharge, should be less than 2.0 ng/ml. In some bitches, the proestrus can be prolonged, making breeders anxious that they are going to miss their opportunity to breed the bitch. They tend to force breedings upon bitches who are not receptive and males who know better.

The second phase of the cycle, estrus, the fertile period within the estrous cycle, typically lasts for 3 to 5 days. The vulva is soft but swollen, there is a clear to straw colored vaginal discharge, and the bitch is normally very receptive to the male. She may stand solidly for him or make advances including play bows and mounting the male if he is reluctant to breed. Care must be taken to interpret signs carefully because not all bitches are receptive, not all males are willing to breed, and not all bitches have lost the bloody color of their discharge. It is easy to wait too long assuming she is not yet ready to breed. This is where vaginal cytology, vaginoscopy, and progesterone testing become invaluable. The vaginal cytology should show 70 to 100% cornified epithelial cells – large darkly-staining irregularly shaped cells without nuclei, with few bacteria, white blood cells, and red blood cells in the background. Vaginoscopy shows crenulated vaginal folds. Progesterone levels rise from the baseline of less than 2.0 ng/ml to 5.0 ng/ml at ovulation, and into the 20s and 30s ng/ml post-ovulation.

Diestrus immediately follows estrus and lasts from 56 to 58 days after ovulation. The vulvar swelling diminishes and there is little discharge. The bitch is no longer receptive to males, but may continue to be attractive to inexperienced males. Vaginal cytology shows non-cornified epithelial cells, many white blood cells, some bacteria, and no red blood cells. Vaginoscopy shows pale mucosa with no crenulation. Progesterone levels remain high throughout, not uncommonly from 20 to 50 ng/ml or higher.

Anestrus is the period between estrus cycles, typically lasting 2 to 9 months. There is no vaginal swelling or discharge. She is not receptive to the male and the male is not interested in her. Vaginal cytology shows non-cornified epithelial cells. Progesterone levels remain at or below 2.0 ng/ml. The uterus undergoes involution.

The ideal age and frequency of breeding

Veterinarians and breeders have different views regarding the ideal age and frequency of breeding. The veterinarian devotes a great deal of time and energy to helping clients maximize the fertility of their bitches and stud dogs. The breeder has performance based goals (putting titles on their bitches) and screening based goals (screening for diseases, some of which cannot be ruled out until a certain age).

Many veterinarians advise breeding as early as the bitch's second birthday. Fertility is at its peak and she is structurally and mentally mature enough to handle a pregnancy and maternal duties. Most pre-breeding screening tests can be completed by this age. At one time, the recommendation was to wait until she had 1 successful litter before breeding with frozen semen. Many veterinarians now advise using frozen semen on these young bitches. Most bitches will have their largest and healthiest litter at the first or second breeding. Litter size typically decreases after the third litter. Bitches over age 5 have smaller litters than younger bitches.

Many veterinarians now recommend breeding the bitch back-to-back, without taking a season off. There is no advantage to uterine health by skipping seasons. Each non-pregnant cycle ages the uterus irreversibly. Some think the uterus is healthier pregnant than non-pregnant.

Non-pregnant cycles, when the uterus is under the 2 month influence of progesterone, lead to uterine pathology such as CEH-pyometra. The recommendation is to breed the bitch as many times as the breeder considers reasonable, then retire and spay her. The breeder may have other reasons to skip estrous cycles including market demand for puppies and the need to breed other bitches in their program. If bred too frequently the bitch may become nutritionally depleted.

The number of C-sections that can be tolerated is based on medical and non medical considerations; the medical question has more than one answer. There is a great deal of individual variation between how bitches tolerate the surgery, how much they enjoy raising puppies, and how well the uterus and abdominal wall hold up. Many clients complain that their veterinarian told them the bitch should not have any more pregnancies because the uterus is "paper-thin." It is normal for the uterine wall to be thin at full-term pregnancy. Only the breeder can answer the non-medical questions. Some have opinions on how many surgeries their bitch can have. There is no standard answer to the upper limit to the number of C-sections a bitch can have. Her fertility, individual uterine health and the breeder's preference are the limiting factors.

Maximizing litter size

Many factors influence litter size, and the male has little to no control over it. His influence is all-or-none – either he delivered enough sperm to produce a litter or he did not.

There are 3 broad categories of causes of apparent infertility: 1. Failure for fertile semen to reach fertile ova, 2. Failure to conceive, and 3. Failure to maintain the pregnancy.

Unlike other "production" animals such as cattle and swine, few dog breeders have selected for ease of breeding, ease of whelping, litter size, lactation, and maternal skills. There are non-genetic factors as well as the concern that if only one trait is selected for, other valuable traits will be bred out of the breeder's lines.

Small litter size

This discussion will focus on the bitch that successfully achieves a pregnancy but does not produce the number of viable fetuses anticipated for her breed.

Overall health

A bitch cannot perform at her maximal reproductive capacity if she is not physically healthy, is not in great physical condition or has a heavy parasite burden. A pre-breeding physical examination, fecal analysis, Brucella and heartworm tests should be considered prior to breeding. This is also an opportunity to discover and discuss inherited physical abnormalities and their impact on her suitability as a brood bitch. A CBC and chemistry profile for all bitches undergoing surgical insemination is advisable. Consider this protocol for other bitches to assure that the breeder is not imposing a pregnancy on an already metabolically abnormal bitch.

Oviduct and uterine pathology

There are no practical procedures for detecting or treating oviduct patency in dogs. Scar tissue or inflammation may obstruct the oviduct, preventing fertilization and passage of the fertilized ova into the uterus. Endometritis, inflammation of the uterus, does not allow for implantation and fetal development. Cystic endometrial hyperplasia, if advanced enough, does not allow adequate surface area for implantation and fetal development to occur. Although these conditions can be diagnosed by uterine biopsy, the changes cannot be reversed with treatments available at this time.

Nutritional health

The plane of nutrition is essential to the bitch's ability to conceive and carry a maximal litter to term. Place the bitch on an ideal diet for pregnancy prior to breeding. Either a diet designed for pregnancy, puppy or a performance diet should be used. Do not under or overfeed. Start feeding this diet several weeks prior to the anticipated onset of estrus because follicles are recruited several weeks prior to ovulation, and some nutrients such as folic acid need to be at increased levels prior to conception to maximize their effects.

Frequency of breeding

This relates directly to the bitch's nutritional health. Body store depletion of nutrients occurs during pregnancy and lactation and may take up to 8 months for the bitch to fully recover. Frequently, after a large litter, the bitch will produce a smaller litter, and conversely, after a small litter, the next will be larger.

Dietary components that influence reproductive capacity

Protein, carbohydrates and fats must be in the correct ratios. The ratio of Omega 6 to Omega 3 fatty acids is important for maximal fertility as well as fetal brain and eye development. Appropriate levels of minerals such as copper, zinc, and manganese have been related to litter size. Folic acid should be in appropriate levels prior to breeding to reduce the incidence of cleft palates. Beta-carotene and tyrosine have have positive effects on hormone production and heat detection. (Royal Canin June 20, 2009 Dr Bretaigne Jones, D.V.M.)

Timing of the breeding

If the bitch is bred too early, the sperm are too old by the time the ova are ready to fertilize. If she is bred too late, either the eggs are aged or the cervix will have closed, preventing the passage of sperm into the oviducts for fertilization.

Fewer breedings per cycle, particularly if not performed on the ideal date, will result in smaller litters.

Type of semen

Vaginal deposition of fresh semen leads to a 15% reduction in litter size compared to natural breeding. Litter size is reduced by 15% using chilled semen and 25% with frozen semen. In general, fresh semen survives 5 to 7 days (dependent upon the quality of the semen and ejaculate), chilled semen survives 3 days, and frozen semen survives 1 day in the female's reproductive tract.

Type of semen deposition

Natural semen deposition has a high success rate achieving maximal litter size. Surgical AI, regardless of semen type, achieves the maximal litter size and success regardless of the type of semen (fresh, fresh chilled, or frozen) used. When frozen semen is used, either TCI or surgical insemination is necessary.

Genetics
Her breed
Statistically, smaller bitches have fewer pups per litter and larger bitches have more pups per litter.

Her inbreeding coefficient

The more closely line-bred the litter is, the fewer pups produced. Many breeders use computer programs to do this calculation. Line breeding with too high an inbreeding coefficient can lead to fatal gene combinations, causing early embryonic death and resorption or apparent infertility.

Family traits

Some family lines ovulate fewer eggs than others. There may also be familial tendencies toward uterine pathology.

Age and parity, and environment

(See Chapter 5)

History and clinical findings in the infertile bitch
Diagnostic workup for the infertile bitch

(See Appendix D-6, A-10, D-15, and B-1)

Use of a pre-written questionnaire, complete systematic physical examination and thoughtful diagnostic work-up will help keep the busy clinician from overlooking the obvious. Although no protocol or algorithm can be all-inclusive, consistent and thorough evaluations can keep the work-up from derailing.

Remind the client to bring all the available breeding records, including prior breedings, stud dog performance, test results, and medications to the appointment. If the bitch has traveled for the breeding, she may have left the care of your hospital so this may leave gaps in the information in her medical file at your hospital.

The technician or doctor should take a complete breeding history. This should include:

Identification of the patient, including her breed, call name, microchip or tattoo number, date of birth and date of the assessment;

A general health history of the bitch including health, illness, surgical and vaccine history, diet fed, current medications, supplements given, and description of housing including lighting and concentration of dogs housed;

Health screening history;

Previous diagnostics – CBC/Chemistries/UA/Progesterone – Brucella testing – dates and results/ Thyroid/Lyme/Ehrlichia/Anaplasma/Ultrasound;

Information on her lifestyle and travel history;

History of all estrous cycles – from the first one to the most recent;

All successful breedings for this bitch, ages when bred, number of pups, method used for timing and breeding, pregnancy and delivery details;

All unsuccessful breedings for this bitch, dates of estrous cycles, ages when bred, method used for timing and breeding (natural/AI/Fresh chilled/Frozen), method used for pregnancy diagnosis, stud dog used, his breeding history and semen analysis including Brucella testing;

Perform a complete physical examination; including a vaginal examination and evaluation of the mammary glands

If there was questionable timing or semen quality, plan the next breeding with both to be improved;

If there was good timing and good semen quality, draw blood for progesterone level, other tests based on physical examination findings, and consider testing for herpesvirus and brucellosis;

Consider ultrasound to evaluate for uterine and ovarian pathology;

Consider either surgical insemination or surgical uterine biopsy if there was good timing and good semen quality.

Client history form
(See Appendix A-10)

Planning the next breeding
Two of the most important steps in breeding a bitch are planning ahead and having great communication with the owner of the stud dog. This communication also includes the bitch and stud dog owner's veterinarians if there will be veterinary intervention.

The bitch owner should select a stud dog and contact the owner well in advance of the estrous cycle at which she is planning to use him. This is regardless of the method of breeding. Even if the stud dog has frozen semen stored at the same facility the bitch owner uses for veterinary care, the stud dog owner needs advance notice – paperwork needs to be signed by the stud dog owner. If fresh chilled semen is to be used, the stud dog's veterinarian should have shipping kits, extender, and the skills to collect and ship the semen. Access to a teaser bitch on the stud dog's end of the shipment can be instrumental in colleting the stud dog, especially if the stud dog or collecting veterinarian are inexperienced. The shipping arrangements should have been discussed, taking into account weekend and holiday plans.

Use of a veterinary clinic with experience in handling breedings is strongly recommended, particularly if using fresh chilled semen, frozen semen, or if either dog has a history of infertility. All veterinarians need to get experience somewhere. However, starting with fertile stud dogs and bitches with uncomplicated breeding plans is recommended over starting with complex breedings.

Abnormal estrous cycles
(Figure 9-1 and 9-2).
Failure of the bitch to cycle
For some breeds and some individuals, it may be normal for a bitch under the age of 24 months to not have had an estrous cycle. This bitch should be closely evaluated to assess her external genitals. If the vulva has a mature appearance, she probably had a silent heat cycle that the owner failed to detect. This is less likely if there are male dogs in the same facility.

If she has a prominent os clitoris or has characteristics more typical of a male of her breed, she should be evaluated for intersex by karyotyping or exploratory laparotomy and biopsy of the genitals. If the vulva has an immature appearance, it is probable that she has not yet reached sexual maturity. No treatment or diagnostics are indicated until she is over 2 years of age.

Genetic intersex
There are several combinations of defects in sexual differentiation described in dogs over two years of age. This can be diagnosed by karyotyping the DNA to evaluate the presence of X and Y chromosomes, or by biopsying the gonads and performing histopathology to detect the presence of ovarian and/or testicular tissues.

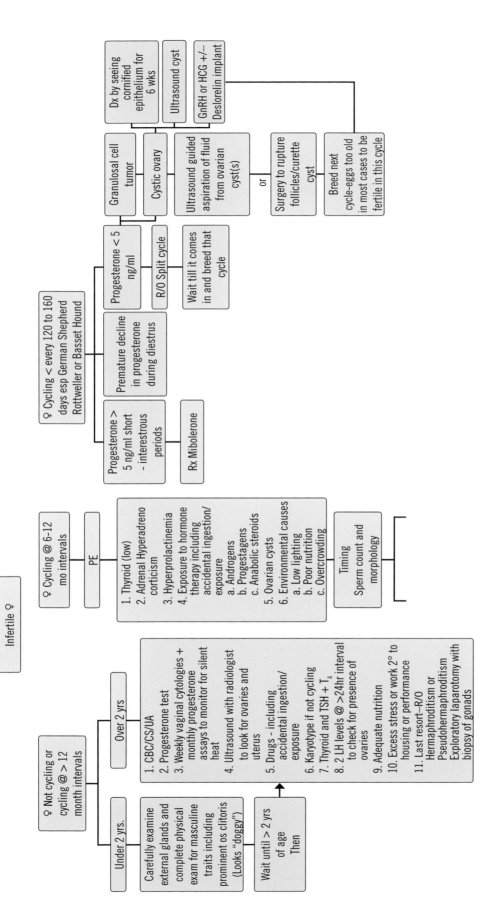

Figure 9-1.
Page 1. Female infertility

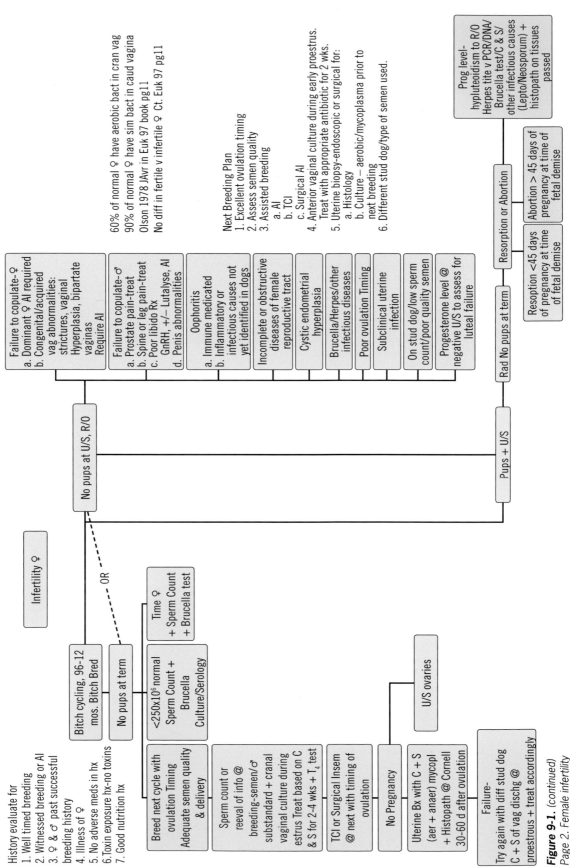

History evaluate for
1. Well timed breeding
2. Witnessed breeding or AI
3. ♀ & ♂ past successful breeding history
4. Illness of ♀
5. No adverse meds in hx
6. Toxin exposure hx-no toxins
7. Good nutrition hx

Infertility ♀

No pups at U/S, R/O

OR

Bitch cycling, 96-12 mos. Bitch Bred

No pups at term

Time ♀ + Sperm Count + Brucella test

<250x10⁶ normal Sperm Count + Brucella Culture/Serology

Breed next cycle with ovulation Timing Adequate semen quality & delivery

Sperm count or reval of info @ breeding-semen/♂ substandard + cranal vaginal culture during estrus Treat based on C & S for 2-4 wks + T₄ test

TCI or Surgical Insem @ next with timing of ovulation

No Pregnancy

U/S ovaries

Uterine Bx with C + S (aer + anaer) mycopl + Histopath @ Cornell 30-60 d after ovulation

Failure-
Try again with diff stud dog C + S of vag dischg @ proestrus + treat accordingly

Failure to copulate-♀
a. Dominant ♀ AI required
b. Congenital/acquired vag abnormalities: strictures, vaginal Hyperplasia, bipartate vaginas Require AI

Failure to copulate-♂
a. Prostate pain-treat
b. Spine or leg pain-treat
c. Poor libido Rx GnRH, +/- Lutalyse, AI
d. Penis abnormalities

Oophoritis
a. Immune medicated
b. Inflammatory or infectious causes not yet identified in dogs

Incomplete or obstructive diseases of female reproductive tract

Cystic endometrial hyperplasia

Brucella/Herpes/other infectious diseases

Poor ovulation Timing

Subclinical uterine infection

On stud dog/low sperm count/poor quality semen

Progesterone level @ negative U/S to assess for luteal failure

60% of normal ♀ have aerobic bact in cran vag
90% of normal ♀ have sim bact in caud vagina
Olson 1978 JAvr in Euk 97 book pg11
No diff in fertile v infertile ♀ Ct. Euk 97 pg11

Next Breeding Plan
1. Excellent ovulation timing
2. Assess semen quality
3. Assisted breeding
   a. AI
   b. TCI
   c. Surgical AI
4. Anterior vaginal culture during early proestrus. Treat with appropriate antibiotic for 2 wks.
5. Uterine biopsy-endoscopic or surgical for:
   a. Histology
   b. Culture – aerobic/mycoplasma prior to next breeding
6. Different stud dog/type of semen used.

Rad No pups at term

Pups + U/S

Resorption or Abortion

Resoption <45 days of pregnancy at time of fetal demise

Abortion > 45 days of pregnancy at time of fetal demise

Prog level-hypluteoidism to R/O Herpes tite v PCR/DNA/ Brucella test/C & S/ other infectious causes (Lepto/Neosporum) + histopath on tissues passed

Figure 9-1. *(continued)*
Page 2. Female infertility

True hermaphrodites may occur with the presence of ovarian and testicular tissues. This has been described in many breeds of dog. The true hermaphrodite chimeras have either XX/XY or XX/XXY chromosomes. These affected females have external female genitalia with an enlarged clitoris and a combination of ovarian and testicular tissue.

A pseudohermaphrodite has the external genitals of one sex with the gonads of the opposite sex. They should be classified male or female based on the sex of their gonads, not the external genitals. The female pseudohermaphrodite has XX chromosomes and ovaries but the external genitals are male. This condition is seen in many breeds. The male pseudohermaphrodite has testicles, usually retained, but female external genitals. They have a karyotype XY. There is no treatment, so surgical neutering is generally recommended.

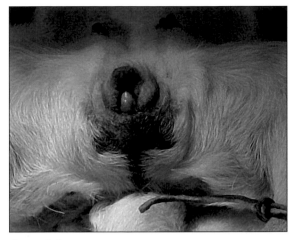

Figure 9-2.
Female external genitals with enlarged clitoris, genetic intersex.

XX sex reversal occurs when the gonadal sex does not agree with the XX chromosomal sex. This has been reported in the American Cocker Spaniel, Beagle, Chinese Pug, Kerry Blue Terrier, Weimaraner, and German Shorthaired Pointer.

Ovariohysterectomy
A bitch may have been ovariohysterectomized by a prior owner and sold without incomplete veterinary records. To determine this, a paired LH test can be performed. LH is canine specific, and must be done with the Synbiotics ICG Status-LHR assay kit or at a referral laboratory using the canine test. LH is secreted by the pituitary gland. If no ovaries are present, there is no feedback, so the LH is persistently elevated. If 2 consecutive LH tests have a high result, the bitch has been ovariohysterectomized.

Ovarian aplasia or agenesis
This is a rare cause of anestrus.

Previously cycled, now fails to cycle
Silent estrous
This is defined as ovarian activity with ovulation occurring but with no typical signs such as vaginal swelling or discharge. This is a common cause of apparent infertility. To detect silent heats, weekly vaginal cytologies can be collected by the owner and submitted to the veterinary staff for microscopic examination. Alternatively, progesterone levels can be assessed monthly, with a progesterone rise above 2 ng/ml as diagnostic of functional luteal tissue.

Pharmacologic interference
Several drugs can block the estrous cycle. Some, such as mibolerone, are intentionally used to prevent estrous. Others such as corticosteroids, androgens, and progestagens (Megestrol Acetate), may have this effect. Deslorelin implants, if used in proestrus, may also block estrous.

Illness
Bitches with many systemic illnesses may fail to cycle. A thorough clinical history and physical examination, as well as a CBC, chemistry panel, and urinalysis should be performed to assure that

the bitch is in good physical condition with no apparent underlying disorders. Disorders such as diabetes mellitus, hyperadrenocorticism and hepatic and renal failure may interfere with fertility. Bitches with diseases such as hepatic and renal failure should NOT be bred because the added metabolic load from the pregnancy is likely to accelerate organ failure. Bitches with diabetes mellitus are very challenging to manage during pregnancy.

Hormonal abnormalities
Both hypothyroidism and hyperadrenocorticism are suspected of interfering with normal estrous cycles. Typically, an affected bitch will have clinical symptoms of this disorder. Testing should be done if either disorder is suspected. Test results should be carefully interpreted as there are several causes for test results to be outside the normal range. Consider using a laboratory with endocrinology interpretation of the results available. Some causes of thyroid disease are thought to be heritable, so the breeder should be counseled regarding the wisdom of including a confirmed hypothyroid bitch in a breeding program. The heritability of hyperadrenocorticism has not been established.

Functional ovarian cysts
Luteal ovarian cysts that are secreting progesterone may cause a failure to cycle. This may be diagnosed with progesterone testing and ultrasound. The treatment of choice is surgical removal of the cyst.

Environmental causes
Environmental causes include high stress levels, high concentration of dogs housed, bitches who are very athletic and/or are worked hard, bitches that have inadequate nutrition for their activity level, low lighting conditions, and bitches who are housed with highly dominant bitches.

If the bitch is competing at a high level, is on the road most of the time, or is under a great deal of mental or physical stress relative to her temperament, returning her home or to a lower stress housing situation may allow her to cycle more normally. Housing a bitch with other cycling bitches may also induce estrous – similar to what is described in humans as the "convent" or "dormitory" effect.

Similarly, increasing the nutritional plane of a bitch with a body condition score that is less than ideal for fertility may allow her to begin to cycle spontaneously. Crowded housing or housing with low light levels may also interfere with regular estrous cycles; improving her environment, may allow for a spontaneous return to fertility.

Careful evaluation of the bitch's lifestyle, demeanor, and body condition may suggest an environmental cause, thus recommendation of a modification of lifestyle.

Infertile estrous cycles
A minimum of 4 months is required between estrous cycles for the bitch to be fertile. It is thought that endometrial repair is necessary, and too short an inter-estrous period does not allow for adequate uterine health to support pregnancy.

There is breed variation, with German Shepherds, Labrador Retrievers, American Cocker Spaniels, and Rottweilers, showing the shortest time between cycles. The interestrous time period may be an inherited trait.

Bitches with cystic endometrial hyperplasia seem to have shortened inter-estrous cycles. Endometrial hyperplasia can only be confirmed with uterine biopsy.

Another cause for short inter-estrous cycles is a functional ovarian cyst secreting estrogens.

These should be treated immediately. These bitches are infertile and long-term exposure of the uterine lining to high estrogen levels may predispose them to CEH-pyometra complex and bone marrow suppression, resulting in non-regenerative anemia. Diagnosis is best made by ultrasound, recognizing hypoechoic cyst(s) larger than 1 cm on the ovary/ovaries. It is possible to surgically remove the cyst(s) (via laparotomy or laparoscopy). Alternatively, a skilled ultrasonographer may be able to aspirate the fluid from the cysts with an ultrasound-directed needle. Treatment with HCG or GnRH used to be recommended, but there is strong evidence that this predisposes the bitch to a pyometra within several weeks of treatment.

In the absence of functional ovarian cysts, cycles closer together than 4 months require treatment to restore fertility. Mibolerone used daily is the only drug with historical label indications to treat this condition. Mibolerone, previously known as Cheque® drops when manufactured by Upjohn, is now only available as a controlled substance through compounding pharmacies. Mibolerone, a testosterone derivative, blocks the release of LH from the pituitary gland. This negative feedback blocks maturation of the follicles, interfering with ovulation.

Mibolerone use may cause an elevation in liver enzymes. A liver panel should be run prior to the onset of therapy, and every 6 months during treatment. This drug may cause increased epiphora, heavier coat and musculature, and a sticky vaginal discharge similar to that of a puppy with vaginitis (Figure 9-3). All handlers must be aware that this is not a vaginal discharge associated with pyometra so she will not be inadvertently diagnosed with a treated for a non-existent pyometra. Mibolerone should never be used prior to the first estrous and not for more than 2 consecutive years. Some reports suggest that mibolerone should not be used for longer than 3 consecutive months. Treatment with mibolerone should be initiated 30 days prior to the anticipated estrous cycle. The average time between stopping therapy and the onset of the next cycle is 70 days, but the range varies widely. The bitches should be bred on the first cycle after the cessation of mibolerone treatment, because it is common for the bitch to relapse to short inter-estrous cycles after treatment.

Short inter-estrous cycles must be distinguished from split heat cycles. In split heats, the bitch fails to become attractive to males, there is no cornification of vaginal cytology, and no rise in progesterone.

Prolonged inter-estrous cycle

A prolonged inter-estrous cycle is defined as failure to cycle within 10 to 18 months after the previous estrous.

This may be associated with silent heat cycles, systemic illness, hypothyroidism, hyperadrenocorticism, or recent pregnancy. It may also be typical for the Basenji, Dingo, and wolves and wolf-hybrid dogs.

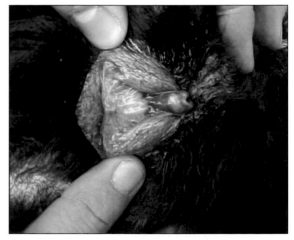

Figure 9-3.
Bitch on mibolerone showing enlarged clitoris and sticky mucoid discharge typical when on this medication. Should not be confused with appearance of discharge pyometra.

Confirm that the bitch has not had an undetected estrous prior to treatment. This can be done by progesterone assay – a progesterone level of less than 2 ng/ml suggests that the bitch has not recently (within the last 60 to 90 days) cycled. She should also receive a complete physical examination and accompanying lab work to rule out the possibility of hormonal abnormalities or illness.

The bitch may be treated with cabergoline and Deslorelin® as described under "Inducing Estrous."

Split heats

Split heats are defined as "successive short proestrous signs, at intervals of 2 weeks to 2 months, associated with short interestrus intervals."

Most bitches with a split heat cycle are young, stressed by travel during estrus, or Northern breeds. They will start in proestrus, but fail to have a progesterone rise that exceeds 5ng/ml. They generally will not be receptive to males and will have vaginal cytologies that begin to cornify, then return to non-cornified cells. They frequently go out of heat, return to proestrus within 4 to 6 weeks, and have a normal ovulatory cycle that is usually a fertile. No cystic structures will be seen on the ovaries on an ultrasonogram. No treatment is indicated for split cycles. They do not cause infertility.

Prolonged estrous cycle

A prolonged estrous cycle is generally defined as a cycle that exceeds 30 days from start of the proestrus. By contrast, most normal fertile bitches will ovulate, based on behavior, vaginal cytology, and rising progesterone levels (that exceed 5 ng/ml) within 21 days of the onset of proestrus. If a bitch fails to ovulate within 21 to 30 days of the onset of proestrus, she is unlikely to conceive. If she is having a split cycle, she may conceive when she had her next normal estrous cycle.

Prolonged estrous cycles can be caused by a functional ovarian cyst, an ovarian tumor, the use of exogenous estrogen creams, or they can appear to be a split heat cycle (Figure 9-4).

Functional ovarian cysts are a relatively common cause of prolonged proestrus in older bitches. If a functional ovarian cyst is suspected, ultrasound to confirm the cyst and rule out an ovarian tumor is recommended. Success in finding the ovary to assess for a tumor or cysts varies and depends on the skill of the ultrasonographer and quality of the equipment. An ovarian cyst usually exceeds 11 mm in diameter and has a thicker capsule, usually filled with hypoechoic or anechoic fluid, than a normal ovulatory follicle. An ovarian tumor is usually larger and has a more complex internal structure than a cyst.

Treatment of the cyst should begin by day 21 of proestrus. The most common treatment is a series of 3 hCG (Human chorionic gonadotropin) injections dosed at 10 IU/pound body weight/day IM, once daily for 3 consecutive days. This can be repeated if there is no response within 1 week. If the bitch has not ovulated by day 21 to 30 of her cycle, it is unlikely that she will have a fertile cycle because of the age of the ova. It is theoretically possible for a bitch to develop anaphylaxis from the use of hCG, but there are no reports to support this. hCG stings when administered IM.

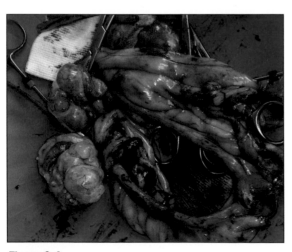

Alternatively, GnRH can be used 3.3 mcg/kg/day IM for 3 consecutive days. Bitches that develop a cystic ovary during one estrus cycle may have a recurrence. There is no breed predilection for ovarian cysts.

If the bitch fails to respond to medical treatment, surgical drainage and curettage of the cyst can be used. This can be done via laparotomy or laparoscopy. Closely evaluate both ovaries for evidence of a tumor. Unless neoplasia is suspected, it is not necessary to remove the ovary. If there are no plans to use the bitch in future breedings, ovariohysterectomy is recommended.

Figure 9-4.
Ovaries with cystic structures.

Bitches treated for ovarian cysts are at increased risk of developing pyometra following a prolonged estrous cycle. The patient should be closely monitored. Inform the client of the risk and discuss the medical versus surgical treatment options.

Ovarian neoplasia, particularly granulosal cell tumors, must be included in the differential diagnosis of bitches with prolonged proestrus. This tumor type produces estrogens, thus leading to prolonged estrus. If ultrasound is unavailable or non-diagnostic, and the bitch fails to respond to hCG or GnRH, encourage the client to consider surgical exploration. Many ovarian tumors are benign, and often can be successfully resected if found early. Radiation and chemotherapeutic protocols have not been extensively evaluated in the bitch.

Exogenous estrogen creams and gels prescribed for post-menopausal women may also cause symptoms of prolonged estrous in dogs. They may be ingested (licking the application site on the arm or chewing up a tube of cream) or absorbed transdermally. This is common in small breed dogs with thin hair coats on the abdomen when in close contact with a patient using these creams and gels. This may be an uncomfortable question, but it should be asked when taking a history.

Anovulatory cycles

Failure to ovulate was reported as 1% in one study. Here, the progesterone failed to rise above 3.5 ng/ml. When followed, 45% of the bitches had a normal ovulatory cycle during their next estrous. For the bitches who do this recurrently, treatment with GnRH or hCG may be used on subsequent cycle.

Missed breedings

The most common cause of missed breeding, as a cause of apparent infertility, is thought to be breeding at the wrong time; that is failure to deliver the semen into the oviducts 2 to 3 days post-ovulation. The second most common cause is poor semen quality. A third cause in the cycling bitch is abnormal estrous cycles, suggesting ovarian or uterine pathology. There are many other causes. Some result in failure to conceive and some result in pregnancy loss (See Figure 9-2).

Infertility

There are 3 basic assessments to consider when a bitch fails or appears to fail to conceive and complete a pregnancy?

1. Did fertile sperm get to a fertile egg?
   a. Was semen with a normal count, mortality and morphology deposited in the bitch's reproductive tract?
   b. Did the bitch ovulate?
   c. Was the semen deposited at the right time?
   d. Did viable semen get to the oviduct?
   e. Did a viable egg get to the oviduct?

2. Did the bitch conceive?
   a. Did the sperm successfully fertilize the egg?
   b. Did the fertilized egg survive and become an embryo?
   c. Did the embryo successfully implant and form a placenta?

3. Did the bitch successfully maintain this pregnancy?
   a. Was a healthy fetus with a healthy placenta maintained?
   b. Were the fetuses successfully delivered at full term?

Ultrasound for pregnancy 4 or more weeks after breeding can help to distinguish between failure to conceive and failure to maintain pregnancy. Palpation is not useful in distinguishing viable from non-viable feti. Blood testing lacks specificity, cannot be reliably used before day 28 of pregnancy, and cannot accurately distinguish viable from non-viable feti. Encourage the client to have the bitch ultrasounded in the range of days 24 to 28 or later. This is particularly important for bitches that have previously missed breedings.

When evaluating for infertility, start with a complete history, including the previous breeding history of both the male and female, how timing of the breeding was determined, sperm quality, and physical examination of the bitch (See Appendix D-6, A-9 and A-10).

No pregnancy – No pups seen on ultrasound

As obvious as this seems, a bitch is often presented for evaluation for pregnancy or infertility when no breeding has been witnessed. Unless the breeder was present and witnessed a tie, **failure to copulate** must be considered. The female may not have been receptive because the male and female were not left together at the correct time.

There can be psychological causes for failure to copulate. Sometimes, the female is very aggressive toward the male and intimidates him, or she may be shy or timid. At times, the male may not be assertive enough. Sometimes, the bitch or dog may have personal preferences and not like the mate the breeder has chosen for her or him.

There can be physical reasons for an inability to copulate. The male may have pain associated with his prostate, back, hips or stifles. He may have a penile frenulum, a hair ring, or other penile pathology making copulation impossible. He may not be tall enough to mount the bitch; she may be too tall or too short for the male. Her vulva may be too small or too far cranial for the male to reach. She may have a stricture, septum, mass, foreign body, vaginal hyperplasia or other vaginal pathology making copulation impossible. These anatomical abnormalities may be congenital or acquired from difficult whelping, mating trauma, or a poorly healed episiotomy. These abnormalities may be surgically correctable if planned for between estrous cycles.

Artificial insemination, using quality semen and accurate timing, is often an appropriate option for the next cycle with a young healthy bitch and male dog. If there are greater issues, such as an aging bitch or stud dog, or poor semen quality, more aggressive treatment options may be offered.

Timing

Poor timing is the most common cause for missed breedings. The incidence of apparent infertility caused by missed timing ranges between 40% and 80% of all bitches presented for fertility evaluations. This is a management issue, not infertility.

There is great variation between bitches and even between cycles of the same bitch for breeding. Many breeders believe that their bitches are ready to breed on day 12. However, it is clear from progesterone timing and successful outcomes that some bitches are ready to breed on day 3 and some on day 30.

Many breedings today are more complicated than in years past. Breeders who have historically used 2 dogs within their kennel or geographic proximity could rely on the stud dog and bitch to do their own timing, because the semen was viable for long enough to make their timing look good. We now have higher expectations that we will be so successful, we will always produce a litter.

Because we now use bitches with questionable fertility, aging stud dogs, shipped semen, and/or frozen semen that cannot be replenished, accuracy in timing is increasingly important.

When presented with a bitch for apparent infertility, simply reviewing how the timing, if any was done, and using vaginal cytologies, progesterone testing, and good quality semen on the next cycle will often be all that is necessary for a successful outcome.

Failure to ovulate

Some bitches will appear to cycle, but may fail to ovulate, either because of split cycles or cystic ovarian disease. Careful monitoring of their cycle, with vaginal cytology, observation of the behavior of the bitch and stud, and progesterone testing will usually detect this failure.

Poor semen quality

Inadequate sperm at the breeding is the second most common reason for apparent infertility.

Opinion varies regarding the minimum number of normal viable sperm required to successfully impregnate a bitch; the range is from 50 million to 250 million viable normal sperm. Calculations must include the total sperm count, and the number of forwardly motile morphologically normal sperm. The number of normal spermatozoa with normal morphology and progressive motility is the important factor, not the volume of the ejaculate. An accurate sperm count is an essential component of the fertility workup.

The typical male dog produces 10×10^6 (10 million) sperm per pound of body weight. This is 1 billion sperm for a 100 pound dog. This far exceeds the number known to be necessary for successful fresh and frozen semen breedings. In general, 100 to 200 million sperm are used for a frozen semen breeding, although it may be possible to use fewer in a small breed or young healthy bitches.

Sperm counts can be done manually with dilutions in a Unopette™, with a sperm counter calibrated for use in the dog, or at a commercial laboratory (See Appendix A-8).

Microscopic evaluation for forward motility and morphology can be done easily and quickly using a warmed microscope slide with the sample under low power.

Although it is desirable to have 80% or more normal motile sperm in an ejaculate, stud dogs with much lower percentages of normal sperm can still sire litters if the sperm count is high enough and the bitch has good fertility. For example, if a stud dog has 1 billion sperm (1×10^9), with only 10% normal, he still has 100 million sperm potentially eligible to fertilize the ova.

It is useful to know if this stud dog has been successful at impregnating other females within a short time period prior to or following the bitch you are examining.

A stud dog is classified as fertile if there are 100 million to 200 million or more viable forwardly motile normal appearing sperm. If the stud dog the breeder wants to use does not meet these criteria by the time the bitch is ready to breed, the veterinarian may suggest that the owner select an alternative stud dog. Some breeders will opt for a different stud. Some are so committed to the original selection that they are willing to use a stud with marginal fertility; they prefer to risk missing the breeding than to compromise their stud dog selection.

Bacterial vaginitis

Vaginitis can lead to infertility. It seems to be an under-diagnosed condition, with no distinguishing clinical signs. If white blood cells are seen on vaginal cytology during proestrus or estrus, an appropriate antibiotic regimen may be considered.

Semen delivery – Oviduct disease – Obstruction, inflammation

Semen delivery may be impaired by any obstructive lesion along the bitch's reproductive tract, including the vagina, uterus, cervix, or oviduct. It may be a congenital segmental aplasia, or acquired secondarily to inflamation, infection, trauma, aging changes, or surgery on the reproductive tract.

Evaluation of the oviduct for disease is under-evaluated. Although it is likely that scarring, obstruction, neoplasia, and inflammatory changes interfere with the delivery of semen to the oviduct, we have no current practical methods for imaging, diagnosing, or treating this disorder.

Immunologic infertility

This is not well documented in the bitch. On submission of a uterine biopsy to Dr. Schlafer at Cornell, the author has had one clinical case of infertility where this was suspected.

Failure to implant

Fertilization occurs approximately 3 days after ovulation. After the sperm fertilizes the egg, cell division occurs, and the developing embryo implants and forms a placenta approximately 18 days after ovulation. There are no diagnostic tests for detecting pregnancy prior to implantation. It is probable that many more bitches conceive than are confirmed pregnant, even with ultrasonography. This cause of infertility or pregnancy failure cannot be diagnosed.

Failure to form and maintain a healthy placenta

Failure to form and maintain a healthy placenta cannot be determined prior to 24 to 28 days post-ovulation.

Ultrasonography can be used to confirm pregnancy, detect fetal resorption, fetal death, and abortion. In some cases, only part of the litter is lost; in others the entire litter is.

If fetal loss occurs prior to approximately day 45 of pregnancy, resorption occurs. If fetal loss occurs after approximately day 45 of pregnancy, stillborn pups pass.

Resorption is a common event in the dog, with up to 33% of conceptions resorbing.

Failure to maintain pregnancy – Pups seen on ultrasound, pregnancy lost – Resorption

Early embryonic death, resorption, abortion, stillbirth, and neonatal mortality have many causes. Some causes cannot be determined but there are many infectious and noninfectious causes for which we have good diagnostic, treatment and preventive protocols (Figure 9-5).

Brucellosis

Canine brucellosis, caused by Brucella canis, is the only documented infectious bacterial cause of infertility in the bitch. The bacterium is nearly impossible to eliminate from the infected dog and it can cause a long-term infectious disease in the human (Figure 9-6).

Recently there has been an increasing number of outbreaks throughout the United States, particularly in commercial breeding operations. As infected dogs move out of these facilities and co-mingle with other dogs as breeding stock and rescued dogs, brucellosis may easily spread into other breeding facilities and client's homes. Dogs may be exposed by routes other than venereal transmission, such as through casual contact with urine and genital discharges at dog events and breeders who rescue dogs from breeding facilities. Veterinarians and breeders must be less complacent about testing for this important and devastating disease.

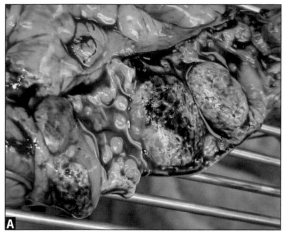
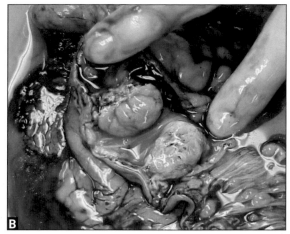

Figure 9-5.
*Cystic endometrial hypoplasia (small white cysts) with sterile fetal resorption sites (large, beige plaques) attached to the uterine lining, close up view **A**, with CEH **B**.*

Canine brucellosis as a zoonotic disease

Canine Brucellosis in humans can be serious and difficult to diagnose. It is frequently overlooked by physicians. Symptoms in humans include recurrent fever, lung and heart disease, and bone infections. It is more likely to occur and cause serious symptoms in the immune-compromised patient (children, the elderly, patients on chemotherapy, patients on corticosteroids or organ rejection drugs, patients with HIV-AIDS, and those with chronic diseases such as diabetes or leukemia). Although few human cases have been reported, we have a responsibility to educate and protect our clients and staff.

Human exposure to <u>Brucella canis</u> can be by ingestion, mucus membrane contact, skin wounds, or inhalation of the organism. Masks, goggles and gloves should be worn by personnel handling suspected animals, bedding or tissues.

If a client or staff member is exposed or may have symptoms of brucellosis, he or she should contact their physician. Early symptoms include intermittent (undulant) or prolonged fever; body, muscle and back aches; loss of appetite; headaches; sweats; fatigue; other flu-like symptoms and enlarged lymph nodes. Early treatment with appropriate antibiotics is usually effective.

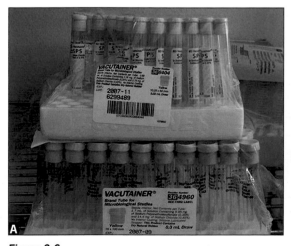
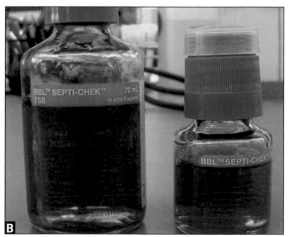

Figure 9-6.
*A. Blood tubes for Brucella canis culture. **B.** Media used to culture Brucella canis.*

Symptoms of canine brucellosis in the bitch and puppies

Symptoms in the bitch include apparent infertility due to early fetal death, resorption, abortion, and the delivery of weak or sick pups. Late term abortion after 45 to 60 days of pregnancy is common. Abortion is accompanied by a long-standing vaginal discharge. Aborted pups often show signs of decomposition. Pups born alive may die soon after birth, or show signs of illness. The sick pups may have enlarged lymph nodes, recurrent fevers, and uveitis. Affected bitches may also have fevers of undetermined origin, diskospondylitis, and uveitis.

Testing dogs for canine brucellosis

All dogs and bitches that have direct sexual contact with each other, dogs that will have their semen frozen, and all dogs and bitches with symptoms of brucellosis should have screening blood tests.

1. Brucella testing is frequently done as a serologic test. The most common screening test is a rapid slide agglutination test (RSAT). (D-Tec CB® from PZoetis). When the kit is available, the RSAT test can be done at the veterinary clinic, or at a reference laboratory. It is a test that can be done in a few minutes, after the blood is drawn and serum is harvested. It is inexpensive, sensitive, and 99% accurate. It also detects antibodies within a few weeks of infection. False positives are in the range of 1% to 10%. The false positives are due to other bacteria that cause cross-reaction. A second test is included in the kit,the 2-ME step. The addition of 2-mercaptoethanol reduces false positives. A negative test result indicates that either the dog does not have an active brucellosis infection or that it was exposed in the past 8 to 12 weeks.

2. The agar gel immunodiffusion (AGID) test is more specific and used to rule brucellosis in or out for dogs positive on the RSAT test. It is only available at the veterinary diagnostic laboratory at Cornell University.

3. Isolation of <u>Brucella canis</u> by culture can be done at a reference laboratory. The advantages are 1) There are no other bacteria that can cross-react and give false positive test results, 2) The test will detect infections earlier than the RSAT and AGID tests and 3) the test is not expensive to run. The disadvantages are 1) Long turn-around time, up to 4 weeks, 2) the test is only available at reference labs 3) sample handling is more labor-intensive and 4) <u>Brucella</u> is a difficult organism to grow in culture so the diagnosis can be missed. Costs for these different tests are similar.

   Samples that may be submitted for brucellosis testing are blood collected sterilely, aborted fetal tissues, urine, ejaculated fluid or tissues from the male or female reproductive tract. <u>Brucella</u> is a difficult to culture and is easily overgrown by contaminants.

   Blood cultures must be taken sterilely into bacterial culture vacuum blood tubes with a surgical prep on the skin. This tube has a yellow stopper, and contains SPS and ACD. Other blood collection tubes cannot be substituted. Multiple tests may be needed to confirm the patient's negative status.

   Aborted fetuses should have stomach contents submitted for culture; pups that are born alive and die soon thereafter should have internal organs and lymph nodes submitted for culture. If a dog or bitch suspected of having brucellosis is euthanized, lymph nodes, spleen, liver, testes, prostate, uterus, and placenta should be collected sterilely and submitted for culture.

4. Iowa State University now offers a PCR test for canine brucellosis. Urine from males, vaginal swabs from females, or tissues are the preferred samples. PCR tests detect the DNA of the bacteria, not the antibodies developed in response to the infection. For this reason, PCR testing can identify infected dogs earlier in the course of the disease. The test is hoped to provide earlier and more accurate results.

	Iowa State PCR	Synbiotics RSAT
Advantages	Accuracy – no false positives. Detects DNA of the bacterial agent.	Accuracy – no false negatives unless very early after exposure.
	Assurance of quality control when sharing results with other breeders and veterinarians.	Speed – in house, results in under 1 hour.
Disadvantages	Speed – takes up to 3 weeks.	Many false positives which require verification at outside reference lab.
		Old technology.

Transmission of canine brucellosis
Transmission of brucellosis dog-to-dog may occur venereally. However, other routes of transmission are more common – these include ingestion or inhalation of aborted materials, transplacental transmission, and contact of any bodily secretions with the mucus membranes. One of the first documented human cases (1966) was an air conditioner repairman who was exposed under a porch where a bitch whelped a litter of infected pups.

Prevention of an outbreak of canine brucellosis in a kennel
Once a year, test all breeding stock in the kennel. Keep newly introduced dogs isolated from breeding stock. Test all dogs prior to introduction into a breeding colony twice at 4 to 6 week intervals. Females that abort should be assumed positive and should be isolated until proven otherwise.

Managing an outbreak of canine brucellosis
In many states, canine brucellosis is a reportable disease. This means if you confirm a brucellosis case, you must contact your state veterinarian. You only need to report a positive test result on the RSAT that is confirmed on either blood culture, PCR, and/or the AGID test. These veterinary authorities may dictate the management of testing and culling infected dogs and those in contact with infected dogs.

Euthanasia of all CULTURE positive dogs is frequently recommended. This is recommended because antibiotic regimens are not curative and the disease has zoonotic potential.

During an outbreak, all dogs in the kennel should be tested monthly for 3 months until the all the dogs housed in the kennel are negative on 2 successive tests. All females should be separated at birthing to reduce transmission in the kennel.

If an individual dog is infected, he or she must be sexually altered (ovariohysterectomized or castrated) and placed on long-term antibiotic therapy or euthanized. Antibiotic regimens that have been described include minocycline (25 mg/kg po SID x 14 days) with dihydrostreptomycin (5 mg/kg IM BID x 7 days) and tetracycline (30 mg/kg po BID x 21 days) with streptomycin (20 mg/kg IM SID x 14 days). Dihydrostreptomycin is no longer available; as a substitute, gentamycin or rifampin have been proposed but the side effects are considerable, including renal failure due to prolonged use of gentamycin. There is great cost associated with long-term antibiotic therapy, ongoing testing for monitoring resolution of the disease, and side effects associated with treatment.

Spayed females pose little risk of disease to family members after they are ovariohysterectomized. However, brucellosis can be harbored in the prostate, so it may not be possible to clear the male dog from this disease even with castration and long-term antibiotic therapy. The zoonotic risk of the disease must be discussed with the client, particularly in households with young children or immune-compromised members.

If one or more individual dogs in a group housing situation are infected, the entire colony must be euthanized or tested and culled multiple times. The following protocol has been recommended:

Confirm brucellosis is present based on PCR, blood cultures or cultures from infected tissues;

Report the disease as required by state laws;

Strictly limit movement of dogs in or out of the kennel, for any reason;

Identify ALL infected dogs. Try to determine the source of infection and all dogs in contact with infected dogs. Blood cultures are the recommended test;

Cease breeding;

Test all animals in the facility, and cull all infected animals. This often means euthanasia of large groups of dogs;

Separate groups of dogs to minimize transmission;

Retest all animals in the facility every month. Continue to cull infected animals;

The facility is not considered clear of brucellosis until all the animals have tested negative for 3 consecutive months. This may require 5 to 7 months of testing and culling;

Unless the kennel is closed to incoming and outgoing dogs and breeding is temporarily ceased, the kennel may never be cleared of brucellosis.

Preventing a canine brucellosis outbreak in a household or kennel of breeding dogs
Breeders have a great deal at stake every time they breed naturally or introduce a new dog into their household or kennel. Many have spent a lifetime developing their genetic lines; an outbreak of canine brucellosis could destroy a lifetime of work in a moment of oversight or poor judgment.

All dogs and puppies the breeder is exposing their dogs to should have a negative canine brucellosis test. This is particularly important if they are introducing a rescue dog from a breeding kennel into the household or kennel.

Require that any stud dog or bitch the breeder uses for breeding have a negative brucellosis test. To protect your bitch and kennel, it is reasonable to require a stud dog be tested before *each* breeding, not just on a bi-annual basis as many breeders choose to do. This includes stud dogs having semen shipped as fresh extended semen and stud dogs prior to collection semen for freezing. Freezing preserves <u>Brucella canis</u>.

Other infectious agents
Other bacteria reported to have caused fetal loss include: <u>Camyplobacter</u> and <u>Salmonella spp.</u> (from raw meat diets); <u>Listeria</u>; <u>Leptospirosis brataslava</u>; <u>Coxiella burnetti</u> (Q fever); and Chlamydia.

Canine herpesvirus
The mere mention of canine herpesvirus will strike fear into the hearts of most experienced dog breeders. For them and many veterinarians, this term is synonymous with certain death of an entire litter.

Canine herpesvirus (CHV) is a viral infection reported world-wide in 6% to 88% of the canine population.

In the adult dog, it causes mild respiratory symptoms, and is of little consequence. It is most devastating in pregnancy and the neonate, frequently causing resorption, abortion, and early death if contracted in the last 3 weeks of gestation through the first 3 weeks of life. There is no zoonotic potential for canine herpesvirus.

Symptoms

The primary symptom in puppies over 6 weeks of age through adulthood is mild upper respiratory disease, similar to mild kennel cough. If transmitted sexually, there may be pustular lesions on the mucus membranes of the vulva and penis and prepuce. These may be referred to as "dog pox".

Infection of an immunologically naïve bitch <u>prior to</u> 6 weeks of pregnancy can cause apparent infertility or reduced litter size, depending on the percentage of fetuses lost. Typically, the affected bitch has no clinical signs of illness.

Infection <u>after</u> 6 weeks of pregnancy often leads to placentitis, a secondary drop of progesterone, premature labor, delivery of stillborn pups, and premature delivery of sick or weak pups that die shortly after birth. Typically, the affected bitch has no clinical signs of illness, other than premature labor.

Pups may also be infected during birth by exposure to active vesicular lesions in the vulva, or shortly after birth from oro-nasal and vaginal secretions from their mother, littermates, or other dogs in the household.

Canine herpesvirus, like the human herpesvirus, tends to live on the mucus membranes of the oro-nasal and genital regions. CHV thrives at slightly lower-than-core body temperatures. Because puppies cannot thermo-regulate, they tend to have body temperatures between 96° and 99° F. This, combined with a naïve immune system, predisposes neonates to the systemic effects of CHV not seen in the older pup or adult dog.

Pups from the same litter may be born prematurely and die soon thereafter, be born healthy and become sick and die soon thereafter, or be born healthy and thrive.

Pups that are stillborn, born prematurely and fail to thrive, or that become ill within 1 week of birth were probably exposed in utero. Pups that were born healthy and become ill within 1 to 3 weeks of age were probably exposed in the immediate post-partum period.

CHV can look like many other diseases that cause abortion, stillborns, and "fading" puppies. Canine Herpesvirus is considered a common cause of neonatal death, from the pre-partum period up to 6 weeks of age.

Pups are most vulnerable from 9 to 14 days of age. Symptoms range from sudden onset of persistent crying (mewing), respiratory distress, abdominal pain and bloating, hypothermia, depression, anorexia, diarrhea, and weakness. This often progresses to death within 4 to 24 hours.

Testing for canine herpesvirus

Confirmation of canine herpesvirus can be difficult. If the bitch failed to conceive or resorbed her litter, herpes is one possible cause.

Serology testing in the bitch is ideally done with paired serum titers, with a 4 fold rise over a 10 to 14 day period. However, this testing is often not possible if serum samples were not collected from the bitch early in the course of the disease. CHV is poorly immunogenic, so titers do not rise much and fall quickly. Alternatively, any titer of greater than 1:2 when seen with resorption, abortion, or neonatal death is suggestive of herpes. Titers for CHV are available at several veterinary referral labs.

PCR testing is also available at a limited number of veterinary referral laboratories. Molecular detection by PCR is rapid, specific and highly sensitive. Sampling requirements for PCR testing are swabs (from vesicles, the nasopharynx, conjunctiva, or trachea), whole blood in EDTA (lavender top tube) or ACD (yellow top tube), or fresh or frozen tissues from the neonatal post mortem. PCR in the bitch will only remain positive transiently, so it is easy to miss a positive case.

A definitive diagnosis can be made on post mortem examination of aborted fetuses or dead neonates using PCR or histopathology. The classic gross lesions of herpes in the neonate are regions of focal necrosis and petechial hemorrhages on the surfaces of the liver and kidneys, caused by marked thrombocytopenia. These organs have a speckled appearance on the serosal surface.

PCR on neonatal tissues can be definitive. In the bitch with a suspected diagnosis of CHV, PCR testing is most useful when paired with a positive antibody titer. When combined testing and clinical signs demonstrate an active viral infection and an immunologic response, it is strongly suggestive of CHV.

Viral culture is not a routine method of diagnosis due to the labile nature of the virus.

Transmission
CHV infection can be transmitted by sexual contact, transplacentally, via direct exposure to pustules during birth, or via the oro-nasal route by direct or aerosol transmission. The virus can replicate and be shed, even in the presence of circulating antibodies.

The virus is poorly immunogenic and does not produce enough maternal antibodies in a previously exposed bitch to protect subsequent litters.

During periods of stress, such as at whelping, the latent virus reappears. This can allow large numbers of virus to be shed shortly after whelping, when the pups are most susceptible. Passive immunity, usually from colostrum or from injected plasma, is the most successful method of managing disease in the neonate. If vaccine is available, boostering during each pregnancy may be indicated to protect the pups. The antibodies appear to disappear in as little as 3 months, allowing the virus to reactivate (Merial website Canine Herpesvirus).

Managing an outbreak
There is no known treatment during pregnancy. Treatment of the neonates is largely supportive (See chapter 8). This includes 1) an environmental temperature of 90° to 95° F to keep the pups rectal temperatures at or above 99° F. 2) supplemental oxygen 3) nutritional support, including tube feeding if there is no vomiting 4) fluid therapy, via SQ, IV, IO, or PO route 5) antibiotics to reduce secondary invaders 6) serum or plasma transfusion for passive immunity 7) Vitamin K if there is hemorrhage 8) basic hygiene and assistance with eliminations and 9) any other supportive care, including butorphanol, deemed helpful in keeping the pups comfortable. There are anecdotal reports of successful treatment with Acyclovir.

Raising the ambient temperature can be used as an adjunct to treatment. Canine Herpesvirus lives preferentially on the mucus membranes of the extremities where the temperature is slightly below body temperature. This appears to be the main reason that CHV is more serious in the neonate than in a mature animal with a body temperature over 100° F. Increasing the ambient temperature may aid in preventing and/or treating affected or exposed neonates. Care is needed to prevent overheating and dehydration.

Prevention
There is no vaccine or pharmaceutical agent available for treatment or prevention of CHV in the United States. Some breeders attempt to reduce exposure of the pregnant bitch by staying home with all their dogs from dog events during the bitch's pregnancy and the pup's early neonatal period.

In Europe, a commercial vaccine is available for use in pregnant bitches. Use of the vaccine has been reported to produce increased litter size, higher birth weights, and lower neonatal death rates from Canine Herpesvirus.

Two doses of the vaccine are given during pregnancy, and need to be repeated during each pregnancy. It appears unlikely that this vaccine will be approved for use in the United States.

Other viral infections

Other viral infections can cause resorption, abortion and neonatal death. These include canine distemper virus, canine adenovirus, the canine minutevirus or parvovirus 1, canine parvovirus type 2 (CPV-2), and probably a multitude of others that are too rare or hard to confirm.

Most bitches who are adequately immunized against canine distemper virus and canine parvovirus 2 (the parvovirus routinely used in commercial vaccines) and have mounted an appropriate immunologic response will be protected. The pups should be protected through the transplacental and colostral transfer of antibodies.

Canine parvovirus 1 or the Minutevirus is another significant cause of apparent conception failure, birth defects, and early neonatal death. Symptoms of parvovirus 1 are vomiting, diarrhea, respiratory distress, constant crying, and sudden death. It is clinically indistinguishable from Canine Herpesvirus. Supportive care as used for Canine Herpesvirus (See chapter 8) is the only treatment, but is often unsuccessful. Diagnosis is confirmed at post-mortem.

Subclinical bacterial uterine infections and mycoplasma/Ureaplasma

During estrus and whelping, the cervix opens. This provides the opportunity for the same bacteria found in the cranial vagina during proestrus and estrus to ascend into the uterus. Many aerobic bacteria can be found in the uterus of fertile bitches. The most common uterine bacterial infections are coliforms, pasteurella, staphylococcus, and streptococcus species. The other potential route of infection is through hematogenous spread. Anaerobic bacteria and mycoplasma found in the uterus may be pathogenic.

Any bacteria found in pure culture or high numbers in the uterus or carefully collected aborted fetuses (kept sterile, from stomach contents or organs) are considered significant. The author has had 1 case reported by Dr. Casal at the University of Pennsylvania where Serratia sp. were recovered from inside the body cavities of multiple puppies in one litter that were aborted.

To obtain clinically significant cultures, samples can be taken by high vaginal culture at abortion (using a guarded swab), at C-section, by surgical biopsy, from aborted fetuses, placentas, or at the onset of the next estrous cycle on the first day vaginal discharge is noted (using a guarded swab).

It is possible for an apparently healthy bitch to have a subclinical bacterial infection of the uterus which would interfere with carrying a pregnancy full term. This type of infection is different from the bacterial component of pyometra.

Mycoplasma and ureaplasma organisms are found in the reproductive tract of normal and infertile bitches' reproductive tract. Their significance is unknown.

It is tempting to reach for antibiotics to attempt to solve infertility problems in the bitch and in the stud dog. Unless the patient has a documented bacterial cause for infertility, this is not recommended. It is normal to have a mix of bacteria, mycoplasma, and ureaplasma organisms in the vagina. Like in the gut and on the skin, these resident bacteria play a role in protecting this area from pathogenic invaders. Unjustified use of antibiotics, which will upset the normal flora, is likely to cause bigger problems, not resolve them. Unless there is a culture showing a subclinical or clinical bacterial disease in the uterus, vaginitis, a bacterial cause of abortion from a previous litter, an active bacterial endometritis or placentitis, or a pure culture of bacteria from a guarded high vaginal culture taken during proestrus, antibiotics should not be used.

Parasitic infections

Neospora caninum, Toxoplasma gondii, and other parasites are reported to cause ocular or neurologic disease in the neonate. These are rare unless the bitch has been fed a raw meat diet during or prior to her pregnancy. These disorders should be investigated if suggested by the history or symptoms.

Hypoluteoidism

Hypoluteoidism occurs when the level of progesterone, supplied by the luteal tissue in the ovary, is too low to maintain pregnancy. Progesterone is the only hormone necessary to maintain pregnancy. It is a rare condition. The Bullmastiff, German Shepherd, and Rottweiler appear to be overrepresented, but it may occur in bitches of any age and breed.

Routine supplementation of progesterone should be avoided unless determined to be necessary based on progesterone testing. Exogenous progesterone can cause masculinization of female fetuses. Progesterone supplementation must be stopped at approximately 61 days of pregnancy calculated from ovulation to allow for normal parturition. Placental aging past this time will not support the fetus and will lead to fetal death in utero.

The minimum level of progesterone shown to maintain a normal late term pregnancy in the bitch is 2.5 ng/ml. Levels below 5.0 ng/ml are inconsistent in preventing abortion. Levels below 5 ng/ml prior to day 55 of pregnancy may indicate hypoluteoidism and may require treatment. Bitches who have previously lost pregnancies should have progesterone levels monitored every 5 to 7 days during the last 5 weeks of pregnancy to allow for intervention to save the litter. If test results will not be available for 24 or more hours after submission, it may be necessary to initiate treatment at levels above 5 ng/ml. Whelpwise™ is another useful tool for managing high risk pregnancies.

Progesterone levels rise from a baseline of 2.0 ng/ml prior to ovulation, to 5.0 ng/ml at ovulation and may reach 15 to 80 ng/ml in the first few weeks after ovulation, whether the bitch is pregnant or not.

Hypoluteoidism may be primary, where the bitch's ovary fails to support the pregnancy, or secondary to a failing pregnancy and imminent abortion. It may be difficult to distinguish the difference. Regardless of the cause, if viable pups are seen on ultrasound, the progesterone level is below 5 ng/ml and the client opts to attempt to maintain the bitch's pregnancy despite the risks, progesterone supplementation may be necessary.

When to treat

The first decision is whether to attempt to save this litter. If the pups are deceased and the owner does not intend to breed the bitch again, ovariohysterectomy with IV fluid support at surgery may be indicated. If the bitch is ill, other supportive care should be instituted. Treatment is similar to that for pyometra.

If all pups have been aborted, or appear dead on ultrasound, and the bitch is to be bred again, progesterone supplementation should not be given. The bitch, if left untreated, is likely to pass all the fetal tissues barring oversized or emphysematous fetuses. Judicious use of Lutalyse® may aid in this but requires low doses and careful monitoring. If the bitch is sick or cannot deliver the pups, the equivalent of a C-section, removing fetal and placental tissues, saving the samples for histology and culture, flushing the uterus and treating appropriately, may be done.

If one or more pups are viable, progesterone supplementation may be considered. There is the risk of losing the litter, but there is also the opportunity to spare the remaining pups and the bitch's reproductive tract for future breedings. A successful pregnancy and delivery can coexist with a pyometra and/or otherwise failing pregnancy.

If the cause is primary hypoluteoidism, the bitch will require frequent ultrasounds and progesterone testing on all subsequent pregnancies. If the cause is secondary to a disease such as herpes, future pregnancies are likely to be normal.

Treatment of hypoluteoidism
There are 2 kinds of progesterone that can be used for supplementation. There are pros and cons to each, and often the choice is based on personal preference or availability. Both are available as equine preparations, not labeled for use in the dog.

Progesterone in oil
This is usually available through compounding pharmacies. It is measured on progesterone blood tests; the advantage is that you can evaluate the efficacy of treatment based on the progesterone level; the disadvantage is that you cannot determine the need to repeat the dose or if the treatment was even necessary. The dose is 1 mg/lb of body weight administered IM every 1 to 3 days until day 61 post-ovulation, or more frequently if supported by progesterone testing or tocodynometry. The preparation stings when administered. The more frequently the bitch needs to be supplemented, the more likely it is to be a secondary hypoluteoidism.

Altrenogest, ally-trenbolone or Regumate is available through Hoechst-Roussell. Because it is a synthetic hormone, it does NOT cause elevation of progesterone on blood tests; the disadvantage is that you cannot evaluate if the dose you are using is sufficient to prevent abortion; the advantage is that you can determine the need to continue or discontinue therapy. The dose is 0.088 mg/kg administered orally once daily, no later than 61 days post ovulation.

Many bitches with increased uterine contractility will respond quickly to the administration of either form of progesterone to quiet the uterus, even in cases where the progesterone levels are considered high enough to support pregnancy. This treatment has initiated pyometra in experimental models, so use with caution.

Antibiotic therapy
This should not be routinely administered during pregnancy, but it should be instituted if one or more fetuses have been expelled or there is an active vaginal discharge. Antibiotics are useful in treating primary metritis or secondary ascending vaginal infections. Normally the cervix should remain closed and prevent ascending uterine infections. However, once the cervix has opened, the risk of bacteria ascending into the uterus increases greatly.

The antibiotic chosen should be one known to be safe during pregnancy and one the bitch is known to tolerate well. Clavamox®, cephalexin, enrofloxacins, and trimeth-sulfa are good choices as they are broad spectrum, safe during pregnancy, and well tolerated by most bitches who are not allergic to them. They should be administered at the labeled doses based on the pregnant weight of the bitch and continued to term.

The only way to determine if the cervix is open or closed is with rigid endoscopy. It is not possible by digital vaginal examination due to the length of the vaginal vault.

Terbutaline
This is a human asthma drug, given orally or by SQ injection which has in some cases been used

successfully as the sole therapy to quiet uterine contractions. Cardiac arrhythmias are a potential risk in humans, suggesting caution if used in the bitch.

Combination of therapy

This can be used if the owner wishes to attempt to save the litter. Progesterone, terbutaline, and antibiotics in combination can be used based on progesterone levels, tocodynometry and clinical response. Treatment should be discontinued 61 days from ovulation. Metoclopramide can be started at day 61 from ovulation to assist with lactation as progesterone therapy will suppress lactation. Antibiotics should be administered if any fetuses have been expelled or there is an active vaginal discharge that is anything more than clear mucus. An Adaptil® collar will help the bitch develop maternal skills.

Pharmaceutical and nutritional supplements causing infertility

There are pharmaceutical agents and nutritional supplements that can cause fetal death or expulsion of fetuses from the uterus.

These may need to be used if the bitch has a life-threatening condition with no other treatment options available and owner consent.

Many drugs cause teratogenic effects or death of the fetus. A complete history is needed to uncover these, because owners may consider them to be routinely used and harmless.

Prior to the use of any drug with a luteolytic effect, ultrasound must be used to assure that no pregnancy exists. Prior to day 45 of pregnancy, a radiograph cannot distinguish between an early pregnancy and a pyometra. These 2 conditions may co-exist and in some cases can be treated successfully. Overzealous use of luteolytic agents can cause the expulsion of viable premature fetuses.

Any product containing a corticosteroid, including topicals such as ear and eye drops, as well as oral and injectables, luteolytic compounds – (Lutalyse®, Estrumate®), Aglepristone, and Raspberry tea leaf preparations can cause expulsion of fetuses.

Genetic incompatibility

Genetic incompatibilities, or fatal genes, have been documented in humans and dogs. Confirmation can be made on post mortem. If suspected, use of a different unrelated stud dog may be advisable. Litter sizes increased when out-crossed lines were compared to line-bred litters. This suggests partial loss of a litter in those with some genetic incompatibilities.

Oocyte quality also decreases with age, with bitches over age 4 being affected, and worsening by age 8. Although this is not treatable, it should be considered as a differential during a diagnostic work-up.

Uterine pathology – CEH, Fibrosis, Neoplasia

Uterine pathology (metropathy) is common in the intact bitch. Metropathy includes cystic endometrial hyperplasia (CEH), fibrosis, neoplasia, endometritis, pyometra, and subclinical uterine infections.

Each time the bitch is in estrous, the uterus is subjected to 60 to 90 days of progesterone influence. This causes irreversible pathology, suspected by some to damage the uterus more than pregnancy (Figure 9-7).

Fertility decreases by 33% in bitches over the 6 years old. The reduced fertility is probably due to aging of the oocysts, but some is also due to metropathy.

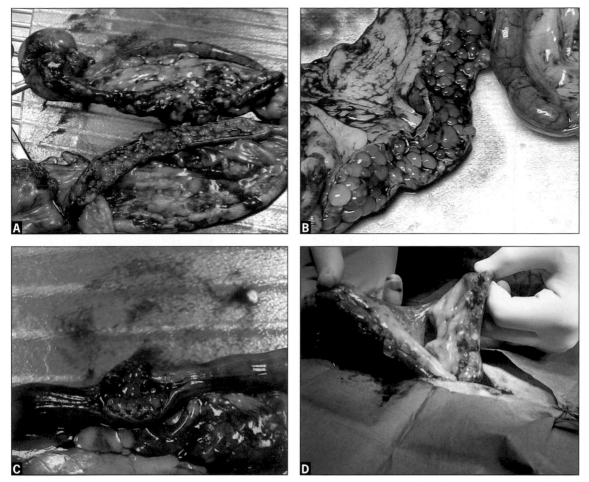

Figure 9-7.
A and B. Uterine lining with marked cystic endometrial hyperplasia. C. Uterine lining with marked cystic endometrial hyperplasia. Note the distended appearance of the intact uterine horn. D. Cysts on the serosal surface of uterus. These do not have a negative impact on fertility.

Ultrasound is useful in detecting significant ovarian and uterine lesions, such as severe cystic endometrial hyperplasia or uterine or ovarian neoplasia. Some pathology is visible grossly and on palpation of the uterus at surgical insemination. However, some changes are so subtle that they are only detected by uterine biopsy.

Uterine biopsy for histopathology and culture (aerobic, anaerobic, and mycoplasma/ureaplasma) can provide invaluable information. Infectious endometritis is a treatable cause of infertility. Some bitches have become pregnant on the subsequent estrous cycle using appropriately selected antibiotics.

Sometimes the biopsy results are only helpful for prognosis. The endometrial changes may be so severe that pregnancy is impossible and the best option is to stop trying. Sometimes the changes are reversible, and sometimes the prognosis is good because there is no pathology.

Uterine biopsy should NOT be attempted at the same time as a surgical breeding because of the associated inflammation. If a metropathy is suspected or confirmed at C-section, uterine biopsy, molecular pathology, and culture with histopathology and placental histopathology can be a useful service to offer the client.

If a bitch is bred with quality semen at the appropriate time based on progesterone testing, and is not pregnant based on ultrasound at 4 weeks post-ovulation, **AND** nothing in her history or on physical examination suggests a cause for her infertility, a surgical breeding at her next cycle or surgically obtained uterine cultures and biopsies should be considered. This is recommended only **IF** the breeder is committed to achieving a pregnancy. The procedures are invasive, require general anesthesia and cannot be combined. Surgical breeding may lead to a pregnancy. Surgical biopsy, may provide a prognosis and diagnosis. If surgical breeding with good semen and good timing is unsuccessful, surgical biopsy at the end of diestrus should be done to determine the cause. The decision is made by the client in consultation with the veterinarian and is influenced by the age of the bitch, availability of high quality but replenishable semen, previous attempts to breed, and the way that the client makes decisions. In some cases, uterine cytology samples can be collected using a transcervical catheterization collection technique which is a less invasive option than surgical biopsy.

The ideal time for uterine biopsies is near the time the bitch would whelp, 60 days after ovulation, if she had gotten pregnant. This is the time of maximal progesterone influence, the time which should demonstrate the greatest pathological changes in the uterus (Figure 9-8).

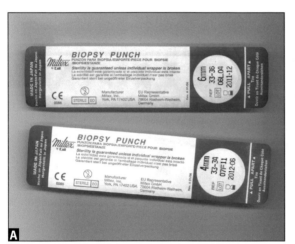
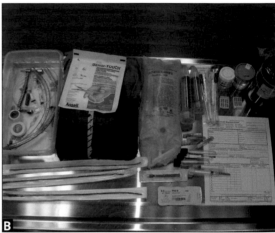

Figure 9-8.
A. Uterine punches used to collect full thickness uterine biopsies. **B.** Surgical instruments and supplies used to collect histology and microbiology samples surgically, as part of an infertility work – up in a bitch.

Uterine biopsy technique
There are 3 steps to the uterine biopsy technique.

Collect uterine tissues in Bouin's solution and formalin for histopathology.

Collect uterine tissues and fluid from inside the uterus for aerobic, anaerobic, and mycoplasma/ureaplasma culture.

Flush the uterus through the biopsy sites with the hope that if adhesions or other pathology is present, there may be some therapeutic value.

The specifics of these techniques are laid out in the Appendix D-11 along with the supplies needed and the sequence of events. This format is very helpful to the veterinary staff so that they are organized and can be certain all samples are collected and handled correctly.

The surgical biopsy procedure can be done by laparotomy or laparoscopy. Some clinicians collect samples endoscopically using TCI. Endoscopic biopsies are mucosal samples, not full thickness biopsies as obtained at laparotomy. Using general anesthesia and a routine prep and abdominal approach, the uterus and ovaries are identified. The ovaries should be palpated and if possible visually inspected, but not disrupted or traumatized. If ovarian pathology is suspected, the affected ovary(ies) may need to be exposed and the bursa opened, taking care to avoid trauma to the oviduct. If cystic structures are found, they should be aspirated (save the fluid), opened and curetted, and/or biopsied. If there are suspicious lesions, a biopsy of the ovary should be obtained. The bursa should be sutured closed and the ovary repositioned. If ovarian neoplasia is strongly suspected, the affected ovary may be removed surgically. This may be done by removing only the affected ovary, by unilateral ovariohysterectomy. Submit the fluid for cytology and progesterone assays.

Inspect the uterus for pathology. If free fluid is palpated, pack off the uterus with moistened lap towels prior to opening. Aspirate the free fluid and save it for cytologic examination (slides and lavender top), and culture (aerobic, anaerobic, mycoplasma). Plan the biopsy site prior to incising the uterus. The biopsy site should ideally look and/or feel like it has pathology, but be in a location that can be closed without compromising the lumen of the uterus or pathway from the cervix to the oviduct. The biopsy may be taken as a wedge with a scalpel blade or with 1 or more adjacent punch biopsies (Miltex punch biopsy) in a 2, 4 or 6 mm size. This decision is based on the size of the uterus and amount of tissue to be collected. The tissue samples should be divided between formalin, Bouin's solution, and culture solutions. Prior to placing in fixative solution, those tissues to be fixed should be placed in the foam-filled cassettes provided for tissue samples to keep them flat to minimize tissue distortion during fixation.

Lavage the uterus after all the samples for cytology, histopathology, and culture are collected. The abdomen should be well packed off with absorbent lap towels to keep uterine contents out of the peritoneal cavity. Insert a sterile red rubber feeding tube of appropriate size into the incision site(s) of the uterus, hold the uterine wall around the tube with one hand. Lavage with warmed Lactated Ringer's or normal saline, creating gentle distension. This is not only to flush the uterus, it may (optimistically) help open any mildly obstructive lesions in the tract.

Carefully close the uterus to minimize stricture formation that can interfere with future semen transport and placentation. If possible, close the incision perpendicular to the long axis of the uterus, not longitudinally to keep the lumen patent. Use a continuous suture in the Utrech inverting continuous pattern (See Figure 6-10) with 5-0 PDS for closure. Avoid penetration into the uterine lumen. Lavage the abdomen with warmed Lactated Ringers or normal saline, and close routinely.

You need to maximize the chances of a diagnosis with excellent tissue samples. Meticulous sample and tissue handling is critical to ensure that the bitch has the best chance of a return to fertility.

Cornell's veterinary diagnostic laboratory is the preferred location for biopsies of any reproductive tissues, for both bitches and dogs. (http://diaglab.vet.cornell.edu/). Dr. Schlafer prefers tissues preserved in Bouin's solution. Although this solution is more difficult to obtain than formalin, the histologic results are better. Store Bouin's solution carefully. If it dries out into a powder, it is reported to have explosive tendencies.

Fixation

Tissues fixed in Bouin's solution should be changed to 70% ethanol after 4 to 48 hours (less than 24 hours is optimal). If the tissues are fixed longer than this they tend to become brittle and difficult to section. (NOTE: long term storage in 70% ethanol can lead to shrinkage of the tissue)

Establish a treatment plan based on the biopsy and culture results. If there is evidence of bacterial infection, antibiotics should be chosen based on the culture and sensitivity results. If there is cystic endometrial hyperplasia (CEH) causing implantation failure, mibolerone may improve the uterine health enough to allow a pregnancy to go to term.

If indicated, use 30 mcg of mibolerone per 25 pounds of body weight once daily for 6 months

(Appendix C-5). Breed the bitch on the first estrous cycle after the drug is withdrawn. If neoplasia is present, ovariohysterectomy is recommended. Fibrosis or other inflammatory changes may respond to low doses of corticosteroids used just prior to the expected onset of estrous and discontinued at the time of breeding.

Hormonal alteration of estrous

Inducing estrous

There are several effective protocols to induce estrous in the bitch. The veterinary staff should encourage breeders to be certain that they have a stud dog or semen lined up and ready to go prior to the induction of estrus. The range is 3 to 17 days from the start of the medication until the bitch is ready to breed. Once the commitment to induce an estrous cycle is made, there will not be adequate time for "plan B" breedings.

Convenience is arguably the weakest reason to induce estrous. However, it makes arranging live breedings much more manageable. This can be arranged around show schedules, stud dog and bitch availability, and the special scheduling needs of clients.

Failure to cycle is an important reason to induce estrous. A thorough diagnostic work-up should be performed prior to an attempt to induce estrous.

Prolonged inter-estrous. If greater than 12 months, there is no reason for concern except that the breeder may be ready to breed the bitch. This is reason enough for some breeders to request this service.

Induction technique

Currently available pharmacologic agents induce estrous by removing what is inhibiting the cycle, rather than by attempting to drag the bitch into heat. Cabergoline and bromocriptine are dopamine agonists, which work by exerting a direct inhibitory effect on the secretion of prolactin by the pituitary. Pregnancy rates may be lower in induced cycles than in naturally occurring estrous.

Cabergoline is preferred over **bromocriptine** because it has a longer duration of action and is less likely to cause vomiting. **Deslorelin** is also used to induce estrous in the dog. Deslorelin increases the levels of endogenous luteinizing hormone (LH), thereby inducing ovulation.

Cost for treatment with either cabergoline or Deslorelin is similar for the moderate sized dog. Cabergoline must be compounded for dogs under 25 pounds. There is a liquid product containing 50 mcg/ml of cabergoline labeled as Galastop available in Europe.

Cabergoline, or Dostinex®, is given orally once daily at 5 mcg/kg for 10 days. If the bitch has not started her estrous cycle by day 10, it is continued at 5 mcg/kg every other day for 10 additional days. Approximately 70% of the bitches treated will show signs of estrous within 30 days of starting the drug. This is a human drug, available through the pharmacy. It is not labeled for use in the dog.

Deslorelin, or Ovuplant®, is a drug pellet, inserted under the mucus membrane of the lip of the vulva with local anesthesia. Ovuplant® is an equine product, not labeled for use in the dog. The dose is 1 pellet per bitch, regardless of size. Check the serum progesterone prior to placement to be sure the bitch is not in early proestrus. If the progesterone is greater than 1 ng/ml, the drug will block, not induce, estrous. Once the progesterone has been tested and is baseline (<1 ng/dl), the implant may be placed. It is best if a standard protocol is established for location of the pellet. The author (right-handed) uses the inner lip of the right labia, halfway between dorsal and ventral commissures. This is significant, because knowing the location of the implant will make removal easier following ovulation. The implant must be removed after ovulation (Figure 9-9) (Appendix D-2).

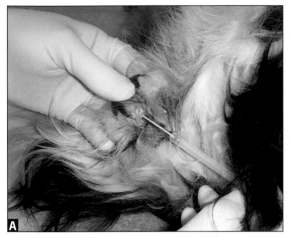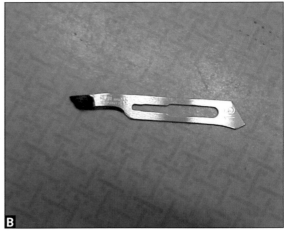

Figure 9-9.
A. Placement of ovuplant showing hand and needle position. B. The ovuplant can be removed using local anesthesia and either a scalpel blade or laser incision. In most cases, the ovuplant can be lifted out as a pellet.

No shaving is necessary. Position the patient with her right side down, so there is easy access to the inner right labia. Have 1 assistant hold the head and forelegs, and a second hold the right rear leg with 1 hand and the tail with the opposite hand. With Nolvasan®, prep the inner lip of the vulva. Instill the lidocaine mixed 10:1 with sodium bicarbonate with a TB syringe into the labia near the mucocutaneous junction, halfway between the dorsal and ventral commissures. Put on sterile gloves and re-prep the region with Nolvasan®. Open the Ovuplant® taking care to keep the applicator sterile. Carefully position the drug pellet into the needle before inserting the needle under the mucosa, as this will make placement require less force. Be careful not to push the pellet out of the needle or allow it to drop out during positioning. With a gauze square in the left hand, gently pull the tip of the vulva toward the bitch's feet, separating the lips. The implant must be placed with the needle directed from dorsal to ventral to reduce the chances that the pellet will dislodge while the tissues are sealing over. Directed ventrally and bevel up, the needle should be inserted near the dorsal commissure of the right labia and slid just under the mucus membrane ventrally. The goal is to see the pellet through the mucus membrane as it slides into place, with the final destination halfway between the ventral and dorsal commissures, adjacent to the mucocutaneous junction. To control bleeding, a cotton ball or portion of one can be placed inside the vulvar lips. This will dislodge during urination. She is discharged to the care of the breeder.

The estrous cycle usually starts within 3 days following placement of the Deslorelin implant. The bitch must be monitored closely because the proestrus will be shortened. Rather than starting progesterone testing on day 6 of the estrous cycle, these bitches should be started on day 3. It is best to keep the bitch at home until she is in estrous. Most bitches who fail to cycle with Deslorelin are the ones who have been sent directly to the stud dog after implantation. The typical bitch will be ready to breed on approximately day 6 to 15 after insertion of the drug. Because of the shortened proestrus and predictability of the breeding, counsel the client to have their schedule cleared and a stud dog or semen available prior to starting the protocol. Progesterone testing and timing the breeding then proceeds as with a spontaneous estrous cycle. The author places a fluorescent sticker in the patient's file so all staff is aware that the Ovuplant® needs to be retrieved after breeding.

(See Appendix D-2)

Supplies for insertion of the Ovuplant®:
1. Ovuplant®
2. Sterile gloves – 1 pair
3. Sterile gauze squares
4. Nolvasan® surgical prep
5. Lidocaine
6. Sodium bicarbonate
7. TB syringe
8. Cotton balls
9. Ovuplant® stickers
10. Vetrap® or hair clips to control hair on long-coated bitches
11. 2 assistants to hold dog

Once the progesterone rises above 5 ng/ml and the breeding is completed, whether naturally, by AI, or surgically, remove the Ovuplant®.

A client handout for managing the induced heat cycle and breeding is in Appendix C-4.

If the bitch is bred naturally, the Ovuplant® can be removed after the final breeding. In this way there is no unnecessary discomfort from the incision during the tie with the stud dog. If bred by AI, remove the Ovuplant® BEFORE the AI so restraint of the bitch does not contribute to semen escaping the reproductive tract. If bred surgically, remove the Ovuplant® prior to recovery from anesthesia. If the Ovuplant® is in place for over 14 days, recovery can be difficult as the pellet tends to fragment and is difficult to find. If the pellet cannot be located, leaving it in will may not interfere with conception and pregnancy.

To remove the Ovuplant®, the bitch is again positioned with her right side down with 2 assistants restraining her. No clipping is necessary. The hair should be managed again with hair clips or Vetrap®. The Ovuplant® should be identified on visual inspection and palpation of the right labia. This must be done prior to injection of the lidocaine bleb because the bleb will obscure the pellet and make removal more difficult. The Ovuplant® pellet is usually visible as a small white raised area near the placement site. If not visible, palpate the right and left labial lips and compare to determine the location. Prep the labia with Nolvasan®, and inject a 10:1 mixture of lidocaine:sodium bicarbonate mixture. Sterile gloves are donned, a second prep is applied, and a small 2 to 3 mm incision is made just over the Ovuplant®. The incision can be made with a scalpel blade or a cutting laser. Using the cutting laser makes removal easier (the Ovuplant® sparks when located) as well as less pain and blood is noted. In some cases, the Ovuplant® can be lifted out intact with the tip of the scalpel blade. In other cases, the Ovuplant® must be gently scooped out in fragments. Flush the region with saline to remove any remaining fragments. No suture is necessary, but 4-0 Vicryl® can be used if the incision is extended. A cotton ball or portion thereof can be placed in between the lips of the vulva to reduce bleeding. It will be flush out when the patient urinates (Appendix D-3).

(See Appendix D-3)

> **Supplies to gather to remove the Ovuplant®:**
> 1. Sterile scalpel blade and curved mosquito forceps
> 2. Sterile gloves – 1 pair
> 3. Sterile gauze squares
> 4. Nolvasan surgical prep
> 5. Lidocaine
> 6. Sodium bicarbonate
> 7. TB syringe
> 8. Cotton balls
> 9. 3 cc saline flush
> 10. Vet-rap or hair clips to control hair on long-coated bitches
> 11. 2 assistants to hold dog

Preventing estrous

Mibolerone is one of two non-surgical option/pharmaceutical option currently available in the United States to prevent estrous cycles. The other non-surgical option is megestrol acetate. The other alternative is surgical alteration by ovariectomy or ovariohysterectomy.

Mibolerone, previously marketed by Upjohn as Cheque® drops, is now a controlled substance available only on a case-by-case dispensing basis from several compounding pharmacies throughout the U.S. You must be careful to assure that your client receives the product you ordered at the dose you prescribed from the compounding pharmacy. Removal of Mibolerone from the market was apparently an economic, not a medically based decision. The DEA has placed mibolerone in a class of controlled substances because of human abuse of this anabolic steroid. Due diligence is a duty of the prescribing veterinarian to assess the drug and pharmacy before prescribing.

The use of mibolerone in the breeding bitch is controversial. It was originally labeled by Upjohn as not for use in the breeding bitch. Some argue that sparing the uterus from cycling and the influence of progesterone on the uterus is beneficial to good uterine health and improved fertility. Others argue that long-term use (1 year or more) will thin the endometrium and reduce fertility.

Indications for the use of mibolerone
Client handout in Appendix C-5

Short inter-estrous cycles
Mibolerone is the drug of choice to extend the time between estrous cycles. The uterine lining requires at least 120 days between estrous cycles to return to a state healthy enough to support a pregnancy. For bitches who cycle more frequently than at 4 month intervals with no evidence of ovarian pathology, mibolerone is the only treatment option. There is also some indication that bitches with CEH cycle more frequently than bitches with normal uterine linings, so this may spare her uterine health and allow her to be bred successfully after treatment.

Pyometras
If successfully treated for pyometra, and the bitch will not be bred her on her next cycle, consider mibolerone to prevent her from coming into estrous for up to 2 years, or until 2 to 3 months before the client is ready to breed her. Some reports suggest once a bitch has had a pyometra, she will have one on every cycle. Based on clinical observations, veterinarians know this is not always the case. However, no one can predict which bitches will have a recurrence at the next cycle and which will not, so mibolerone may be used as a precaution.

Convenience
For many breeders, particularly if they have multiple bitches and stud dogs, minimizing the number of cycling bitches can be very helpful.

Competition
Control of estrus is useful when competing in conformation, field trials, agility, and other events. Bitches in season are barred from competing in some events. Many breeders delay breeding their high-performing bitches until they are retired and can stay home to raise puppies. As the ovaries and uterus age, the likelihood of a successful pregnancy diminishes. Resting the uterus by preventing heat cycles and the influence of progesterone on the uterine lining may be an option that appeals to the breeder.

Guidelines for mibolerone use
Mibolerone is a valuable but potent hormone, and must be used carefully.

Never use the product prior to the first estrous cycle. Estrogen is necessary for growth plates to close and use of mibolerone in a pre-pubertal bitch can alter the process.

Side effects
Vaginal discharge
This is a sticky discharge, similar to that of puppy vaginitis, caused by hormonal influence. It is NOT A PYOMETRA – it is not possible for a bitch on mibolerone to have a pyometra. Be certain everyone who provides care for this dog is informed of this. If the dog is with a handler, and away from her regular veterinarian, be certain they know so that an attending veterinarian does not mistake this for pyometra and whisk her off to surgery.

Epiphora
Tearing reported in 1%, but is probably higher. This is not clinically significant.

Enlarged clitoris
From the influence of testosterone. May be irritating to the bitch, but is not of great concern.

Increased muscle mass and tone, and better coat
This can actually be beneficial for bitches in competition.

Never use Mibolerone for more than 2 consecutive years. If long-term use is indicated, she should come off, have 1 cycle, and reinitiate treatment. There are reports of thinning of the uterine wall with prolonged use, so inform the client of this.

Run a liver panel prior to starting the drug and every 3 to 6 months while she is on this product. Liver enzymes often become elevated, but this does not appear to be clinically significant. It is recommended that Mibolerone not be used in Bedlington terriers or bitches with a history of liver disease.

Be sure the client is aware that mibolerone must be given EVERY day. Follow the dosage schedule carefully and remember, German Shepherds require a higher dose than other breeds.

Mibolerone must be started at least 30 days prior to the onset of estrous – once the bitch is in estrous, the product will not interrupt it.

Mibolerone can only be ordered from a compounding pharmacy on a case-by-case basis. The DEA will not allow it to be purchased in bulk quantities for dispensing out of the veterinary clinic's pharmacy. Choose your compounding pharmacy carefully – there is a big difference in reliability and quality. The product can be expensive (Table 9-1).

Table 9-1 Dosages for mibolerone		
lbs	kgs	mcg/day
1-25	0.5-12	30
25-60	12-25	60
50-100	25-45	120
> 100	> 45	180
German Shepherd		180

Never use this product if a bitch may be pregnant because it will cause masculinization of the female fetuses.

The average bitch will cycle 70 to 90 days after withdrawal of mibolerone. She may safely be bred on the first cycle. After all, that is why she was on it in the first place. The range of time to cycle is 7 to 240 days after withdrawal. If the bitch fails to cycle when desired, the author has initiated cabergoline or Deslorelin treatment after waiting 30 to 180 days, and successfully induced fertile estrous cycles.

Cats – **never** use this in cats as they are reported to develop fatal liver or thyroid disease.

Megestrol acetate or Ovaban®, has been removed from the veterinary market, but can be purchased as a human product. It was originally marketed as a drug to prevent estrous. It acts by blocking or reducing GnRH release from the hypothalamus. It may induce histologic lesions of CEH, predisposing bitches to the development of pyometra. On the other hand, some practitioners theorize that megestrol acetate may protect bitches from pyometra by blocking estrous cycles that precede pyometras. There are also reports of mammary neoplasia and diabetes mellitus linked to the use of megestrol acetate.

Megestrol acetate can be used to prevent estrous with one of two protocols:
1. 2.2 mg/kg PO SID for 8 days if started within the first 3 days of estrus (92% efficacy).
OR
2. 0.55 mg/kg PO SID for 32 days if started 7 or more days prior to the onset of proestrus.

This should not be repeated more often than every 6 months.

GnRH agonists and antagonists may have a place in estrous control in the future.

Prolonged estrous
There are several reasons for prolonged estrous. These include split heats, cystic ovaries, ovarian neoplasia and inadvertent exposure to exogenous estrogen creams. Ultrasound is recommended for early detection of ovarian or uterine neoplasia, in any bitch over the age of 4 who has a change in her estrous cycle.

Pseudopregnancy
Hormonally, EVERY bitch has a pseudopregnancy for the 2 to 3 months following her estrous cycle unless she is pregnant. Progesterone levels rise and remain elevated for 60 to 90 days after ovulation, whether the bitch is pregnant or not. Some bitches are clinically affected and some are clinically asymptomatic. The clinical signs vary in severity and the type of syndrome noted.

Prior to treatment, verifiy with ultrasound or radiographs that the bitch is not pregnant with a single pup or a litter so small it may be undetected. Most pseudopregnancies do not require any treatment. However, if the symptoms are so severe that it is problematic for either the bitch or her owner, treatment should be initiated. Bitches spayed during certain phases of the estrous cycle, specifically during diestrus, may also exhibit symptoms that merit treatment.

Symptoms of false pregnancy are more related to the progesterone drop than rising levels of estrogen and prolactin, and may be better described as false whelping than false pregnancy.

Symptoms of false pregnancy are:
Engorgement of the mammary glands with lactation
    Secondary mastitis – rare
Nesting and whelping-like behaviors
Maternal behaviors, such as collecting soft toys and mothering them

---

Treatment of false pregnancy/False whelping

Water and food should be mildly restricted for several days. Avoid manipulation of the mammary glands that may stimulate lactation. Use of an Elizabethan collar or dressing the bitch in a t-shirt may reduce licking and self-stimulation of lactation. Cabergoline and bromocriptine are drugs that block prolactin secretion. **Bromocriptine** is less expensive than **cabergoline**, but is more likely to cause vomiting. It is a human drug, dosed at 10 mcg/kg tid for 16 days po. **Cabergoline** is a human drug, dosed at 5 mcg/kg/day once daily for 5 to 7 days po. Avoid the use of **acepromazine**, **metoclopramide**, and other dopamine antagonists because these will exacerbate lactation. Ovariohysterectomy can be performed prior to the next estrous cycle if the symptoms are severe and there are no plans to use the bitch again for breeding.

Diagnosis and treatment of pyometra

(Appendix D-17)

The typical bitch with pyometra is an intact middle aged to older (9 to 12 years of age), who was in heat in the last 6 to 9 weeks. In some cases, the owner may not have recognized her estrous cycle or may not mention it unless questioned about it. Pyometras can occur at any time in an intact female, so should be on the rule out list for any sick female. She may present with a varied combination of symptoms, including feeling sick, lethargic, <u>without</u> a fever, with increased water consumption, increased urination, dehydration, loss of appetite, and sometimes vomiting and/or diarrhea. She may just seem vaguely unwell with no specific symptoms because the onset is gradual and insidious. Rarely, she may have a history of recent treatment with estrogen or progesterone hormones (mibolerone cannot cause pyometra). Golden Retrievers, Collies, Rottweilers, Bernese Mountain dogs, and Airedale and Irish Terriers appear to be over-represented. It is most common in the older bitch that has never produced a litter. By 10 years of age 25% of all female dogs will develop pyometra. Pyometra may be suspected in a female with a poorly documented medical history pertaining to her ovariohysterectomy status and has been reported in male pseudohermaphrodites (Figure 9-10).

If the cervix is closed – closed pyometra – there is no vaginal discharge indicating pyometra. She tends to be sicker than her counterpart with an open cervix.

If the cervix is open – open pyometra – there can be a scant to copious muco-purulent to bloody vaginal discharge, often with a foul odor. She has probably been licking her perineum for several hours to several days. On vaginal cytology, there is an overwhelming number of toxic white blood cells, frequently with phagocytized bacteria, usually rods.

Some patients will have an elevated white blood cell count (70%), sometimes as high as 50,000, while 25% will present with a WBC of only 12,000 WBC,. Some will have a classic left shift (25%), some will not. Some may have leukopenia (an unusually low WBC).The left shift is less likely if the bitch has endotoxic shock or an open cervix. Some will have a high BUN and elevated creatinine

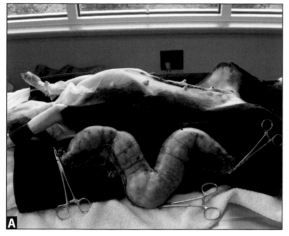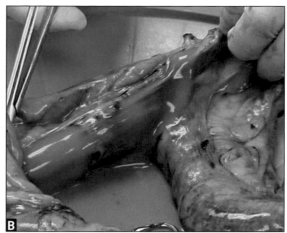

Figure 9-10.
A and *B.* Pyometra.

(30%), but some will not. Some will be borderline anemic, some will not. Some will have isothenuric urine. Most (50 to 75%) will have an elevated SAP, but some will not.

Some bitches will present with prerenal azotemia and dehydration despite their PU/PD status. She may also be hyperproteinemic (from dehydration) and hyperglobulinemic (from antigenic stimulation). If she presents with endotoxemia, she may have decreased GFR and be isothenuric. She may already have a secondary membranous glomerulonephritis associated with the antigen-antibody complexes against E. coli. Proteinuria, if present, may be predictive of renal failure.

Many savvy breeders will suspect a pyometra, even if the cervix is closed. If they haven't had a bitch with pyometra, they are knowledgeable about them by association with someone who has. They will refer to it as a "pyo", which then quickly becomes a verb ("pyoing" or a variation on this). If the owner presents a bitch to you with this suspicion, do not dismiss it until you are certain you have ruled it out. Pyometras come in all sizes and shapes. They can occur after the first estrous cycle. They can present a few days after a heat cycle, or up to 12 weeks later. They do not always conform to what we think of as "typical".

One cause of pyometras is probably due to prolonged progesterone influence on the uterine lining, and associated bacterial invasion. Whether the bacterial invasion is primary or secondary is controversial. The pathogenesis involves estrogen stimulation of the uterus, followed by bacterial invasion, progesterone influence creating endometrial proliferation, uterine glandular secretions, closure of the cervix, and decreased myometrial contractions. The uterus retains fluid and has decreased inherent immunity at this time. Any uterine pathology complicated by a bacterial invasion, ascending or hematogenous, may lead to pyometra. Because of the multitude of causes, pyometras may occur at any time in the bitch's cycle.

The same E. coli found in the gut of the patient is commonly found in her uterus. In less than 10% of cases, the E. coli release cytotoxin necrotizing factors – these are the sickest bitches, presenting with hypothermia and septic shock. Staphylococcus aureus, Streptococcus spp., Pseudomonas spp., and Proteus spp. are sometimes found in the uterus; there are no sterile pyometras. Whether cystic endometrial hyperplasia (CEH) and pyometra are always found together or if they are two different diseases is controversial. This is probably more important in theory than in practice. Pyometra is a separate disease entity from mucometra and post partum metritis.

Diagnosis of pyometra

Physical exam findings, history, CBC, chemistry panel, vaginal cytology and imaging may all be needed to confirm a pyometra. Collection of urine by cystocentesis should be avoided, because it could lead to uterine rupture or abdominal contamination. Open-cervix pyometras are easier to diagnose. Abdominal ultrasound, showing an anechoic or hypoechoic fluid filled uterus, either with a consistent diameter or segmental loops, is invaluable in confirming a diagnosis. An ultrasound of the ovaries is valuable to rule out an ovarian cyst or neoplasia. Ultrasound is also essential to confirm that there is no concurrent viable pregnancy.

A pyometra can be difficult to visualize on abdominal radiographs; additionally, films cannot be used to distinguish a pregnancy from a pyometra if the bitch is less than 45 days from ovulation. It is possible that an owner may not realize that an unwitnessed breeding occurred.

If there is a possibility the bitch is bred and ultrasound is not available, referral to a veterinary hospital where ultrasound is available should be offered. Many clients will prefer the option for referral to having an ovariohysterectomy as the only option.

Medical treatment versus surgical treatment

One of the most consistent sayings in veterinary school is "never let the sun set on a pyometra." This is now considered outdated due to advances in diagnosis and treatment and increased awareness of the need to stabilize patients pre-operatively. In the interest of full disclosure, medical treatment as an alternative to surgical treatment should be discussed. Many patients may be more safely treated medically than surgically, and go on to produce litters.

There is no one-size-fits-all approach to treatment for pyometra. Each case requires consideration of both treatment options. Neither the medical nor surgical option is 100% safe. There are complications seen with both, with a 4% mortality reported.

Closed cervix pyometras are suspected in many intact bitches presented 1 to 2 months after their heat cycle and not feeling well. While this is certainly appropriate to include in the differential, don't assume that she has a pyometra until the diagnosis is confirmed. Many other conditions, including pregnancy, can mimic the clinical signs of closed-cervix pyometra. Open-cervix pyometra tends to be a more straight-forward diagnosis, but there are other conditions with similar symptoms (Figure 9-11).

It may appear obvious that surgical alteration is a better choice if a bitch is not to be used for breeding. But this is not always the case. The main advantage of surgical treatment over medical treatment is that the opportunity for recurrence is eliminated. There are several advantages to medical therapy.

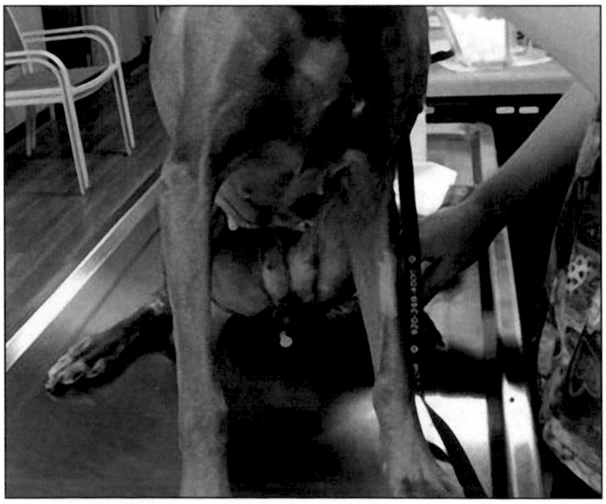

Figure 9-11.
Vaginal discharge associated with an open pyometra.

The following factors should be considered prior to instituting a treatment plan:

Is the bitch pregnant with a normal litter but isn't eating or feeling well because she is pregnant? The most common clinical indicators of pregnancy are loss of appetite and mucoid vaginal discharge. Lab values often show a mild elevation of the white blood cell count which is normal in the pregnant bitch should not be construed as a response to an infection. Be CERTAIN that she is not pregnant before proceeding with treatment.

Is she pregnant with viable fetuses concurrently with her pyometra?

Is she a candidate to breed in the future?

Does she appear to be a good candidate for surgery in her current condition?

Other than breeding, is there any other reason the owner prefers to leave her intact?

Is she clinically ill or does she have a muco-purulent vaginal discharge as her only symptom?

Is there evidence the illness and/or vaginal discharge is a pyometra and not some other disorder that mimics pyometra? Diabetes mellitus can make a bitch PU/PD or can co-exist with pyometra and pregnancy. Uterine or ovarian neoplasia can look like or cause pyometra. Vaginal masses and foreign bodies can cause muco-purulent vaginal discharge.

Is the bitch currently on or been recently treated with mibolerone?

How old is the bitch?

What other organs appear to have pathology based on a current blood chemistry panel? Does she have a normal liver and kidney profile? Is she losing protein in her urine? Does she have diabetes mellitus?

What other health conditions does she have? Cardiac function? Neoplasia? Coagulopathy? DIC? Other health issues?

Can you improve her condition with supportive care and medical management of her pyometra and take her to surgery later when she is a better surgical candidate?

Will the owner approve the surgical procedure? The medical procedure? Euthanasia?

Have you discussed the pros and cons of both medical and surgical options? You should discuss both options, but it is your responsibility to guide the client to a medically appropriate treatment plan.

Will she ever be a candidate for surgery?

Treatment of pyometra

Treatment can be surgical, medical, or a combination of both. There is some difference of opinion regarding medical treatment particularly with closed-cervix pyometra. There are many reports supporting successful medical treatment of closed-cervix pyometras, with the bitches going on to produce litters. Remember that the drugs given to induce luteolysis will also soften and open the cervix, allowing the uterus to drain.

The client should always be advised that neither medical nor surgical treatment of pyometra can be guaranteed to have a successful outcome. Success is defined as a bitch that lives through treatment. A subsequent successful pregnancy is a bonus.

Medical treatment should be considered for the young to middle aged (under 6 to 8 year old) valuable breeding bitch, for those who are too sick for anesthesia and surgery, or for owners who refuse surgical treatment. The cost of medical treatment may be similar to or even exceed the cost of surgical treatment. The value is the possibility of preserving the bitch for future breeding or delaying surgery until the patient's medical condition has stabilized enough to make her a better surgical candidate.

Surgical treatment should be considered for bitches who have no breeding potential or who are aged, <u>and</u> are good surgical candidates. Surgical treatment requires a longer anesthetic and surgical period, additional diagnostics, additional days in the hospital, additional fluid therapy, and additional medications with at least 1 week of antibiotics post-op, making the cost of treatment much higher than that for a routine ovariohysterectomy.

Medical treatment followed by surgery after stabilization should be considered for patients who are not good surgical candidates at presentation. Even in bitches with closed-cervix pyometras, there is little question that some are too sick for surgery at presentation but can be supported medically until stable. All bitches should be stabilized pre-op with IV fluids and broad-spectrum antibiotics. Many will benefit from fluids, antibiotic therapy, and luteolytic treatment (Lutalyse® or aglepristone) for several days to stabilize them and reduce the volume of purulent material in the uterus prior to surgery.

Medical treatment requires multi-drug treatment, a minimum of a 5 day stay in the hospital, fluid therapy, careful observation, hand-walking, repeated lab tests and ultrasounds.

Medical management of pyometra

Lutalyse® is the backbone of pyometra therapy, but MUST be used concurrently with antibiotics. The drug has multiple effects – it is luteolytic, lysing the corpus luteum which is producing progesterone; it increases smooth muscle contractions to help evacuate the uterus; and it aids in relaxing and opening the cervix to allow drainage. Lutalyse® is not a drug labeled for use in the dog, but there are many reports indicating that it is being used within the standard of care. Because of its effect on all smooth muscles, it can cause bronchospasm, vomiting, and diarrhea. Brachycephalic patients are at increased risk of respiratory distress; therefore many avoid the use of prostaglandins in these breeds.

<u>Lutalyse® should be handled with caution to minimize risks to the staff.</u> It has abortifactant and bronchospasm effects, even when the drug is in direct contact with the skin or is aerosolized. Precautionary protocols should be established and followed specifically. These may include: not allowing women of child-bearing age to handle the drug, particularly if pregnant; not allowing individuals with asthma or other restrictive respiratory disease to handle the drug; only using luer-lock syringes, not slip-tip syringes, to reduce the possibility of the needle dislodging and aerosolizing the drug during injection; immediate disposal of the needle and syringe into a sharps box to avoid accidental needle sticks; wearing gloves and/or a mask and not dispensing the drug to clients.

Lutalyse® has the side-effect of causing not only the smooth muscle of the uterus to contract, but also all smooth muscles. Using the following techniques can make the treatment easier on the bitch and the veterinary staff.

Time the use of Lutalyse® so that it is not administered with anything given orally to minimize the likelihood she will vomit the oral medications and food – usually 1 hour between the injection of Lutalyse® and administration of any oral medication is sufficient.

Walk the bitch for 15 to 20 minutes after each injection to minimize the abdominal cramping, vomiting and diarrhea she may experience with the first few injections.

Start with a lower dose of Lutalyse® (10 mcg/kg) and slowly increase to the therapeutic dose (50 mcg/kg) within 48 hours. Less that 15% of patients will experience side effects with this protocol. The side effects may include vomiting, diarrhea, panting and salivation.

Dilute the Lutalyse® with saline to a final volume of 2 to 10 ml – this will slow absorption and reduce abdominal cramping, vomiting, and diarrhea. Administer the drug subcutaneously.

Include atropine or metoclopramide if needed to reduce side effects.

One commonly recommended protocol administers Lutalyse® at a starting dose of 10 mcg/kg (0.01 mg/kg) SQ for the first 24 hours, increasing the dose to 25 mcg/kg SQ for the second 24 hours, reaching a maximum dose of 50 mcg/kg per dose SQ for 3 days. The dose for a 45 pound (20 kg) dog is 0.2 cc of Lutalyse® 3 to 5 times a day at the maximum dose.

Continue treatment for a minimum of 5 days or until the vaginal discharge becomes scant and ultrasound shows that the uterus is reduced by at least 50% in diameter. Ultrasound should be repeated every 2 to 3 days to monitor treatment success. Treatment can take up to 3 weeks. The bitch may come into estrous 1 to 2 months sooner than expected.

If medical treatment is unsuccessful, ovariohysterectomy may be indicated.

Sometimes treatment is recommended for 5 days, resting the bitch (at home if possible) for several days, and continuing treatment for an additional 5 days. This seems to diminish the uterus's tendency to become refractory to treatment. The WBC may lag behind the clinical response as the uterus empties and monitoring the CBC can be misleading.

There are other medications that can be used in place of Lutalyse®, depending on availability and familiarity with these products. Lutalyse® is the most commonly used drug for treating pyometras.

Alternative medications

Cloprostenol (Estrumate®) is labeled for use in large animals only. Administer 1 to 5 mcg/kg (0.001 to 0.005 mg/kg) subcutaneously once a day for 7 to 14 days. Side effects at this dose are greater than Lutalyse®. The side effects and precautions for humans handling the drug are comparable to Lutalyse®. The advantage is once daily dosing. It is not as effective in creating the uterine contractions essential for emptying, thus requiring a longer treatment protocol.

Aglepristone is not currently available in the United States and is relatively expensive. It blocks progesterone receptors, creating the effect of lower progesterone levels. For the treatment of open or closed-cervix pyometra, anti-progestins cause virtually no side effects, while prostaglandins produce a well known cascade of side effects. This protocol is only useful if the bitch presents with a progesterone level of 2 ng/ml or higher. An intact uterine wall should be confirmed prior to starting treatment. Aglepristone opens the cervix, allowing the uterus to empty. Since it does not create uterine contractions, some practitioners combine aglepristone with prostaglandins.

Dosage of aglepristone is 10 mg/kg administered on day 1, 2, 8, 15, and 29. It can be combined with cloprostenol (at 1 mcg/kg subq once a day from day 3 to day 7) to increase uterine evacuation. For closed-cervix pyometra, the cervix opened on an average of 26±13 hours following the first dose. A success rate of 90% is reported after 28 days.

Aglepristone can be used to prevent pyometra recurrence if the bitch is not bred on the next cycle(s).

Antibiotics are essential to treating pyometra, but are insufficient if used alone. Start immediately upon diagnosis. E. coli is the most common organism found and is usually sensitive to most routinely used antibiotics. Culture and sensitivity testing are frequently recommended but are seldom enlightening and antibiotic therapy should not be withheld pending these results. Clavamox® is most commonly used. Amoxicillin and Cephalexin are also frequently prescribed, but are not preferred because they do not penetrate the uterine lumen well. The enrofloxacins are also recommended, but offer little that Clavamox® or cephalexin do not. Oral antibiotics are usually tolerated well. Injectable cefazolin, Baytril® or Unasyn® may be used for the first few days if the bitch is initially unable to tolerate oral medications due to the vomiting induced by Lutalyse®. These are all used at standard label doses. Antibiotic therapy should continue for 4 weeks beyond the end of Lutalyse® therapy.

Bromocriptine or cabergoline aid in luteolysis, rapidly dropping progesterone levels, and can be useful in patients with progesterone levels over 2 ng/ml at the initiation of therapy. This accelerates cervical relaxation and uterine evacuation by several days. Some treatment protocols include one, but not both of these drugs.

Bromocriptine is less expensive than cabergoline and is more readily available at most human pharmacies. It does, however, cause more vomiting than cabergoline.

Bromocriptine (Parlodel®) is dosed at 10 to 25 mcg/kg BID to TID po for the first 8 days of therapy. The tablets are 2.5 mg (2500 mcg), and for smaller bitches, should be dissolved in 10 cc of water (to make 250 mcg/ml), and stored in the refrigerator in a dark amber bottle. Shake the bottle to resuspend before administereing.

Cabergoline (Dostinex®), is dosed at 5 mcg/kg once daily po. These tablets are difficult to divide and may need to be compounded in oil at a professional compounding pharmacy to make the dose needed for most smaller breeds. There is a liquid product containing 50 mcg/ml available in Europe.

Fluid therapy is almost always indicated for pyometra patients, if they are dehydrated, depressed, toxic, septic, anorectic, and/or vomiting when treatment begins. IV fluids are recommended for sick bitches. The dose and type of fluids are based on patient condition.

For patients that appear well-hydrated and are not vomiting until medications are initiated, subcutaneous fluids may be sufficient. IV fluid therapy may be initiated if the bitch becomes more depressed, is not drinking well, or does not tolerate subcutaneous fluids well.

For patients who never feel sick, are able to drink and eat well, and tolerate all medications well, fluid therapy may not be required.

Metoclopramide by injection can be useful in reducing nausea and vomiting. The dose is 0.2 to 0.4 mg/kg SQ TID and can be injected at the same time as Lutalyse®.

Misoprostol can be instilled intravaginally (as far cranially as possible, to be close to the cervical os) at a dose of 1 to 3 mcg/kg once daily concurrently with Lutalyse® to help open the cervix (Tables 9-2 through 9-4).

What to expect during pyometra therapy and how to monitor treatment success

The patient should be monitored closely and supportive treatments provided. In exceptional cases, such as a client with profound financial restrictions and a patient who appears stable, outpatient therapy may be appropriate using cloprostenol and antibiotics. This is not ideal and the client should be advised of the risks.

Table 9-2 Pyometra treatment for a typical 9 hour veterinary hospital							
	Time						
Drug	8 am	9 am	11 am	12 noon	2 pm	3 pm	5 pm
Lutalyse® SQ, walk 20 min	x		x		x		x
Metoclopramide SQ if vomiting	x			x			x
Bromocriptine (tid) or cabergoline (sid) PO		x		x		x	
Antibiotic PO or by injection		x		X (if TID)			x

Table 9-3 Pyometra treatment for a patient in a typical 12 hour veterinary hospital							
	Time						
Drug	7 am	8 am	10 am	1 pm	2 pm	4 pm	7 pm	8 pm
Lutalyse® SQ, walk 20 min	x		x	x		x	x	
Metoclopramide SQ if vomiting	x			x			x	
Bromocriptine (tid) or cabergoline (sid) PO		x			x			x
Antibiotic PO or by injection		x			X (if tid)			X (if bid)

Table 9-4 Pyometra treatment for a patient in a 24 hour veterinary hospital												
	Time											
Drug	7 am	8 am	11 am	12 noon	3 pm	4 pm	5 pm	7 pm	9 pm	11 pm	2 am	3 am
Lutalyse® SQ, walk 20 min	x		x			x			x			x
Metoclopramide SQ if vomiting	x			x						x		
Bromocriptine (tid) or cabergoline (sid) PO		x			x					x		
Antibiotic PO or by injection		X (if bid or tid)					X (if TID)	X (if bid)		X (if tid)		

The typical hospitalized patient should be on fluids, antibiotics, and prostaglandins, and may also be on cabergoline and anti-emetics. She should begin to show clinical improvement with increased appetite and decreased side effects within 48 hours. Her vaginal discharge should significantly increase within 24 to 48 hours. Blood and urine chemistries should be monitored. The WBC will slowly return to normal, but typically lags 7 to 14 days behind clinical improvement and may initially worsen.

Uterine size should be reduced by at least 50% within 3 to 5 days. If this is not noted, administer additional medical therapy or consider ovariohysterectomy. An underlying cause such as an ovarian tumor may be the reason for a poor response to therapy.

Summary

Diagnosis
History

CBC, Chemistry Panel, +/– coagulation panel to assess for DIC

Vaginal cytology

Ultrasound – be sure she is not pregnant

Progesterone level – to determine if she will benefit from luteolytic therapy with bromocriptine or cabergoline

Treatment
Lutalyse® or other luteolytic agent – walk the bitch

Antibiotics

Fluid therapy

+/– Bromocriptine or Cabergoline

+/– Anti-emetic

+/– Misoprostol

Monitoring therapy
Ultrasound – treat until the uterus is 50% size originally treated. Repeat 2 weeks after completion of prostaglandin therapy.

Monitor volume of vaginal secretion

+/– CBC

Antibiotic therapy for 4 weeks

Surgical treatment risks
The risks of surgical treatment include anesthetic complications including death, peritonitis, renal failure (which may become apparent up to several weeks post-op), DIC; and incision dehiscence. Myocardial injury may occur secondary to endotoxemia, inflammation, septicemia, or infarction and may contribute to unexpected deaths.

Medical treatment risks
The risks of medical treatment include uterine rupture, peritonitis, inflammation of the oviducts, renal failure, DIC and death.

Although DIC has been associated with pyometra and treatment with heparin subcutaneously have been utilized to treat pyometra, there are no reports supporting the use of this protocol.

Recurrence rates are not well documented, in part because new therapies have not been adequately evaluated and because of the variety of clinical presentations. The incidence may be no higher for the affected than unaffected bitch. Fertility rates in bitches who responded rapidly (less than 5 days) also appear to be unaffected.

One report showed a 93% rate of clinical resolution of pyometra after treatment with prostaglandins, with 38 of 44 whelping healthy pups.

These patients are often valuable older bitches and they should be bred on each subsequent cycle as appropriate. Ovariohysterectomy can be considered if medical therapy fails, she becomes febrile, she relapses, pyometra reoccurs, if she later fails to become pregnant, or she is at the end of her breeding career.

If it is more appropriate to delay breeding a young dog, mibolerone or other novel therapies to delay estrous may be utilized.

Miscellaneous disorders of the female reproductive tract

Miscellaneous disorders of the female reproductive tract associated with vaginal discharge

There are many causes of vaginal discharge in both the intact and spayed bitch. Although pyometra should always be a priority to diagnose early, other causes should not be overlooked. Bitches who may be or are pregnant deserve careful assessment to avoid an overzealous attempt to diagnose pyometra (Table 9-5).

Ovarian neoplasia

Ovarian pathology exists in up to 29% of ovaries examined histologically according to one study from 1960 (Figure 9-12).

It is often undetected because many types of ovarian pathology have no clinical signs, with the exception of infertility or atypical estrous cycles.

There are several kinds of ovarian neoplasia. It is relatively uncommon in the bitch. The most common types of ovarian tumors are: adenocarcinoma, papillary adenomas and cystadenomas (50%), and granulosa-cell tumors (40%) (GCT). Some are benign and some are malignant. The average age of diagnosis is approximately 6 to 8 years of age. Some may occur bilaterally; if unilateral, they tend to cause the opposite ovary to become inactive. Boxers, Boston Terriers, German Shepherds, and English bulldogs may be predisposed to GCT; English pointers may be predisposed to adenocarcinomas. DES hormonal therapy may predispose bitches to carcinomas.

Table 9-5 Miscellaneous disorders of the female reproductive tract		
Abortion	Ovarian neoplasia	Urinary tract disease
Brucellosis	Ovarian remnant syndrome	Uterine neoplasia
Estrous	Pregnancy	Uterine stump pyometra
Hypoluteoidism	Prolonged estrous with ovarian cyst	Vaginal foreign body
Intersex	Pyometra	Vaginal hyperplasia
Metritis	Puppy vaginitis	Vaginal neoplasia
Mibolerone use	SIPS	Vaginal polyp
Mucometra	Transitional cell carcinoma	Vaginitis

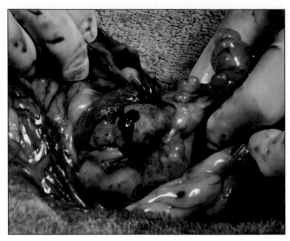

Figure 9-12.
Ovarian neoplasia.

In general, ovarian neoplasia has a low metastatic rate (30%), with the exception of teratomas and adeonomcarcinomas.

Patients with ovarian tumors may be asymptomatic or may have anestrus, atypical estrous cycles (prolonged or increased frequency); pyometra; lactation; hair loss; non-regenerative anemia or thrombocytopenia; or show signs of abdominal distension, abdominal distress, vomiting, diarrhea, and weight loss.

Diagnosis is best done by a skilled ultra-sonographer. These masses may be as large as 30 cm. If a mass is found, fine needle aspirate is NOT recommended, as this can lead to metastasis. Ovarian masses may also be found during routine ovariohysterectomy. Any suspicious-looking ovarian or uterine tissue should be submitted for laboratory evaluation and discussed with the owner.

Suspicious ovarian tissue should be handled with care to minimize seeding the abdominal cavity. Some ovarian neoplasias are functional, secreting hormones, and some are not. Even the metastatic lesions are sometimes functional. Metastasis may have already occurred by the time of diagnosis. The prognosis is better if the neoplastic tissue is contained within the ovarian bursa. Some are so advanced or so invasive at the time of diagnosis that resection is not possible.

Teratomas, although not common, are the most dramatic neoplasia of the female reproductive tract. They are more commonly seen in younger dogs. They can reach massive size by the time of diagnosis. The most common symptom is abdominal distension, which can be mistaken for pregnancy. The tumor usually contains tissues from 2 to 3 embryonic cell lines, and may contain grotesque accumulations of hair, skin, other epithelium, fat, bone, teeth, and muscle. The prognosis is poor because of the high metastatic rate.

Surgical treatment starts with careful resection of the abnormal tissue at ovariohysterectomy. Handle the resected tissues carefully to reduce exfoliation of tumor cells. Lavage the abdomen and remove as much fluid as possible prior to closure.

If a breeding bitch has a unilateral tumor that is not a teratoma, unilateral ovariectomy may be considered. The prognosis for pregnancy is guarded, both because the contralateral ovary may be non-functional and because there is a risk of developing CEH-pyometra. Uterine biopsy at the time of ovariectomy should be discussed with the client. There are reports that bitches treated with unilateral ovariectomy have become pregnant.

Treatments for neoplasia are updated frequently. Referral to a veterinary oncologist should be offered to all clients.

Uterine neoplasia

Uterine neoplasia is rare, accounting for less than 1% of cases in dogs, and is usually but not always benign. The most common tumor types are leimyoma (found in 3 forms – intramural, intraluminal, or expansile from the serosal surface); fibroleiomyoma, lipoma, fibroma, adenocarcinomas, hemangiosarcomas, and lymphomas (Figure 9-13).

It is most common in the intact bitch, but is reported to occur at the uterine stump.

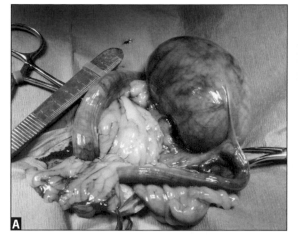

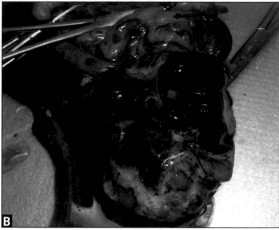

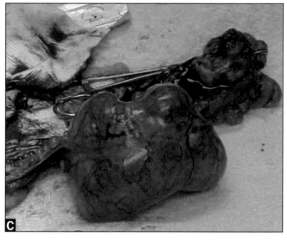

Figure 9-13.
A. *Uterine polyp at surgery.* **B.** *Uterine polyp with uterine wall opened, showing mass diagnosed as uterine polyp on histology. The bitch presented with a fever and leukopenia.* **C.** *Lymphoma in a uterine horn. The bitch presented as in estrus.*

Bitches with uterine neoplasia usually present with a vaginal discharge which may be mistaken for estrous. The diagnosis may be made on abdominal palpation, or imaging with radiographs or abdominal ultrasound.

Treatment starts with ovariohysterectomy which may be unilateral, if the bitch is to be used for breeding. The prognosis for benign neoplasia is excellent. The prognosis for future reproduction remains guarded.

Patients with malignant neoplasia should be referred to a veterinary oncologist.

Ovarian remnant syndrome

Ovarian remnant syndrome is suspected when a dog that has undergone complete bilateral ovario-hysterectomy shows symptoms of a heat cycle. Symptoms include a bloody vaginal discharge and behavioral signs of being receptive and attractive to male dogs. Vaginal cytology at the time of the discharge should show cornifying epithelial cells and the associated red and white blood cells typical of a bitch's cytology in estrus. The presence of an ovarian remnant can be confirmed by waiting several weeks and running a serum progesterone test. If the test results exceed 2 ng/ml, some remaining ovarian tissue is present. This can be from incomplete excision of the ovary, intentionally not removing one or both ovaries, or ectopic ovarian tissue not appreciated during surgery (Figure 9-14).

It is important to determine if the bitch is indeed intact, and to rule out bladder infections, or discharge from the anal sacs that can attract male dogs. Vaginal cytology LH and progesterone

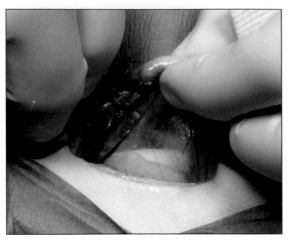

Figure 9-14.
Ectopic ovarian tissue along the ovarian ligament (in a cat).
Without careful examination, this could easily be left behind
at an ovariohysterectomy.

testing can confirm or rule out these disorders. LH testing (canine specific) can also be done to detect ovarian tissue which may not have been removed or to determine if a female is intact prior to surgery. Two LH tests, run 24 or more hours apart, both with positive results, will confirm the presence of functional ovarian/tissue.

Treatment consists of exploratory laparotomy and excision of remaining ovarian tissue. Exploratory laparotomy during estrus or diestrus makes locating the ovarian remnant(s) easier. A non-surgical alternative is to use mibolerone or GnRH agonists, but this should be reserved for non-surgical candidates.

Mucometra and hydrometra

Mucometra is an accumulation of sterile mucus in the uterus. Hydrometra is an accumulation of sterile fluid in the uterus. These are frequently diagnosed at routine ovariohysterectomy in the mature bitch. The incidence is unknown and is probably of little clinical significance. This may be the precursor to CEH- pyometra complex, when complicated by bacterial invasion.

If a bitch is diagnosed with this at uterine biopsy or ultrasound for an infertility work-up, she can be treated with Lutalyse® or cloprostenol as the only drug, at the doses recommended for pyometra treatment. This can be differentiated from pyometra based on the bitch's normal clinical appearance, degree of uterine distension, vaginal cytology showing few bacteria and WBCs, and normal CBC. The prognosis for return to fertility has not been reported.

Post-partum metritis

Pyometras differ from metritis in the timing – metritis occurs as a post-partum infection and inflammation, usually associated with a difficult delivery, or retained pups or placentas. There is no predisposing or preexisting metropathy. The patient tends to be acutely ill, febrile, and has a foul odor to her vaginal discharge. Treat with an appropriate antibiotic, Lutalyse® or cloprostenol if indicated to expel retained placentae, and surgically if there are retained pups. An ovariohysterectomy may be needed if she is toxic or the uterus is in poor condition (See metritis, Chapter 7).

SIPS

Subinvolution of placental sites or SIPS is failure of the placental attachment sites to heal completely. It is most common in bitches after their first litter. The only symptoms are an ongoing vaginal discharge with blood or bloody mucus past 3 weeks post-partum. The bitch and pups do not show signs of illness; the vaginal discharge is bloody but does not look cloudy or have an odor; and the delivery was usually normal.

Diagnosis is usually based on vaginal cytology showing red blood cells, with only a few morphologically normal white blood cells and a few bacteria. A CBC with a normal red blood cell, white blood cell and platelet count will assure the veterinarian and owner that she is not anemic, thrombocytopenic or suffering from metritis.

There is generally no indication for medical or surgical treatment. It is a self-limiting disease that resolves spontaneously and probably will not recur at future whelpings. If the disorder becomes problematic, prostaglandin F2 alpha can be used at 50 mcg/kg subcutaneously twice daily until the red blood cells disappear on vaginal cytology. IF the prostaglandin F2 alpha is dispensed for administration at home, carefully discuss the risks to human handling the product with the client. If the bitch is ovariohysterectomized for another reason near this time, bands of green tissue may be noted in the uterine lining. Ovariohysterectomy for SIPS is rarely indicated. (See Chapter 7).

Segmental aplasia

Segmental aplasia of the uterus is a rare condition in dogs. It occurs when a portion of the uterus is not fully formed, leaving a blind pouch in the proximal uterine horn. When found, it is most commonly seen in the right horn, and in West Highland White Terriers and related breeds. Most veterinarians know this as "white heifer disease", the equivalent in cattle (Figure 9-15).

Diagnosis may be on ultrasound when evaluating a bitch for infertility or pyometra, or at routine ovariohysterectomy or C-section. The affected horn may contain an accumulation of mucoid fluid. The opposite horn is usually normal. Treatment is by complete ovariohysterectomy for a non-breeding bitch, or unilateral ovario-hysterectomy for a bitch with reproductive potential. Bitches can be successfully bred following unilateral ovariohysterectomy.

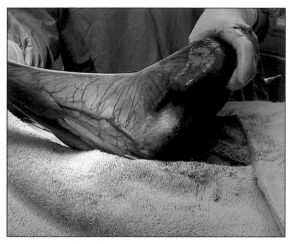

Figure 9-15.
Bitch at C-section with segmental hyperplasia and pyometra in one uterine horn and viable fetus in opposite horn. The affected horn was removed at surgery but the pregnant horn was not removed. The bitch went on to produce a litter of 4 pups at her next breeding.

Uterine torsion

Torsion of a pregnant uterine horn can occur in late stage pregnancy. If dystocia is recognized early and treated surgically with C-section, the prognosis for puppy and bitch survival and sparing the uterus is very good. Many cases are mild and cause only dystocia. The typical labor pattern is the bitch that starts into stage 1 labor, begins to progress, and then stops.

Overzealous use of oxytocin or delays in C-section may lead to uterine rupture, loss of life of the fetuses, loss of the uterus, and potentially the loss of the bitch's life as well.

There is no specific method for diagnosis of this condition. Early recognition of abnormal labor patterns, care in handling a patient with dystocia, and early surgical intervention are key to a good outcome. If the horn is necrotic from ischemia, the affected horn or the entire uterus may need to be removed.

Uterine prolapse

Uterine prolapse is less common in small animal medicine than in large animal medicine. It is rare in dogs and slightly more common in cats. It most common when reported in the immediate post-partum period. Great care must be taken to assure that the bladder is left undamaged or that damage found is addressed. Tissue trauma and swelling often make repositioning the uterus into the abdominal cavity impossible, even with laparotomy. Ovariohysterectomy is the treatment of choice. (See Chapter 7).

Vaginal fold prolapse or Hyperplasia

During proestrus and estrus, some bitches may have such marked edema of the vaginal folds that this tissue will prolapse through the lips of the vulva. The amount of tissue exposed can be quite startling. This has the appearance of a large red doughnut, with varying amounts of tissue exposed. This should not be mistaken for a tumor or other form of neoplasia (Figure 9-16).

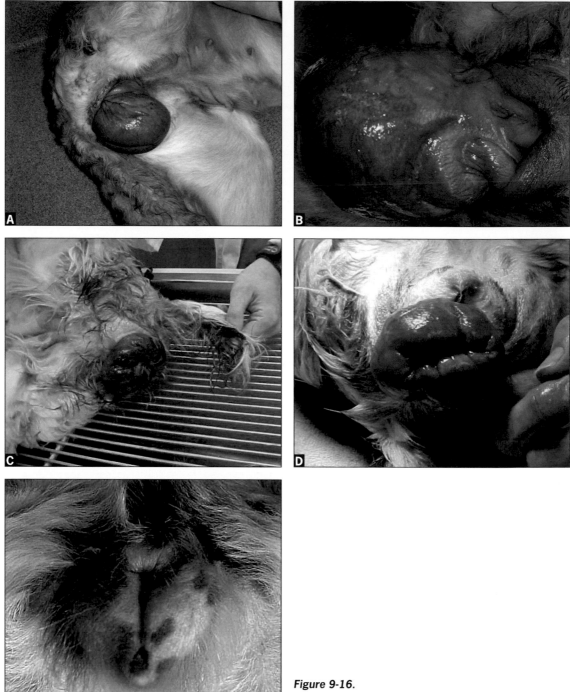

Figure 9-16.
A-D. *Vaginal hyperplasia.* **E.** *Vaginal hyperplasia after repair.*

This is the vaginal tissue's response to estrogen. It typically resolves as the bitch enters diestrus, and on rare occasion will recur near whelping. If the hyperplastic tissue reappears at whelping, a C-section may be required.

Treatment consists of protecting the tissues from trauma and excessive licking. Gently clean the exposed tissues. House the bitch where particulate matter such as gravel or shavings do not contact the exposed tissues. Using a water-soluble gel such as K-Y Jelly® or witch hazel and a pair of boxer shorts, turned to place the bitch's tail through the fly is usually sufficient. Elizabethan collars may create more trauma than they prevent by the bitch rubbing the edge of the collar on the exposed tissues. Hormonal intervention to induce ovulation does not speed resolution and may increase the risk of pyometra development.

Rarely, if the tissues do not spontaneously diminish in size, the excess may need to be resected surgically. Mattress sutures, placed circumferentially, are an effective technique for surgical resection. Preserving the integrity of the urethra should be foremost. It can be identified and managed by inserting a urinary catheter pre-op. Spaying during this cycle will not speed resolution and may have associated risks.

This is common in the Boxer, but is also seen in other brachycephalic and giant breeds. Occurrence on one cycle predicts to recurrence at subsequent cycles.

Vaginal fold prolapse does not interfere with fertility. However, if the tissues do not diminish in size by ovulation, vaginal AI may be required. Following resolution, the bitch may develop an unusual vaginal discharge several weeks after the start of diestrus as the fluid trapped upstream is permitted to escape.

Dysuria is rare despite urethral displacement. Several clues help to differentiate vaginal fold hyperplasia from tumors. First is the age of the bitch – vaginal fold hyperplasia is most common in young females and tumors such as leiomyomas and fibromas are more common in older bitches. Second, vaginal fold hyperplasia usually originates on the ventral floor of the vagina (assessed with a gloved finger manipulation). Third, vaginal fold hyperplasia will usually regress after the bitch enters diestrus. Fourth, bitches with vaginal fold hyperplasia often have a family history of the condition.

Vaginal masses
Neoplasia of the vagina is relatively rare, representing 2.5% of all canine tumors, with 70% of these masses being benign. Leimyoma is the most common benign mass of the vagina. Transmissible Venereal Tumor (TVT), a venerally spread condition, is most common in young promiscuous bitches. TVTs are seen regionally, in warm or tropical climates.

Vaginal masses occur in both intact and spayed dogs. Symptoms include a visible vaginal mass, perineal swelling, vaginal discharge, and difficulty urinating. These differ from vaginal fold prolapse in that the prolapse is seen in proestrus and estrus and resolves spontaneously. They also differ in appearance – the masses are usually smooth and pedunculated whereas the fold prolapses are usually doughnut-shaped. The TVT is often ulcerated and irregular on the surface.

Surgical resection, usually with an episiotomy, with histopathology is diagnostic for most vaginal masses. The prognosis and treatment varies with the type of mass. Infrequently, a transitional cell carcinoma can occur caudally enough to cause vaginal discharge and dysuria.

Vaginal foreign bodies
Any unexplained vaginal discharge should be evaluated for vaginal foreign bodies. This can be done by digital examination, or by vaginoscopy using a rigid endoscope used for TCI, a sterile

anoscope, or a sterile tip on an otoscope. The vaginal vault is much longer than most veterinarians would suspect, and during some stages of estrous may be very convoluted. Sedation or general anesthesia may be required for most bitches, particularly if they are not in estrus.

Although not common, foreign bodies should part of the differential. Objects may be introduced accidentally, iatrogenically during veterinary procedures, or intentionally as seen in animal abuse cases.

Puppy vaginitis

Puppy vaginitis is very common in the pre-pubertal bitch. The typical patient is a normal healthy bitch puppy at a wellness veterinary visit. The owner may mention the symptoms, but it often goes unnoticed by the owner, until it is pointed out during the wellness visit (See Figure 8-15).

There is a sticky yellow vaginal discharge from the vulva, which is also frequently pasted in the surrounding haircoat. She may lick her vulva, and have urinary accidents or the puppy will be normal clinically. Diagnosis is made on vaginal cytology, vaginoscopy, and physical examination. Frequently the culture is unremarkable.

In mild cases, when neither the pup nor owner are affected, benign neglect (i.e. no treatment) may be the best option.

Treatment of the puppy with no urinary signs is accomplished by instilling antibiotics in the vaginal vestibule, inserted gently with a syringe, and sending her outside for 10 minutes to keep the carpet clean. Treat for a maximum of 5 days to prevent development of a secondary fungal infection. The alternative treatment is hormonal – the disorder is caused by an immature vaginal lining. Premarin dosed at 20 mcg/kg twice a week or every 4 days for 2 weeks will relieve symptoms. Long-term therapy is avoided because of the risk of anemia. Reserve oral antibiotics for pups with signs of urinary tract infection (based on culture) or severe symptoms that fail to respond to topical antibiotics and premarin.

A good option is to allow the puppy to have 1 estrous cycle prior to ovariohysterectomy. The first heat cycle will allow the vaginal epithelium to mature and symptoms will resolve. Many bitch puppies have an inverted vulva. The first heat cycle frequently changes the external anatomy of the vulva, allowing it to develop a mature confirmation. Allowing the bitch to go through puberty can lead to valuable permanent anatomical changes that cannot be replicated pharmacologically or surgically. Allowing the bitch to experience one heat cycle predisposes her to a negligibly increased risk of developing mammary tumors as she ages. Spaying prior to the first estrous may condemn her to a lifetime of vaginitis, dermatitis, and/or chronic urinary tract disease.

Uterine stump pyometra

This occurs in the previously ovariohysterectomized bitch. The bitch typically presents with a muco-purulent vaginal discharge and may also be ill with depression, loss of appetite and elevated WBCs. Closed-cervix uterine stump pyometras can be difficult to diagnose without abdominal ultrasound, and should be included in the differential for any sick female dog. Uterine stump pyometra is often very near the bladder. One half to three quarters of the affected bitches have residual ovarian tissue – the cause for the changes in the uterine wall that allow the pyometra to develop.

Treatment is surgical and requires removal of the affected uterine tissue, remaining non-absorbed suture material, and residual ovarian tissues. Resection of the uterine stump is sometimes complicated by adhesions to the urinary bladder.

Some practitioners prefer ovariectomy to ovariohysterectomy. It is a less complicated procedure with a faster post-op recovery. In many practices, it is now done laparoscopically. If done with complete removal of both ovaries, there is no increase in the rate of uterine stump pyometra over the traditional ovariohysterectomy.

Other findings

Determining all the causes of infertility is not possible. There are almost certainly infectious causes that have not yet been determined. Assessing patency of the oviducts is not a technique available. Many causes of uterine pathology still have not been fully explored.

There are aberrant findings that may or may not be tied to infertility. Visceral larval migrans, can cause unusual and suspicious lesions, but is probably not a cause of infertility. More study is needed to determine the etiology of these lesions (Figure 9-17).

The accidental breeding

Clients frequently ask for assistance when they have witnessed an accidental breeding or suspect that one took place in their absence.

The first thing the client can do is have vaginal cytology done to determine the stage of her estrous cycle and to look for sperm. Progesterone testing should also be considered. The presence of cornified vaginal epithelial cells, a progesterone between 3 ng/ml and 30 ng/ml, and/or the presence of sperm all suggest a possible pregnanancy. A lack of sperm cannot assure the client that the bitch will not conceive. No treatment should be administered at this time.

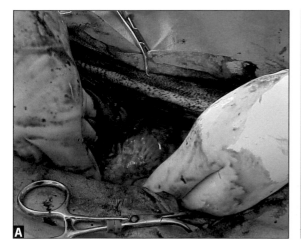
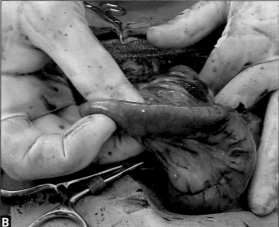
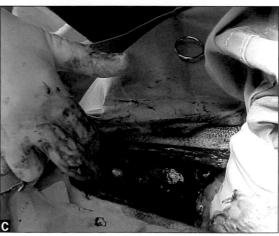

Figure 9-17.
Visceral larral migrans lessions. **A.** *Ascarid lesion on the kidney.* **B.** *Ascarid intestinal lesion.* **C.** *Ascarid lesion on the liver.*

In a study done by Autumn Davidson, only 60% of all bitches with 1 witnessed breeding were confirmed pregnant. The current recommendation is to wait until 28 days, assess for pregnancy on ultrasound, and develop a treatment plan based on the results.

Estrogenic drugs have historically been administered within 72 hours of breeding as a "mis-mate" shot. The risks associated with this treatment protocol are great and it is no longer recommended. Side effects include pyometra, pregnancy that continues despite treatment, and death due to bone marrow suppression caused by the estrogens. Better alternative treatments are available.

Options for the brood bitch

If the pregnancy is confirmed on ultrasound at day 26 to 28, 3 options can be offered to the client

1. Allow the bitch to carry the litter to term. This can be an opportunity for her to learn to care for pups. Some clients will be open to this – particularly if she is pregnant with a litter of pups from her breed or if she was intended to be bred to that male, just at another time.

2. Offer an ovariohysterectomy shortly after pregnancy is confirmed. The disadvantage is that the bitch will end her breeding career. For bitches who were not intended to be bred, who are likely to have a difficult pregnancy, or who are pregnant with mixed-breed pups, this may be a reasonable option.

3. Interrupt the pregnancy pharmacologically with a luteolytic drug. The protocal is a safe and effective alternative to ovariohysterectomy.

Interrupting the unwanted pregnancy

Luteolytic agents have changed the treatment options for clients who find themselves with a bitch pregnant with an unwanted litter.

Lutalyse® has been used for many years as an abortifactant. Although it is very effective, it has side effects that will make the bitch temporarily ill, requires hospitalization, and is therefore costly to the owner. The dose ranges from starts at 10 mcg/kg and is increased to 50 mcg/kg 3 to 5 times a day given subcutaneously for a minimum of 5 days.

Treatment may take up to 12 days in young large breeds with large litters. Use ultrasound to assess the bitch for the treatment endpoint. Advise clients prior to the start of treatment that they may see fetuses pass.

Lutalyse® has some potential risks for the staff handling the drug and predictable side effects to the patient (See Pyometra earlier in this chapter).

Cloprostenol (Estrumate®), is an effective alternative and is less costly. It should be used instead of Lutalyse®, not along with it. Although the side effects are similar to those of Lutalyse®, it is easier on the bitch because only need 2 or 3 doses are needed and no hospitalization is required.

The protocol is as follows:

On day 26 to 28 from breeding, the bitch should be scheduled for abdominal ultrasound. If she is pregnant, the first dose of cloprostenol is given – the dose is 1.0 to 2.5 mcg/kg IM, with large breed bitches, Labradors, Rottweilers, and bitches pregnant with large litters receiving the upper end of the dose. Diluting the drug with sterile water will minimize side effects. The bitch should be walked for 15 to 20 minutes following the injection, prior to traveling, to minimize the side effects of vomiting and diarrhea. She does not need to be hospitalized. Advise the client that fetuses may be seen to pass if treatment is initiated late in pregnancy.

Four to five days later, the bitch should return for a second ultrasound and progesterone testing. Administer the second injection of cloprostenol at the same dose and with the same precautions as for the first. IF the fetuses still look round and healthy on ultrasound AND IF the progesterone level is over 2 ng/ml, she should return for a 3rd injection in 5 more days. IF the fetal structures look like they are collapsing inward and the progesterone is less than 2 ng/ml, treatment is completed with only 2 injections.

If the progesterone at the second visit was greater than 2 mg/dl, five days later, the bitch should return for a 3rd ultrasound, progesterone testing, and 3rd injection. If her ultrasound and progesterone levels suggest she is still carrying a viable litter, cabergoline or bromocriptine should be added to the protocol. Although this is seldom necessary, in some large bitches pregnant with large litters, this may be indicated.

The third option is cabergoline OR bromocriptine alone, or combined with Lutalyse®. The cabergoline only protocol causes the least severe side effects but is not consistently effective in terminating a pregnancy.

At 26 to 28 days, when the pregnancy is confirmed, oral cabergoline or bromocriptine treatment can be started. The dose is 5 mcg/kg once daily until ultrasound confirms that the pregnancy is terminated. For small bitches, cabergoline can be compounded in oil by a compounding pharmacy. Pups typically pass 5 to 7 days into treatment. Lutalyse® or oxytocin may be added to aid in passing the pups. Aglepristone is an effective alternative but is not an FDA approved drug in the US.

Special breedings

The American Kennel Club recently began to accept registrations of litters as purebred AKC registerable puppies even if the pups were sired by 2 or more fathers. This would not be possible without DNA proof of paternity.

This policy includes breedings done intentionally with the semen of 2 or more fathers as well as from breedings planned by the dogs but not their owners.

DNA must be collected and submitted on all pups, the mother, and all potential fathers. As the DNA is collected from the pups, some form of permanent identification must be used so the correct father's name is on the pup's registration. Although microchips are not labeled for use in pups this young, this is a successful means of permanent identification. No microchip migration problems were noted when pups at 10 days of age were microchipped.

The samples are submitted for testing at an AKC-approved laboratory, and the results can be deciphered by the breeder or by AKC for an additional fee. If the pups are found to be from more than 1 father, there is a special form and an additional fee to register the litter. More information is available at the AKC website – www.akc.org and by going to "downloadable forms".

Mammary tumors

Most mammary tumors are discovered by the client, the veterinary staff, or the veterinarian on digital examination of the mammary chain (Figure 9-18).

Mammary tumors are the second most common neoplasia in female dogs, second only to skin tumors. They represent 42 to 50% of all tumors seen. Approximately one half are histologically malignant and one half of the malignant tumors metastasize. Ten years is the average age when the tumor is noted.

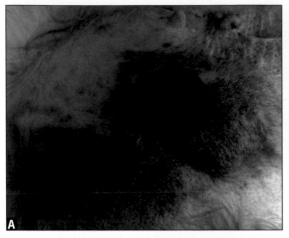
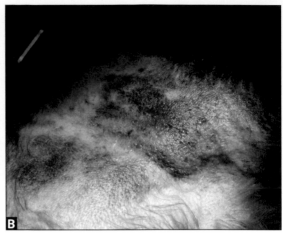
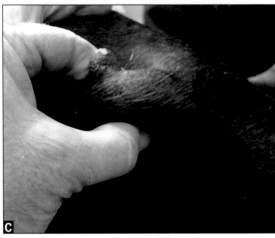

Figure 9-18.
A. and *B.* *Inflammatory mammary carcinoma. This tumor carries such a poor prognosis that excision should not be attempted.* *C.* *Adenocarcinoma. This tumor has a guarded prognosis.*

There are 2 basic types of mammary tumors: 1) the solitary mass or masses, in varying sizes, shapes, and textures, located anywhere along the mammary chain and 2) the inflammatory mammary carcinoma.

An inguinal hernia may be confused with a mammary mass. Other mammary pathology includes: fibrous hyperplasia, seen after an estrous cycle pseudopregnancy/pseudowhelping; galactostasis; mastitis; abscesses; foreign bodies; granulomas; and other non-mammary neoplasias. Mammary hypertrophy or fibroadenomatous hyperplasia is seen in young cats. Most mammary pathology is diagnosed and treated surgically with one very important exception, the inflammatory carcinoma:

Inflammatory mammary carcinoma

This is a devastating, highly malignant form of mammary cancer that is rarely seen in dogs. Bitches with this disease will present acutely ill. They have warm painful diffuse nodular or rash-like dermal lesions, often covering the entire mammary chain. Regions may be ulcerated. Although the mammary chain is uniformly firm, there are no discrete masses like those seen in most patients with mammary tumors. Clinically this may mimic mastitis, but is usually seen in an older bitch who is not postpartum or even intact. Frequently they have edema to the rear limbs, associated with blocked lymphatics and had previously had one or more benign or malignant mammary tumors diagnosed.

By the time they present, 100% of the affected bitches have lymph node metastasis. By presentation, 32% have metastases to the lungs, visible on thoracic radiographs. Many present in DIC with petecchial hemorrhages visible. This is a grave disease, with only a 25 day average survival time. Surgical resection is NEVER indicated, because they will die of the disease prior to surgical recovery. Average survival time of patients taken to surgery to resect inflammatory carcinoma is 48 hours! Confirmation of disease may be done, if necessary, by biopsy of a small sample and histopathology. The only therapy is palliative – anti-inflammatory and pain medication. Piroxicam has been reported to lead to a longer survival time than doxorubicin.

Primary mammary tumors

Most mammary tumors are diagnosed on physical examination. The owner often finds the mass during inspection at home. Sometimes, the mass(es) are discovered during a comprehensive physical examination. All bitches, whether intact or spayed, should have a complete palpation of the mammary chain during wellness visits, at presentation for illness, or while under anesthesia for other procedures.

When discussing mammary tumors with clients, you may find when you use the term mammary tumor or mammary neoplasia, you get a blank look from your client(s). Substitution of the term "breast cancer" will not only improve the client's understanding of the disorder, but will move them to action. This small difference in terminology can save your patient's life.

Palpation is the basic method of detecting mammary tumors. Although fine needle aspiration of the tumor is often suggested for diagnosis, this is primarily of value for ruling in other mammary diseases, not ruling out mammary tumors. The mammary tumors seen in dogs are often heterogeneous, and the small sample taken by needle aspirate or biopsy will not be representative of the mass – only 67.5% of FNAs are accurate. This may mislead the veterinarian into believing there is no evidence of neoplasia. Each mammary mass must be individually evaluated because each individual tumor has a 50% chance of being malignant. The preferred method of diagnosis of mammary gland disease is to remove each gland for submission to a pathologist.

Most mammary tumors in dogs are of epithelial origin, with half being malignant and half being benign. As a rule of thumb, small dogs with small tumors have the lowest malignancy rate and large dogs with large tumors have the highest malignancy rate. Some of the more malignant types originate from other cell lines; tumors such as sarcomas or mast cell tumors should always be considered malignant.

Risk factors

There is strong evidence in the dog that early ovariohysterectomy is protective.

Other risk factors include previous mammary tumor – 65% of bitches with 1 tumor will have a second tumor; obesity – the risk is increased when the bitch is obese; progestins – there is an increased risk when the bitch has been treated with progestins; and size of the mass – the larger the mass, the more likely it is to be malignant (Table 9-6).

There is no sparing effect of pregnancy and lactation in the dog, as is seen in women.

Table 9-6 Incidence of mammary tumors associated with ovariohysterectomy	
Age of ovariohysterectomy	Incidence of mammary tumors associated with ovariohysterectomy:
Prior to the first estrous	0.5%
Prior to the second estrous	8%
Prior to the third estrous	26%
After the third estrous	No protective value

(adapted from Schneider R, Dorn COPYRIGHT, Taylor DO: Factors influencing canine mammary cancer development and postsurgical survival. J Natl Cancer Inst 1969; Dec; 43(6): 1249-1261.)

Diagnosing and staging mammary tumors

Most mammary tumors are firm, round to oblong nodular structures. The masses can vary in size, shape, and number of nodules in each mass. They can occur anywhere along the chain, but most masses are closer to the nipple than the periphery of the gland. The caudal mammary glands tend to have a higher number of masses than the cranial glands.

Over 50% of bitches affected have multiple mammary tumors; 1 study has shown that 37% of bitches with multiple mammary tumors had both benign and malignant lesions. For this reason, fine needle aspiration and/or biopsy of the tumor often produces misleading results. Complete excision and submitting the entire mass for histology will lead to a more accurate prognosis.

Determining the type of tumor and staging the tumors: (modified Owen)

The following are the types of mammary tumors described in the literature:
Adenocarcinoma
Anaplastic carcinoma
Inflammatory carcinoma
Squamous cell carcinoma
Malignant Mixed Mammary Tumor
Carcinosarcoma
Sarcoma

Ideally, the following diagnostics are recommended to stage a bitch with mammary tumor(s):

CBC/Chemistry panel/urinalysis (if collected by cystocentesis, be careful to avoid placing the needle through a mass) and coagulation profile. A coagulation profile should be performed in dogs suspected of having inflammatory carcinoma or that have a high risk of metastasis because of the associated risk of disseminated intravascular coagulation (DIC).

Abdominal radiographs or ultrasound to assess regional lymph nodes, particularly the sublumbar lymph nodes.

Thoracic Radiographs, with 3 views. Although CT has a slightly higher yield in detecting metastases, the WHO staging protocol still relies on radiographic detection.

Palpation of regional lymph nodes.

As with all veterinary diagnostic and treatment plans, the client's resources must be factored into this decision. If the client can't afford both the staging and the surgery, their money will probably be better spent on surgical excision and histopathology. Ideally, the treatment plan including surgical excision would follow complete staging. Staging and referral to a veterinary oncologist should be offered to owners of dogs with all but the least complicated disease.

Treatment of mammary tumors

Due to the frequency of mammary tumors, most veterinary practitioners are very familiar with this type of neoplasia. With early intervention and appropriate surgical technique, the prognosis can be good. Surgery remains the mainstay of mammary treatment. The general practicing veterinarian, not the oncologist, will provide first-line treatment for most bitches with mammary gland disease.

The patient may present with a large tumor that has ulcerated the overlying skin due to the mass outgrowing its blood supply. Appropriate treatment dictates that all ulcerated or necrotic tumors must be surgically removed in their entirety. Although the prognosis tends to be poorer for this large tumor size, the skin over the ulcerated tumor will never heal whether treated medically or with conservative therapy (attempting to close the wound). IF an owner does not consent to surgery, euthanasia should be discussed as the most humane alternative.

Surgical therapy

Ovariohysterectomy should be done before tumor removal to prevent seeding the abdominal cavity with cells from the mammary neoplasia. The abdominal incision should be placed away from the site of a tumor for the same reason.

Dogs have 5 pairs of mammary glands and cats have 4 pairs, in most cases. They are numbered from cranial to caudal. The lymphatic connections between the glands, including crossing the midline, vary between patients. There is an extensive blood supply to the mammary glands that tends to anastomose. A surgical anatomy book should be consulted prior to surgery if the surgeon is uncertain of the regional blood supply. Carcinomas tend to spread between glands via the lymphatics, while mesenchymal tumors tend to spread via the bloodstream.

Prior to surgery, cabergoline or bromocriptine (higher incidence of vomiting) are useful in reducing the size of the tumor. This can be very helpful in patients with medium to large tumors, who are lactating, or with bloody fluid in the gland. Cabergoline should be dosed at 5 mcg/kg once daily for 5 to 8 days pre-op. By making the tumor smaller, the surgery is easier on the patient (smaller incision), the surgeon, and the client (less expense).

The surgeon should plan an aggressive surgical approach. The entire affected mammary gland should be removed if possible. The primary post-op concerns in aggressive surgical procedures are a difficult recovery (tension on the sutures), post-op pain and lymphedema. Some of the post-op concerns in humans do not apply to the dog – the post-op bitch does not have a body image concern.

The following principles of surgical oncology should be applied to removal of mammary tumors, and to other potential neoplastic tissues:

Change gloves and instruments if additional surgical incisions are to be made after the mammary tumor resection to prevent seeding remotes sites with tumor cells.

Plan the biopsy and fine needle aspirate tracts to be excisable and remember to excise all biopsy and fine needle aspirate tracts; because mammary tumors are not uniform in cell distribution, fine needle aspiration and biopsies may lead to an inaccurate diagnosis and prognosis.

Ligate all vessels early, particularly venous supply to minimize metastasis;

Take wide margins;

Keep the manipulation of the tumor minimal and gentle;

In general, drains are contraindicated as they can lead to tumor seeding through the drainage tract.

Some clients need to be reassured that surgical removal of the primary tumor has greater benefits than risks. Recommendations range from performing only a lumpectomy to removal of the entire affected gland (mammectomy) to radical mastectomies. There is ongoing controversy. Current recommendations are to remove the entire affected gland on most patients. There is no evidence supporting that a radical mastectomy provides a longer survival time than a single gland mastectomy. Cancer death in dogs is not thought to be caused by the primary tumor, but by the metastases. The most important factor is to remove all of the affected tissue, plus 1 tissue plane deep to the tumor. "Peeling out" a mammary tumor is poor surgical technique because it leaves the most aggressive components of the tumor behind.

The incision should be carefully planned. This can be done with the dog standing, folding the tissues in your hands. Under anesthesia, positioned on her back, you can determine how much tissue there is when overlapped. Although it is preferred to close the wound, on occasion, a wound that must granulate in is preferable to a wound with tumor cells left behind.

Typically, an elliptical incision is used. The incision should be around the affected gland(s), done with sharp dissection, using excellent hemostasis. Electrosurgery and laser surgery can interfere with the pathologist's ability to assess the margins for complete excision. The incision may be made with a scalpel or scissor to remove the tissue, followed by electrosurgery or laser for hemostasis and pain control. The caudal superficial epigastric artery and vein are the largest blood vessels and supply the 4th and 5th mammary glands. They should be identified and double ligated individually prior to being incised.

Extend the incision through the subcutaneous tissue down to, but not including the body wall unless the tumor involves the body wall. Once the gland is elevated one tissue plane deep to the tumor, the plane of dissection should be completed sharply. This can be accomplished by gliding a sharp pair of Metzenbaum scissors through the tissues in the plane established. The underlying muscle should generally not be incised. Even if the muscle wall requires some excision, in all cases, avoid penetrating the peritoneum. Invasion through the peritoneum may seed the abdominal cavity with tumor cells.

A radical mastectomy as a first surgical procedure is only recommended if so many neighboring glands are involved that they cannot be removed individually. This is especially true when the 4th and 5th glands on the same side are involved. Two surgeries may be needed in some cases to allow for staging of the resection. In this way, enough involved glandular tissue can be removed to attempt to cure the patient, but also to allow closure of the surgical wound.

It is better to remove too much tissue than too little. "One study of dogs with incompletely resected mammary gland tumors revealed that 75% were dead within 2 years of initial presentation".

Even with careful planning, the incision closure can be a challenge, because of the large amount of tissue that must be removed. Drains are best avoided as they are messy for clients to manage, and can allow metastasis along the tract. Other surgical techniques can be used to reduce tension on the suture line. These include the use of skin flaps, releasing incisions, "walking sutures" or including tubing or buttons in the suture to ease tension on the skin. Walking sutures can cause increased post-op pain because of the immobility of the tissues post-op. The reduction in suture tension and seroma formation usually offset the disadvantages. Small suture material, such as 3-0 or 4-0 monofilament absorbable with a taper needle should be used. The technique for walking sutures is as follows:

The suture placement should be sequential from cranial to caudal or caudal to cranial.

The skin is elevated by lifting with a thumb forceps.

The first bite of tissue is taken into the dermis at the deep margin of the undermined skin, well back from the edge of the cut margin of the skin.

The second bite is taken on the body wall side, into the fascia, closer to the center of the wound. A row of sutures can be pre-placed in the same row as far from the skin incision as possible.

Sutures should be placed 2 to 3 cm apart, in 1 row.

Once the row furthest from the incision has all the sutures pre-placed, the knots can be tied.

A second row of sutures can be placed, staggered with the first row, on the same side of the incision, but closer to the cut edge of the skin. Again these can be pre-placed and then all tied.

This can be repeated on the opposite side of the skin incision in 1 to 3 rows as needed based on the extent of the surgical incision.

During placement of the sutures, towel clamps may be used to hold the skin in apposition, to reduce heat loss and drying of the tissues.

After the walking sutures are all placed, a continuous suture pattern of the subcutaneous tissue may be completed. Skin closure is at the discretion of the surgeon. Staples or interrupted skin sutures are recommended.

The patient must be kept well-hydrated and warm throughout the procedure. The extensive size of the incision and length of time in surgery will cause both fluid and heat loss. Continuously infuse warmed IV fluids. The patient should be kept warm with circulating water blankets, warm air circulating heaters, or other techniques, taking care not to cause thermal burns.

Post-op complications

Surgery on the mammary glands is relatively painful. Radical mastectomies lead to very painful recoveries. Treatment should include excellent pre-operative, intra-operative, and post-operative pain management. Drugs often used include opioids, CRI pain medications, Fentanyl® by CRI or patch, local anesthesia, and non-steroidal anti-inflammatories. Cold compresses post-op are also helpful.

Lymphedema – one or both rear limbs may develop edema if the surgical excision is extensive.

Seromas commonly develop at the surgical site. Careful closure of the wound to minimize dead space in the subcutaneous tissues will minimize seroma formation. They are not painful but may delay wound healing. The only reason to aspirate a seroma is to differentiate it from an abscess. If aspiration is attempted, follow aseptic technique to prevent abscess formation. Attempting to aspirate all the fluid is non-productive because it will re-accumulate quickly. Minimizing post-op activity will reduce the formation of seromas. Warm compresses will speed fluid resorption.

Post-op wound infection is associated with fever, pain and wound dehiscence. Antibiotics should be started as soon as fluid is collected for culture and sensitivity testing. The antibiotic can be changed depending on the test results.

Ovariohysterectomy remains controversial. There is no protective effect. The bitch will not benefit by reducing the likelihood of developing more tumors.

The only advantage is that she will not have additional heat cycles, there will be no accidental breedings (remember, dogs do not go through menopause), and she will not have to endure another surgical procedure if she develops some form of uterine or ovarian disease, such as pyometra. Some owners opt to leave the bitch intact because they may plan to breed her again (please leave her some mammary tissue and the associated nipples if this is to be the case) and some owners prefer to leave their bitches intact (for competition, to prevent coat changes seen after spaying and to spare breeds such as the Boxer from urinary incontinence). A recent study showed that intact females with mammary tumors had a 16 times greater incidence of ovarian pathology than those without mammary tumors. This is strong evidence that the bitch will benefit from ovariectomy or ovariohysterectomy at the time of the mammary tumor removal.

If a breeding bitch with a planned surgical insemination has a single mammary mass, a lumpectomy and histopathology is recommended. The nipple should be left if possible to allow for lactation. A mastectomy is not recommended because the surgery would be too prolonged. If there are multiple tumors, the owner should be advised and future breeding plans reconsidered.

Removal of the lymph nodes does not change the prognosis or survival time post-op. However, the inguinal lymph node(s) are frequently included in the inguinal fat pad excised when the 5th mammary gland is resected. The axillary lymph node should only be removed if it is palpably enlarged, and preferably through a separate skin incision.

Medical therapy of the mammary tumor
In almost every case, surgery should be recommended, with other therapies used to augment treatment.

Chemotherapy is only recommended for dogs with the highest grade of malignancy. This includes tumors shown to have vascular invasion, lymph vessel invasion, a high mitotic rate, and/or infiltrative growth. There are no large scale studies to support wide-spread use of chemotherapy in the dog. Cats, by contrast, have much more aggressive tumors, with 85% malignant with metastases. Cat owners should always be referred to a veterinary oncologist.

Referral to a veterinary oncologist for palliative radiation therapy may be considered as an adjunct to surgery to improve local control in dogs with non-resectable lesions.

Tamoxifen has not proven to be effective in veterinary patients with mammary tumors. Most canine tumors (93/100) lack the hormone receptor that is the key to its use. There is some research that suggests GnRH agonists and Aglepristone (a progesterone blocker) may be useful in adjunctive therapy in the future.

There is strong evidence that COX-2 receptors have been found on certain highly malignant mammary tumors. This suggests that COX-2 inhibitors, specifically Piroxicam, may be of use in the treatment of malignant mammary tumors. This is similar to work being done to treat other canine neoplasms (transitional cell carcinoma and squamous cell carcinoma). No work supporting the use of other COX-2 inhibitors such as meloxicam or carprofen available, but they are under scrutiny.

One recommendation is to initiate the use of piroxicam treatment at the time of suture removal and to continue it for the rest of the dog or cat's life. It is theorized that this may reduce the metastatic behavior of the tumors. Piroxicam should be dosed very carefully as the margin of safety is narrow with this drug. The dose for the dog is 0.3 mg/kg once daily. The dose for the cat is 1 mg/cat every 48 hours. Often, these will need to be compounded by a compounding pharmacy because the accuracy of dosing is essential for the safety of the patient. The practitioner should be familiar with the side effects of piroxicam and advise the owner of them prior to starting therapy. Piroxicam should not be given concurrently with other non-steroidal anti-inflammatories or corticosteroids.

Prognosis
Tumor markers are not useful in clinical practice.

Age should not be considered a poor prognostic indicator nor a reason to deny a patient a surgical option. If lung or other metastases are found pre-op, palliative removal of the mammary tumor(s) may still be considered if quality of life is likely to be improved.

In general, small dogs with small tumors have a better prognosis than large dogs or dogs with large tumors. There is a longer survival time in general in dogs with tumors smaller than 3 cm. Dogs with multiple tumors do NOT have a poorer prognosis. Dogs with lymph node involvement have shorter survival times. A cure can be achieved in most cases with complete surgical resection of a benign or low-grade mammary malignancy.

The prognosis should be based on the most malignant mass removed. The general impression is approximately 15% of bitches diagnosed with mammary tumors die of their disease.

Dogs with inflammatory carcinomas, sarcomas, or poorly differentiated carcinomas have a poorer prognosis than dogs with epithelial tumors.

Vascular invasion, lymph vessel invasion, a high mitotic rate, and/or infiltrative growth are all considered in the prognosis. The histologic features of each tumor submitted should be evaluated separately. The pathologist who read the tissues should be contacted regarding the completeness of the resection, or if there are any questions about the histopathology report. A second surgery or a radical mastectomy may sometimes be recommended.

Mammary tumors in cats are very different than in dogs. Cats have an 85% malignancy and metastatic rate. There is a protective effect of spaying – there is a 91% reduction of mammary tumors when cats are ovariohysterectomized by 6 months of age. A cat that presents with a tumor smaller than 3 cm can have a first surgery to remove the lump for histopathology. If malignant, the cat should go back to surgery. Cats with malignant mammary tumors or a tumor(s) larger than 3 cm at presentation should have bilateral radical mastectomies and be referred for chemotherapy.

Summary of surgical recommendations for mammary tumor removal
Explain carefully the gravity of the disease to the client – small tumors become larger tumors, which are more likely to be malignant and life-threatening. Use the words "breast cancer" so the client understands what you are worried about and why they should opt for surgery early on in the course of the disease.

Recommend surgery early. Saying let's "Watch the tumor" is only going to allow you to watch it get bigger. And bigger leads to death of your patient. In the intact bitch, the tumor will frequently grow very quickly at each estrous cycle. Cut early and cut aggressively.

Start the patient on cabergoline pre-op if there are large tumors, the bitch is lactating, or there is a bloody fluid in the gland.

The single most important variable at surgery in reducing post-op survival time is inadequate excision. Excise the tumor widely, taking 1 tissue plane deep to the tumor. Do not peel out the apparently encapsulated tumor. The first surgery represents the best chance to cure the patient.

Use ligatures early in the procedure to minimize vascular metastasis.

Do not use drains. Instead use "walking sutures" to minimize tension and dead space in the incision.

Excise biopsy and fine needle aspirate tracts.

If ovariohysterectomy is planned, perform this first avoiding an incision into any area of potential tumor.

Change gloves and instruments prior to wound closure.

Go back to surgery to perform a radical mastectomy if indicated based on histopathology.

Use excellent pain management for any patient with surgical removal of mammary tumors, particularly for patients who have had radical mastectomies.

Although the surgery is done aseptically, many patients benefit from post-op use of antibiotics. Amoxicillin post-op may reduce post-op inflammation, particularly in the tender-skinned white dogs.

Talk to the pathologist if there is any question in interpreting the report.

Offer a referral to a veterinary oncologist.

Consider the lifetime use of piroxicam in any malignant mammary tumor.

Remember to treat cats differently than dogs.

CHAPTER 10
Infertility and Reproductive Disorders in the Valuable Stud Dog

Breeding soundness evaluation including complete physical examination, history, and semen analysis
(Table 10-1)

Clinical signs suggesting that the male dog has a problem with infertility or a disorder affecting the male urogenital tract include: failure of a bitch to conceive; lack of interest or ability in breeding an estrus bitch; abnormalities in the ejaculate; abnormal testes, scrotum, prepuce or penis; discharge from the penis; abdominal pain; and/or pain or abnormalities on urination or defecation.

A complete physical examination and in-depth history is an important step in evaluation of the stud dog. The evaluation should include information on his libido, ability to copulate and ejaculate normally, and to produce normal semen **(See Appendix A-9 and D-16)**. The Society for Theriogenology has a CANINE BREEDING SOUNDNESS EVALUTION form available on their website for use of SFT members.

Breeding history

A complete history needs to include the call name and registered name of the stud dog, the owner and co-owner names, the names of the parties responsible for making medical decisions, his date of birth and registration, microchip and/or tattoo numbers.

Any history of health concerns should be investigated. Age is an important factor because young dogs may be transiently infertile and older dogs have a multitude of age-related reproductive problems. Previous illnesses and results from diagnostic testing may shed light on the current health concern. Any history of recent thermal insult to the testes or scrotum is particularly

Table 10-1 Summary of causes of infertility or sterility	
Potential cause	Diagnostics and treatments to consider:
General illness	Complete physical examination, CBC, Chem panel, consider ultrasound
Incomplete ejaculate	Alkaline phosphatase on ejaculate, teaser bitch at next attempt
Thyroid disease	Thyroid profile at Michigan State
Fever	History
Hernia – scrotal or inguinal	Physical examination
Intersex chromosomes	Karotype – especially consider for Kerry Blue Terrier, Pug, English Cocker, Beagle, Weimaraner, German Shorthair Pointer.
Trauma or torsion	History, palpation
Orchitis	Physical examination, Brucella test, culture
Autoimmune disease	History, palpation, size, testicular biopsy
Testicular tumor	Palpation, ultrasound the testes
Obstructive disease	Palpation, ultrasound, testicular biopsy, alkaline phosphatase on ejaculate
Retrograde ejaculation	Urinalysis by catheterization post-ejaculation
Stress/work	History of breeding overuse
Adrenal gland disease	ACTH stimulation, and/or low dose dexamethasone tests
Infection	Culture, Brucella test
Prostate disease	Rectal examination, ultrasound, prostate biopsy, CPSE blood test, culture
Medications	History of steroids, cancer drugs, ketoconazole, hormones
Contaminated equipment	Repeat using disposable equipment
Immotile cilia syndrome	Electron microscopy on sperm tails, thoracic radiograph

important. Housing temperature and grooming routines should be included in this history. Any recent inflammation of the testicles or scrotum could cause impairment of spermatogenesis.

If the dog has never sired a litter, congenital causes of infertility should be investigated. If he has sired a litter in the past but not recently, the condition could be either acute or chronic. If the dog has recently sired a litter, acute conditions should be investigated first.

Housing conditions should be evaluated, preferably with a personal visit to the kennel or home. Crowding, stress due to other intact males, or multiple bitches in season in the household may contribute to physical and psychological concerns. Excessive heat and cold conditions in sleeping quarters may cause testicular or scrotal insults. Certain chemical disinfectants used in the kennel as well as shampoos and other topical treatments and chemicals applied to the surrounding areas such as agricultural treatments may cause infertility. Travel, particularly without the owner, may cause stress and decreased spermatogenesis. A complete travel history may suggest exposure to diseases not typically seen in the dog's home area. Marginal nutrition may also lead to infertility.

Trauma to any portion of the urogenital tract can lead to infertility. Scrotal trauma may cause inflammation and increased temperature, interfering with spermatogenesis. Testicular trauma may lead to orchitis and/or epididymitis. Direct trauma to the penis including lacerations, abrasions, bite wounds, foreign bodies (both accidental and malicious) and fractures of the os penis will create pain and/or an inability to copulate.

Several drugs are known to cause male infertility. Corticosteroids, including those administered by oral or injectable routes as well as those applied topically, are known to cause reduced sperm counts. Anti-neoplastic drugs will interfere with spermatogenesis as can accidental exposure to human steroid creams, either from the tube or from the surface of the skin of a member of their household. Ketoconazole and itraconazole can reduce testosterone levels and sperm motility.

If there are related dogs with intersex, abnormal spermatogenesis, early loss of fertility or immune-mediated infertility, these conditions must be considered. Information regarding related dogs may help decide which diagnostics to run first.

Previous semen analysis, use of a teaser bitch, techniques and equipment used to collect and evaluate the semen are important factors. No intact male dog, without an exceptional reason, should be classified as infertile or sterile on one semen analysis alone. Some dogs are reluctant to ejaculate in unfamiliar surroundings or without a teaser bitch. In some instances, contaminants from the dog, urine, or contaminated collection equipment can kill sperm and lead to an inaccurate assumption that the sperm quality is poor. For this reason, several evaluations should be made prior to classifying him as infertile or sterile.

The physical examination should be thorough and begin with the non-reproductive systems. Many apparently unrelated disorders can influence fertility (such as orthopedic disease) or may reveal abnormalities related to fertility (such as alopecia suggesting an endocrinopathy).

The reproductive aspects of the physical examination
Palpation of the scrotum
The scrotal skin should be evaluated for thickening, tumors, or skin lesions. Abnormal contents could suggest an inguinal hernia.

Palpation of the testes
Two testes should be present. They should be firm, oval, and symmetrical in consistency, size and shape. The epididymis should be palpated and should be felt to wrap around the testicle and

smoothly incorporate into the spermatic cord. A spermatocele is palpable as a cystic structure. Any variation in size between the 2 testes should be noted. If one or both are noticeably soft (indicating atrophy) or have a noticeable firm nodule (indicating a mass) or firm texture (indicating acute orchitis or other swelling) within, this should be investigated. The testes should be measured in all 3 dimensions with a caliper to detect subtle differences in size between the 2 testes and to document the size as a baseline as the dog ages. Ultrasound is more sensitive than palpation in detecting changes in the testicular architecture.

Evaluation of the penis and prepuce
The penis should be evaluated in both its erect and non-erect state. The penis should first be palpated through the prepuce. To most completely evaluate the non-erect penis, the dog can be held in lateral recumbency and the non-erect penis can be exteriorized gently. It is best to reflect the prepuce back to the fornix to allow complete examination of the penis for lesions, discharge, or foreign material. The erect penis should also be evaluated on all aspects at the time of semen collection. The os penis should be palpated for evidence of trauma or congenital abnormalities.

Palpation of the prostate and pelvic urethra
A rectal examination should be performed on any male dog presented for breeding, regardless of age. Dogs under the age of 4 usually have a prostate that is palpable in the pelvic canal. As dogs age, the prostate frequently drops cranially into an abdominal position. It is easier to palpate the older dog's prostate by either standing him with his front feet elevated on a stair or chair and/or by placing the opposite hand on the ventral abdominal wall to elevate the prostate toward the finger in the rectum so the size, shape, and the character of the entire prostate can be appreciated. The prostate gland should be approximately walnut sized, firm, symmetrical and have a division between the two lobes notable on palpation.

Evaluation of the mammary chain
The mammary glands should be small and unremarkable.

Collecting the stud dog
Ideally, the stud dog should have a minimum of 5 days of sexual rest prior to semen collection for analysis. If significant abnormalities are noted in the ejaculate and the dog has had prolonged sexual rest, the dog can be collected a second time as a comparison to assess the sperm for aging abnormalities.

Supplies for semen collection and evaluation
A clear plastic disposable artificial vagina with a clear plastic disposable graduated centrifuge tube attached will be needed. Clear artificial vaginas with clear centrifuge tubes allow the collector to assess for the stage, volume, and content of the ejaculate. If urine, blood, or excessive prostatic fluid is being collected, the sleeve can be changed to minimize contamination of the sperm-rich fraction of the ejaculate (Figure 10-1).

Some who collect prefer to use a funnel system and change tubes between the 3 fractions of the ejaculate. Some dogs are easier to fractionate than others, depending on their level of enthusiasm at collection. The supplies needed include:

Artificial vagina with collection tube
Non-latex exam gloves, rinsed with saline to reduce the powder on the surface;
Non-spermicidal lubricant;
Microscope;
Microscope slides and coverslips;
Waterbath, slide warmer, or heating pad;

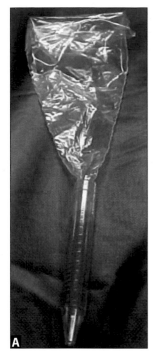

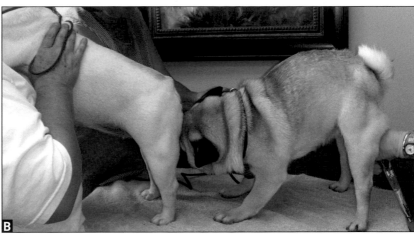

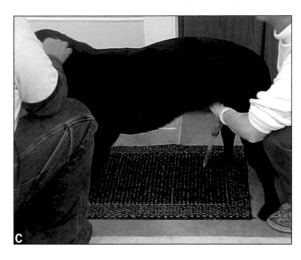

Figure 10-1.
A. The disposable collection sleeve is preferred over reusable sleeves because there is no cross contamination and no danger that disinfectants will alter sperm quality.
B. Small dogs are more easily collected on a table than on the floor if they have secure footing and are accustomed to being handled on a table. *C.* Large dogs, or dogs that are unfamiliar with a table are better collected on a non-slip surface on the floor.

Hemocytometer;
Unopettes® or alternate lysing solution
Sterile saline, replace with a fresh bag or bottle after no more than 24 hours;
Live-dead stain;
Eosin-nigrosin stain
Centrifuge tubes
Centrifuge that can spin at 1000 rpm.

Semen collection by manual ejaculation is a procedure done daily in the busy reproduction-oriented practice. However, there are many other occasions in veterinary practice that this technique is valuable.

The obvious uses for semen collection are insemination, shipment of semen for breeding at remote locations, and semen preservation. Semen collection for fertility evaluation is also a service commonly requested by clients with intact male dogs – sometimes hoping they are still fertile and sometimes hoping they are not. Evaluation of ejaculated prostatic fluid with or without the sperm rich fraction is valuable in any diagnostic work-up when the prostate is to be examined. This includes examining the prostate for benign prostatic hypertrophy, prostatic abscessation, and prostatic malignancy.

Not only can the ejaculate be evaluated for the presence of sperm, it is also useful for determining the sperm count, sperm morphology, sperm motility, semen viscosity, pH, color and the presence of other cells.

In many cases, ejaculation is the best or only way to obtain these samples. Semen cannot be collected directly from the testicle or the epididymis without potentially causing damage to the blood-testicular barrier so necessary to maintain fertility. Prostatic massage produces a substandard sample of prostatic fluid, whether to be used for cytology or culture.

In some cases, the dogs most difficult to collect an ejaculate from are the ones you need a sample from the most. This can be because the dog has had limited sexual experiences, has pain associated with his reproductive organs, or is too ill to focus on the process. It can also be difficult to arrange in advance for a teaser bitch, well known to aid in semen collection by ejaculation, when the demand of the veterinary clinic's schedule does not allow for access on short notice to an estrus bitch. In these cases, the best alternative must be sought.

Location
The following is a description of the "ideal" situation for semen collection. In general, the stud dog should NOT be allowed to urinate just prior to collection for 2 reasons. First, the ejaculate is likely to be contaminated with urine, which will alter sperm motility and longevity. Second, older dogs are less likely to retrograde ejaculate with a fuller bladder.

The ideal location is in a quiet room with good footing. Rugs are used not only for providing good footing under the dogs and a soft place for the person collecting to kneel but also to carry over the odor from the previous bitch in season. These rugs are infrequently laundered to enhance the aroma of the area for the stud dog. It is best to use the same entrance to the hospital and the same room for collections because many dogs quickly identify the reason they are at the hospital making collections easier. For dogs that are easily distracted, telephone ringers, timers and cell phones should be turned off. Staff should not knock on the door or enter during collection of a distractible or shy dog.

Staff and doctors
If the dog has a preference, when possible, the person collecting should remain consistent as this again is psychologically beneficial to the dog. Some dogs develop "white coat syndrome." If the dog is reluctant to collect, removing lab coats and stethoscopes from the collector can improve the dog's level of comfort. Two staff members should be present – one to steady the teaser bitch and one to collect the stud dog.

The audience
Most dogs will do well with the owner or handler present. The handler may stand next to the dog but should be instructed to hold the leash loosely (assuming the dog does not bite) and should keep speaking to a minimum as this can confuse the dog. Many dogs are very "in-tune" with their owners/handlers and talking can be misinterpreted by the dog to mean they are doing something they should not be doing. Other people should not be in the room.

The teaser bitch
This is an essential component of the collection effort. The ideal bitch is of the same breed as the stud dog and in standing heat. Many stud dogs prefer their own breed and even individuals within the breed. If the stud dog's one true love is available but not in season, she may be used if scented with the secretions of an estrus bitch that has been preserved in the freezer and resuspended in saline. In most cases, an estrus bitch will needed. In general, any bitch in standing heat will have to do as most veterinary clinics do not have easy access to a vast array of available estrus bitches. However, a match of size, temperament, color, or body type may improve the level of cooperation of a reluctant stud dog.

If there is contact between the stud dog and bitch, including sniffing or licking secretions and mounting, both must have a current negative <u>Brucella</u> test. Even casual contact is considered an exposure. This precaution should always be taken to reduce liability to the hospital.

It is usually best to have the bitch in the collection room first, well positioned, and restrained prior to introducing the stud dog. The very willing stud dog should be intercepted quickly as he approaches the bitch so that no contact occurs. A mount is acceptable to improve the sample quality as long as the bitch permits it. The shyer stud dog may need a few minutes to meet and court the bitch prior to collection. A shy dog can turn off very quickly if the collector intervenes prematurely.

Step by step semen collection

Exam gloves, either latex-free or rinsed to be free of powder on the outside of the glove are needed for the person collecting the semen. These should be donned prior to the stud dog entering the room. Provide 2 collection sleeves with centrifuge tubes attached, top rolled back, labeled with the stud dog's name. Check the brand of non-spermacidal lubricant with a fresh collection to assure it will not be detrimental to sperm motility.

The comprehensive examination of the stud dog should be completed AFTER the semen is collected. The only evaluation that should be done in advance is to be certain the collection will not be detrimental to him or the bitch. Work in a quiet room with 1 to 2 assistants and 1 collector, 1 <u>Brucella canis</u> negative estrus bitch, with good footing.

The bitch should be positioned in the room prior to the male dog's entrance. She should be facing away from the male, near the front of the rug used for footing so as to leave enough room behind her to allow the male to have all 4 feet on the rug as well. She should be held by the veterinary assistant who is kneeling beside her, 1 arm gently restraining her head from under her neck and the other arm under her abdomen to support her in a standing position. This is best done with the assistant facing a wall, with the bitch between the assistant and the wall; this aids in keeping the stud dog from wandering during collection. If the bitch is likely to object to the stud dog's approach or mount, she should be muzzled.

If the stud dog is trustworthy and unlikely to swing his head around to the person collecting him, the owner may now enter the room with the stud dog on a loose leash to approach the restrained bitch. IF the stud dog does not allow easy handling of his genitals, the owner should not be on the leash. Instead, an experienced veterinary assistant should handle him. This assistant should direct the stud dog's attention to the bitch and protect the person doing the collection. Although it is unusual for most stud dogs to object to this type of handling, there are some that are potentially harmful to the person kneeling beside or behind him. Care should be taken to protect the bitch, the owner, and the veterinary staff.

The semen collector should quietly approach the rear of the stud dog as he approaches the bitch. The stud should be given the opportunity to sniff the bitch. At this point, the confident dog is easily aroused. The stud dog can then be made aware that the collector is present beside or behind him by a gentle touch to his rump; then the sleeve can be slipped onto the penis as the bulb of the penis begins to swell. If this process is delayed, it may become difficult or painful to slide the prepuce caudally to expose the bulb. In most cases, dogs are more comfortable during ejaculation if the prepuce is slid caudal to the bulb of the penis prior to full erection. If his erection is too advanced to allow exposure of the bulb without causing pain, the stud dog should be walked away from the bitch, allowed to calm down, and then handled more quickly on the second approach.

If there is excess contamination in the prepuce, quickly wipe the penis with a non-abrasive saline-moistened towel to cleanse the area.

As the prepuce is slid caudally, exteriorizing the penis with one hand, the collector can slide the collection sleeve over the penis with the opposite hand. Care should be taken to avoid touching the penis to the tube as this can cause superficial hemorrhage. Gentle but firm stimulation of the shaft of the penis proximal to the bulb will increase the stimulation of the male and retain the prepuce caudal to the bulb, helping him to maximize his erection and ejaculate. Once he is stimulated, the collector should firmly encircle the base of the penis proximal to the bulb with the thumb and fingers, simulating a tie, allowing him to complete his ejaculation. Some dogs will thrust vigorously as they ejaculate while others are quietly non-demonstrative.

When possible, only the second portion of the ejaculate, the sperm-rich fraction (the milky-white portion) should be collected. The collection sleeve can be changed between fractions if the dog is standing steadily enough to avoid losing a portion of the sperm-rich fraction. In many cases, the first and second fractions may both be collected. The second fraction containing the sperm is typically between 0.5 ml and 4.0 ml in volume. The first and third fractions vary widely in volume, and may exceed 15 ml in larger dogs. At this point, the dog will often swing his leg over the arm of the collector, directing his penis backwards between his rear legs, as in a normal tie. The third fraction of the ejaculate is usually clear (unless the prostatic fluid is bloody or purulent). During the third fraction, the urethra can be felt to pulsate and the anal sphincter can be seen to contract. As this portion containing only prostatic fluid does not need to be collected, the sleeve should be removed or changed. Clients should be assured that this fluid does not contain any valuable sperm.

Once the sleeve is removed from the penis, a water-soluble non-spermicidal lubricant should be applied to the penis to prevent drying of the mucus membrane because this is painful. Slow walking of the dog away from the presence of the bitch may aid in retraction. The dog may be allowed to lick himself to accelerate retraction of the penis into the prepuce. In some cases, particularly with long-haired or thick-bodied dogs, they may need assistance retracting the penis into the prepuce. Prior to leaving the hospital, the collector should visually assess the dog to assure that his penis is fully retracted and he is comfortable.

Shy dogs should be allowed more time to introduce themselves to the bitch. Sometimes, off-leash courting can help his confidence. Care should be taken though that the bitch is not so outgoing as to frighten him. This is when a temperament mis-match can be a problem.

After the less confident stud dog has had the opportunity to familiarize himself with the bitch, she should be steadied by an assistant and he should again be allowed to approach her. In some cases, the assistant can assist the male by holding the bitch with an arm under her rear legs; but in other cases, this is a deterrent to the male to approaching or mounting the bitch.

Some stud dogs are easily collected with no bitch in the room – these are the dogs who are confident and familiar with the routine. However, the sperm count will generally be much higher if a bitch is present. Some stud dogs are content to sniff the bitch and collect well this way. Other stud dogs must mount the bitch once or multiple times before they will collect. This often requires patience on the part of the people collecting. There is a fine line when too little or too much patience becomes a deterrent to the stud dog to collect so there are times the collector's experience will signal that it is time to end these efforts. Everything possible should be done to prevent the stud dog from having a negative experience that will interfere with his next efforts at collection.

There is a small population of dogs, often those with shy temperaments, those who have been trained not to collect, and those with an associated medical condition that causes them discomfort when they mount or ejaculate, that are difficult or impossible to collect. There are several options for dogs with reluctance to collect. These include:

1. Having the handler or owner leave the room, and changing the veterinary staff or way the staff is assisting, including the person doing the collection. A more experienced collector may be able to finesse the dog into relaxing and ejaculating.

2. Using a different bitch, in case the bitch used is not to his liking – dogs do have preferences.

3. Changing locations – a different room in the veterinary hospital, or outside if the weather permits. Leaving the room with either the dog or bitch and reintroducing them.

4. Pharmaceutical and hormonal intervention. This can include a prostaglandin or GnRH injection to improve the quantity of sperm in the ejaculate. Lutalyse® can be administered subcutaneously 15 minutes prior to collection. This is thought to both help to improve libido in the stud dog and to increase peristaltic movement of sperm through the epididymis.

The prostaglandin dose should be carefully calculated, with the lower end dose used for the larger dogs to minimize side effects of vomiting and nausea. Use of Lutalyse® at the first visit or routinely for dogs who collect well without should be avoided because of the negative psychological effects it may produce. It is most helpful for the young or nervous dog on a second or subsequent visit. The dose is 0.05-0.1 mg/kg sq 15 min prior to collection. Lutalyse® is most effective when used with an estrous teaser bitch. Nausea and vomiting are a common side effect, and can be reduced by walking the dog between the time of the injection and the time of the collection. In addition to vomiting, the collection volume may be smaller (but with a good sperm count) and the dog may ejaculate without an erection. Care should be taken in patient selection and handling the drug. It should not be given to elderly patients or those with airway disease such as asthma or brachycephalic patients. To limit potential liability, the drug should not be handled by women of child-bearing age who could potentially be pregnant, or around staff with a history of respiratory disease including asthma. Lutalyse® is an extra-labell use in the dog, and owners should be advised of this prior to administration. The effect of Lutalyse® is short-lived and can be repeated at the next collection. Lutalyse® coupled with the presence of a teaser bitch is reported to have an additive effect, meaning its greatest effect was when an estrus bitch was present in the room.

GnRH increases libido in the male dog by increasing the release of endogenous testosterone. It can be administered at 3.3 mcg/kg IM once daily 60 minutes prior to collection (typically found as 50 mcg/ml). GnRH should be used with caution in males with testosterone-related disorders such as benign prostatic hypertrophy and perianal gland tumors. GnRH can be used daily during a breeding cycle or once weekly preceding breeding.

Exogenous testosterone, or testosterone as a supplement, should never be administered to increase libido, as it will cause negative feedback on the pituitary, reducing endogenous testosterone release, eventually reducing the sperm count and causing testicular degeneration.

5. Pain management in aged dogs with orthopedic pain, treatment with an appropriate non-steroidal anti-inflammatory can be helpful. The delay in response may mandate the next attempt be rescheduled after the drug has begun to relieve inflammation. In aged dogs with prostate pain, appropriate management may require days to weeks for a response.

It is recommended to collect only the 2nd of the 3 ejaculate fractions – that which is the sperm-rich fraction. The pre and post-ejaculate consist largely of prostatic fluid and sometimes urine, both of which are detrimental to semen survival. In some dogs, particularly those who collect with great enthusiasm, splitting the fractions without losing a portion of the sperm rich fraction can be difficult. As a result, it may be necessary to dilute the ejaculate with normal saline and centrifuge the ejaculate after collection to remove the supernatant.

Sperm count and morphology
(Appendix A-6)

A complete semen analysis includes evaluation of the semen volume and gross appearance, sperm count, sperm motility, and sperm morphology. A trained veterinary assistant can perform the entire analysis with a centrifuge, microscope, Unopette® and hemocytometer. The mere recognition of sperm in the ejaculate is not sufficient to determine if the dog is fertile or subfertile.

The semen analysis should be performed as soon after collection as possible. While the semen is awaiting analysis, it should be maintained at room temperature. If there is a delay in using the sperm, it should be covered with Parafilm®, kept away from any chemicals, centrifuged if necessary, extended and refrigerated. The semen motility evaluation must be done when the semen is still fresh and warm or has been carefully rewarmed. Although the semen should not be kept warm for an extended time prior to evaluation, it is best to keep it at a constant temperature and to rewarm at least 1 drop on a microscope slide prior to evaluation. There are several techniques for warming the semen. These include a slide warmer (free-standing or on the microscope stage), a water bath, a heating pad set low with a towel over it, or holding the sample against a body surface. One drop of semen should be placed on the warmed microscope slide, a warmed coverslip applied, and evaluated immediately. If the slide begins to cool, it should be rewarmed and re-examined. If the slide dries, repeat the process with another drop.

Semen volume

The volume of the ejaculate is simple to determine, particularly if the semen is collected in a sleeve with a clear plastic graduated centrifuge tube attached. When possible, only the sperm-rich fraction should be collected. The typical dog's sperm-rich fraction varies from 0.5 ml to 4.0 ml. Some dog's total ejaculate volume, when all of the prostatic fluid is saved, can exceed 30 ml. A larger volume of ejaculate does not correspond to greater fertility. Many clients expect to see a greater volume and are disappointed that their stud dog "didn't do very well" if only the 1ml of sperm-rich fraction is collected. The volume should be recorded on the semen evaluation form to use for calculation of the total sperm count.

Gross appearance of the ejaculate

The normal sperm-rich fraction of the ejaculate should be a dense milky white color. It should not be thick or viscous. A faint cloudiness suggests a low sperm count; clear yellow suggests urine; cloudy yellow suggests white blood cells; and red, brown or copper color suggests blood. Blood can be the result of trauma to the penis, prostatic disease or a neoplasia in the urogenital tract. Blood in the ejaculate of the dog does not interfere with fertility, but the underlying cause such as prostatic disease can.

Sperm count

This is an essential part of the semen evaluation. There are several techniques for performing a sperm count: manual with a hemocytometer, by spectrophotometry using a sperm counter, and by computer assisted technology. The presence of sperm is not sufficient to determine fertility; an actual sperm count with motility and morphology is necessary to assess the male's fertility. As a corollary, the absence of sperm in a single ejaculate is not sufficient to classify a male as sterile; he may have had sperm at a previous time or in the future.

A normal dog should have 10 million sperm per pound of body weight in the total ejaculate. The concentration is dependent on the volume of the ejaculate and does not correlate with fertility. The average semen dose considered to be adequate for a fertile breeding is 100 to 250 million sperm. There are anecdotal reports of lower doses successfully achieving a pregnancy.

The least expensive but most time-consuming method of counting sperm is manually with a Unopette™ and a Neubauer hemocytometer. Unopettes™ are being discontinued and other methods of diluting and lysing the other cells in the ejaculate are being proposed and should be a viable option in the future. To perform a manual sperm count, the collection should be covered with Parafilm® and tilted several times to evenly distribute the sperm in the ejaculate. The capped top of the diluting chamber is used to pierce the No. 5853 Unopette™, and rotated to make a wide opening in the sealed chamber, taking care not to flex the cap so much that the interior pipette is broken. This uses 20 microliters of semen diluted into 2 ml of diluent. The evenly mixed semen is drawn up into the pipette by capillary action. With one hand holding the chamber and the other holding the pipette, the chamber is gently squeezed. The pipette is slid through the newly made opening in the chamber, and the pressure on the chamber is released as the pipette is firmly engaged into the top of the chamber. Taking great care to squeeze gently, the chamber is squeezed several times to rinse the semen out of the pipette and uniformly distribute it into the chamber. Squeezing too hard will create a spout out of the top of the chamber and lead to an inaccurate sperm count. Both chambers of the hemocytometer should be loaded (first place the calibrated coverslip on the slide chamber with the diluted solution immediately or if there is a delay, the solution should be swirled to make certain the sperm are evenly distributed. The hemocytometer should rest for 5 minutes to allow the sperm to settle into the same visual plane.

After the hemocytometer has rested, it should be placed on the stage of a microscope, with the stage moved down to allow the objective to clear the coverslip. Because the hemocytometer is much thicker than a regular glass slide, care must be taken to avoid hitting the coverslip with the objective. One of the central squares comprised of the 25 small squares should be moved under the objective. At 200x magnification, all the sperm in the 25 square grid should be counted, with sperm falling on the upper and left lines counted and those falling on the lower and right lines not being counted to avoid counting the same sperm twice. A hand-held counter can make this process more efficient. This should be repeated for the opposite 25 square grid. The two numbers should be averaged. If the difference between the 2 counts exceeds 10%, repeat the count. Multiply the averaged number by 10^6 to get the final concentration per ml. The concentration per ml should be multiplied by the volume of the ejaculate to calculate the total sperm count.

Sperm motility

Place a drop of semen on a warm glass microscope slide, apply a warm coverslip, and evaluate under 100x magnification with a microscope using a low light setting. Perform as soon as possible after collection with a warm slide and coverslip. A normal evaluation should show 80% or more sperm moving forward.

There are 2 components to the motility evaluation. The first is the <u>percentage</u> of sperm that are motile in a direct forward motion. This should be done as a percentage. Sperm that are coiled or otherwise abnormal but moving should not be included. If a high percentage of the sperm appear to be gently curved and are moving in a circular pattern, the semen should be rewarmed and reevaluated because this is often the motion of cool sperm. The second component is based on how <u>fast</u> the sperm are moving forward. This is frequently done on a scale from 1 to 4, with P1 moving slowly forward and P4 moving rapidly and deliberately forward. If the semen is very concentrated on the slide, diluting the sample with the dog's prostate fluid or 0.9% saline will improve visibility of individual sperm.

Live-dead stain can be used to help distinguish between dead and imomotile sperm.

Computerized technology has been developed for evaluating sperm count, motility and speed. Although this may be appealing, expensive technology is not necessary to do an accurate semen evaluation nor can it replace the human element so necessary for a complete semen evaluation.

Sperm morphology

Morphology of the sperm cells is an important component of male fertility evaluation. A stud dog is considered "normal" if his sperm cell morphology is 80% or more normal. When the percent of normal sperm drops below 60%, fertility is impaired. The morphology should be performed on unstained semen allowed to cool enough to render them immotile. Unstained semen is best evaluated for morphology using phase-contrast microscopy. Staining the sperm cells may cause some artifacts but will allow the examiner to detect defects not visible in an unstained sample. Eosin-nigrosin stain is preferred for this application. Once the sperm are immotile, 100 sperm cells should be counted with the following defects noted: head abnormalities, acrosome abnormalities, midpiece abnormalities and tail abnormalities.

Sperm cell defects can be classified by either the area of the testicle in which the defects develop or by the significance of the defect. Clinically, the significance of the defect is more applicable: major defects which interfere with fertility and minor defects which do not impair fertility. Defects that occur in the testicle during sperm cell production are considered a primary or major defect. These include altered head size or shape, bent midpieces, and detached heads. Defects that occur as the sperm are maturing in the epididymis, during transport through the vas deferens, or in sample handling are considered secondary or minor defects. These defects include bent or coiled tails, and distal cytoplasmic droplets.

A normal dog spermatozoa should be straight or gently curved with a normal head, midpiece and tail. Sperm with proximal droplets may be immature sperm or may represent a morphological abnormality. If the dog has been recently collected and the sperm motility appears normal, there may be no reason for concern. The dog should have another semen analysis after sexual rest. If the proximal droplets are still present in large numbers, the motility is slow and deliberate, or the dog has a history of infertility, these droplets probably represent a defect and not a lack of time in the epididymis to mature. Semen that is abnormal at collection but motile may not chill and ship or freeze well but may still produce a pregnancy in the bitch when used as a fresh breeding.

A rapid Wright's Geimsa stain (DiffQuik®) or eosin/nigrosin stain (SFT stain) can be used. The Wright's stain is used as for a blood smear – the semen is placed on the slide, a second slide is used to smear it, and it is stained in each of the solutions for 5 minutes. After rinsing and drying, the slide may be evaluated under oil emersion. The eosin/nigrosin stain is used by placing 1 equal sided drop of each sperm and stain on one end of a slide. These 2 drops are mixed, and made into a smear. The slide should be dried quickly on a slide warmer to prevent artifacts.

When the Wright's stain is used, sperm will appear purple on a clear background. When the eosin/nigrosin stain is used, normal (live sperm when collected) will appear white against a dark background. Sperm that are abnormal (dead when collected) will appear pink against a dark background in some species. This live-dead ratio has not been correlated with fertility in dogs.

To evaluate the stained sperm, 100 spermatozoa should be counted using oil immersion. The abnormal sperm should be classified by defect: primary defects including defects that occur during spermatogenesis (defects in head shape, detached heads, bent midpiece, persistent proximal cytoplasmic droplet, and doubling of any portion of the spermatozoa) and secondary defects including defects that occur during epididymal maturation or staining (persistent distal cytoplasmic droplets, and bent tails). There is a poorly defined correlation between specific defects and fertility in dogs.

The semen should also be assessed for the presence and quantity of red blood cells, white blood cells, and bacteria. Epithelial cells are often normal. Neoplastic cells are seldom identified.

Sperm agglutination

Sperm occasionally cluster together by their heads. This agglutination is due to development of anti-sperm antibodies which are thought to develop as the result of disruption of the blood-testicular barrier, allowing sperm to be exposed to the immune system. This leads to the development of antibodies, causing agglutination. Trauma and testicular infections may lead to antibody development. Dogs with this condition should be tested for <u>Brucella canis</u>. Because these sperm have reduced motility and an alteration in penetrating the zona pellucida, fertilization may be compromised. Intrauterine insemination may improve fertility.

Semen pH

The pH of the semen can be useful if there is poor semen motility or quality. This can be measured by placing 1 drop of semen on pH paper (do not immerse the paper into the semen). The normal pH of semen should be between 6.5 and 7.0; any alteration from this could reflect a prostatic infection and be useful in determining the antibiotic of choice.

Longevity

If semen is to be extended and refrigerated or shipped for use within a few days, assess with a test chill using the specific extender. The type and ratio of extender used should be recorded. The progressive motility should be assessed at 24 and 48 hours after warming a drop of semen. Some extenders are reported to retain semen viability for up to 10 days.

When the semen is aspirated or extender is added to the ejaculate, it should be done slowly to avoid mechanical damage or shock to the sperm cells.

Diagnostic workup for the infertile stud dog
Endocrinopathies and hormonal diseases

(See Appendix D-16)

Several endocrine disorders can interfere with normal sperm production. These include a hormone-secreting testicular tumor, thyroid disease, hyperadrenocorticism (Cushings), hypoadrenocorticism (Addison's), Diabetes Mellitus and corticosteroid administration.

A hormone – secreting testicular tumor

There are 3 kinds of testicular tumors: the Sertoli cell tumor (most commonly found in the abdominal retained testes, which can secrete estrogen), the seminoma (the most common type in subcutaneously retained testes) reported to cause paraneoplastic syndrome, and the interstitial cell tumor (which can secrete testosterone). Any or all can occur in the same patient, even in scrotal testes. Larger tumors are palpable, some are too small to palpate but can be seen on ultrasound, and some can only be diagnosed by biopsy or fine needle aspirate. They are seldom malignant. Unilateral or bilateral castration is usually curative. Unilateral castration should only be considered in a valuable breeding dog and if the opposite testicle appears normal on ultrasound. Because a unilateral testicular tumor can cause poor semen quality, the decision to remove only the neoplastic testicle should not be determined by semen quality at the time of the tumor diagnosis (Figure 10-2).

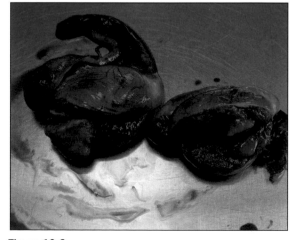

Figure 10-2.
Testicular tumors in both testes. Both testes from this dog had multiple tumor types.

Thyroid disease

Is often discussed and implicated as a cause of infertility in both the male and female dog. However, the literature does not support this as a common cause of infertility. Dogs that are profoundly hypothyroid may exhibit lower libido, but not diminished sperm production. "It appears that euthyroidism supports optimal reproductive performance, but clinically significant reproductive dysfunction is manifested only under certain uncommon conditions of thyroid disease in dogs and cats." Johnson CA Clin Tech Small Animal Practice 2002 Aug; 17(3): 12932

So it appears supplementation of thyroid hormone will not resolve poor semen production. "Although animals and people with thyroid disorders may also have reproductive disorders, usually disorders other than thyroid disease are the cause of reproductive abnormalities."

A link between autoimmune thyroiditis and orchitis has been suggested. However, there is value in knowing the thyroid status of an individual dog; if he has lymphocytic thyroiditis or another form of congenital hypothyroidism thought to be inherited, the breeder may consider eliminating him from their breeding lines based on this and his other qualities.

Hyperadrenocorticism (Cushing's Disease), Hypoadrenocorticism (Addison's Disease) and Diabetes Mellitus

All 3 of these endocrine disorders can be implicated as a cause of infertility. Low dose dexamethasone suppression testing or ACTH stimulation testing may help determine the underlying cause. Abnormally high or low levels of glucocorticoid may alter the metabolism of hormones, leading to deterioration of the seminiferous epithelium.

Corticosteroid administration

There are many undocumented references indicating that corticosteroid administration may interfere with spermatogenesis, particularly if administered for long periods at high doses. Only betamethasone and boldenone undecylenate have specific references to decreased sperm production.

Oral, injectable or topical corticosteroids should be used judiciously in any valuable stud dog.

Disorders of the prostate

(See Appendix D-14)

Clinical signs and the 4 disease processes of the prostate often overlap, making a definitive diagnosis difficult without advanced diagnostics. Diagnostics include: complete physical examination including rectal palpation, CBC, chemistry panel, urinalysis, cytology and culture of prostatic fluid (collected by ejaculation and prostatic massage), x-rays, ultrasound, an ELISA test, and ultrasound-guided needle biopsy.

Prostatic fluid is secreted continuously in the intact male dog, with secretions either flowing into the urethra externally or retrograde into the urinary bladder.

BPH – Benign Prostatic Hypertrophy

Benign Prostatic Hypertrophy (BPH) is the most common disorder of the prostate gland. Most (80 to 100%) intact male dogs who are middle-aged to older are affected but many are asymptomatic. BPH is part of aging and alterations in hormones, with both an increase in cell number and increase in cell size contributing to the enlargement of the gland.

Diagnosis of BPH

The most common presentation to the veterinarian and most startling symptom to the owner is dripping blood from the penis of an intact male dog independent of urination. Other symptoms include: blood in the urine or ejaculate, poor semen quality, infertility, straining to defecate, and flattened stools. Dogs rarely have difficulty urinating. The CBC and chemistry profile are typically normal. The urinalysis may be normal or may show hematuria (and sperm).

A presumptive diagnosis can be made on rectal palpation – a patient with BPH has a prostate that is symmetrically enlarged, often positioned in the abdomen rather than the pelvic canal (requiring the veterinarian to place their opposite hand on the ventral abdominal wall to direct the prostate caudally to meet their opposite finger in the rectum). It is seldom painful. Radiographs show only an enlarged prostate. Ultrasound is more useful; on ultrasound, the prostate can be seen to be uniformly enlarged, of uniform echogenicity (somewhat greater echogenicity than most abdominal organs) with no mineralization, and with few to no cystic structures. Ultrasound can be used to distinguish BPH from cysts inside the prostate and paraprostatic cysts. The only way to definitively confirm that the dog has BPH and not neoplasia is by biopsy: a skilled ultrasonographer with specialized equipment can collect an ultrasound-guided prostate biopsy sterilely with a needle biopsy from an anesthetized patient. There are several different approaches to needle biopsy – including transrectal and transabdominal. The ultrasonographer will base the technique on their particular expertise. Prior to biopsy, the patient should be assessed to assure a normal coagulation status. Surgical biopsy for histology and culture via laparotomy is another alternative to confirm a diagnosis. An ELISA test to distinguish BPH from other causes of prostatic disease is available in Europe.

A biopsy is not essential prior to instituting treatment for BPH if clinical signs and diagnostics suggest BPH. If the patient fails to respond to therapy for BPH, diagnostics should be initiated.

Cytology by evaluation of the third fraction of the ejaculate, prostatic massage or prostatic wash may be useful but cannot confirm that the patient has BPH. Ejaculation is the easiest, least expensive and least invasive of these three procedures. The third fraction of the ejaculate may also be submitted for culture to distinguish the patient with BPH from the patient with prostatitis or a prostatic abscess.

Technique for prostatic massage
Under general anesthesia, pass a urethral catheter into the bladder to remove all urine. A urinalysis may be run on this reserved sample. Flush the bladder with 5 ml sterile physiologic saline solution and save the fluid. Label this specimen Sample 1. Retract the catheter tip and align it with the caudal pole of the prostate gland (positioning is determined via rectal palpation). Massage the prostate gland for 1 minute, with care to avoid possible rupture of a prostatic abscess. Flush 5 ml sterile physiologic saline solution slowly through the catheter while the urethral orifice is occluded around the catheter to prevent retrograde loss of the sample. Advance the catheter into the bladder as fluid is aspirated. Save the fluid and label Sample 2. Submit for cytology and culture. Quantitate bacterial numbers in both specimens to ascertain significance of bacterial growth in prostatic fluid specimen (Sample 2). Perform a culture and sensitivity test on the sample collected.

Treatment of BPH
Castration is curative but is not the only treatment option available. The prostate is usually half its pre-castration size within 3 weeks, and will continue to involute. A follow-up rectal exam is recommended at 3 weeks post-op. If the prostate does not respond to castration or one of the medical therapies, other causes of prostatic enlargement should be considered.

Many dogs are valuable as breeding dogs and their owners may wish to delay castration. Antibiotics are not useful in treating uncomplicated BPH. If urinalysis supports a diagnosis of cystitis, appropriate antibiotic therapy is recommended in addition to medical treatment of BPH.

Medical treatment of BPH

There are several drug therapies that can reduce the size of the prostate and simultaneously maintain the stud dog's fertility. These drug therapies include progestational compounds and antiandrogens.

The most commonly used and available synthetic progestin drug in the U.S. is megestrol acetate. This can be dosed at 0.25 mg per pound once daily for the first 21 days of therapy, then at 0.25 mg per pound once a week.

Megestrol acetate can be used on a long-term basis. This will reduce the volume of the ejaculate but not the semen quality. The drug should not be used just prior to collection, so when a breeding or collection is scheduled, the drug schedule should be adjusted. Other progestational compounds may be available in other countries.

Antiandrogens, such as finasteride, reduce the size and secretions of the prostate. Finasateride works by manipulating 5 alpha-reductase, the enzyme that metabolizes testosterone to dihydrotestosterone, which affects the prostate. Finasteride, available for human use in the U.S. can be dosed at 0.1 to 0.5 mg/kg once daily PO. Tablets are available in 1 mg and 5 mg sizes.

Osaterone, a progesten and anti-androgen, is labeled and marketed to treat BPH in countries outside of the US. This drug will not alter libido or semen quality and can be used long term.

Relapse will occur as soon as either mediation is discontinued. It is essential that you as the prescriber give notice to the owner to restrict the handling of tablets to only people who could not be pregnant as finasteride can harm the male fetus. Liver disease is a contraindication to use in humans.

Both drugs uses listed are considered extra-label uses. There are no reports showing harm to the fetuses sired by dogs on anti-androgens.

Response to treatment can be monitored by clinical signs, rectal examination, serial semen evaluations, and serial measurements of the prostate by ultrasound. Due to side effects, estrogen therapy is not currently recommended.

GnRH agonists are under investigation but cause infertility and/or sterility, so their use is not recommended in dogs who have an active reproductive future.

Bacterial prostatitis and prostatic abscesses

Along with age-related hyperplastic changes in the prostate gland, cysts may develop in the body of the prostate gland. Bacterial prostatitis or abscesses may occur secondarily to these age-related alterations of the prostate gland. Other causes of prostate inflammation include trauma, stricture, uroliths, and neoplasia. Prostate infections can either cause or result in urinary tract infections and infections of the testicle and/or epididymis. Aerobic bacteria are most commonly implicated, with E. coli being the most common. Staphylococci, Streptococcus, Proteus, Klebsiella, Brucella, and Pseudomonas spp are also found. Anaerobic bacteria, fungal and mycoplasma prostatic infections are rare. Blastomycosis and cryptococcosis causing granulomatous prostatitis are rare but do occur (Figure 10-3).

Acute prostatitis

Dogs affected by acute prostatitis are often very ill systemically. This is often due to sudden inflammation of the prostate caused by bacterial infection. This may develop from a recent or long-standing prostate infection or from a hematogenous spread. These dogs can be acutely and

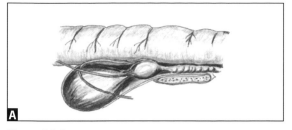
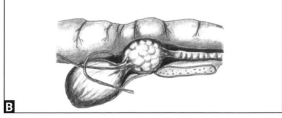

Figure 10-3.
A. Normal prostate with the pelvis cut away. B. Prostate with benign prostatic hypertrophy with the pelvis cut away.

profoundly ill. It is possible for septicemia to develop or for prostatic abscesses to rupture and cause peritonitis. Symptoms at presentation include depression, anorexia, vomiting, fever, stiff gait, urinary incontinence, hindlimb pitting edema, and caudal abdominal pain. Some patients may have fluid or blood dripping from the penis independent of urination. There is usually an associated infertility, either because of diminished semen quality or because of reluctance of the male to breed.

Chronic prostatitis
Dogs with chronic prostatitis may present without symptoms suggesting that the prostate is involved. Some may be lethargic, reluctant to move, or vaguely ill; others may present with fever, pain, and signs of septic shock. Many will present with symptoms of recurrent cystitis, fluid dripping from the penis independent of urination, or blood in the urine. Dependent upon which area of the prostate is involved, the dog may present with difficulty passing stool or urine. Some may present due to a history of infertility, either due to diminished semen quality or reluctance of the male to breed. Many will present with no clinical signs, making a diagnosis of chronic prostatitis difficult. Often the prostate will be enlarged, asymmetrical and with variable consistency but non-painful.

Diagnosis of acute and chronic prostatitis
Diagnosis is typically based on history (intact older male dog), physical examination findings (which should <u>always</u> include a rectal examination), lab results, imaging, and response to treatment.

In acute prostatitis, the CBC often reveals an elevated WBC, often with a left shift; in chronic prostatitis, the WBC is usually normal. In acute prostatitis, blood chemistries are often normal but an elevated alkaline phosphatase may be noted. Some will have elevated bilirubin and up to 40% will have hypoglycemia. Dehydration with pre-renal changes may be noted. In both acute and chronic forms, urinalysis will usually show bacteria, WBCs, RBCs and protein in the urine.

Ejaculation and evaluation of the sample may be useful in dogs with chronic prostatitis, but dogs acutely ill from prostatitis are usually too painful and too sick to ejaculate. The small risk of causing peritonitis by ultrasound-guided FNA should be considered prior to recommending this procedure. Urine and ejaculates should be submitted for culture, with more than 10,000 CFU per ml of prostatic fluid or urine diagnostic for prostatic infection. The same organism is usually found in the urine and the prostate fluid. If Blastomyces prostatitis is suspected, the sample should not be submitted for culture due to the risk to lab personnel. The current diagnostic test of choice is to test for Blastomyces antigen in the patient's urine.

Imaging
Radiographs may be normal or may show poor radiographic contrast, an enlarged symmetrical or asymmetrical prostate, or enlarged sublumbar lymph nodes. Ultrasound may show an enlarged prostate with increased echogencity of the prostate. Cysts, abscesses and paraprostatic cysts may be noted. It is not possible to differentiate BPH from prostatitis or neoplasia on ultrasound or radiograph.

Medical therapy for prostatitis

Treatment of acute prostatitis should include hospitalization on IV fluids, and IV antibiotics for the first 24 to 48 hours of therapy. Fluoroquiniolones are an appropriate antibiotic choice while culture and sensitivity results are pending. Based upon clinical response and antibiotic sensitivity results, the patient may be switched to oral antibiotic therapy. During the acute phase of prostatitis, the blood-prostate barrier is not usually intact so antibiotic selection may be based on sensitivity results alone. Antibiotic therapy should be continued for 4 to 6 weeks. Appropriate antibiotic choices for treatment after the blood-prostate barrier is reestablished include trimethoprim-sulfonamide, erythromycin, fluoroquinolones, and clindamcyin, with side effects considered. Fungal prostatitis can be treated with itraconazole at the normal recommended dose.

Re-evaluation of the patient should be performed twice, at 1 and 4 weeks after the completion of antibiotic therapy. The follow-up should include a complete physical examination including a rectal examination, urinalysis, urine culture, and culture and cytology of the prostatic fluid. The importance of this ongoing evaluation should be stressed to the owner as one way to minimize the development of chronic prostatitis. Castration should be considered as it may improve the long-term prognosis. However, castration should be delayed until the patient has been on a minimum of 5 to 7 days of antibiotics, both to stabilize him and to reduce the likelihood of post-op development of scirrhous cord. Hormones to manage BPH are an alternative to castration.

Acute prostatitis may also be associated with blood in the ejaculate, orchiepididymitis, and immune-mediated orchitis (Figure 10-4).

There may be a decrease in morphologically normal sperm due to an alteration in the quality of the prostatic fluid.

Although patients with chronic prostatitis are not as ill as patients with the acute form, the treatment is more difficult because the blood-prostate barrier prevents adequate penetration of antibiotics. Both penetration and sensitivity results must be taken into account when an antibiotic selection is made. Antibiotics that can penetrate the blood-prostate barrier include trimethoprim-sulfonamide, erythromycin, fluoroquinolones, and clindamcyin. Treatment should continue for 4 to 6 weeks, with follow-up 1 and 4 weeks after the cessation of antibiotic therapy. The re-evaluation should include a complete physical examination including a rectal evaluation of the prostate and culture of the prostatic fluid. This is to assess for resolution of chronic prostatitis. Either castration once the

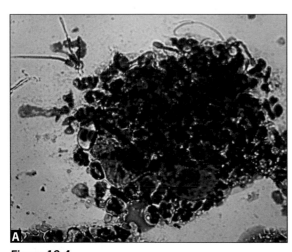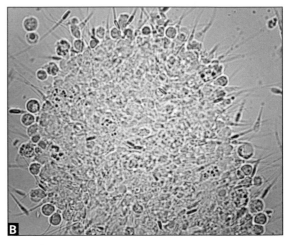

Figure 10-4.
A. A stained sample of ejaculate of a dog with prostatitis, showing a large clump of white blood cells, epithelial cells and sperm. **B.** Unstained appearance of a large clump of white blood cells and sperm coalesced, typical of a dog with prostatitis at semen evaluation.

patient is stable or treatment with one of the previously described drugs to modify the size and secretion of the prostate (antiandrogen or progestational) should be considered. This is thought to improve the prognosis by resolving the underlying BPH. Antibiotics alone may be insufficient to resolve prostatitis.

Prostatic abscesses

Prostatic abscesses have a poor short-term and long-term prognosis with a survival rate of approximately 50%. In addition to IV fluids, other supportive care as indicated, and long-term appropriate antibiotic therapy, drainage of the abscess is indicated. Drainage techniques include surgical insertion of a Penrose or tube drain, marsupialization of the prostate gland, and ultrasound-guided aspiration of the contents of the abscess. Blood cultures and cultures of the abdominal fluid may be indicated. Samples of the prostate and associated fluid should be collected for cytology and culture at laparotomy. Complications include septic shock, peritonitis, urinary incontinence, recurrent urinary tract infections, and recurrence of abscesses. Long-term antibiotic use, castration, and follow-up evaluations at 1 and 4 weeks post-op will reduce long-term complications.

Cysts and paraprostatic cysts

The prostate may be affected by two different types of cysts. Cysts may either be within the prostate gland (retention cysts), or adjacent to the prostate (paraprostatic cysts).

Cysts within the gland may be caused by BPH or be secondary to squamous metaplasia caused by estrogen-secreting Sertoli cell tumors. Up to 5% of dogs with prostatic disease may have paraprostatic cysts (Figure 10-5).

Neither prostatic nor paraprostatic cysts cause clinical signs unless they become large enough to interfere with urination or defecation or unless they abscess. On physical examination, they may be palpable through the abdominal wall or rectally. CBC and chemistry panels are not diagnostic unless an abscess is present. Ultrasound is more useful than x-rays in identifying cystic structures.

Treatment

Ultrasound-guided or surgical drainage, omentalization, and/or marsupialization are the treatments of choice for retention or paraprostatic cysts. Castration may be useful in preventing recurrence but alone is not likely to be curative. Alternatively, medical therapy with finasteride or megestrol acetate may reduce recurrence and the need to repeat drainage.

Paraprostatic abscesses, like prostatic abscesses, may cause sepsis and an associated poor prognosis.

Neoplasia of the prostate

Unlike other pathology of the prostate, neoplasia occurs 4 times more frequently in neutered male dogs than intact male dogs. It is the most common prostatic disease diagnosed in dogs neutered as adults. It may be hormonally related, but does not only involve testicular hormones. Like many other neoplastic conditions, the cause of prostate cancer is unknown and occurs most commonly in the aging dog.

The most common tumor of the prostate is malignant adenocarcinoma. The prognosis is uniformly poor. It tends to metastasize early to the regional lymph nodes, the regional vertebral bodies and the lungs. Even if no metastatic lung lesions are noted, 40% of patients have metastases by the time of diagnosis. Other rare types of malignant prostate neoplasia include transitional cell carcinoma, metastatic lymphosarcoma, hemangiosarcoma, and squamous cell carcinoma.

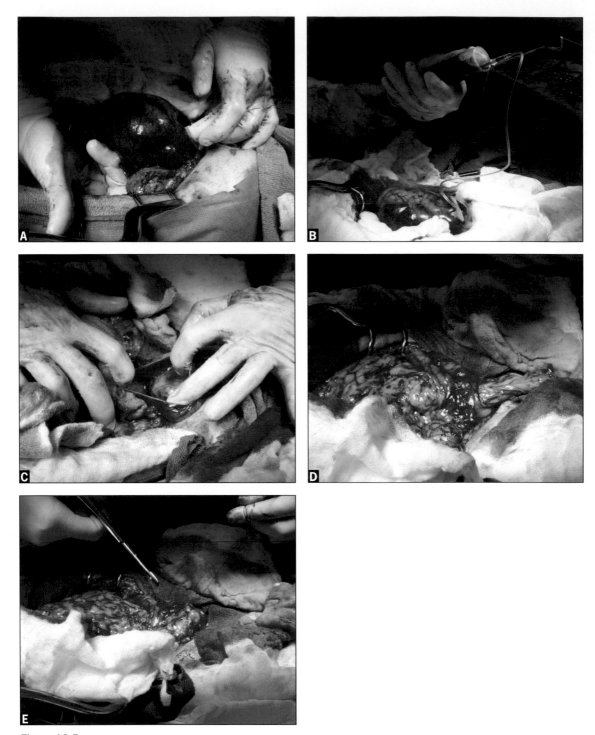

Figure 10-5.
*A. The appearance of a paraprostatic cyst, in situ, at exploratory laparotomy. **B.** Aspirating the fluid from a paraprostatic cyst in preparation for omentalization. **C.** The paraprostatic cyst after the fluid was aspirated in preparation for omentalization. **D.** The paraprostatic cysts, after the omenum has been introduced to create drainage. **E.** Closing the repair of the paraprostatic cyst.*

The typical patient with adenocarcinoma is a medium to large breed dog with a mean age of 9 to 10 years. Clinical signs suggesting prostatic neoplasia include difficulty urinating and/or passing stools; rear limb stiffness, pain, and weakness; anorexia; weight loss; and bloody discharge from the penis. Physical examination findings include a prostate that is oversized for a neutered male dog of his size with one or more firm irregular immovable nodules palpable on rectal exam, sometimes with pain on palpation. He may be febrile and depressed. The CBC may reflect a normal leukogram or a left shift. Approximately 20% have a mild non-regenerative anemia. The chemistry panel may show an elevated alkaline phosphatase with an elevated BUN if there is urinary obstruction. The urinalysis frequently reveals blood, and some may have WBCs and tumor cells that have exfoliated into the urine. Secondary bacterial prostatitis may complicate the diagnosis. There is no canine form of blood test to detect the tumor marker (PSA) as there is in humans.

Imaging
Radiographs of the abdomen may show an asymmetrical irregularly shaped enlarged prostate. Lysis of the vertebrae may be noted. The normal prostate should not exceed 50% of the width of the pelvic inlet on a ventrodorsal radiograph. Prostatic enlargement of >90% of the pubic brim-sacral distance indicates that prostate neoplasia, prostatic cysts, or a prostatic abscess is present.

Both ultrasound and x-rays may show mineral densities. Ultrasound may show an irregular prostate with hyperechoic regions. Metastatic lesions in the lungs, long bones, vertebrae, ribs, pelvis and digits suggest a diagnosis of prostate cancer.

Prognosis
Unless a voided urine cytology reveals tumor cells or metastatic lesions are noted, a biopsy is necessary to differentiate prostatic neoplasia from other forms of prostate disease such as paraprostatic cysts and prostatic abscesses. This differentiation is important because of the difference in treatment and prognosis of prostate cancer.

Most patients with prostate cancer are euthanized within a few months of diagnosis due to declining quality of life. Surgical excision of the tumor is usually not possible because of the rapid progression of the disease and the severe complications related to excision. Intra-operative radiation therapy is the current treatment of choice. Castration may actually increase the rate of growth of the tumor and is not recommended. No chemotherapy protocols have been developed. Hormonal therapy is under investigation.

Disorders of the testes
Unilateral and bilateral cryptorchidism, ectopia
Cryptorchidism or ectopic testicles is the failure of one or both of the testes to descend into the scrotum by 6 months of age. The ectopic testes can be located anywhere from the caudal pole of the kidney to the subcutaneous region just cranial to the scrotum. This is considered to be congenital, with an inheritance pattern that has not yet been determined.

Testicular descent should occur in puppies by 3 to 10 days of age. Careful palpation should reveal the testes presence in the scrotum by 3 to 4 weeks of age. If the testes are not initially palpable, the pup should be placed back with his littermates, allowed to relax, picked up again without touching him in the abdominal or inguinal region or startling him, and palpated again. At a young age (6 to 8 weeks), such as when initial health checks and vaccination are given, even normal pups are likely to have their testes move along the ventral abdominal wall transiently when handled. If the testes are not palpable in the scrotum by 10 weeks of age when the pup is relaxed, the pup may have delayed testicular descent at best, or may be tentatively considered to be cryptorchid.

The retained testicle(s) in dogs are predisposed to testicular neoplasia at a rate 14 times that of the normal dog. These include sertoli cell tumors in testes retained in the abdomen and seminomoas in testes retained in the inguinal canal. Additionally, the undescended testicle is at increased risk of developing torsion of the spermatic cord. The retained testicle cannot produce sperm but can still produce testosterone. If both testes are retained, the dog is likely to be sterile. If only one testicle is retained, he may still be able to sire litters. Like other congenital defects with a hereditary basis, the affected dogs and their parents and siblings may not be ideal candidates for breeding. All factors influencing testicular descent are not known. This, of course, must be balanced against other genetic traits.

Medical and surgical treatment of cryptorchidism is considered unethical by the breed registries. Medical therapy for cryptorchidism has largely fallen out of favor. The most common and successful treatment uses serial injections of hCG, dosed at 100 to 1000 IU IM twice a week for a series of 4 injections. In a group of 22 cryptorchid dogs under 16 weeks of age, 21 responded with complete descent of the testes. In the control group, all 28 puppies remained cryptorchid (Feldman). If medical therapy is successful, the affected pup is spared the more invasive surgical procedure of locating and removing the retained testicle. Surgical translocation of the retained testicle may be possible if the spermatic cord is long enough. However, this is considered unethical and use of such dogs in a breeding program may lead to an increased incidence of cryptorchidism in future generations.

Because of health risks, dogs with one or both retained testes should have the retained testicle surgically removed, preferably prior to age 3. The retained testicle may be located by palpation or imaging by a skilled ultrasonographer. X-rays are unrewarding.

Prior to and after anesthetic induction, careful palpation may reveal the retained testicle present in the subcutaneous region near or in the inguinal canal. Surgical techniques are based on the location of the retained testicle. If the testicle is suspected to be subcutaneous or inguinal, this region should be explored. If the testicle is located in the abdominal cavity, routine laparotomy should be performed. The abdominal testicle(s) is usually dorsal and slightly lateral (on the retained side) to the urinary bladder. If not present there, the vas deferens can be located as it passes over the ureter and followed to locate the ectopic testicle. Each testicle should have its blood supply and spermatic cord identified and ligated/transfixed routinely, spermatic cord transected and testicle removed, followed by routine abdominal wall closure.

Ectopic testicular tissues
Ectopic testicular tissue is rarely found after both testes have been surgically removed. This tissue can become neoplastic or the testosterone it produces can cause secondary health concerns such as benign prostatic hypertrophy or feminization. This possibility should be investigated if a swelling is noted at the site of the original prescrotal incision or in the scrotum, or the testicle was intra-abdominal at the time of the original surgery.

Agenesis
Actual failure of one or both testes to develop is very rare in the dog. These patients should be considered cryptorchid until agenesis (monorchidism or anorchidism) is proven.

Hypoplasia of the testes
Testicular hypoplasia results from abnormal development of the seminiferous tubulular germinal epithelium. Based on the degree of the lack of tubules, both decreased testicular size and fertility will be noted after the dog reaches sexual maturity. This can be unilateral or bilateral. There is no treatment.

Aplasia of the testicular duct system

This is the failure of any part of the testicular duct system to develop. It may be unilateral or bilateral. It is frequently undiagnosed if it is unilateral and its location does not cause fluid accumulation with secondary testicular degeneration. If bilateral, the patient will be sterile. Surgical correction is not practical.

Testicular tumors

Testicular tumors are relatively common in the male dog; they are second only to skin tumors in frequency. Testicular tumors are far more common than prostate tumors. Tumors can occur both in descended and undescended testicles, but with different frequencies. The three most common types tend to occur at approximately equal frequencies in the descended testicles. In the retained testicle, Sertoli call tumors account for 60% of all tumors and seminomas account for 40%. All three occur within the body of the testicle.

Tumors in descended testes are easier to diagnose than in retained testicle because they are readily visible and palpable; despite their accessibility, few clients notice that they are present.

Sertoli cell tumor

Sertoli cell tumors are the most common type of tumor in the retained testicle. This type is found in highest incidence in testes retained within the abdomen. They arise from the cells that support developing spermatogenic cells and secrete hormones. They may either secrete no hormone or may secrete estrogen, causing feminization.

They are firm and nodular and on the cut surface, they are pale yellow to gray. They are slow-growing and tend not to be invasive but up to 20% may be malignant, spread to local lymph nodes and metastasize to distant sites (lungs and spleen).

Seminoma

Seminomas are the second most common type of tumor in the retained testicle. This type is found in highest incidence in the testicle retained subcutaneously in the inguinal canal. They arise from the cells that form mature spermatozoa. They do not secrete hormones, but a poorly understood paraneoplastic syndrome has been reported. They are usually soft and lobulated and on the cut surface, they are gray to white. They are slow-growing and non-invasive. Up to 10% may metastasize to local and distant sites (reports include metastases to abdominal and thoracic viscera, brain, eye and lung).

Interstitial cell tumor

Interstitial cell tumors are also called Leydig cell tumors. They are almost always found in scrotal testicles and arise from interstitial cells that surround the seminiferous tubules. They may secrete testosterone or estrogen, causing a paraneoplastic syndrome.

They are soft on palpation and on the cut surface, they are brown-orange. Again they tend to be slow-growing, non-invasive and of low malignancy.

Other tumors found in the testes

Tumors such as hemangiosarcomas, fibrosarcomas and embryonic carcinomas are rare in the testes.

Diagnosing testicular tumors

Most tumors in the scrotal testicle are found on routine physical examination or at a fertility evaluation. The client occasionally presents the patient for evaluation of an enlarged testicle in the scrotum. The primary physical exam finding is that one or both testes are abnormal in size. Semen quality and quantity can be profoundly or mildly affected at the time of diagnosis. This can be distinguished from orchitis and torsion of the spermatic cord by the lack of swelling, heat, and discomfort of the affected testicle(s). If the tumor has metastasized or is secreting estrogen, symptoms related to these conditions will also be noted.

Frequently, there is one enlarged and one smaller testicle. The smaller is usually the non-neoplastic testicle, having atrophied due to altered hormonal feedback and increased local temperature. On occasion, both testes can have a tumor, often of different types. Even less often, more than one tumor type is found in the same testicle. Ultrasound should be used to assess the testicles prior to surgery if removal of only the affected testicle is an option the client wishes to pursue – the attending veterinarian needs to assure they are removing the affected testicle and that the contralateral testicle is indeed normal.

A retained testicle that is subcutaneous or inguinal may also be found on a thorough physical examination or as a presenting complaint by the client. If the retained testicle is intra-abdominal, detection of the tumor and cause of the dog's illness is more difficult. He may present with signs of a mass occupying lesion in the abdomen, signs of metastatic disease traceable to the testicular tumor, or signs of paraneoplastic syndrome related to excess estrogen production by the tumor. Abdominal radiographs may reveal an intra-abdominal mass. Ultrasound is more useful because a skilled ultrasonographer may locate not only the retained testicle, but also the tumor(s) within the testicle and evidence of abdominal metastases.

Signs related to estrogen secretion by Sertoli cell tumors or less commonly by interstitial cell tumors include a combination of: estrogen-induced pancytopenia, bilaterally symmetrical alopecia of the trunk and flanks, hair loss, enlarged mammary glands, an enlarged prepuce, an enlarged prostate and becoming sexually attractive to intact male dogs. The paraneoplastic syndrome associated with testosterone secretion includes BPH, perineal hernia, perianal adenoma and perianal and tail gland hyperplasia.

Treatment

Relatively few intact male dogs have retained abdominal testes because veterinarians have been successful in encouraging clients to surgically remove the retained testicle prior to the age when this syndrome typically develops.

Removal of the affected testicle(s) is the treatment of choice for all types of testicular tumors. Bilateral castration is recommended for most patients without future value as breeding dogs. Unilateral castration may be very useful for dogs considered valuable breeders. His semen quality and quantity usually improve within 3 months of removal of the affected testicle. Ultrasound confirmation to assure that the affected testicle is the one to be surgically removed and that the contralateral testicle is normal at the time of the study is recommended if the client opts to retain one testicle in a dog with future value as a stud dog. The entire testicle is removed (or both testes), not just the tumor from the testicle. The prognosis is good if there are no metastases and the affected testicle(s) is removed.

Dogs with Sertoli cell tumors and associated paraneoplastic syndrome have resolution of clinical signs beginning 3 weeks after neutering. Dogs with bone marrow suppression related to the excess estrogen levels have a much more guarded prognosis and need additional supportive care.

The ideal pre-operative evaluation for patients undergoing surgical removal of one or both testes with tumor(s), whether intra-abdominal, subcutaneous, or scrotal, should include, a CBC and serum chemistry profile, all 3 radiographic views of the thorax to check for metastatic disease, abdominal ultrasound or radiographs to look for abdominal metastases and lymph node involvement and any other assessments routinely done by the hospital. Biopsies of the tumors prior to castration tend to be of little use. All testicular tissue removed should be submitted for pathology.

If metastatic disease is present, current information regarding chemotherapy and/or radiation should be sought.

Orchitis/Epididymitis – Inflammation or Infection

Orchitis is inflammation and/or infection of the testicle; epididymitis is inflammation and/or infection of the epididymis. There are many causes. Bacterial infections of the testicles or epididymis can originate from bacterial cystitis, prostatitis, bacterial septicemia, or trauma including puncture wounds. Brucellosis should always be a differential in patients with orchitis and/or epididymitis. Autoimmune disease causing inflammation can be primary and associated with other immune mediated disorders such as lymphocytic thyroiditis or secondary to infection or trauma that disrupts the blood-testicular barrier. Other causative organisms include Blastomyces and Mycoplasma.

On physical examination, the acutely affected testicle(s) and/or epididymis is swollen and painful. The patient may resist palpation and manipulation of the testes. The patient is often febrile in the acute phase. Diagnostics include CBC and chemistry panel, Brucella testing, cytology and culture of the ejaculated semen (if not too painful), ultrasound and FNA of the affected testicle and/or epididymis. Ultrasound is useful in differentiating orchitis from torsion of the spermatic cord. Cultures should be taken for aerobic and anaerobic bacteria, and Mycoplasma. Urine testing for blastomycosis can be considered. Positive culture is useful in antibiotic selection but does not aid in localizing the source of the bacteria. FNA can be submitted for culture and cytology. A large number of PMNs supports a diagnosis acute orchitis and/or epididymitis.

Treatment in the acute phase with broad-spectrum antibiotics for a minimum of 3 weeks may save the affected testicle. Some patients are septic and should be hospitalized for IV fluids and IV antibiotic therapy. Antibiotics should be started while cultures are pending. The antibiotics of choice at initial therapy include trimethoprim-sulfa, cephalosporins, or oxacillin.

Pain can usually be managed with non-steroidal medication but corticosteroids may be considered. Castration should be considered for dogs without future value as stud dogs. To reduce the risk of scirrhous cord, castration should be delayed until the infection is controlled and the patient is stable. Unilateral orchiectomy may be considered if the owner opts to retain him as a stud dog. Removal of the damaged testicle may be protective to the remaining normal testicle. Because the contralateral testicle was also insulted, fertility may not return to normal for 2 to 6 months. Nutritional supportive care may be useful in returning him to stud service. (See section later in this chapter).

Immune-mediated orchitis

Damage to the blood-testicular barrier from trauma or infectious diseases can expose spermatozoa antigens to the immune system. This leads to invasion of the interstitial tissues by lymphocytes and plasma cells, followed by deterioration of the seminiferous epithelium and sterility. Prednisone and/ or other immunosuppressive drugs may be beneficial.

There is a possible link between autoimmune thyroiditis and orchitis, and a non – thyroid related familial tendency toward immune – mediated orchitis has been proposed. Some dogs with immune – mediated orchitis are younger than expected when fertility problems develop. These dogs may be so young as to have never sired a litter. They tend to have testes that are smaller and softer than their age-matched counterparts. Diagnosis is made by FNA or biopsy of the testicle.

Thermal damage

The testes and scrotum are susceptible to extremes of both heat and cold. The owner is often unaware of the risk and damage. Frostbite or necrosis of the scrotal skin can occur at or below freezing. If the damage is mild, supportive care may lead to recovery. If the damage is severe, castration may be the only option. Heat trauma can include heat absorbed by the testes when the dog is resting on asphalt in hot climates or from frequent hot baths and hot blow-dryers.

Either extreme of thermal damage can lead to the production of sperm with detached heads/tails. If the testes are not permanently damaged, they may return to fertility with supportive care.

In addition, any elevation of the temperature of the testes (fever from systemic illness or inflammation) or any interference with normal thermoregulation of the testes can transiently or permanently interfere with spermatogenesis. Careful questioning of the owner may reveal a previously undiscovered cause.

Trauma

Blunt trauma or punctures (from bite wounds, hunting accidents, and other sources of trauma) to the testes may lead to immune-mediated orchitis and epididymitis. Early intervention and supportive care may allow an eventual return to fertility. Symptoms include swelling of the testes, pain, inappetance and a reluctance to walk normally.

Encircling foreign bodies, inadvertently or intentionally applied around the scrotum, can cause irreparable harm to the blood flow to the testes. Careful inspection may be required to locate these if there is a long coat or they are deeply imbedded into the tissues.

Torsion of the spermatic cord

This condition is casually referred to as testicular torsion. Although it is more common in the retained testicle, it is easier to diagnose in the scrotal testicle. There is no breed predilection (Figure 10-6).

An intrascrotal spermatic cord torsion will present with an acutely enlarged and painful testicle, edema of the scrotum, a palpable thickened spermatic cord, and a discolored and cold scrotum. Ultrasound with color Doppler may be useful to confirm the diagnosis and assess blood flow. The position of the epididymis may be useful on palpation and ultrasound to confirm that the torsion is present. Differentials include inguinal hernia, orchitis/epididymitis, and testicular neoplasia.

If the duration and degree of torsion are not too great, and the owner wants the dog to retain both testes, the intrascrotal testicle can sometimes be salvaged. Testicular fibrosis and atrophy is a common complication, even with detorsion. Surgical correction involves general anesthesia with appropriate pre-operative assessment, a surgical approach to the testicle, detorsion, and a pexy to prevent the spermatic cord from torsing again. The testicle can be pexied after repositioning by a full through and through suture from 1 side of the scrotum to the other and back, then placing a spacer on either side of the scrotum to avoid the suture cutting through the scrotal skin. The suture can be run through a 20 or 22 gauge needle so it can be placed with minimal trauma to the already compromised testicle. The testicle will need at least 90 days to recover its ability to produce sperm.

Intra-abdominal torsion of the spermatic cord is more difficult to diagnose than an intrascrotal torsion, particularly if the dog is bilaterally cryptorchid and there is a vague history of castration. A dog with a retained testicle typically will present with an acute abdomen. Symptoms include vomiting, abdominal distress, shock, lethargy, loss of appetite, and stilted gait. Although retained testes that have enlarged due to a tumor are more commonly involved in a torsion, even young puppies with an immature retained testicle can suffer from a torsion. Other symptoms may relate to the testicular neoplasia such as a mass that is palpable in the abdomen, an enlarged prostate, and other signs related to paraneoplastic syndrome.

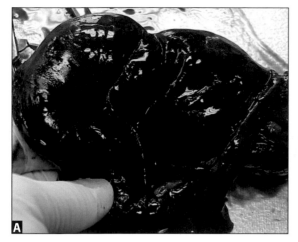
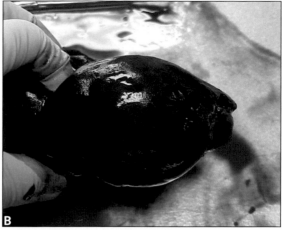
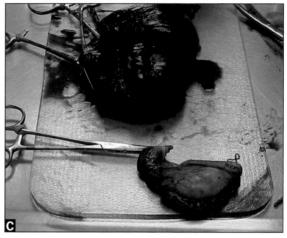

Figure 10-6.
A. and *B.* A long – standing testicular torsion, showing the testicle removed surgically. *C.* The same testical in (A and B), showing the contralateral testical removed surgically.

Diagnosis of spermatic cord torsion can only be confirmed by exploratory laparotomy. Diagnosis is supported by CBC, chemistry profile, abdominal radiographs and abdominal ultrasound. Surgery will reveal either an enlarged abnormal testicle or a small necrotic testicle. Bilateral castration is recommended. Histology of the abnormal testicle is useful in confirming the diagnosis and developing a prognosis.

Sperm granuloma/Spermatocele

A spermatocele is a localized area in the epididymis that retains sperm. A sperm granuloma is an area of the epididymis with retained sperm that causes an inflammatory response, which is palpated as swellings along the caudal epididymis. This may result from trauma or infectious causes. Diagnosis is confirmed by surgical biopsy. If the granuloma is unilateral, the dog is likely to be fertile; if bilateral he is likely sterile with no therapy currently available.

Scrotal hernia

A scrotal hernia results when abdominal contents are contained in the scrotum. They can occur when abdominal contents pass through the inguinal canal or directly through the abdominal wall into the scrotum. They may be unilateral or bilateral. Clinical signs include intermittent or continuous swelling of the scrotum. If the abdominal contents become trapped, the dog will show signs of an acute abdomen. Differential diagnosis includes testicular neoplasia, torsion of the spermatic cord, and orchitis. Careful palpation and ultrasound may differentiate these conditions from a hernia. Surgical correction is the treatment of choice.

Varicocele

A varicocele is a dialated spermatic vein that develops a thrombosis. This disrupts blood flow and temperature regulation of the testes. Although the thrombosis is usually unilateral, the contralateral testicle may be affected due to changes in thermoregulation within the scrotum. Diagnosis can be made by a skilled ultrasonographer. Unilateral castration to remove the affected may allow the unaffected testicle to return to normal.

Testicular degeneration and senile atrophy

Degeneration and atrophy of the testes occur for many reasons. Often there are no presenting clinical signs other than a smaller softer testicle (unilateral or bilateral) and a report of recent infertility. Causes include fever, trauma, infectious and non-infectious inflammation of the testes and/ or epididymis, and neoplasia. Senile atrophy is a common change with aging. In many cases, even with a complete history and physical examination, no etiology can be found. FNA or testicular biopsy may be useful in determining an underlying cause and offering a prognosis. If cytology reveals no active spermatogenesis, the prognosis for return to fertility is poor.

Drug or Radiation therapy

A small number of drugs are known to interfere with spermatogenesis or libido. These include certain corticosteroids, anabolic steroids, testosterone, progestogens, estrogens, ketoconazole, amphotericin B, cimetidine, GnRH agonists and antagonists and anti-neoplastic agents. Radiation therapy in the region of the genitals will also interfere with spermatogenesis. The prescribing veterinarian should review the literature for contraindications to the use of all new drugs in the active stud dog. The veterinarian should always discuss the risks and benefits in a situation where the owner is faced with saving the dog versus saving his fertility.

Accidental or inadvertent topical or oral exposure to estrogen creams used by owners can cause a hormonal imbalance. Careful history taking may reveal this.

Bilateral castration

On rare occasion, the patient history may lack the information needed to determine if the dog is bilaterally cryptorchid or if he has been castrated. A skilled ultrasonographer may be able to locate one or both testicles if they are retained in the abdomen or inguinal canals, keeping in mind that they may be very small. Testosterone levels alone are often not diagnostic. As an alternative, a hormonal stimulation test may be useful.

Protocol for testorerone stimulation test

Draw a baseline testosterone blood sample prior to hormone use. Contact the lab in advance to determine if plasma or serum is requested;

Administer GnRH (50 mcg SQ) or hCG (100 IU IM);

Draw additional samples at 12 and 24 hours post-injection;

A 2 to 4 fold increase of the testosterone level from baseline suggests the dog has retained one or both testes.

Diagnosis of testicular disorders

Ultrasound of the scrotal testes of the intact male dog is a relatively simple process. The dog can be standing, or in lateral or dorsal recumbency. Sedation is not usually needed and no clipping is necessary. Gel is applied to the scrotum. Either a 5.0 or 7.5 MHz transducer can be used. The normal testicle should have a coarse and homogenous echogenicity. Both testes should be approximately the same size and shape with the same echogenicity. The mediastinum testes is usually visible centrally in the testicle as a hyperechoic band. If a tumor is present in the testicle, it will be visible as a discrete region that has an altered echogenicity (hyper or hypoechoic or multiloculated cystic areas within the testes) as compared to the rest of the testicle.

The epididymes are dorso-lateral to the testes. They are normally hypoechoic when compared to the testes.

Fine Needle Aspiration (FNA)of the testicle and/or epididymis to collect samples for cytology and culture can be used to confirm or rule out disorders with minimal expense to the owner and minimal trauma to the testicle and epididymis.

Cytology can reveal the presence or absence of live motile sperm, inflammatory cells, neoplastic cells, bacteria, and fungal elements. Culture for aerobic and anaerobic bacteria as well as Mycoplasma can also be performed on this sample.

FNA technique
Brief general anesthesia or sedation is recommended. Gently apply a surgical prep on the scrotal skin over the area of the testicle and/or epididymis to be aspirated. Use a 22 or 23 g butterfly needle or a 22 or 23 g needle with an extension set attached to a 60 cc syringe. The operator should direct the needle into several areas of the testicle carefully without pulling out of the testicle several times while an assistant applies strong suction on the syringe, but should release suction prior to the operator removing the needle from the testicle. Remove the needle from the syringe, pull air into the syringe, reapply the needle, and blow the contents of the needle onto a slide for cytology or culturette for culture. To aspirate the epididymis, perform the same procedure in only one location.

Stain the slides for cytology. A normal testicle should have many sperm cells, many without tails during spermatogenesis. If only sertoli cells are found, this testicle is sterile and will not produce sperm cells. If normal sperm are found but none are noted in the ejaculate, blocked efferent ducts may be the cause and may transiently respond to prednisone therapy. If bacteria and inflammatory cells are found, the patient should be treated with an appropriate antibiotic, based on culture. Bacterial cultures should be prepared from the remaining sterile sample.

Testicular biopsy
Biopsy of one or both testes can be a useful diagnostic tool but is not without risk to future fertility. The blood-testicular barrier is disrupted at biopsy, potentially leading to immune-mediated orchitis and progressive testicular degeneration. Hematoma formation is also a risk. The risk for both is greater with biopsy than for FNA. On the other hand, for some patients with a poor prognosis for return to fertility, the value of a specific diagnosis and treatment plan may outweigh the risks. If both testes appear to be equally affected, only one should be biopsied, to reduce the risk of irreversible damage to the contralateral testicle.

Procedure for testicular biopsy
After appropriate pre-surgical evaluation, place the dog under general anesthesia and position in lateral or dorsal recumbency, based on the surgeon's preference. Gently clip and surgically prepare the pre-scrotal area as if for a neuter. Make a small skin incision through the pre-scrotal skin and advance the testicle to be biopsied to the incision site.

For a Tru-Cut biopsy, pass the biopsy punch into the portion of the body of the testicle of interest, taking care to avoid the epididymis. Collect the sample and place in Bouin's solution. Reserve a portion for culture if indicated. The tunic, subcutaneous tissue and skin should be closed routinely.

For a wedge biopsy, incise the testicular tunic, remove the portion of the testicle that is bulging with a scalpel blade (or remove a wedge if the testicular tissue does not bulge), and place in Bouin's solution, reserving a portion for culture if indicated. Close the tunics separately with 4-0 absorbable suture, then close the subcutaneous tissue and skin routinely.

Submit the samples to a pathologist familiar with testicular pathology. Bouin's solution is preferred to formalin for preserving testicular architecture.

The primary advantage of testicular biopsy over FNA is the opportunity to evaluate the testicular architecture.

Unilateral castration
Unilateral castration is discussed in multiple sections in this chapter. This is a viable option for owners of a dog with future value as a stud and should always be discussed with the owner prior to surgical intervention. This option is more appealing to an owner of a dog unaffected by other testosterone-dependent disorders such as BPH or perianal tumors.

The procedure is the same as any other orchiectomy, with the primary difference that the testicle to be spared should be evaluated by ultrasound for abnormalities in advance of the procedure and should be carefully protected from trauma at and following the procedure. Even testes that do not show normal fertility pre-op may be able to produce sperm within 2 to 6 months post-op. Removal of the offending testicle may eliminate the source of inflammation, allowing the remaining testicle to recover. The remaining testicle often compensates, producing sperm at a quantity of 75% of what would normally be anticipated based on the dog's weight. With this type of recovery, many dogs can be maintained or returned to use as a successful stud dog.

Culture from different parts of the urogenital tract
Culturing different fractions of the ejaculate or use of multiple FNAs from the testes, epididymis and prostate may be useful in determining the source of a bacterial nidus. The 1st and 3rd fractions of the ejaculate are from the prostate, the 2nd fraction is from the testes. Careful fractionation may demonstrate the source. Urine collected by cystocentesis and cultured may support a diagnosis of bacterial prostatitis or cystitis.

Scrotal disorders
Scrotal dermatitis
The scrotum can be irritated by trauma, thermal exposure, both hot and cold, generalized dermatitis, chemicals on the surface or secondarily by acute orchitis. Chemicals and disinfectants used to clean kennels may be the cause, taking a detailed history may reveal the problem. Treatment of the underlying cause should allow a resolution. Use of topical therapy (cream, not ointment) and an Elizabethan collar may accelerate healing.

Scrotal tumors
Like any other area of skin, the scrotal skin can be affected by neoplasia. The most common 3 types of skin tumors of this region are: squamous cell carcinomas, melanomas, and mast cell tumors. The treatment of choice for all 3 is wide surgical excision and histopathology of the lesion. Castration may be necessary to attain wide surgical margins. Consultation with an oncologist may be indicated if additional therapy is sought by the owner.

Scrotal trauma
Trauma to the scrotum may lead to bacterial invasion, orchitis and epididymitis, and self-mutilation. Supportive care should be provided to protect the testes. Symptoms may be mild or may include excessive licking and an abnormal gait.

Disorders of the penis

Hypospadia

Hypospadia is a congenital abnormality in the formation of the penile urethra, penis, prepuce and/or scrotum. Diagnosis is based on the abnormal position of the urethral opening. This results in a ventral opening in the urethra in a variety of locations: perineal (most common), glandular, scrotal, or penile. This congenital defect may be genetic or caused by hormonal influences on the fetus during gestation. They can be diagnosed by visual evaluation of the urinary tract. Although some males may not be affected by this defect, it may be the reason for urinary incontinence, urinary tract infections, and urine scalding (Figure 10-7).

The degree of malformation can vary greatly. Severe cases are obvious at birth and may require either euthanasia or surgical correction when the pup is considered to be a surgical candidate. When surgical correction is required, it may be best done by a referral to a surgeon. Depending on the location of the defect, it may be closed by reconstruction or require penile urethrostomy. Dogs so affected should be castrated at correction and not be included in a breeding program.

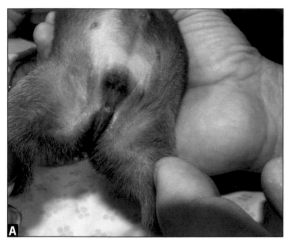 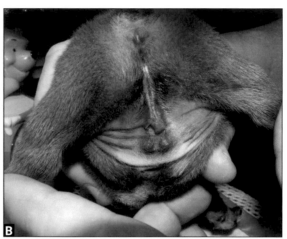

Figure 10-7.
*A. A newborn pup, ventral view, with hypospadia, a failure of the midline to close. **B.** A newborn pup, caudal view, with hypospadia, a failure of the midline to close.*

Penile hypoplasia

This is a congenital abnormality where the penis is abnormally short. It is a contributing cause to irritation of the prepuce. It may be associated with female pseudohermaphrodism. It is most commonly reported in the Great Dane, Collie, Doberman Pinscher, and Cocker Spaniel.

Persistent penile frenulum

A penile frenulum is a thin band of tissue that joins the ventral penis to the prepuce or to the body of the penis. It may be of little to no clinical significance in the sexually inactive dog, neutered dog, or dogs not intended for breeding. Some dogs will exhibit signs of excessive licking of the penis and unusual urinary patterns and urine scald on the skin (Figure 10-8).

In breeding dogs, the penile frenulum interferes with normal erection and copulation, as it is exaggerated with erection, forcing the erect penis into a ventral or lateral position. It may first be noted at a fertility evaluation of a stud dog with a history of being unable to copulate normally. All male dogs with an inability to insert the penis into the bitch should be evaluated for this condition. It is easily detected by visual examination of the exteriorized penis.

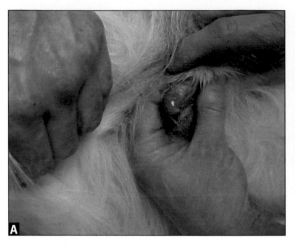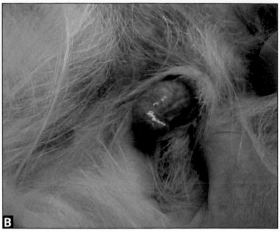

Figure 10-8.
*A. The penis, exteriorized, showing a penile frenulum, the band of tissue along the surface. **B.** The same penis showing that the further the penis is exteriorized, the more obvious the deviation of the penis due to the penile frenulum.*

Correction is simple, painless and straightforward. If the band of tissue is not vascular, it may be snipped without anesthesia. If it is thick or vascular, brief anesthesia may be used to allow transection. An inherited tendency is suspected.

Os penis deformity
Deformity of the os penis may cause an inability to copulate or retract the penis into the prepuce.

Penile trauma and foreign bodies
Trauma to the penis can result from a breeding accident, a bite wound, trauma caused by reflecting the prepuce in the field, hair rings, malicious application of rubber bands or other restrictive devices, or general body trauma. Clinical signs include pain, bleeding, difficulty urinating and penile paralysis.

If the penis is traumatized when erect, the high vascularity of the organ can allow for significant hemorrhage. Rapidly reducing the erection (by general anesthesia if necessary) will minimize blood loss.

Thorough inspection of the exteriorized penis is indicated, with sedation if necessary. If present, remove the foreign body. Lacerations of the penis can be sutured like any other mucus membrane. Twice daily exteriorization of the penis will diminish the likelihood that it will adhere to the lining of the prepuce. Appropriate topical and antibiotic therapy as well as pain management may be indicated. The patient should be carefully monitored to ensure that normal urination is possible; catheter placement may be required. House the patient where sexual stimulation is minimal. In severe cases, penile amputation may be indicated.

Os penis fracture
This is a rare sequella to trauma. The affected dog may either present at the time of the injury or later if healing is difficult. Clinical signs may include pain, difficult urination or urinary obstruction, or penile deviation. Treatment consists of relieving the urinary obstruction. Repair of the penis and associated other trauma may be indicated.

Preputial stenosis
The excessively small preputial orifice may cause an inability to exteriorize the penis with associated infection. In rare cases, it may cause neonatal septicemia and early death.

Phimosis

Phimosis is the inability to exteriorize the penis. It may be caused by preputial stenosis or be secondary to trauma, hair, inflammation or neoplasia. Young patients may develop urine scald and urinary obstruction. Older patients may be unable to copulate. Patients of any age may show pain. Removal of the hair and/or surgical correction of the preputial opening will resolve the problem.

Paraphimosis

Paraphimosis is the inability to retract the non-erect penis completely into the prepuce. This is a genuine and relatively common emergency; immediate care is needed to prevent permanent injury to the penis. The blood flow to the penis is rapidly compromised, leading to necrosis (Figure 10-9).

Paraphimosis occurs most commonly after sexual stimulation or copulation. It can also be caused by neurologic disease. The longer the penis is exteriorized, the greater the damage. Treatment consists of repositioning the penis in the prepuce. Sedation or anesthesia may be indicated. If the mucosal surface of the penis has been damaged, it should be cleansed and foreign material removed from the surface. Gentle cranial traction on the prepuce and lubrication of the penis and/or hypertonic dextrose may aid in reducing the swelling and improving reduction. If the penis cannot be repositioned into the prepuce, the preputial opening may be surgically enlarged. The patient should be anesthetized, the prepuce prepped and an incision made on the ventral midline. The prepuce should be sutured by opposing mucosa to skin on the right and left sides (not crossing the midline) to maintain a slightly larger opening.

After reduction, a pursestring suture can be placed at the preputial opening, whether it was surgically enlarged or not, to protect the tip of the penis from exposure. If the surface of the penis is ulcerated, the penis should be exteriorized twice daily to reduce the likelihood of adhesion to the prepuce. Antibiotic therapy and lavage of the prepuce may aid in healing. Rarely the urethra may be compromised. If the damage is severe or the patient is unable to urinate, either catheterization or in extreme cases, penile amputation may be indicated. The patient may need to wear an Elizabethan collar to reduce the chance of severe self-mutilation. To prevent recurrence, minimizing sexual arousal may be required.

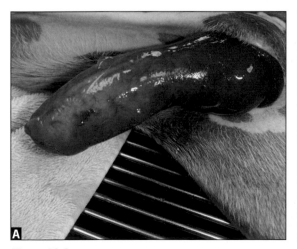 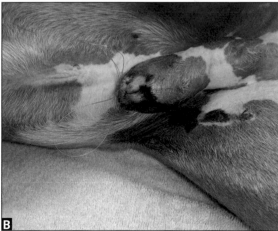

Figure 10-9.
*A. Paraphimosis of several hours duration. Note the ulceration of the mucosa from prolonged exposure and trauma. **B.** After the penis was returned to the prepuce, done with lubrication and patience, the prepuce was temporarily closed to protect the penis from trauma until the decreased swelling reduced the chance of recurrence.*

Urethral prolapse/Eversion

Urethral prolapse frequently presents with intermittent bleeding, especially when sexually aroused, from the tip of the penis of a young dog, usually under 2 years of age. This may also be seen in neutered males. The diagnosis may be difficult as the prolapsed tissue may not be visible unless the dog's penis is erect. Manipulation of the tip of the penis or manual ejaculation allows the prolapsed tissue to be visualized to confirm the diagnosis. Pexy of the prelapsed tissue should be curative. Following recovery, the dogs may be used for breeding, although most affected dogs are castrated at pexy.

Neoplasms of the penis

Penile neoplasia is rare. If found, Transmissible Venereal Tumors (TVTs) and squamous cell carcinomas are the most commonly seen. Other tumors include mast cell tumors, plasma cell tumors, and chondrosarcomas of the os penis. Diagnosis is made based on visualization of the mass as it protrudes from the prepuce, distension of the prepuce, hemorrhage from the penis, and pain or inability to copulate. TVTs are spread venereally and can also cause mass lesions in bitches. Surgical excision should be considered for all tumors of the penis. TVTs may be treated with vincristine.

Balanitis, posthitis and balanoposthitis

This is an assortment of inflammation of the penis (balanitis), prepuce (posthitis) and both at the same time (balanoposthitis). It is characterized by licking of and yellow-green thick discharge from the prepuce. The bacteria found are usually normal flora. In its mild form, it is common in many young male dogs, comparable to puppy vaginitis. In its more severe form, it may require lavage (with saline or dilute betadine), topical and/or systemic antibiotic therapy. Underlying causes such as allergic dermatitis, foreign bodies, neoplasia and structural congenital abnormalities should be ruled out based on complete examination of the prepuce and exteriorized penis.

Lymphoid follicular hyperplasia

The base of the penis may be affected by multiple small follicles on the mucosal surface. The etiology has not been determined. They are of little clinical significance.

Failure to achieve sexual maturity and intersex

There are many combinations of disorders of chromosomal sex. Although the different syndromes are interesting, they usually have few clinical symptoms and are almost always infertile. They may be identified only when presented for neutering or spaying or for a fertility evaluation. Diagnosis is confirmed based on careful gross and microscopic evaluation of the urogenital tract and/or karyotyping.

Disorders of erection

Pain from any source including prostate, testes, penis, back and orthopedic pain can cause erectile dysfunction. Pain from many sources can impact the stud dog's willingness and ability to breed a female. If a formerly willing stud dog begins to show resistance or fails to mount and breed a bitch, his reproductive organs, limbs and back should be evaluated as a source of pain. His penis should be exteriorized and examined, including at the base to assess for masses and hair rings. His testes and prostate should be palpated for swelling and other changes. Not as obvious are sources of orthopedic pain. Back pain or bilateral orthopedic disease may be sufficient to prevent his willingness to mount and tie with a bitch, but may not be lateralized enough to cause lameness. If suspected, evaluate the hips, stifles, hocks, feet and lumbar spine for pain. Radiographs may be indicated to assess for non-palpable disease. Blood tests may be required to diagnosis other disorders such as Lyme disease and rheumatoid arthritis.

Detecting and treating the cause of the pain may restore his normal libido and improve performance. Use of non-steroidal anti-inflammatory drugs may reduce pain quickly enough to allow him to mate during the current estrus cycle. Megestrol acetate may also reduce the size and discomfort of the prostate as well as the amount of blood in the ejaculate in only a few days, making his use during the bitch's intended estrus cycle plausible. Both non-steroidal anti-inflammatories and megestrol acetate can be used without compromising semen quality. Other causes of pain such as orchitis or prostatitis may not be able to be corrected quickly enough to allow him to breed to the bitch during her current estrus. Additionally, the white blood cells and bacteria in the ejaculate of a dog with orchitis and/or prostatitis may be so undesirable that an alternative stud dog (or the selected dog with frozen semen) may be sought.

If the affected stud dog has sufficient semen quality and libido but is merely unable to mount and tie, and his underlying condition does not eliminate him as a stud dog (i.e. hip dysplasia severe enough to prevent him from being physically able to breed would likely eliminate him as a genetically appropriate mate), manual collection of the semen and artificial insemination would be appropriate.

Care should be taken when collecting semen from every stud dog to prevent any negative experience from interfering with his future willingness to breed or be manually ejaculated. Some dogs are psychologically more delicate and need to be handled with care when approached and touched. Dogs who are inherently shy or who have been taught not to become sexually aroused are more difficult to teach to be collected. There is a learning curve for the dog when he is allowed to breed or be collected for the first time. Some dogs require several visits to the veterinary clinic and carefully selected bitches with gentle temperaments to learn that sexual behavior is acceptable in certain settings.

Some dogs, even those with experience, can have a painful or frightening experience that will negatively impact their willingness to be manually collected. The penis should be handled with care to prevent trauma while stimulating to ejaculate and it is exteriorized. Drying, and hair catching as it retracts into the prepuce should be avoided to prevent possible unwillingness to be handled at future collections. When using a teaser bitch, she should be carefully selected and restrained to prevent physical and/or psychological trauma to the stud dog. If the dog is unwilling to develop an erection and/or ejaculate, he should be allowed to relax prior to a second attempt. If he fails at the second try, it is best to stop and assess the timing of the bitch and his physical condition to be certain he is not psychologically impacted in a manner that would interfere permanently with future collections.

Disorders of ejaculation

Retrograde ejaculation caused by bladder sphincter incompetence

Retrograde ejaculation of semen into the bladder is an infrequent cause of low sperm numbers in the ejaculate. This is diagnosed by collection of urine by voiding or catheterization immediately after semen collection and comparing the number of spermatozoa in the urine to the number in the collected ejaculate. This is more commonly seen in older dogs. Causes include weakening of the bladder sphincter with age, neurological disorders, and hypothyroidism. Correction of the hypothyroidism with supplementation does not correct the retrograde ejaculation.

Treatment consists of not allowing the dog to urinate prior to collection, to increase pressure in the bladder and the use of sympathomimetic drugs. The drugs include Phenylpropanoloamine at 3 mg/kg PO BID or pseudoephedrine at 4 to 5 mg/kg PO TID, repeated several hours prior to collection or breeding can be used.

Collection of the urine followed by centrifugation to concentrate the sperm and adding an extender to protect the sperm from the toxic effects of urine has not successfully resulted in pregnancy.

Infections of the prostate, testes or epididymis

An infection in the reproductive tract can lead to decreased sperm quantity and quality. Scarring in the epididymis may lead to irreversible obstruction of outflow paths for sperm. Active infection may lead to pain and unwillingness to ejaculate.

The correlation between finding white blood cells and bacteria in the ejaculate and positive cultures is not strong enough to eliminate infection as a possibility based on microscopic examination of the ejaculate for white blood cells alone. White blood cells in the ejaculate may be considered a normal finding because semen is not sterile. Culture of the ejaculate and growth of more than 10,000 bacteria per ml of semen is the basis of a definitive diagnosis.

Infections of the male reproductive tract are not generally considered to be a cause of disease including pyometra in the bitch. Brucella canis is an exception.

Sexual immaturity

The age of sexual maturity varies between breeds as well as individuals within a breed. The size of the testicles corresponds to sexual maturity.

Several products, some available in countries outside the United States, will reduce spermatogenesis, some to the point of causing apparent sterility. The GnRH vaccine, will transiently cause aspermia. Other products include the deslorelin drug pellet implant, radiation therapy, chemotherapy, and hormone exposure that may be inadvertent. A complete drug and vaccine history may reveal the previous use of the drugs.

Sexual overuse

Sexual overuse can cause depletion of sperm reserves, resulting in lower sperm numbers per ejaculate. As few as 5 consecutive daily ejaculations can result in depletion in normal healthy dogs. Maximal total sperm output is achieved when dogs are ejaculated every 4 to 5 days. This information is particularly valuable when applied to dogs collected frequently for cryopreservation.

Orthopedic/Arthritis/Back pain as causes of copulation failure

Use of non-steroidal anti-inflammatories, pain medications including tramadol, heat, veterinary spinal manipulation therapy, acupuncture, and artificial insemination as an alternative to natural mating may allow an affected patient to remain an active stud dog. The client should be counseled to consider if they may be perpetuating a heritable disease.

Disorders of sperm production, classification, diagnostics and treatment

(Appendix D-6) (Table 10-1)

Infertility evaluation and treatment

Stud dog infertility can be classified as dogs with normal sperm with low to no libido, normal to low libido with low sperm counts (oligospermia), normal to low libido with abnormal sperm (teratospermia), normal to low libido with no sperm (azoospermia), normal to low libido with blood in the ejaculate (hematospermia), normal to low libido with abnormal sperm motility (astheno-zoospermia) and normal to low libido with abnormal ejaculate components including red blood cells, white blood cells, and tumor cells;

Treatment protocols

These conditions may appear individually, overlap and occur simultaneously, or noted singly in the same patient over the course of time. In the dog, 62 days are necessary to produce and release a spermatocyte, with another 15 required for transport through the epididymis. The process cannot be altered or rushed – it may take 3 or more months to determine if treatment for the condition has been successful. Infertility is defined as lowered fertility. Sterility is defined as permanent loss of reproductive capacity.

Normal sperm from a stud dog with low to no libido

If the stud dog has no libido, a semen analysis may be very difficult. A urine sample to see if the dog has sperm in his urine is the easiest way to begin the work up. A catheterized sample or sample collected by cystocentesis may have less sperm than a voided sample. If sperm is present, he is not azoospermic.

Low libido may have many causes. A complete history including medication the dog is on or has been on in the recent past should be taken. These medications include hormonal agents that decrease testosterone levels.

The first step is to collect the stud dog using an estrus teaser bitch. If an estrus bitch is not readily available, the humane society or local dog club may be able to assist in locating one. If a teaser bitch was used, and he still has little interest, there are several possible causes. The teaser bitch was not at the right stage of her estrous. Many experienced stud dogs will not put forth the effort to ejaculate if the timing is not perfect. The stud dog may not like that particular female – some dogs have breed, size, color, or behavior preferences. If that individual bitch was too aggressive previously, he is likely to be timid. Different people have different approaches to handling dogs and some dogs develop preferences. They may also have had a previous bad experience with that collector, particularly if the collector is the dog's regular veterinarian (white coat syndrome). If the person accompanying the dog has instructed the dog to avoid sexual behavior in the past, the dog may continue to have low libido (observer or handler preference). Some dogs have location experience and prefer different footing, a different room, or to be outdoors rather than indoors (location preference). Treatment requires determining the underlying problem and attempting to offer the dog an alternative.

Pain

If the dog appears to favor the teaser bitch and surroundings but is still reluctant to ejaculate, pain associated with collection should be considered. This pain could be in his back, limbs, prostate, or genitals. A complete physical examination including a digital rectal examination should be performed. His testes should be palpated for pain or other irregularities. His penis should be exteriorized with the prepuce reflected to look for foreign bodies, hair rings, and other abnormalities. Radiographs may be necessary to evaluate the size of the prostate and his back and limbs for arthritis or other causes of pain. The source of pain should be identified and the underlying cause treated. Dogs with orthopedic or back pain should be pretreated with an appropriate anti-inflammatory before future breedings. Prostate pain associated with benign prostatic hypertrophy or prostatitis should be treated appropriately to reduce the size and inflammation of the prostate.

Some dogs who have previously been successful at breeding but are now reluctant to breed naturally will be found to have developed a preference for manual collection over natural breeding. Recommended treatment is to offer the male a suitably cooperative bitch.

Sertoli cell tumors can produce sufficient estrogen to interfere with libido and spermatogenesis. In addition to palpation, ultrasound of the testes can help assess if there are testicular abnormalities. In rare cases, there could be a tumor present in the testes that are too small to detect with ultrasound. If the opposite testicle is normal, the affected testicle can be removed. Castration is recommended if the condition is bilateral.

If the dog has no libido and has no history of ever having normal libido, a karyotype should be considered. Intersex dogs that have male genitals have been reported in the Kerry blue terrier, pug, English Cocker, beagle, Weimaraner, and German Shorthair Pointer. There is no treatment for this condition.

Stud dog with low to normal libido but a low sperm count (Oligospermia)

A normal sperm count for a healthy mature stud dog in good health should be 10 million per pound of body weight. This calculates to be approximately 1 billion for the stud dog of 100 pounds, and 500 million for the stud dog of 50 pounds. Too frequent or too recent collection(s) may make a dog with normal fertility appear oligospermic. The history should include information on when and how frequently the dog was collected. Some clients will ejaculate the dog just prior to the veterinary visit in an attempt to "clean out" the stud dog – this often leads to a collection at the veterinary clinic with an abnormally low sperm count.

If a teaser bitch was not used, another attempt with an estrous bitch is the next step. Many of the above conditions apply including stage of estrous; bitch, collector, handler, and location preference. Pain during collection or the hormonal alterations caused by testicular tumors may also cause a lower sperm count. Collecting the dog 60 or more days after the last use of corticosterois or anti-neoplastic drugs may result in an improved semen quality.

A complete physical examination should be performed after ejaculation. Evaluate for testicular tumors, prostatic disease, and orchitis/epididymitis.

Hypothyroidism may cause low sperm counts, however, the thyroid levels must be profoundly low for an extended time period. Hyperadrenocorticism (Cushings disease) may also cause low sperm counts. Treatment of the underlying endocrine abnormality may allow improvement in semen quality. Some causes of hypothyroidism may be heritable which should be considered prior to using this stud dog.

Immune-mediated testicular disease can initially cause the sperm count to drop, and later cause an absence of sperm in the ejaculate. Young dogs with small soft testes are suspected of having this disorder but it can only be confirmed on testicular needle aspirate or biopsy. Prednisone may be useful early in treating the condition but can be a double-edged sword because it may also interfere with spermatogenesis.

Concurrent or resolving orchitis is another cause of low sperm counts. The causes of orchitis can include infection, including Brucella canis, trauma, thermal damage, and torsion. Treatment of the cause may improve the sperm count. Bacterial culture of the ejaculate may reveal a pure culture; appropriate antibiotic therapy may resolve the bacterial component of the disease. A mixed culture of commonly found bacteria suggests normal flora. Mycoplasma is frequently incriminated as a cause of infertility in the male but this has not been documented. Mycoplasma may be a secondary invader.

Dogs with brucellosis should be euthanized or castrated and treated with an extensive course of an appropriate antibiotic.

If trauma or thermal damage is suspected, sexual rest and recollection in 90 or more days may allow the sperm count to recover. Testicular tumors are common causes of low sperm counts; the testes should be palpated carefully. Ultrasound can be used to assess testicular architecture, looking for tumors, atrophy, spermatoceles or sperm granulomas. Unilateral castration to remove the abnormal testicle may improve the sperm count if the opposite testicle is found to be normal on palpation and/or ultrasound. If an offending drug is the cause, it should be withdrawn if medically appropriate.

If no underlying cause can be determined for a low sperm count and the stud dog is scheduled to be bred soon, use of a teaser bitch, GnRH (at 1 to 3.3 mcg/kg IM 1 hour prior to collection with or without hCG at 1600 IU IM) or Lutalyse®, and restricting collections to times when the bitch is fertile can improve the count and preserve the semen that can be collected. This protocol has not been evaluated with controlled studies. It has been shown to anecdotally produce results within 1 hour and can be used for long-term improved libido and sperm counts.

Additionally, careful timing of the breeding and intrauterine insemination of the bitch with either TCI or surgical breeding can improve the chances of a pregnancy.

Stud dog with normal to low libido and abnormal sperm morphology (Teratozoospermia)

Abnormal sperm morphology is known as teratozoospermia. There are 2 general underlying causes: congenital and acquired. It can be difficult to determine if the cause is congenital. Acquired causes include: inflammation of the testes (tumor, trauma, fever or other thermal damage, and orchitis), and underuse and overuse of the stud dog. A thorough history and complete physical examination may help discover the underlying cause. Ultrasound can be used to assess testicular architecture, looking for tumors, atrophy, spermatoceles or sperm granulomas.

Test for <u>Brucella canis</u>. Culture of the ejaculate may detect a bacterial cause of orchitis. Unilateral castration may improve the dog's sperm count if the opposite testicle is normal on palpation and/ or ultrasound. If an underlying cause is found, such as thermal damage exposure, overly hot or cold surfaces or the use of a blow dryer should be avoided.

Stud dog with normal to low libido with no sperm (Azoospermia)

Azoospermia is an absence of sperm in the ejaculate. A dog should not be considered sterile based on one azoospermic sample. There can be physical as well as psychological causes.

The psychological cause should be evaluated first. The stud dog should be collected at another visit, using a teaser bitch that he is attracted to, a location with good footing that is private, and staff that he is comfortable with. Treat any underlying medical causes. Like many other skills our dogs have, this too can be enhanced by training.

Examine the collection microscopically to determine sperm presence. Some collections are turbid enough to create the impression, on gross examination, that sperm are present. Turbidity is usually due to epithelial cells, tumor cells, and white blood cells that are present in the collection. If any sperm are present, the sample should be classified as oligospermic rather than azospermic.

If no sperm are present in the ejaculate, an alkaline phosphatase level should be run on the ejaculate. This level is most accurate if run only on the second fraction of the ejaculate. Collection of the entire ejaculate containing largely prostate fluid may be less accurate because the prostatic fluid will dilute the fraction in question and lead to an artificially low reading. The same equipment that is used to run alkaline phosphatase on serum and plasma samples can be used. Accurate measurement may require serial dilutions if the level is high enough to be outside the linear range of the equipment. For samples submitted to a reference laboratory, the sample source should be listed on the requisition form; send enough sample for multiple samples to be run.

A complete ejaculate from a normal dog with normal testicles should have an alkaline phosphatase level greater than 5,000 U/L; it can exceed 20,000 U/L. A sample with an alkaline phosphatase level below 5,000 U/L (often below 2,000 U/L) indicates that the dog either failed to fully ejaculate, ejaculated only prostatic fluid with no fluid from the testes (pain or psychological reasons) or has a bilateral outflow blockage of the ducts (a physical outflow obstruction). If it is suspected the dog failed to fully ejaculate, he can be collected additional times, addressing reasons for failure to ejaculate by manipulating the environment. Lutalyse® or GnRH, may be used to maximize his opportunity to collect fully.

Once the ejaculate is determined to be complete, history and physical exam findings become the focus of the investigation **(See Appendix D-6)**.

If the dog has been on medications that impair fertility and it is medically appropriate to discontinue the offending drugs, he should be evaluated 90 or more days after medication is stopped. If there has been recent trauma, illness, or thermal insult, reevaluation 90 or more days later may reveal improved fertility. If hernias are detected, surgical correction and reevaluation 90 or more days after recovery may reveal improved fertility. If only one testicle is found to be normal on palpation and ultrasound, removal of the abnormal testicle (tumor, atrophy, spermatocele) may allow the contralateral testicle to recover and regain fertility. A Sertoli cell tumor may cause azoospermia by local inflammation, a rise in the intratesticular temperature of both testes, and/or an increase in estrogen secretion interfering with sperm production in both testes.

If the SAP is high (>5000 U/L), pre-testicular and testicular causes should be pursued first. If the SAP is low (<5000 U/L), post-testicular causes are more likely. Azoospermia may occur if there is bilateral outflow obstruction. This can be caused by bilateral spermatocele, sperm granuloma or segmental aplasia of the epididymis.

If there is an endocrine disturbance, fertility may return once the underlying problem is managed. A dog with confirmed Brucella may need to be euthanized. A dog with a culture result with one predominant bacteria may respond to appropriate antibiotic therapy. Mycoplasma is often isolated from the ejaculate but may not be the primary cause of infertility; it may only be a marker indicating another underlying cause. Testicular biopsy results may suggest an underlying treatable cause. If the karyotype indicates an intersex dog, there is no treatment to initiate fertility.

Stud dog with normal to low libido with blood in the ejaculate (Hematospermia)

Blood in the ejaculate commonly originates from the prostate or trauma to the penis or other reproductive organs. Careful observation during collection can usually distinguish whether the source is from the prostate (blood mixed with the ejaculate) or from the penis (fresh blood from the exterior surface of the penis). Care during collection and avoiding contact between the penis and any rigid semen collection equipment will minimize the likelihood of trauma. Minor trauma during collection does not appear to cause discomfort.

Unlike in some other species, blood in the ejaculate does not interfere with fertility unless present in such large volumes that blood clots interfere with sperm motility. If large quantities are noted, fresh sterile saline should be added immediately to the ejaculate to minimize blood clotting.

Benign prostatic hypertrophy is a common cause of hematospermia in the middle-aged to older dog. A presumptive diagnosis is made based on clinical signs and rectal palpation. It can only be confirmed by biopsy of the prostate, preferably ultrasound-guided by an experienced ultra-sonographer or the CPSE blood test. This condition frequently responds well to medical therapy. (See section on Disorders of the Prostate earlier in this chapter.)

Stud dog with normal to low libido with abnormal sperm motility (Asthenozoospermia)

Asthenozoospermia is defined as sperm motility that is less than 70% of normal. Some astheno-zoospermic dogs can still successfully impregnate a bitch, but the semen does not ship or freeze as well as normal semen. The causes are similar to those of teratozoospermia (abnormal sperm morphology) and include testicular tumors, infection of the reproductive tract, collection equipment contaminated with disinfectants or glove powder, and immotile cilia syndrome.

A complete history and comprehensive physical examination should follow collection. The history should include when the condition was noted, the reproductive history of the stud dog, and information regarding the type of equipment used to collect and inseminate. The stud dog should be collected at the clinic where the evaluation is being done. If the client has been handling breedings without veterinary assistance, the equipment and supplies being used should be gathered and brought to the appointment for evaluation. What seems to be of little significance to the breeder client may reveal an important non-medical cause of apparent infertility.

If sperm motility is low, centrifuge the semen to remove any possible urine or prostatic contamination. An appropriate semen extender should be added, the sample carefully warmed, and re-evaluated microscopically. If this corrects the condition, the procedure should be repeated at each collection.

If motility remains poor, test the dog for Brucella canis and culture the ejaculate. If the dog is brucellosis positive, euthanasia may be an option. Appropriate antibiotic therapy may be indicated based on culture results.

Electron microscopy can be done at some reference laboratories to evaluate the sperm tail in cross-section. If there are no motile sperm, immotile cilia syndrome may be a differential. In affected dogs, there are no motile cilia in the respiratory tract and sperm. The dog generally has a history of respiratory disease. Some will also have situs inversus, where the organs are reversed right-to-left.

Stud dog with normal to low libido with abnormal ejaculate components including red blood cells, white blood cells and tumor cells

Any semen sample collected at the clinic should be examined microscopically. Bacteria, exfoliated epithelial and other cell types may be seen in addition to sperm. The semen containing this group of cells may look normal or be grossly abnormal in appearance. The ejaculate should be evaluated microscopically both before and after centrifugation.

A normal stud dog can have up to 2000 white blood cells (WBCs) per ml and be normal. White blood cells in the ejaculate do not always mean there is an infection; this may be an inflammatory process or they may be from the prepuce and not reflect any infection. It is possible to see WBCs and be unable to culture any bacteria. It is also possible to culture bacteria without finding WBCs in the ejaculate. If the culture produces more than 10,000 CFU per ml of semen, it is considered significant. Normal bacterial flora is found in parts of the urogenital tract.

Blood may be noted microscopically and/or grossly in many ejaculates. If present in large amounts, it can trap sperm in clots and prevent them from being delivered into the bitch's reproductive tract. Blood commonly results from trauma to the penis during collection or from the prostate. If from the penis, it is seldom of any significance in that it will not interfere with successful breeding of the bitch and it will not usually reflect any pathology in the male. It is usually bright red and the source of the trauma on the penis is often noticed at the collection. If blood is from the prostate, it is often a darker color and mixed uniformly with the ejaculate. The RBCs do not interfere with fertility, but the character of the prostatic fluid may be altered by prostatic disease, reducing sperm motility and longevity. The affected stud dog should be evaluated to determine the cause of the prostatic disorder and treated accordingly. RBCs can also originate from other locations in the urogenital tract.

Although rare, cells exfoliated from a tumor anywhere in the urogenital tract may be seen in the ejaculate. If suspect, these can be prepared and submitted to a reference laboratory for evaluation.

If confirmed, a complete evaluation of the urogenital tract is required to locate the source of the abnormal cells.

Blastomyces organisms can be shed into the ejaculate from the prostate. Blastomyces is potentially hazardous to laboratory personnel and samples should not be submitted for culture if it is suspected. Testing the urine for Blastomyces antigens is a better choice.

Treatment protocols for the infertile stud dog

Treat the underlying cause of infertility if it can be determined. Spermatogenesis takes approximately 62 days, and an additional 15 days is required for transit through the epididymis. It therefore takes a minimum of 90 days for the stud dog to return to normal spermatogenesis. There is no shortcut. Less than 10% of stud dogs who no longer produce sperm will be returned to fertility.

In addition to removing or treating the underlying cause, or if no cause can be found, a nutritional approach to improving semen quality may be considered. For many clients, this is very appealing. And at the least, you are doing something during the long 90 day wait-and-see period.

Nutritional supplements may help to improve semen quality but there are few published reports to support their efficacy in managing fertility problems in males or females. Supplements should be evaluated by the attending veterinarian to assure safety and that there are no contraindications to their use.

Commonly used supplements
Glycosaminoglycans
This is the most common nutraceutical category used for improving sperm quantity and quality. It is found in many formulations by many manufacturers. Many, like International Canine Semen Bank's CF- Plus®, contain perna (green-lipped) mussels as the primary active ingredient. Anecdotal reports suggest improved semen quality in bulls, horses, and dogs. The the mechanism of action, according to Dr. Roger Kendall, is enhanced cellular reactions and amino acid uptake.

There is no documentation to support the use of this product in the dog. The dosage for this application has not been determined; there are dosage regimens for the use of these products for other purposes such as improving joint mobility. Unless there is an allergic response, it is unlikely that this product will cause any harmful side effects.

Anti-oxidants
These typically include Vitamins C, E, beta carotene, and selenium among others. They are available from many manufacturers over-the-counter. They appear to act by removing free radicals, thus protecting the cells. Greater sperm numbers have been reported in the ejaculate following their use. There is no documentation to support the use of this product. There are anecdotal reports that semen concentrations are improved, that there are fewer head and acrosomal abnormalities when used, and semen tolerates cooling and freezing better when patients are on this type of product. Some components can be harmful if used in excess, so care should be taken when this is prescribed.

Fatty acid supplements
These are available from many manufacturers over-the-counter. Anecdotal reports indicate that there is improvement in semen morphology when the dog has a high percentage of proximal droplets. The components and ratio of omega 3 to 6 fatty acids should be assessed to ensure that it is supplied in an anti-inflammatory ratio.

L-Carnitine
This nutritional supplement alters fat metabolism. It is available from several manufacturers and is

found in some senior dog diets. Anecdotally, it is reported to improve sperm motility. The mechanism of action has not been determined. It is included in some commercially available dog foods to aid in weight loss and should be used with care to avoid excessive weight loss in the patient.

No commercially available dog food has been documented to improve semen quality, morphology, motility, or quantity.

Technical advances in canine reproduction

Business and technical advances during the last forty years have allowed us to provide breeders services not previously possible. These advances include:
The successful use of frozen canine semen;

The successful use of fresh chilled shipped canine semen;
International shipment of fresh and frozen semen;
Rapid results from blood tests, and the ability to use very small blood samples for neonates
 including in – house CBC's, Chemistry profiles and progesterone levels;
Ultrasound;
Improved anesthetic protocols and pain management;
New drugs – prostaglandins, prolactin inhibitors, GnRH agonists and antagonists;
Overnight courier service;
Fax and email communication;
 Internet websites;
 Mapping of the canine genome;
Expanded data bases for OFA, development of CERF and PennHip and others;
DNA health screening;
DNA parentage testing;
Endoscopic procedures;
Telemedicine;
Vaccine advances.

CHAPTER 11
Special Breedings — Working with Fresh Chilled and Frozen Semen

Introduction

Semen freezing is a unique service available at a limited number of veterinary hospitals and non-veterinary facilities throughout the U.S. and the world. Many veterinarians are less familiar with this procedure than their clients. This chapter serves only as an introduction to the process and is not intended to be comprehensive enough to substitute for training in how to freeze, store, and use canine semen. Veterinarians interested in learning this are encouraged to seek hands-on training from one of the semen freezing franchises or at a theriogenology conference (Figure 11-1).

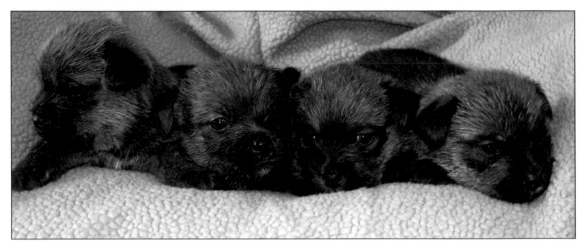

Figure 11-1.
A litter of 4 puppies produced from semen that was over 25 years old.

Who and why?

Who are the clients and dogs that semen freezing would be useful for? First, the clients, because they make the decisions. The client may be any breeder interested in expanding their genetic opportunities outside of their chronological or geographical area without traveling a long distance. Line breedings are no longer limited by the lifespan of the dog. Outcrosses are no longer limited by the part of the world the bitch lives in. Any breeder who is willing to go to the additional time, trouble and expense is a candidate for semen freezing. Collecting semen for freezing and using it for breeding is more costly than using fresh semen, but provides options not otherwise available. Frozen semen can be collected from and used to inseminate any healthy sexually mature dog who has passed the appropriate genetic screening tests for that breed, exhibits good temperament, is a superior specimen of the breed or shows promise of longevity.

Terminology

To clarify terminology, the following terms will be used. This is to ensure accurate communication on what techniques are planned.

Fresh semen

Semen collected at the time to be used and inserted immediately. Both dog and bitch on premises.

Fresh chilled extended semen

Semen: collected 24 to 48 hours prior to insemination, transported from the location of the male to the location of the bitch. The stud dog must be alive and available. The advantage is the stud dog and bitch may be at very remote locations from one another but can still be bred without shipping the dogs or traveling.

Frozen semen
Semen collected at any time in advance of use frozen and stored in liquid nitrogen until used, thawed and immediately inseminated using specialized insemination techniques. The stud dog does NOT have to be available.

Surgical breeding
A routine invasive surgical procedure useful when the bitch has a history of infertility or the semen is compromised by freezing, chilling or infertility.

Transcervical Insemination (TCI)
An invasive but non-surgical endoscopic procedure requiring specialized skills and equipment to place semen directly in the uterus.

When to collect
Collections from a young, healthy adult male are preferred. Ages 2 to 5 years are ideal. Even young dogs who have not completed their performance titles should be considered candidates for freezing if the owner predicts they will accomplish great things. It is preferable to have some or all of their health screening completed.

Any age male that is still able to produce viable sperm can be collected, but in some cases, older dogs tend to have semen that does not tolerate freezing as well.

Under some circumstances, semen can also be frozen from a dog's testicles removed at neutering or from any intact male within 24 hours of death if kept cool. If the patient dies acutely or is neutered, the spermatic cords should be ligated using sterile technique, the testes placed in a zip-top bag, and transported in a chilled container, avoiding freezing, to a veterinarian who can harvest and freeze the semen within 24 hours of castration or death.

We recommend that you freeze early and freeze often.

When to inseminate
The most successful outcomes result when frozen semen is used during a normal estrus cycle in a young to middle-aged healthy bitch. Precise timing is required for success.

Where to freeze
Semen freezing requires specialized training, supplies and equipment. Using frozen semen for a breeding is a skill many veterinarians can master with some assistance from the shipping veterinarian and their staff (Figure 11-2).

How to freeze
Semen thawing and surgical technique is described in Chapter 4 (Appendix B-3).

The AKC registration or other registry papers, DNA profile (can be collected at the appointment if not previously done), current Brucella test results and a consent form, including information for who controls the use of the semen if the owner becomes unavailable, should be available at the appointment to freeze.

The oldest frozen canine semen is approximately 40 years old. Bovine semen pre-dates canine semen by approximately 20 years. Both are still successfully producing pregnancies. Because frozen semen uses minimal energy, it is expected to last for many more years.

The semen must remain frozen until ready to use. Semen is stored and shipped in liquid nitrogen or nitrogen vapor, at a temperature of -322° F or -70° C. Even brief exposure to room air will cause permanent damage to the semen. Once thawed, it cannot be refrozen. The frozen semen is shipped in specialized tanks known as dewars. These dewars are expensive to purchase, maintain and ship. They have a limited lifespan. They work by absorbing liquid nitrogen into the liner; the nitrogen then creates a vapor in the chamber to keep the semen frozen. Some may maintain the semen from 7 days up to 14 days. No commercial shipper in the U.S. will allow free liquid nitrogen to be transported due to its hazardous nature, so all semen shipped must be in a vapor shipper. The vapor shipper must be properly charged and drained to avoid excess liquid nitrogen from being spilled in transit (Figure 11-2D).

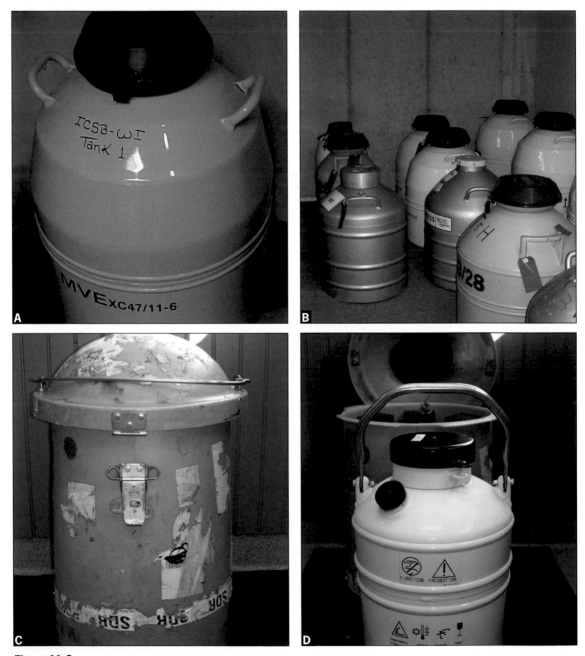

Figure 11-2.
A. and B. Storeroom with liquid nitrogen tanks storing frozen canine semen. C and D. Reusable nitrogen vapor shipper for shipping frozen semen overnight.

Frozen canine semen is most frequently packaged in either straws or pellets (Figure 11-3). They are each frozen using different techniques. Veterinarians who freeze semen have preferences, but both have been used for 40 years with success. In either form, the number of viable sperm after thawing should be known so that the correct "dose" of semen is available at thawing. Both forms need to be maintained in liquid nitrogen from the time they were frozen, through shipment, until moments before thawing. Shipping dewars can maintain the semen in a frozen form for up to 7 days without adding more nitrogen, so even veterinary clinics that do not have storage tanks can provide this service. There is usually a small additional charge to keep the shipping tank – because many veterinary clinics need their shippers returned for another shipment, this should be arranged in advance.

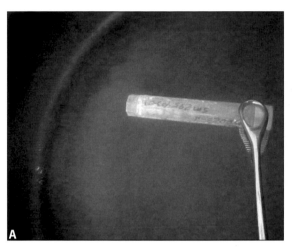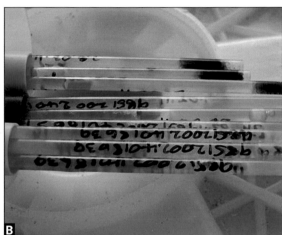

Figure 11-3.
A. Pellets of extended frozen semen in a cryo vial. B. Semen frozen in straws.

Liability
Every facility that freezes and/or stores frozen semen should carry insurance and have a contract with the semen owner to limit their liability in case of semen loss or damage.

Breeding a bitch with frozen semen
Breeding with frozen semen is less forgiving, more complicated, and more expensive than other breedings. It can also be very rewarding utilizing the genetics of stud dogs of a by-gone era or in a remote location (Appendix B-5).

REMEMBER THESE IMPORTANT POINTS

You are using semen that is expensive and is likely limited in availability. Use this finite resource wisely.

Timing the bitch's cycle must be precise, and the insemination window is approximately 12 to 24 hours. This requires the veterinary staff to breed on the bitch's schedule, not theirs. This means that breeding is often added to the schedule on short notice and/or is outside of regular office hours.

Anesthesia and surgery are used for most frozen inseminations. Consider the benefits versus the risks before embarking on this.

As with any breeding, encourage the client to assure that the bitch has current vaccinations, has her pre-breeding screening, and is in good health. You may wish to do this type of breeding only with a young bitch who has successfully completed a pregnancy. Aged bitches tend to release fewer eggs and have decreased fertility. A breeding history should be taken and vaginal exams and cultures done if indicated. A <u>Brucella</u> test should have been run with a negative result within 3 months.

Arrange for the frozen semen to be released prior to the start of the bitch's heat or early in her cycle. The owner of the semen, usually the stud dog owner, must sign a release form. Shipping costs from the storage facility must be paid prior to shipping and can usually be paid with a credit card. The owner of the bitch will usually pay the release fee, overnight shipping to the inseminating veterinary clinic, portable semen shipping tank rental, and return shipping of the tank to the storage facility.

Instruct your client to contact the inseminating veterinary clinic at the <u>FIRST SIGN</u> that their bitch is in heat. It is best to schedule her first appointment in the first 6 days of her estrus for a vaginal cytology to confirm that she is early in her estrus. Plan for sequential vaginal cytologies and progesterone testing based on this cytology and her reproductive history.

Progesterone tests should be run approximately every 24 to 72 hours as ovulation nears. An LH level can also be run if requested in advance. LH levels can be helpful in timing the bitch but must be run every 24 hours and can be costly.

If required by the hospital protocol, pre-surgical blood work should be drawn at one of these visits in preparation for anesthesia.

Once the date of ovulation is confirmed, it is time to schedule the bitch for anesthesia and surgical insemination or TCI. If using surgical insemination, advise the client that their bitch will receive general anesthesia. A midline incision is made similar to that for a spay, the uterus is exteriorized, and examined, semen is placed in the lumen, the uterus repositioned into the abdomen, and the abdominal wall and skin closed. She will be recovered from anesthesia and discharged the same day. The entire visit typically takes about 2 to 3 hours from admission to discharge. She should rest for several days post-op (See Chapter 4).

Perform an ultrasound at day 24 to 28 after breeding, for early diagnosis of pregnancy and provide the client with a pre-natal care handout.

Because the stakes are higher when working with frozen semen, consider a C-section to maximize puppy survival rates.

Developing an interest in canine reproduction can be very rewarding. There have been and will continue to be many advances made, providing new challenges. The clients hold themselves and veterinarians to a high, but usually realistic standard. The clients understand a great deal about the business and practice of veterinary medicine. They seek ongoing education. The patients are usually well-bred, well-trained, and exceptional examples of their breeds. Providing a unique service to allow dog breeders to follow their dreams is one way to find an area of medicine that is professionally satisfying.

BEST WISHES FOR GREAT FERTILITY.

References

Adams, Ana. "Increasing Conception Rates and Litter Sizes." Western Veterinary Conference, Las Vegas, 2004.

Battaglia, Carman: Breading Better Dogs.

Bell J S, Cavanagh K E, Tilley L P, Smith F W K, eds.: Veterinary Medical Guide to Dog and Cat Breeds; Jackson, WY: Teton NewMedia, 2012.

Bouchard G, Plata-Madrid H, Youngquist RS, Buening GM, Ganjam VK, Krause GF, Allen GK, Paine AL: Absorption of an alternate source of immunoglobulin in pups. Am J Vet Res. February 1992; 53(2):230-233.

Brower, Alexandra. "Canine Brucellosis." Richfield WI, 3 Nov. 2007.

Copley K: Parturition management: 15,000 whelpings later: An outcome based analysis. Theriogenology 2009; Vol. 1, Number 2: 297-307.

Davidson, Autumn. "Neonatology." Theriogenology. Albuquerque, 28 Aug. 2009.

Drost Project

Feldman EC, Nelson RW. Canine and Feline Endocrinology and Reproduction. Philadelphia: Saunders; 2001, pg 494.

Fontbonne, Alain. "Infertility in the Bitch." World Small Animal Veterinary Association World Congress, Prague, 11 Oct. 2006.

Fontbonne, Alain. "Pathology of the ovaries and of the uterus in the bitch." ESAVS, Zurich, 12 Sept. 2007.

Fontbonne, Alain. "Infertility in the Bitch and in the Dog." World Small Animal Veterinary Association World Congress, Sydney, 21 Aug. 2007.

Freshman, Joni L. "Complementary Medicine in Reproduction." Western Veterinary Conference. Las Vegas, 2005.

Freshman, Joni L. "Wake the Baby! The Latest on Neonatal Resuscitation For The Dog And Cat." VIN Online. 9 Nov. 2008.

Hess, Milan. "Documented and anecdotal effects of certain pharmaceutical agents used to enhance semen quality in the dog." Theriogenology , Volume 66 , Issue 3, 613-617.

Hoskins, Johnny D. "Small Animal Pediatric Medicine." Tufts Animal Expo. North Grafton MA. 2002.

Hoskins, Johnny D. "Veterinary Pediatrics of the Puppy and Kitten."Atlantic Coast Veterinary Conference. Atlantic City, 2005.

Hutchison, Robert: "Canine Reproduction, Whelping and Neonatal Care." Lakeshore Pembroke Welsh Corgi Club. Crystal Lake, IL. 25 March 2005

International Canine Semen Bank

Johnston SD, Root Kustritz MV, Olson PNS: Canine and Feline Theriogenology. Philadelphia: Saunders; 2001;.

Jones, Bretaigne. "Variables That Influence Litter Size." Lomira WI, 20 June 2009.

Kazacos, KR: "Treatment and Control of Gastrointestinal Helminths." Western Veterinary Conference. Las Vegas. 2002.

Kampschmidt Kit: "Drug Use in the Neonatal Pediatric Small Animal Patient." Western Veterinary Conference. Las Vegas. 2006.

Kampschmidt Kit. VIN online posting. 24 May 2005.

Lopate, Cheryl. SFT list, 15 April 2007.

Macintire, Douglass K. "Pediatric Emergencies." Western Veterinary Conference, Las Vegas, 2004.

Mauldin, G. Neal. "Mammary Gland Tumors." Atlantic Coast Veterinary Conference Atlantic City, 2006.

OFA website, www.offa.org

Philibert JC, Snyder PW, Glickman N, Glickman LT, Knapp DW, Waters DJ. "Influence of host factors on survival in dogs with malignant mammary gland tumors." J Vet Intern Med. 2003 Jan-Feb;17(1):102-6.

Plumb DC: Plumb's Veterinary Drug Handbook. Seventh Edition. Pharma Vet Inc. 2011.

Romagnoli, Stefano. "Canine Pyometra: Pathogenesis, Therapy and Clinical Cases." World Small Animal Veterinary Association, Granda Spain, 2002.

Ronsse V, Verstegen J, Thiry E, Onclin K, Aeberlé C, Brunet S, Poulet H. Canine herpesvirus-1 (CHV-1): clinical, serological and virological patterns in breeding colonies; Theriogenology, Volume 64, Issue 1, Pages 61-74.

Root Kustritz MV. Small Animal Theriogenology. St. Louis: Elsevier. 2003;.

Root Kustritz, Margaret V. "Canine Brucellosis." Western Veterinary Conference, Las Vegas, 2007.

Verstegen J, Dhaliwal G, Verstegen-Onclin K. Mucometra, cystic endometrial hyperplasia, and pyometra in the bitch: Advances in treatment and assessment of future reproductive success. Theriogenology, Volume 70, Issue 3, Pages 364-374.

Verstegen J, Dhaliwal G, Verstegen-Onclin K: Canine and feline pregnancy loss due to viral and non-infectious causes: a review. Theriogenology: 2008; 70: 304-319.

Appendices

Appendix A: For technical staff

A-1. *APGAR scores for newborns*

Proposed APGAR index for neonatal dogs and cats			
Parameter	0 pts	1 pt	2 pts
Activity, muscle tone	Flaccid	Some tone in extremities	Active movements
Pulse, heart rate	Absent – < than 110 bpm	110 – 220 bpm	> 220 bpm
Reflexes when stressed	Absent	Some movement	Crying out
Mucous membrane color	Pale or cyanotic	Slightly cyanotic	Pink
Respiratory rate	Absent	Weak, irregular	> 15/min, rhythmic

Interpretation:

Total points	Vitality
0 – 3	Weak
4 – 6	Moderate
7 – 10	Normal

The views and opinions expressed in this page are strictly those of the page author. (Root-Kustritz)
The contents of this page have not been reviewed or approved by the University of Minnesota.

CHECKLIST FOR FRESH CHILLED SEMEN SHIPMENT

Name of stud dog owner_____ Date_____

Address to ship kit to (owner or veterinarian)_____

_____

Name of recipient bitch owner_____

Call name of bitch_____

Credit card number of recipient bitch's owner: _____ exp_____ MC/VISA

Route to be shipped: UPS/FedEx/Midwest Express/Other

Special Shipping Instructions or Destination _____

TO INCLUDE WITH SHIPMENT:

☐ Extender 1 tube per shipment 2 cc each tube–have at room temp or thawed – use in a 1:2 to 1:4 ratio semen to extender

☐ Plastic conical tube -1 per shipment with blue cap, labeled with name of stud dog & owner and bitch & owner (to package semen)

☐ 2 whirlpacks per shipment, (to double bag semen)

☐ 1 large piece of Parafilm per tube (to seal top of blue tube – prevent leakage)

☐ 1 Shipping box per shipment with insulation either Styrofoam lined – can tape together and ship as 1 package

☐ 2 Gel packs per shipment – 1 frozen and 1 refrigerated

☐ Newspaper to put under tubes and to fill box

☐ Semen Evaluation form

☐ 2 Artificial vaginas (clear sleeve) with clear centrifuge tube to collect dog in to

☐ Shipping label addressed to our hospital

☐ 3M Freeze indicator if outdoor temp is below 32° or has had trouble with semen arriving in poor condition

☐ Instruction form (how to pack box) and how to handle semen

☐ AKC Registry Litter Registration form for Fresh Extended AI (to register litter)

FEES:

☐ Puppy Pack (package to ship in)

☐ Shipping cost

☐ Charges applied to credit card at time of shipment_____(Staff initials)

☐ Additional charges applied to credit card_____(Staff initials)

☐ Tech handling shipment_____(Staff signature)

Crumpled newspaper

Semen/media in screw-cap tube in Whirl-pak.

1/2 inch folded newspaper

Refrigerated cold pack*

Frozen cold pack*

Cut away view of prepared shipping kit

* DO NOT SUBSTITUTE OTHER COLD PACKS FOR THE ICSB PACKS THAT COME WITH THIS KIT.

A-3. *Intraosseous fluid administration set up*

Intraosseous catheter placement – Set-up

1. Needle – 20 gauge. Spinal needle with stylet is preferred if available.
2. Stylet – from IV catheter or smaller needle to clear lumen of needle if plugged.
3. Gauze squares
4. 1 inch white tape
5. Saline flush
6. Sterile gloves – depends on doctors size
7. Nolvasan surgical scrub
8. Antibiotic or betadine ointment
9. Injection port

Laboratory services, vendors, and other services				
Pre-Breeding Health Screening/Registry	PennHIP	www.pennhip.org	Hip x-ray evaluation	215-573-3176
	OFA	www.offa.org	Hip, Elbow, Shoulder x-ray evaluation, thyroid, cardiac and patellar registry	573-442-0418
	CERF	www.vmdb.org	Eye certification	217-693-4800
Laboratories	Marshfield Laboratory	www.marshfieldlabs.org	Laboratory, wide range of services	1-800-222-5835
	Cornell	www.diaglab.vet.cornell.edu	Laboratory, wide range of services including AGID Brucella testing, Coagulation testing and histology with specialty in reproductive and neonatal pathology	607-253-3900
	Michigan State	www.animalhealth.msu.edu	Endocrinology specialty laboratory services	517-353-0621
	MMI	www.mmigenomics.com	Parentage evaluation	800-311-8808 Ext. 3021
Breed Registries	AKC	www.akc.org	Parentage registry	919 233 9767
	UKC	www.ukcdogs.com	Parentage registry	269-343-9020
Health Registry	CHIC	www.caninehealthinfo.org	Bundles of testing recommended by breed clubs	573-442-0418
Shipping	UPS	www.ups.com	Overnight package shipping services	800-742-5877
	FedEx	www.fedex.com	Overnight package shipping services	800-463-3339
Breeding Supplies	MOFA	www.minitube.com	Vendor - semen extenders and semen evaluation equipment	800-646-4882
Blood Products	HemoPet	www.hemopet.org	Blood products including fresh frozen plasma for neonates	714-891-2022
Whelping Services	WhelpWise™	www.whelpwise.com	Tocodynometry (uterine contraction monitoring)	888-281-4867
Breeding Supplies	International Canine Semen Bank	www.ik9sb.com	Semen freezing and extenders	503-663-7031
	Synbiotics	www.synbiotics.com	Semen freezing and extenders	800-228-4305
	CLONE	www.innovativecaninereproduction.com	Semen freezing and extenders	215-489-2620
	Camelot Farms	www.camelotfarms.com	Semen freezing and extenders	800-254-8837
DNA Testing	VetGen	www.vetgen.com	DNA Testing	800-483-8436
	Optigen	www.optigen.com	DNA Testing	607-257-0301
	University of Pennsylvania	www.med.upenn.edu/genetics	Genetic Testing	814-865-7696
	PennGen	www.upend.edu/penngen	Genetic Testing	215-898-8894
	Washington State University	www.vetmed.wsu.edu	MDR and other genetic testing	509-335-2988
Laboratory	Michigan State	www.animalhealth.msu.edu	Iohexol clearance testing	517-355-0281

C-section SET-UP

Paperwork:
☐ Patient Record must be available
☐ Surgery consent form – owner needs to sign
☐ Anesthesia form
☐ C-section surgical report
☐ C-section discharge sheet

Induction/IV setup:
☐ Mouth gag
☐ Endotracheal tube
☐ Bland eye ointment
☐ IV catheter
☐ IV injection port
☐ Endotracheal tube gauze or other tie
☐ 1" white tape for IV catheter
☐ *Lidocaine and cotton swab for cat only*
☐ Saline flush for IV flush
☐ Laryngoscope
☐ Butorphanol or Buprinex injectable
☐ Propofol injectable

Surgery Room Set-up:
☐ Heating pad – wrap around warmed Lactated Ringers for abdominal flush to keep warm
☐ Lactated Ringer or Normal Saline 1 liter heating in microwave for 90 sec., then on heating pad for abdominal flush
☐ Colloids – hetastarch if necessary
☐ Surgery table
☐ V-tray
☐ Heating source for bitch (turned on) – be careful to avoid anything that could cause thermal burns
☐ Have towels ready to support rear of bitch if needed
☐ Suture for closing the uterus, abdominal wall, subcutaneous tissue and skin
☐ Scalpel blade (15)
☐ Lap towels – 2 large and 4 small
☐ Set of 4 towel clamps
☐ Surgery gown – 1 per person scrubbing in
☐ Surgery caps and masks for all in the surgical suite
☐ Surgery pack
☐ Serrated straight Mayo scissors for episiotomy
☐ Surgery gloves – 2 pair for each person scrubbing in
☐ Duct tape to keep long coated hair away from the incision site
☐ Puppy ID towels – 1 set of each colored sterilized/non-sterilized
☐ Oxytocin from refrigerator
☐ Preferred post-op pain medication injectable
☐ Atropine injectable
☐ Metoclopramide injectable (Reglan)
☐ Butorphanol or Buprinex injectable

Puppy Set-up:

- ☐ Non-sterilized set of colored towels matching sterilized set
- ☐ Heating pads
- ☐ Puppy scale (weight in kilograms preferred)
- ☐ Stethoscope
- ☐ Laryngoscope
- ☐ Otoscope with large tip
- ☐ Sterile umbilical pack (needle holder and hemostat)
- ☐ Suture for umbilical cords
- ☐ Laundry baskets
- ☐ Bulb syringes
- ☐ DeLee mucous traps
- ☐ Dopram – 0.1 cc per pup - label
- ☐ Epinephrine
- ☐ Atropine
- ☐ Dexamethasone
- ☐ Lasix injectable
- ☐ Vitamin K injectable
- ☐ Endotracheal tubes suitable for puppies – Cole tube, tom cat catheters, red rubber feeding tubes cut and end smoothed to allow for ventilation (prepare these in advance, clean and can be reused)
- ☐ Stylet for endotracheal tube
- ☐ End to adapt endotracheal tube to fit oxygen hoses or Ambu bag
- ☐ O_2, with regulator turned on
- ☐ Fish tank or O_2 chamber
- ☐ Lasix injectable

Additional Set up to keep work area clean and safe:

- ☐ Place non-slip mat where Dr.'s feet will be
- ☐ Place towels in work area and around surgery table
- ☐ Place waste basket and steel surgery pail where doctor can drop , gauze, and used linen
- ☐ Place incubator or warmed box or basket in an area to move pups when stable
- ☐ O_2 on in treatment area
- ☐ Anesthetic machine in surgery for bitch with O_2 on

Sequence:

- ☐ Arrival of the bitch with possible or confirmed dystocia
  - ☐ Exam room
  - ☐ Heated basket for pups
  - ☐ Towels
  - ☐ Blanket for bitch to nest on during evaluation
  - ☐ Supplies and drugs as listed for neonatal resuscitation
  - ☐ Preparation for possible radiograph
  - ☐ Examination glove and lubricant (KY, Nolvalube, J-lube, etc)
  - ☐ Technician to take history and assist with examination
- ☐ Assess the bitch
  - ☐ Palpation/vaginal digital exam
  - ☐ Episiotomy if indicated (pup trapped in vagina by stricture) should be done ASAP
  - ☐ PE/TPR/Blood pressure
  - ☐ Radiograph and or ultrasound as indicated
  - ☐ Pre-Surgical blood panel with protime if available/Progesterone if available
  - ☐ Doppler to assess pups heart rates if available
- ☐ Owner sign consent form to allow anesthesia and surgical procedure after discussing options and risks

- ☐ Dose bitch with atropine injectable (1 cc per 20 pounds) and Reglan injectable at 0.3 cc per 10 pounds
- ☐ Place IV catheter & start fluids – stabilize before proceeding if indicated
- ☐ Administer antibiotics only if indicated by condition of bitch and pups
- ☐ Shave abdomen before anesthesia
- ☐ Move bitch to surgery room
- ☐ Start oxygen by face mask pre-oxygenate 5 mins
- ☐ STOP! LOOK AROUND TO BE SURE ALL SUPPLIES AND STAFF ARE IN PLACE AND READY TO MOVE QUICKLY
- ☐ Induce anesthesia with Propofol at 1 cc/5 pounds (start with 1/2 to 2/3 and give as needed)
- ☐ Mouth gag
- ☐ Bland eye ointment apply to protect
- ☐ Intubate and inflate cuff/secure tube with gauze
- ☐ GO!
- ☐ Place bitch on surgery table with left side slightly rolled down
- ☐ Attach anesthetic machine and monitors
- ☐ Start IV fluids at rate on chart per hour
- ☐ Scrub the site with Nolvasan and alcohol alternating preps or routine surgical prep per your hospital protocol
- ☐ Roll her onto back and secure in final position as doctor prefers – be sure she is in a comfortable position with her head and neck level, avoid tipping head down (avoid gastric reflux which can cause irreparable damage to esophagus
- ☐ Prep again in case final positioning contaminated surgical field
- ☐ Open supplies – gown/gloves/surgery pack/blade/towel clamps/drape/suture/lap towels/puppy towels

Bitch	Pups
☐ Increase anesthetic gas if light or titrate with Propofol	☐ Suction with bulb syringe or DeLee
☐ Metacam after last pup is out at 0.18 ml/10#sq	☐ Monitor/assist with respirations
☐ Oxytocin p r n	☐ Stethoscope to check for heart beat if not obvious
☐ Suture uterus	☐ Oxygen as needed – face mask or chamber
☐ Belly flush and eliminate soiled lap towels	☐ Dopram and/or caffeine to stimulate respirations
☐ Re-glove	☐ Acupuncture if needed
☐ Closure	☐ Intubate trachea if needed
☐ Discharge instructions	☐ Check for cleft palates and other defects/treat
☐ Make up meds for owner to take home – Metacam/Reglan/Nemex/Tincture of Iodine	☐ Ligate umbilical cord/treat with tincture of iodine
☐ Remove IV catheter IF OK	☐ Identify pups corresponding to map of uterine location
	☐ Weigh pups and record
	☐ Place in oxygen/incubator or warmed basket
	☐ Photographs

A-6. *Canine semen report for owner and receiving veterinarian*

Clinic name, address and contact information

CANINE SEMEN REPORT for Owner and Receiving Veterinarian

From:

Client Name:_____ Client Phone: _____

Dog's call name:_____ Age:_____

Dog's Registered Name:_____ Proven: Yes/No

Registration Number:_____ AKC/UKC/OTHER

Breed:_____

For:

Client Name:_____ Client Phone: _____

Dog's call name:_____ Age:_____

Dog's Registered Name:_____ Proven: Yes/No

Registration Number:_____ AKC/UKC/OTHER

Breed:_____

Semen Analysis: Date_____

Volume collected:_____ Concentration per ml _____

Total sperm count:_____ x 10^6

(MULTIPLY VOLUME IN ML x CONCENTRATION PER ML = TOTAL SPERM COUNT)

Centrifuged? Yes/No Color_____

Volume extender added: _____ Total volume shipped:_____

Extender used: ICSB/Synbiotics/ Minitube _____/Uppsala/Other:_____

Percent motility_____%   Speed of Progression: 0   1   2   3   4   5

Immature___% Bent___% Coiled ___% Detached___% Droplets ___% Other_____

<u>Other:</u> White Blood Cells _____ per 400x   Red Blood Cells ____ per 400 x

Abnormal morphology _____%   Normal Morphology _____%

(MULTIPLY SPERM COUNT /ML X % NORMAL = TOTAL NORMAL SPERM COUNT)

TOTAL NORMAL SPERM CELLS _____ x 10^6

Comments _____

_____

Processed by:_____

Whelping Calendar (from date of ovulation to due date +/- 24 hours)

Jan	Mar	Feb	Apr	Mar	May	Apr	Jun	May	July	Jun	Aug	July	Sep	Aug	Oct	Sep	Nov	Oct	Dec	Nov	Jan	Dec	Feb
O	W	O	W	O	W	O	W	O	W	O	W	O	W	O	W	O	W	O	W	O	W	O	W
1	5	1	5	1	3	1	3	1	3	1	3	1	2	1	3	1	3	1	3	1	3	1	2
2	6	2	6	2	4	2	4	2	4	2	4	2	3	2	4	2	4	2	4	2	4	2	3
3	7	3	7	3	5	3	5	3	5	3	5	3	4	3	5	3	5	3	5	3	5	3	4
4	8	4	8	4	6	4	6	4	6	4	6	4	5	4	6	4	6	4	6	4	6	4	5
5	9	5	9	5	7	5	7	5	7	5	7	5	6	5	7	5	7	5	7	5	7	5	6
6	10	6	10	6	8	6	8	6	8	6	8	6	7	6	8	6	8	6	8	6	8	6	7
7	11	7	11	7	9	7	9	7	9	7	9	7	8	7	9	7	9	7	9	7	9	7	8
8	12	8	12	8	10	8	10	8	10	8	10	8	9	8	10	8	10	8	10	8	10	8	9
9	13	9	13	9	11	9	11	9	11	9	11	9	10	9	11	9	11	9	11	9	11	9	10
10	14	10	14	10	12	10	12	10	12	10	12	10	11	10	12	10	12	10	12	10	12	10	11
11	15	11	15	11	13	11	13	11	13	11	13	11	12	11	13	11	13	11	13	11	13	11	12
12	16	12	16	12	14	12	14	12	14	12	14	12	13	12	14	12	14	12	14	12	14	12	13
13	17	13	17	13	15	13	15	13	15	13	15	13	14	13	15	13	15	13	15	13	15	13	14
14	18	14	18	14	16	14	16	14	16	14	16	14	15	14	16	14	16	14	16	14	16	14	15
15	19	15	19	15	17	15	17	15	17	15	17	15	16	15	17	15	17	15	17	15	17	15	16
16	20	16	20	16	18	16	18	16	18	16	18	16	17	16	18	16	18	16	18	16	18	16	17
17	21	17	21	17	19	17	19	17	19	17	19	17	18	17	19	17	19	17	19	17	19	17	18
18	22	18	22	18	20	18	20	18	20	18	20	18	19	18	20	18	20	18	20	18	20	18	19
19	23	19	23	19	21	19	21	19	21	19	21	19	20	19	21	19	21	19	21	19	21	19	20
20	24	20	24	20	22	20	22	20	22	20	22	20	21	20	22	20	22	20	22	20	22	20	21
21	25	21	25	21	23	21	23	21	23	21	23	21	22	21	23	21	23	21	23	21	23	21	22
22	26	22	26	22	24	22	24	22	24	22	24	22	23	22	24	22	24	22	24	22	24	22	23
23	27	23	27	23	25	23	25	23	25	23	25	23	24	23	25	23	25	23	25	23	25	23	24
24	28	24	28	24	26	24	26	24	26	24	26	24	25	24	26	24	26	24	26	24	26	24	25
25	29	25	29	25	27	25	27	25	27	25	27	25	26	25	27	25	27	25	27	25	27	25	26
26	30	26	30	26	28	26	28	26	28	26	28	26	27	26	28	26	28	26	28	26	28	26	27
			May																				
27	31	27	1	27	29	27	29	27	29	27	29	27	28	27	29	27	29	27	29	27	29	27	28
	Apr																						Mar
28	1	28	2	28	30	28	30	28	30	28	30	28	29	28	30	28	30	28	30	28	30	28	1
							July										Dec						
29	2			29	31	29	1	29	31	29	31	29	30	29	31	29	1	29	31	29	31	29	2
					Jun				Aug		Sep		Oct		Nov						Jan		Feb
30	3			30	1	30	2	30	1	30	1	30	1	30	1	30	2	30	1	30	1	30	3
31	4			31	2			31	2			31	2	31	2			31	2			31	4

O = Ovulation date
W = Whelping date

A-8. *Equipment and vendor list*

Equipment	Vendor
Microscope slides and cover slips	MWI/Butler/Midwest
DiffQuick® Stain	MWI/Butler/Midwest
Dip Quick Stain (JorVet)	MWI/Butler/Midwest
Guarded culturettes	Reproductive Resources 1-800-331-0195
Norm Ject 10 cc syringes (Latex Free)	MWI/Butler/Midwest
Cooled semen shipping kits and extender	ik9sb.com International Canine Semen Bank, MOFA
Cotton swabs, 6 inch	MWI/Butler/Midwest
Non-latex exam gloves	MWI/Butler/Midwest
Surgery gloves	MWI/Butler/Midwest
Normal saline, sterile, new package	MWI/Butler/Midwest
20 g IV catheters	MWI/Butler/Midwest
Tom cat catheters	MWI/Butler/Midwest
Parafilm®	VWR International 1-800-932-5000
Whirl-Paks®	Nasco/MWI
Pasteur pipettes	MWI/Butler/Midwest
Centrifuge tubes	MWI/Butler/Midwest
D-Tec CB Brucella Test (Synbiotics)	Zoetis
Porta-Cul tubes for Brucella cultures	www.bd.com 201-847-6800
Aimes culturettes	Your prefered reference lab
DNA kits from AKC	akc.org
Witness® LH kits (Synbiotics)	synbiotics.com
Status Pro Progesterone test kits	synbiotics.com
Camelot Farms Progesterone	camelotfarms.com
Ovucheck Premate (Synbiotics)	synbiotics.org
Relaxin test kits – ReproCHEK® or Witness®	synbiotics.org
SnuggleSafe®	snugglesafe.ca
DeLee mucus traps (Whelp Wise)	whelpwise.com
Equidone	equitoxpharma.com
Canipro Thaw and Insemination Media	MOFA 1-800-646-4882
Canipro Frozen Semen Extender	MOFA 1-800-646-4882
Canipro chilled Semen Extender	MOFA 1-800-646-4882
Sperm counter (Spermacue)	MOFA 1-800-646-4882
AI Collection Sleeves (ICSB)	ICSB 1-503-663-7031
CF Plus Fertility (ICSB)	ICSB 1-503-663-7031
Freeze Vials (ICSB)	ICSB 1-503-663-7031
Thaw Media (ICSB)	ICSB 1-503-663-7031
Freezing Media (ICSB)	ICSB 1-503-663-7031
Fresh Chilled Media (ICSB)	ICSB 1-503-663-7031
Cryo Media (ICSB)	ICSB 1-503-663-7031
Fresh frozen plasma	Hemopet.org
MWI - mwivet.com	1-888-722-2242
Butler - accessbutler.com	1-888-329-3861
Midwest Veterinary - www.midwestvet.net	1-800-449-0208
ICSB - ik9sb.com	1-503-663-7031
RICA Surgical Products - Incubator	www.ricasurgical.com 800-889-3218
TE Scott	www.scottsdog/thewhne.html

Information about your plans to breed your male:

Your name: _____ Your pet's name: _____

Co-owners names: _____ Your pet's registered name: _____

Registration #_____ DNA completed Y/N _____

Do you have an appointment scheduled? Yes/No   Do you want an appointment? Yes/No

What are your preferred appointment dates? Monday/Tuesday/Wednesday/Thursday/Friday/Saturday

What are your preferred appointment times? Early AM/Late AM/ Noon hour/ Early PM/ Late PM

Best way to reach you? Phone (list times available and numbers) _____ (home)

_____ (cell) _____ (work) E mail_____

Have we seen you as a client before? Yes/No Have we seen this pet before? Yes/ No When?_____

Pet Information: Age:_____ weeks/months/years or Date of Birth_____

Dog/Cat Breed:_____ Sex: Male/ Neutered Female/ Spayed

Breeding Plan:

Date this cycle began: _____ Is AI being done at our clinic? Y/N

Type of insemination planned: Natural /Vaginal #_____ /TCI # _____ /Surgical

Type of semen planning to use: Fresh/Fresh Chilled/Frozen

Date of last Brucella test_____ Test run – RSAT/Culture   Vaginal culture?_____

Name of Owner/Stud dog/Bitch to be bred to_____

Location of bitch's Veterinarian _____ Phone_____

SHIPPING ADDRESS_____

BILLING ADDRESS_____

Shipping plan: FedEx/UPS/Post office/other

SHIPPING BOX PROVIDED BY: Shipping Veterinarian/Recipient

History:

MALE: First breeding/Date previously bred on _____ Natural/ AI/ TCI/ Surgical

Outcome_____

Timing: None/ Male/ Vaginal cytology/ Progesterone_____

Evaluated on palpation/ultrasound/x-ray Semen analysis results:_____

Has your pet been thyroid tested: Yes/ No Results? _____ Date_____

Other previous diagnostics or treatments? _____

Lifestyle: Indoor/ Outdoor Companion dog/ Performance dog/ Breeding dog/ Service dog

Describe his housing and lifestyle: _____

Does your pet have any allergies to food, vaccines, or medications? No/Yes

   If yes, please describe:_____

Does your pet travel? In state? Out of state? Board? Dog events? Location:_____

Describe your pet's normal diet including treats and table food _____

_____

   List of supplements given: _____

What medications have you given your pet in the past month? Please include over-the-counter medications as well as heartworm preventive and flea/tick control products.

_____

WORMING HISTORY: Y/N product and dates:_____

VACCINATION HISTORY: Current/ None/ due for DHLPP on_____/ RABIES due on _____

Has he had his health screenings done: OFA/ CERF/ Other _____

Is there testing or x-rays from a previous illness or injury? Yes/No_____

Is your pet current on vaccinations and worming/fecal examinations? Yes/No

Do you have pet health insurance? No/Yes Name of provider?_____

Does your pet need any testing done or medications refilled?_____

May we request records from your previous veterinarian? Yes/No

Name of your previous veterinarian? _____ Phone:_____

Do you want a referral letter sent to your local veterinarian? Yes/No Name:_____

Symptoms:

Do you have any concerns about your pet's health? No/Yes IF yes, please review below:

Describe your pet's overall health:_____

When was your pet last normal? _____

What symptoms have you noticed? _____

What symptoms did you notice first? And how long ago? _____

Are the symptoms getting better/ worse/ staying the same?

Has your pet been treated for this condition in the past? Describe medications and responses:

_____

Is your pet acting normally? Yes/No If no, please describe:_____

Is your pet drinking normally? Yes/No If no, please describe:_____

Is your pet eating normally? Yes/No If no, please describe:_____

Is your pet urinating normally? Yes/No If no, please describe:_____

Is your pet vomiting? Yes/No If yes, please describe:_____

Is your pet having normal stools? Yes/No If no, please describe:_____

Has your pet's weight increased/ decreased/ stayed the same?

Is your pet's breathing normally? Yes/No If no, please describe:_____

Are the eyes normal? Yes/No If no, please describe:_____

Are the ears normal? Yes/No If no, please describe:_____

   What medications have you used?_____

Is the skin normal? Yes/No If no, please describe:_____

Are there any lumps? Yes/No Where are the sores, hair loss, or lumps?_____

Are there any abnormalities with the legs, neck or back? Yes/No If yes, please describe:

_____

Do you have any behavior concerns? Yes/No Please describe_____

Are the reproductive organs normal? Yes/No

   Plans to breed:_____

Are there observations or concerns we did not include in the questions above?

_____

Client ID:_____ Date:_____ Staff initials:_____ Dr._____

Information about your plans to breed your female:

Your name: _____ Your pet's name: _____

Co-owners names: _____ Your pet's registered name: _____

Registration #_____ DNA completed Y/N _____

Do you have an appointment scheduled? Yes/No   Do you want an appointment? Yes/No

What are your preferred appointment dates? Monday/Tuesday/Wednesday/Thursday/Friday/Saturday

What are your preferred appointment times? Early AM/ Late AM/ Noon hour/ Early PM/ Late PM

Best way to reach you? Phone (list times available and numbers)_____ (home)

_____ (cell) _____ (work) E mail_____

Have we seen you as a client before? Yes/No Have we seen this pet before? Yes/No When?_____

Pet Information: Age: _____ weeks/ months/ years or Date of Birth _____

Dog/Cat Breed: _____ Sex: Male/ Neutered Female/ Spayed

Breeding Plan:

Is she is season now? Yes/No Date this cycle began: _____ Is AI being done at our clinic? Y/N

Type of insemination planned: Natural/ Vaginal #_____/ TCI # _____/ Surgical

Type of semen planning to use: Fresh/ Fresh Chilled/ Frozen

Date of last Brucella test_____ Test run – RSAT/Culture Vaginal culture? _____

Name of Owner/Stud dog/Bitch to be bred to_____

Location of stud dog's Veterinarian _____ Phone_____

SHIPPING ADDRESS_____

BILLING ADDRESS_____

Shipping plan: UPS/ FedEx/ Post office/ other SHIPPING BOX PROVIDED BY: Shipping vet/ client

History:

FEMALE: Date of last cycle _____ First breeding? Yes/No

Date previously bred on _____ Natural/ AI/ TCI/ Surgical Outcome_____

Timing: None/Male/Vaginal cytology /Progesterone_____

Evaluated on palpation/ ultrasound/ x-ray Stud dog proven? Yes/No/ Evaluated?_____

Has your pet been thyroid tested: Yes/No Results?_____ Date_____

Other previous diagnostics or treatments?_____

Lifestyle: Indoor/ Outdoor Companion dog/ Performance dog/ Breeding dog/ Service dog

Describe her housing and lifestyle: _____

Has she had her health screenings done: OFA/ CERF / Other _____

Does your pet have any allergies to food, vaccines, or medications? No/Yes

  If yes, please describe: _____

Does your pet travel? In state? Out of state? Board? Dog events? Location: _____

Describe your pet's normal diet including treats and table food _____

_____

  List of supplements given: _____

WORMING HISTORY: Y/N product and dates: _____

VACCINATION HISTORY: Current/ None/ due for DHLPP on_____/ RABIES due on _____

What medications have you given your pet in the past month? Please include over-the-counter medications as well as heartworm preventive and flea/tick control products._____
_____

Is there testing or x-rays from a previous illness or injury? Yes/ No _____

Is your pet current on vaccinations and worming/ fecal examinations? Yes/No

Do you have pet health insurance? No/Yes Name of provider?_____

Does your pet need any testing done or medications refilled?_____

May we request records from your previous veterinarian? Yes/No

Name of your previous veterinarian?_____ Phone:_____

Do you want a referral letter sent to your local veterinarian? Yes/No Name:_____

Symptoms:

Do you have any concerns about your pet's health? No/Yes IF yes, please review below:

Describe your pet's overall health:_____

When was your pet last normal? _____

What symptoms have you noticed?_____

What symptoms did you notice first? And how long ago?_____

Are the symptoms getting better/ worse/ staying the same?

Has your pet been treated for this condition in the past? Describe medications and responses:
_____

Is your pet acting normally? Yes/No If no, please describe: _____

Is your pet drinking normally? Yes/No If no, please describe: _____

Is your pet eating normally? Yes/No If no, please describe:_____

Is your pet urinating normally? Yes/No If no, please describe:_____

Is your pet vomiting? Yes/No If yes, please describe: _____

Is your pet having normal stools? Yes/No If no, please describe: _____

Has your pet's weight increased/ decreased/ stayed the same?

Is your pet's breathing normally? Yes/ No If no, please describe:_____

Are the eyes normal? Yes/No If no, please describe: _____

Are the ears normal? Yes/No If no, please describe: _____

    What medications have you used? _____

Is the skin normal? Yes/No If no, please describe:_____

Are there any lumps? Yes/No Where are the sores, hair loss, or lumps? _____

Are there any abnormalities with the legs, neck or back? Yes/No If yes, please describe: _____
_____

    Do you have any behavior concerns? Yes/No Please describe_____

Are the reproductive organs normal? Yes/No

    When was her last heat? _____

    Plans to breed: _____

Are there observations or concerns we did not include in the questions above?
_____

Client ID:_____ Date:_____ Staff initials:_____ Dr._____

Appendix B: For telephone staff

B-1. *Appointment scheduling for breeding problem*

Breeding consultation appointment scheduling	
Reason for appointment	Unsuccessful attempts to breed male and female
Ask client and pet name	Name of both male and female owners – often have both dogs in 1 file from a previous appointment
How Soon to Schedule appt/ **urgency**	Often need to schedule for same day, at least to test female's progesterone level so we don't miss the breeding
Length of appointment	If no progesterone level has been done, the test takes about _____ hours/ days from blood draw to results
Time to schedule	If a progesterone level is needed, do NOT schedule at the end of the shift if running in house
Dr to schedule with	
Request client to **bring** with them to appt	IF THEY ARE PLANNING TO BREED THE DAY OF THE APPOINTMENT, THEY MUST BRING BOTH THE MALE AND FEMALE WITH THEM. Recent Progesterone and Brucella test results. History of past breedings for both male and female
To **ask** client before appt	
Special **instructions** client should know about their appt	If we are unable to collect the stud dog's semen, the stud dog owner must give us consent to administer medication to aid him. If the stud dog proves to be unsuitable, do they have a "back-up" stud dog they can access or bring along?
New client	10 minutes in advance to complete paper work.
Finalizing – Urgency	Repeat Doctor, Time, Date, Phone number, Client & Doctor sense of Urgency and Reason – Emphasize this is ALL they are scheduled for

B-2. *Appointment scheduling for sick newborn*

Sick newborn appointment scheduling	
Reason for appointment	Puppies that are sick, crying inconsolably, having vomiting, diarrhea or coughing, losing weight, dehydrated or dying.
Ask client and pet name	Find out the name of the mother of the puppies and pull the file
How Soon to Schedule appt/ **urgency**	Sick babies are always urgent enough to see the day the client calls.
Length of appointment	30 minutes for 1st patient, 40 minutes for a litter
Time to schedule	Earliest available emergency slot
Dr to schedule with	
Request client to **bring** with them to appt	1. The entire litter, 2. A way to keep them warm and safe in transit, 3. Records on puppies or kittens weights, temps, vaccinations, worming, meds, diet fed etc. 4. ALWAYS BRING ALL THE DEAD PUPS OR KITTENS THEY HAVE FOR EXAMINATION AND POSSIBLE TESTING 5. The mother of the litter 6. Fresh fecal sample
To **ask** client before appt	1. Weights of pups 2. Urine color of pups 3. Rectal temperatures of pups
Special **instructions** client should know about their appt	Keep the live pups or kittens warm in transit by using a heating pad, an ice chest lined and covered with a towel to prop the lid open,
New client	10 minutes in advance to complete paper work.
Finalizing – Urgency	Repeat doctor, time, date, phone number, client & doctor sense of urgency and reason – emphasize this is all they are scheduled for

B-3. *Fee schedule and list of services*

Fee schedule for canine reproductive services	
Male Services	Fees
Pre-breeding exam	
Semen collection and evaluation (not to be frozen or stored)	
Brucella testing	
Teaser bitch fee	
Semen collection, storage, and freezing 1st visit	
1. File preparation – for each stud dog – first visit only	
2. Semen collection and freezing – first 4 breeding units	
3. Semen collection and freezing for each unit over first 4 at 1 visit	
4. Semen storage per year for up to 25 breeding units (pro-rated based on month frozen)	
5. DNA swab (only done if not previously tested)	
6. Brucella testing (must be done in past 6 months)	
7. Microchipping including registry (may be done in advance)	
Total fees for first visit for semen freezing	
Semen collection, storage and freezing subsequent visits	
1. Semen collection and freezing – first 4 breeding units at visit	
2. Semen collection and freezing for each unit over first 4 at 1 visit	
3. Teaser bitch fee	
Fresh chilled semen shipment	
1. Semen collection for fresh chilled	
2. Semen shipping pack for semen including extender	
3. Semen shipping overnight (estimated)	
4. Semen shipping add'l for Sat/Sun delivery (estimated)	
Total fees for fresh chilled semen shipment (range)	
Frozen semen shipment	
1. Semen shipping prep < 5 units	
2. Stat fee same day	
3. Stat fee 24 hour prep	
4. Stat fee 48 hour prep	
5. Nitrogen tank rental	
6. Tank shipping 2 way (estimate – dependent on destination)	
7. Nitrogen tank deposit – for out of country destinations	
Total fees for frozen semen shipment	
Overseas shipments – Requires research	

Female Services	Fees
Pre-breeding exam	
Progesterone testing	
Vaginal cytology	
Vaginal culture	
Brucella testing	
Artificial insemination	
Vaginal artificial insemination	
First AI/TCI	
Subsequent	
Weekend fees – doctor	
Technician assistant fee – for after hours or weekends	
Surgical Insemination	
1. Pre-surgical blood panel	
2. Semen Handling if frozen	
3. Semen Handling for incoming fresh chilled	
4. Semen Handling to collect and evaluate fresh semen at breeding	
5. Weekend fee – Doctor	
6. Technician assistant fee – for after hours or weekend	
7. Surgical breeding including anesthesia, post-op pain meds	
Total for surgical insemination – varies with type of semen, lab work done prior to surgery, add'l fee for weekends and holidays	
Ovuplant (need progesterone level w/in 24 hours pre-insertion)	
1. Insertion of ovuplant	
2. Removal of ovuplant at office visit (after natural or vag AI)	
3. Removal of ovuplant at surgical breeding	
Transcervical Insemination First/Additional	
Prenatal Care	
Ultrasound	
Radiograph for puppy count	
C-sections – includes pre-op lab work, IV catheter, post-op pain meds, neonatal resuscitation, reglan, calcium, wormer	
Post-natal care	
Taildocks and dewclaws – office visit and surgery pack $	
Dewclaws – Office visit and surgery pack $	
Sick puppies – exam fee, then add'l for diagnostics and meds	
Pre-sale puppy care	
Exams without vaccinations litter rate	
Exams with vaccinations litter rate	
Intestinal parasite screening	
Wormings	

Questions for evaluation of the bitch at home or at the hospital indicating the probable need for an Emergency C-section

1. Has the bitch been in hard labor (abdominal pushing) over 2 hours on the first or 1 hour on subsequent pups?
2. Did the bitch initially show good abdominal contractions and stop without producing a puppy?
3. Is there is green vaginal discharge PRIOR to the delivery of the first puppy?
4. Does the bitch seem distressed? Frantic? Sick? Weak or unable to stand? Tremoring? Repeated vomiting?
5. Is this labor pattern different than her previous ones?
6. Has the bitch been unwilling or unable to eat and/or drink for over 12 hours?
7. Has WhelpWise® indicated there is a problem with fetal heart rates (<160 BPM) or uterine contraction patterns?
8. Have any pups been born dead?
9. Did a previous radiograph or ultrasound suggest there could be a problem? (low heart rates on ultrasound or pups without visible heartbeats?) (Malpresented or very large pups)
10. Is a pup palpated on vaginal examination and in an unusual position or not progressing through the birth canal?
11. Did her temperature drop to 98 degrees and rise to normal (over 101.0) and stay there more than 4 hours?
12. Has her pregnancy exceeded 63 days?
13. Does she appear to have a very large or very small litter?
14. Does she have a previous history of dystocia?
15. Is she a breed at risk for maternal or fetal causes of dystocia?
16. Does she have unexplained or unusual discharge from her eyes?
17. Is she having weak or non-productive contractions with multiple puppies left?
18. If oxytocin has been used (more later), has there been a minimal or no response?
19. Does the breeder or veterinary staff member have a feeling that something is going wrong? Trust their intuition.

If the answer to any of these questions is yes, you very likely need to assess the bitch as soon as possible and advise your client that the bitch should proceed to emergency surgery unless you can immediately correct any cause for dystocia.

Your clinic information here

FEMALE   (Initials):_____

Reproduction Telephone Referral   Date/Time of call:_____   _____am/pm

Client Information:

Have we seen your Pet before? **Y** or **N**?   If Established client – **Please verify address, phone numbers and email address**

File #_____ Client's Name:_____

Client's phone # (____) _____ (h w c) Alternate # (____)_____ (h w c)
Available from____am/pm to____am/pm   Available from____am/pm to____am/pm

Mail address:_____   _____   _____   _____
                    Street or PO Box   City   State   Zip

E-Mail Address:_____   Info E-Mailed Y or N?

Referring DVM_____   DVM Phone # (_____) _____

Pet info:

Pet's name:_____ Breed:_____ D.O.B:_____

FEMALE INFORMATION: Is your Female in season **Y** or **N**?

Date Estrus Started?_____ Dates of last Estrus?_____to_____ Maiden ? # of Litters?_____

Type of Repro to be scheduled: Pre-Breeding, Prog/Lab, Natural, A/I, Fresh Chilled, Frozen, TCI, Surgical A/I, Ovuplant, Consult, Other_____

Where is the semen?_____
_____

Date	Time		Result	ng/dl	Laboratory	
		AM/PM		ng/dl		Lab used
		AM/PM		ng/dl		Lab used
		AM/PM		ng/dl		Lab used
		AM/PM		ng/dl		Lab used
		AM/PM		ng/dl		Lab used
		AM/PM		ng/dl		Lab used
		AM/PM		ng/dl		Lab used
		AM/PM		ng/dl		Lab used
Owner notified of date/time of breeding appt.					Ovulation Date Estimated	
					Breeding Planned	
					Whelping Date Estimated	

MALE (Initials):_____

Reproduction Telephone Referral   Date/Time of call:_____   _____am/pm
Client Information:
Have we seen your Pet before? Y or N?   If Established client–Please verify address, phone
                                                                    numbers and email address

File # _____ Client's Name: _____

Client's phone # (____) _____ (h w c) Alternate # (____)_____ (h w c)
Available from_____am/pm to _____ am/pm   Available from_____ am/pm to_____ am/pm

Mail address:_____ _____ _____ _____
                        Street or PO Box   City   State   Zip

E-Mail Address:_____   Info E-Mailed Y or N?

Referring DVM _____   DVM Phone # (_____) - _____ - _____

Pet info:
Pet's name:_____ Breed:_____ D.O.B:_____

Type of Repro to be scheduled: Pre-Breeding Exam, Collect/Analysis, Freeze, Storage,
Other_____

Remind to bring registry, DNA and Brucella test results to appointment

When are you planning to have this done? _____

Shipping Information: Incoming/ Outgoing/ Storage@_____/ N/A **(circle one)**

Ship from/ to Client/ Veterinarian/ Other_____ **Phone:**_____

Name of Facility/ Client_____

Address:_____ _____ _____ _____
                        Street or PO Box   **City**   **State**   **Zip**

Method of Shipment: U.P.S., FedEx, Airline Name, **Tracking #**_____

Brief History:_____
_____
_____

Recommendations/Plan:_____
_____
_____

B-6. *Telephone triage*

Your Veterinary Hospital Name here: Telephone Triage

Client Name:		Date of call:	
Client ID:	New? Y/N	Time of call:	
Pet's Name:		Age/Sex:	_____ M/Y/M/N/F/S
Primary Phone Number:	H/W/C	Available times:	
Alternate Phone Number:	(name) H/W/C	Available times:	
Email preferred? Y/N		Urgency of call:	High Medium Low

Reason for Call/ Symptoms	Last normal on_____ Temp?___ Duration of Symptoms
Attitude	Down/Lethargic/Weak /Not Eating/Not Drinking/ Wt Loss /Pain (1 2 3 4 5) (5=severe)/Normal Describe:
Urinary	Not urinating/PU/PD/Change in Urination: Inc/Dec/0/Blood/ Describe:
Cardiovascular	Distressed/Not breathing normally/Coughing/Sneezing/Discharge/Panting/Fainting Abnormal Noise Describe:
GI	Bloat/Vomiting/Diarrhea/Eating Less/Not Eating/Ate FB, Toxin, other/Constipated Describe:
Eye R/L/Both	FB/Squinting/Red/Rubbing/3rd eyelid/Eyelid/Discharge/Eye protruding/Pain/Blind/ Color change Describe:
Ear R/L/Both	Discharge /Red/Swollen/Pain(1 2 3 4 5)(5=severe) /Odor/L/R/Deaf/ Describe:
Skin	Laceration/Hot spot/Lump/Rash/Lesions/Itchy (1 2 3 4 5)(5=severe)/Fleas/Ticks/Hair loss Describe:
Leg/Back RF/LF/RR/LR	Down/Paralyzed/3 legged Lame/Limping/Hunched/Pain (1 2 3 4 5)(5=severe)/Chiro Describe:
Reproduction	In Labor: Y/N/ Pup stuck?/Pups born # _____ /No pups born yet/Discharge Green/Red/ In labor since _____ /Time last pup born/Number of pups lost_____ Due to whelp: _____ Based on US/Rads/Progesterone? Currently trying to breed:_____ Natural/Fresh AI/Shipped/Frozen Timing done this cycle? Vag Cyt/Progesterone/Stud Date_____ Results___ Planning to breed this cycle & now in heat:_____ Need to ship semen:_____ Planning to breed or freeze in the future:_____ Accidental breeding:_____ Male reproductive problem:_____ Female reproductive problem:_____ Other:
Litters: Born on:_____	Symptoms:_____ Sick since?_____ Number in litter?_____ Any pups/kittens lost?_____ Treatment?_____ Temperature?_____ Urine color?_____ Stool Character_____ Weights taken_____ Water?_____ Feeding since/ what?_____ Worming history_____ Vaccination History_____
Client's Request	☐ Reason for call back: Appointment/Lab Results/US or Rad Results/Surgery/Post-op / Euthanasia/ Refill w Appt/Refill wo Appt/Diet change/Billing/Estimate/Complaint/Other ☐ Phone Call from Doctor/Tech/Repro Department/Receptionist/ Practice Manger/ Individual Requested to return call:_____ ☐ Appointment: ASAP/Specific Date & Time Range Preferred_____ ☐ Client will call us back? _____ ☐ Appointment Scheduled for Date_____ Time_____ ☐ Declined

Appendix C: Client information

Veterinary Clinic Name Here

ARTIFICIAL INSEMINATION USING FRESH CHILLED AND FROZEN STORED CANINE SEMEN

For approximately 40 years, veterinarians have had the technology to freeze or chill semen for insemination at a remote time and/or distance. But for most of this time, our success in turning these breedings into pregnancies has been limited by our ability to pinpoint the exact moment in time that the insemination should occur. Recently, more accurate and more accessible progesterone testing has increased our success in producing pregnancies with distant inseminations.

FRESH CHILLED SEMEN COLLECTION TO BE SHIPPED TO A REMOTE SITE:

1. Contact the veterinarians office as early in the bitch's estrus as possible to assure staff and shipping methods are available when needed. Be sure the recipient's address (typically a veterinary clinic) is available.
2. Confirm the dog and bitch are both in good health, have had health screening, such as OFA and CERF, completed in advance, negative Brucella tests in the past 3 months, and are current on immunizations and preventive worming. Consider having a semen analysis done on the male to be used to assure he is currently fertile.
3. Upon confirmation of the date(s) the semen is to be shipped, call to schedule an appointment. Collections for shipment are best done early in the day to allow adequate time for courier service to arrange for pickup. This will help assure timely delivery of the semen. The semen, once collected, is viable for 24 to 36 hours; delayed insemination reduces the chance of a breeding resulting in a pregnancy. The inseminating veterinarian also needs time to schedule the bitch for insemination.
4. Inform the veterinary clinic if additional semen shipments are requested. Typically, using fresh chilled semen, two collections are made and shipped.
5. DNA testing of the stud dog is now required (if not previously done) to register the litter with the AKC. This test is a simple cheek swab, collected at the appointment. Your signature and payment are required for submission to the AKC. A color DNA certificate, which includes your dog's DNA profile number, will be mailed directly to you.
6. Complete the AKC paperwork for insemination with fresh chilled semen at the first shipment. You will need your dog's registered name and AKC number and, if previously DNA profiled, his DNA profile number. You should provide the AKC registered name and number of the bitch as well.
7. The owner of the bitch usually pays fees for the service of collecting and shipping the semen. This is best handled by credit card and must be paid prior to shipping the semen. Charges are as follows:
    A. Fee to collect the stud dog, handle and evaluate the ejaculate: Fee $____
    B. Fee for specialized packaging and shipping media: Fee $____
    C. Fee for shipping: Usually ship by FedEx or UPS overnight. If the owner of the bitch requests another courier, they will need to contact us directly with arrangements. If same day service is required or necessary, such as on weekend or holidays, the owner of the dog or bitch must make arrangements to transport the semen to the airport and select the airline and flight to be used. Known shipper status is required. The airline should be aware that the box contains canine semen and ice packs (not dry ice), as not all airlines will accept these contents.
    D. Fee for teaser bitch if the stud dog owner does not provide one: Fee if available.

Remember, at times, delays in receiving the semen can occur due to problems with inclement weather, lost or misdirected shipments, etc. Keep in mind, this is an inconvenience and may interfere with a successful pregnancy as the outcome, but at least it was only a lost box and not your prized dog, which was lost or delayed. You can always arrange for an additional shipment if notified of this minor catastrophe and if you ship the replacement counter-to-counter, you can typically make up for the lost time of the original next day air shipment. It is the responsibility of the stud dog or brood bitch owner to track the shipment and make sure it arrives on time. The veterinary clinic will provide you with the tracking number.

FRESH CHILLED SEMEN COLLECTION TO BE SHIPPED TO YOU:
1. Prior to the expected estrus, your bitch should have vaccinations updated, worming completed, and a complete physical examination. A breeding history will be taken, and vaginal exams and cultures done if indicated. A Brucella test should be run within the 3 months prior to breeding. Health screening tests such as OFA, CERF, etc. should have been completed in advance. At the time estrus begins, it is not possible to initiate testing and receive results in time for a breeding. The same should hold true for the stud dog – Brucella testing, OFA, CERF, etc. It is also preferred that he should have recently sired a litter or has had a semen analysis performed.
2. Contact the veterinarian's office at the first sign your bitch is in estrus. It is best to see her in the first 5 days for a vaginal cytology to assess that she is truly early in her cycle and has not come into estrus silently. Plan sequential vaginal cytologies and progesterone testing based on this cytology and her reproductive history.
3. At this time, you can contact the collecting veterinarian to ascertain how the semen will be stored and shipped and provide them with the hospital address and phone number for shipping. In some cases, they will have supplies in stock at their hospital. In other cases, you may prefer having the veterinary clinic send out a semen shipment kit to the stud dog owner's veterinarian. These charges will be put on your credit card.
4. Be sure the collecting veterinarian has experience in collecting semen or if not, contact them with detailed information on semen collection and handling. Be sure your stud dog owner's collecting veterinarian labels the TUBE with their name, the dog's name, AKC number, and date and time of collection. Many clinics receive a number of samples unlabeled and when multiple semen shipments are received on the same day, the clinic need to be able to identify the correct semen is being used on your bitch. Ask the stud dog owner to see the sample prior to packaging if necessary to be sure this is done.
5. At the time ovulation is about to occur (based on a progesterone level of 4 to 8 ng/ml), the veterinarian will advise you to contact the owner of the stud dog to arrange for collection and shipment. On weekdays, an overnight courier service such as FedEx or UPS can be used. On holidays and weekends, airline counter-to-counter or the US Postal Service needs to be used. At shipment, you should request the air bill or tracking numbers should a shipment need to be tracked.
6. Arrange an appointment for your bitch to come in for insemination. The insemination is usually done vaginally and is best repeated in 24 to 48 hours to improve the chances of conception. She should be encouraged to urinate prior to insemination and kept quiet/crated for 2 hours post-insemination.
7. The collecting veterinarian may have a regular courier service established for overnight delivery. If so, it is probably easiest to use their normal system. If they do not routinely use one courier, you may wish to contact several to determine fees, pick up and delivery times, etc. Some to consider are FedEx, UPS, or the US Postal Service
   On holidays or weekends, counter-to-counter at the airlines must be used. You will need to arrange to have the shipment at the airport at least 2 hours prior to departure to get the shipment loaded. All airlines need to be individually checked. Shipper must have known shipper status with any airline you use. You and the owner of the stud dog are responsible for travel to and from the airport.
   Be sure to state, if you are questioned, that you are shipping canine semen in a Styrofoam shipper on ice packs (no dry ice is used – this is a hazardous material). In some situations, the USPS will do weekend and holiday pickups and deliveries, but this is not available at all locations, so you need to call ahead to assess service availability.

8. Twenty four to 28 days post-insemination, we recommend your bitch be palpated and/or ultrasounded to establish is she has become pregnant. This is an important piece of medical information to establish a reproductive history. If she is pregnant, this is the time to change her diet to a high quality performance diet, line up supplies for whelping, arrange for someone to be available for whelping assistance.
9. Fees for this service are as follows:
    A. Serial vaginal cytologies and progesterone levels: Fee per sample $____
    B. Fee for inseminations(s) of the bitch: Fee for the first, Fee subsequent $____
    C. Fee for transcervical insemination: Fee per insemination. $____
    D. Fee for palpation/ultrasound/x-rays to confirm pregnancy: Fee $____
    E. Fee to the collecting veterinarian for collection, shipping medium and packaging, and shipment: varies so ask for a quote.
    F. Brucella test: Fee to draw and run the sample. $____

COLLECTING SEMEN FOR FREEZING:
1. Complete all health screenings for your stud dog including such evaluations as CERF and OFA. Have a recent Brucella test (within the past 3 months or since the prior breeding) and semen evaluation. Have a complete physical examination including a digital prostate exam, to assure he is in good general health. The ideal time to freeze semen is prior to the dog's aging (at 2 to 7 years of age) as semen quality is usually better and will yield a higher quality freeze but older dogs have been frozen successfully.
2. Bring a COPY of the dog's AKC certificate. We will also need a side and front photograph – if you do not have these, take digital photos at the appointment for collection
3. Complete DNA testing for AKC (required) if not previously done. This test is a simple cheek swab. Your signature and a check for are required for submission to the AKC. A color DNA certificate, which includes your dog's DNA profile number, will be mailed directly to you.
4. Contact the office to confirm staff and teaser bitch availability. Schedule an appointment.
5. Fees are itemized as follows:
    A. Complete physical examination if not completed at our office in the past 3 months: Fee $____
    B. Fee to set up the file: Fee to collect the stud dog Fee to handle, evaluate, freeze and store for 1 year Fee for up to 4 vials of semen (total Fee): $____
    C. Fee for each vial above 4: Fee $____
    D. Fee for additional collections: Fee $____
    E. Brucella test: Fee $____
    F. Fee for the teaser bitch if you do not provide your own: Fee if available. $____
    G. Fee for storage of up to 30 vials per dog after the first year: Fee $____
6. To release the semen, you as the stud dog or semen owner MUST contact the office directly. You must have the "Semen Release Form" completed and mailed or faxed back to us at least 3 days prior to the requested shipping date. Only then can the semen be released to the owner of the bitch. In addition, your account must show a zero balance in order for frozen semen to be released for shipment. Notify the veterinarian early in the bitch's estrous cycle to minimize costs.
7. You will also need to contact the veterinarian with the name, address and telephone number of the shipment destination – typically a veterinary clinic. Specify how many vials or straws of semen you want shipped. You will need credit card number from the owner of the bitch to cover the associated costs. Without this, the clinic will either need to bill your account or delay shipping of the semen until fees are paid in full.
8. Fees to release and ship the semen are itemized as follows:
A. Fee for semen release: Fee for up to 5 vials, Fee per vial above 5. $____
B. Additional fee for semen release with less than 3 days notice: Fee. $____
C. Tank rental: Fee for first 7 days. $____
D. Overnight shipment or counter-to-counter shipment of semen in the portable semen tank: Fee $____
E. Second day return shipment of portable semen shipping tank: Fee. Include a return shipping label so return shipping is simplified. $____

F. Insurance on semen tank valued at Fee $____
G. Deposit on semen tank: Fee $____
H. Additional rental for failure to return tank within 7 days: Fee per day. $____

PAYMENT IS DUE UPON RELEASE OF THE SEMEN – NO CREDIT WILL BE EXTENDED FOR THIS SERVICE. The bitch owner usually pays shipping costs, and that can best be handled by credit card. However, the semen owner is ultimately responsible for all costs in the event that the bitch owner fails to reimburse us for the shipping or fails to return the tank.

Remember to regard your frozen semen as a finite and valuable asset. Release it with forethought. It should remain viable for many years – make arrangements accordingly in your will.

BREEDING YOUR BITCH WITH FROZEN SEMEN:
Breeding with frozen semen is less forgiving, more complicated and more expensive than other breedings. It can also be very rewarding utilizing the genetics of stud dogs of a by-gone era.
REMEMBER THESE HIGH POINTS:
- You are using semen that is expensive and is likely limited in availability. Use this finite resource wisely.
- Timing the bitch's cycle must be precise, and the insemination window is approximately 12 to 24 hours.
- Anesthesia and surgery are used for most frozen inseminations. Consider the benefits vs. the risks before embarking on this.
1. As with any breeding, be sure your bitch has current vaccinations, has her pre-breeding screening, and is in good health. You may wish to do this type of breeding only with a young bitch who has successfully completed a pregnancy. Aged bitches tend to release fewer eggs and have decreased fertility. A breeding history will be taken and vaginal exams and cultures done if indicated. A Brucella test should be done in the past 3 months.
2. Arrange for the frozen semen to be released prior to your bitch's heat or early in her cycle. The owner of the semen, usually the stud dog owner, must sign a release form. Shipping costs from the storage facility must be paid prior to shipping and can usually be paid with a credit card. The owner of the bitch usually will pay the release fee, overnight shipping to us, portable semen shipping tank rental, and return shipping of the tank to the storage facility.
3. Contact the veterinarian's office at the FIRST SIGN that your bitch is in heat. Her first appointment should be in the first 6 days of her estrus for a vaginal cytology to confirm that she is early in her estrus. Plan sequential vaginal cytologies and progesterone testing based on this cytology and her reproductive history.
4. Progesterone tests should be run approximately every 48 hours as ovulation nears. An LH level can also be run if requested in advance. LH levels can be helpful in timing the bitch but must be run every 24 hours so can be costly.
5. Pre-surgical blood work should be drawn at one of these visits in preparation for anesthesia.
6. Schedule your bitch for anesthesia and surgical insemination or TCI. For surgical insemination she will receive general anesthesia. A midline incision is made similar to that for a spay, the uterus will be exteriorized, and examined, semen placed in the lumen, the uterus repositioned into the abdomen, and the abdominal wall and skin closed. She will be recovered from anesthesia and discharged the same day. The entire visit typically takes about 2 hours from admission to discharge. You are welcome to wait in the lobby or return later for her. She should be kept quiet and crated for a minimum of 4 hours post-op. She should rest for several days post-op.
7. At day 24 to 28, ultrasound her for early diagnosis of pregnancy (see earlier section on ultrasound)

Emergency milk replacers for puppies and kittens:

The formulas below are specific for either puppies or kittens and one should not be substituted for the other because of differences in nutritional needs. In general, these formulas should only be used as short-term support for the neonates until a commercially available formula can be obtained. The formulas below lack adequate nutritional support for long-term feeding.

Homemade Puppy Milk Replacer Formula

120 ml (4 oz) of cow's or goat's milk, pasteurized

120 (4 oz) ml of water

   2 to 4 raw egg yolks, pasteurized if available

   1 to 2 teaspoonful vegetable oil

   1000 mg calcium carbonate (3-4 tums)

Homemade Kitten formula

   90 ml (3 oz) of condensed milk (canned, not evaporated)

   90 ml (3 oz) of water

   120 ml (4 oz) of plain yogurt (not the low-fat)

   3 large or 4 small egg yolks, pasteurized if available

List of items to take for a C-section

- The pregnant dog in need of the C-section
- Cell phone
- Tarp, shower curtain, or vinyl tablecloth to cover the seats or floor of the car
- Crate large enough for the pregnant bitch to travel in
- Large Vari-Kennel crate with top 1/2 removed, which easily gives you access to the bitch or preferred a baby pool
- 3 Blankets for inside crate or pool. One for the way down, then a clean one for the return home and a smaller one that will go on top of the heating pad. The heating pad is between the blankets. Cover the bitch and puppies with a large towel on the return home everything covered except the bitches head so there are no drafts on the puppies, or you can clip a towel over most of the crate, allowing room for easy access if needed
- Heating pad – take two, one for the crate/pool for the return ride home and one for in the basket. Adapter to plug into
- Hot water bottle – take one just in case something happens and the heating pads don't work
- Plastic laundry basket – to use after puppies are cleaned up and getting ready to leave the clinic
- Towels – plenty of them!! Hand towels and full size bath size towels
- Small garbage bag
- Paper towels
- Kleenex – especially good for wiping puppies
- Cotton balls, Q-Tips, and cotton gauze squares
- Nolvasan (properly diluted and ready to use)
- Puppy formula mixed – in a seal tight container and enough to feed litter if needed before leaving the clinic. If bringing a premixed can, remember a container to heat the formula in, and a lid for the remaining unused portion in the can.
- Feeding tube and syringe (sterilized and ready to use)
- Bulb syringe and DeLee mucus trap – for suctioning puppies if needed
- Hemostat
- Dental floss – incase you need to re-tie an umbilical
- Water
- Water dish for bitch, and or a squirt bottle of water
- Cooler
- Ice (bring ice just in case you have a bleeding dewclaw) or Quick-Stop or Antiseptic powder, or all of the above
- First aid kit

C-4. *Ovuplant and cabergoline client information sheet*
Client Handout for ovulation timing

Deslorelin (Ovuplant®) = NEW Way to Control the Timing of Your Bitch's Heat Cycle

Technology advances again and has now allowed us to either delay or induce estrous (heat) cycles in bitches with more ease and accuracy than ever before.

Ovuplant® (2.1 mg) is a hormone contained in a pellet. It is labeled for use only in horses. This pellet is inserted under the mucosa of the vulva. For this product to be effective in inducing estrous, the bitch MUST have a progesterone level of less than 1.0 ng/dl immediately prior to insertion of the drug pellet or it may block, not induce estrous.

Typically, the patient will come into heat within 3 to 7 days, and be ready to breed 8 to 10 days after she comes into season (11 to 17 days after insertion). The implanted drug pellet MUST be removed to maintain pregnancy. This is a prescription drug and must be inserted and removed by a veterinarian. Approximately 90% of the time, the use of this product allows you to have control over the time you breed. This can be valuable for bringing bitches into heat for travel, specialties, to avoid scheduling conflicts in your personal life, or to produce puppies when you need them, such as for futurities.

Cabergoline (Dostinex®) is a similar product, given orally. Approximately 70% of bitches taking the product will start estrous within 10 to 30 days of starting the drug. This is dosed at 5 mcg/kg once daily for 10 days. In small bitches, compounding may be necessary to scale the dose down.

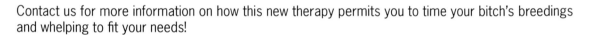

Contact us for more information on how this new therapy permits you to time your bitch's breedings and whelping to fit your needs!

• Please return for removal of the Ovuplant after breeding is completed.

Veterinary Clinic Contact information

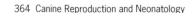

- PREVENTION OF ESTRUS with Mibolerone (formerly marketed as Cheque®) Drops
- Mibolerone drops can be used to prevent estrous. This can be helpful in delaying estrous in bitches who tend to have abnormally short periods between heat cycles or who are competing in dog events and should be kept out of heat to maximize their performance. It can also be used to allow you to time her litters. By preventing estrous cycles, we can preserve the uterine lining of bitches, in many cases allowing them to remain fertile longer than if they were cycling frequently and aging their uterine lining. Mibolerone drops are a testosterone derivative, NOT progesterone.
- This is a prescription drug that must be compounded for your use.

Mibolerone Dosages

Weight in pounds	Mcg/day
1-25	30
25-50	60
50-100	120
>100	180
German Shepherds	180

- The average bitch after going off Mibolerone drops comes into heat after 70 days. The hormone must be administered daily or break-through will occur.
- She should have a liver panel blood test run prior to starting Mibolerone and every 3 to 6 months. Frequently, there is an increase in liver enzymes from the hormone.
- Side effects from Mibolerone drops:
  - One percent tear from the eyes;
  - They tend to muscle up and grow more coat, because it's a male hormone derivative.
  - Frequently, they accumulate mucous around the vulva similar to puppy vaginitis. This can be mistaken as pyometra. However, a bitch on Mibolerone cannot hormonally develop pyometra. If your bitch is on Mibolerone, be sure your vet knows! (dogs with family members and handlers!!!)

- It is safe for a bitch to be bred on the first cycle she has after completing mibolerone therapy.
- Mibolerone should not be used prior to a bitch's first estrous cycle or for more than 3 to 24 months.

- Please return for a liver panel in _____ when on Mibolerone drops.

- The prescribing veterinarian should do Due diligence on the compounding pharmacy compounding this product

C-6. *Puppy weights*

Newborn Puppy Data Sheet for _____ (Date)

Dam: _____ Sire: _____ Born on: _____

Puppy ID	AM Weight	PM Weight	% Change	AM Temp	PM Temp	AM Urine Color	PM Urine Color	Stool character	Feedings?	ENS	Notes

C-7. *Tail dock and dewclaw surgery report*

Taildock and dewclaw surgery report

Date _____ Clinician _____ Staff _____

Client Name _____ Client ID _____ Name of Dam _____

Puppy ID	Temp	Weight	Heart Rate	Resp Rate	MM Color / CRT	Urine Color/ SG	Stool Character	Owner concerns	Feedings/ Therapy Given	PE Findings	Dewclaws Front/Rear	Tail length
1												
2												
3												
4												
5												
6												
7												
8												
9												
10												
11												
12												
13												
14												
15												
16												

Surgical procedure: Sterile pack/ sterile gloves

Taildock – clipped, prepped with Nolvasan/no local anesthesia/local block with _____

Length measured: _____ Scissors vertical/horizontal

Sutured with _____ / Pattern _____

Dewclaws - Sterile pack/ sterile gloves/ closed with nexaband/vetbond/ _____

Technician/Assistant _____

Signature of doctor _____ DVM

Individual puppy data sheet

Puppy ID:		Date of Birth:		Time:	am/pm
Sire:		Dam:			
Registration Number:		Sex:			
Registered Name:		Microchip Number:			
Breed:		Color:			

Day	Date	Weight	ENS	Deworm	Day	Date	Weight	Deworm	Vaccinate
1					17				
2					18				
3					19				
4					20				
5					21				
6					22				
7					23				
8					24				
9					25				
10					26				
11					27				
12					28				
13					35				
14					42				
15					49				
16					56				

Photos:

Head View	Right Side View	Left Side View	Top View

Buyers Information:

Buyer's Names:	
Buyer's Address:	
Buyer's Phone Numbers:	
Buyer's E mail	
Contract? Yes/No	
Summary of contract terms:	

Notes: _____

ITEMS TO HAVE AVAILABLE PRIOR TO WHELPING

1. Whelping box or Whelping Nest Lovett's Heated Whelping Nest®
2. Towels and sheets
3. Newspapers
4. Bulb syringe – to suction mouths of newborns – available at most stores with a pharmacy department.
5. DeLee® Mucus Trap – to suction newborn's airways - available on line from suppliers of midwives or from WhelpWise.
6. Exam gloves, latex or vinyl – to protect breeders from vaginal discharges and placental fluids – available OTC many places.
7. K-Y jelly– to lubricate gloves if vaginal examination is indicated – available OTC many places.
8. Hemostat to clamp off umbilical cords – available from your veterinary suppliers
9. Suture or dental floss– to tie off umbilical cords – available from your suppliers (suture) or OTC many places.
10. Scissors
11. Tincture of Iodine, - to treat the umbilicus at birth, 2 and 8 hours post partum.
12. Chlorhexidine disinfectant solution – to disinfect surfaces in the whelping and nursery areas - available through your veterinary suppliers or local farm stores.
13. Heat source such as heating pads or hot water bottles
14. Ice chest or laundry basket to transport or separate puppies Heating pads, rice bags, or Snuggle Safe – to keep pups warm during sorting – heating pads often have safety shut-offs so are difficult to keep warm. Rice bags are stockinette or socks filled with long-grain white cooking rice microwaved to warm pups. Snuggle Safe® – a microwaveable disc made to warm puppies, available on line.
13. Goat's milk, pasteurized or Puppy formula and
14. Feeding tube and syringe to fit or baby bottle with preemie nipple
15. Cotton balls
16. Thermometer, rectal
17. Thermometer, to check room temperature
18. Gauze
19. Scale in oz or grams
20. Plastic sheets or vinyl tablecloths with flannel backing to cover the floor
21. Ice cream, vanilla for her, your choice of other flavors for humans
22. 25 gauge needle for acupuncture – for stimulation to breath
23. Spray bottle for cleaning
24. Paper toweling
25. Oxygen tank, regulator, hosing and plastic box to serve as oxygen chamber or oxygen concentrator
26. Dopram injections pre-drawn into syringes 1 per puppy anticipated (controversial but better than losing a pup) – to administer to pups that cannot be resuscitated by clearing airways and with mechanical stimulation - available through your veterinary suppliers.
27. Pyrantel Pamoate – to worm the bitch and pups at 2, 4, 6, and 8 weeks post-partum as recommended by CAPC - available through your veterinary suppliers.
28. Stethoscope – to assess newborns for a heartbeat - available through your veterinary suppliers or on line.
29. Fetal Doppler – to monitor fetal heart rates during late pregnancy and whelping - available on line at Whelpwise or some clients have their own.

Letter to client who will be using another clinic for pre-breeding pregesterone testing.

Thank you for contacting us to assist you in breeding your dog.

Prior to breeding, we recommend your bitch be in good physical condition, be current on vaccinations, parasite free, and have her health screenings completed.

Progesterone levels are the backbone of timing bitches for breeding. This is essential for special need bitches with a history of infertility or missed breedings, pregnancies that did not go to completion, or bitches who will be bred using fresh chilled (shipped) or frozen semen. Progesterone testing is also useful in determining when a bitch should be receptive for a natural breeding in cases where either the female or male is reluctant to breed. Additionally, knowing her progesterone levels at the time of breeding allows us to predict within 24 hours when she should whelp. This information can save money, time, and puppies.

As soon as you notice your bitch is in season, please contact us. If you are planning to use frozen or fresh chilled semen, it is helpful if you have notified us in advance. We can assist you in arranging shipment of the frozen semen prior to the start of her heat cycle. We can also help you arrange for supplies and manage the details of shipping fresh semen.

The first progesterone level should be drawn on day 6 of her heat cycle. If she has a history of short cycles, the first progesterone should be drawn at the first sign of estrus. We then recommend you repeat the progesterone testing every 2 to 3 days until her progesterone rises to 3 ng/dl; it should be repeated the next day. A progesterone of 3 ng/dl indicates she is very close to ovulation.

Ovulation occurs when the progesterone is 5 ng/dl. We like to have at least one more progesterone 2 to 3 days after her progesterone reaches or exceeds 5 ng/dl to assure she has completed her ovulation. We typically breed 2 days after 5 ng/dl if using fresh or fresh chilled semen. We typically breed 3 days after 5 ng/dl if using frozen semen IF the progesterone reaches or exceeds 20 ng/dl. Many bitches will have a progesterone level of 15 to 40 ng/dl at the time of the breeding; this is normal. We breed 7 days a week, including holidays, based on your bitch's ideal time for breeding.

We can usually run progesterone levels in our hospital with results available within the hour. If you live a distance away, it is often more convenient to have these drawn and submitted to the lab by your local veterinarian. As we will assist in interpreting the results and timing the breeding, your local veterinarian may prefer not to be involved in any aspect other than submitting the samples for you and providing us with a lab tracking number.

The following are guidelines to assist your veterinarian in submitting blood samples for progesterone levels:

1. Submit the sample to _____ Laboratory for a Canine Progesterone assay whenever possible. Include the date and TIME the sample was drawn on the requisition form. The sample should be placed in a non-barrier tube (not an SST tube), spun down, and the serum transferred into a transport tube. In-office semi-quantitative tests (such as ICG or Camelot Farms) are not accurate enough to use for this situation. You may contact your local human hospital and have a progesterone level run there as they are not species specific. We prefer the results from _____ as they have proven to be reliable and repeatable.

2. Draw and submit the first sample on day 6 of the bitch's cycle. Draw the sample on day 3 of her cycle if she has been brought into heat with medication or has a short proestrus. If the first date is not known, submit at the earliest time you are contacted by the client.

3. Subsequent tests are run approximately every 2 to 3 days but this will vary based on the results and the day of the week upon which this falls. Call us if you have any questions about when to re-sample the patient.

4. Please mark the Laboratory form to fax (or call) the results to us and your clinic as soon as you receive them. Our fax number is _____. Baseline levels, less than 2 ng/dl, can wait until the next working day (use _____ phone or _____ fax). **ANY RESULT OVER 2.5 SHOULD BE CALLED TO US AS SOON AS POSSIBLE (_____) AS THIS REPRESENTS A RISE IN THE PROGESTERONE LEVEL AND SIGNIFIES ACTION WILL BE TAKING PLACE SOON.** We breed 2 to 3 days after the progesterone level begins to rise above 5ng/dl. In many bitches, this rise can be very rapid. As we will need at least 24 hours notice for shipping semen, timely receipt of the results is important. Great communication between our office, your office, and your client is critical at this point to achieve a successful breeding. Your client will appreciate having someone who knows their dog handle the blood testing.

5. The laboratory runs/does not run the tests and reports results even on evenings, weekends and holidays.

6. If the results will be received by your office on a holiday or weekend, **PLEASE CALL _____ WITH THE NAME & PHONE NUMBER OF YOUR CLIENT AND THE lab requisition number SO WE CAN RETREIVE THE RESULTS OUTSIDE OF REGULAR OFFICE HOURS.** This will keep us from having to interrupt your weekend plans.

For ANY bitch that will be anesthetized for a surgical insemination or any non-surgical bitch over 6 or with a history of chronic health problems, we recommend a complete blood panel with chemistries and CBC be drawn in advance of the procedure. If not previously run, we will run this test in house on the day of breeding. We recommend that a Brucellosis test be run prior to breeding **_ANY_** dog or bitch.

It is our goal to make your breeding as simple and successful as possible. Please contact us if you have any questions.

Sincerely,

_____ DVM

your hospital information here:

C-11. *Vaccine recommendations*

Age/Date Next Visit	Examination	Vaccinations	Heartworm Test and Other Lab Tests	Medications	Other
2 and 4 Weeks	As needed	–	–	Pyrantel Pamoate	–
6 to 8 Weeks	Veterinary Puppy Visit #1	DAPP(No Lepto)	Fecal No Heartworm test due	Heartworm preventive with pyrantel q 4 weeks, with pyrantel 2 weeks later Flea/Tick Control*	
9 to 11 Weeks Due	Veterinary Puppy Visit #2	DAPP(No Lepto) Bordetella	Fecal No Heartworm test due	Heartworm preventive with pyrantel q 4 weeks, with pyrantel 2 weeks later Flea/Tick Control*	Obedience Class
12 to 16 Weeks due	Veterinary Puppy Visit #3	DAPP/Lepto 4 way* Lyme* Rabies Canine influenza vaccination*	Fecal No Heartworm test due	Heartworm preventive wormer Flea/Tick Control* Pyrantel pamoate fenbendazole	Vaccinations may be divided so fewer are administered at each visit Large Breed: X-ray hips for laxity
16 to 20 Weeks due	Comprehensive	DAPP/Lepto 4 way* Lyme* Canine influenza vaccination*	Fecal No Heartworm test due	Heartworm preventive Flea/Tick Control*	
2 weeks after last vaccination	Distemper/Parvo Titer Blood test		Titer for Distemper and Parvovirus	Recommended to assess response to vaccination	Repeat boosters if low or no response to previous vaccinations
6 Months or older	Presurgical	Complete series if not yet done	Presurgical blood test, Heartworm test if not on preventive	Heartworm preventiveFlea/Tick Control*	Spay/Neuter – if appropriated medically or dependent on owner's plans. Microchip
15 Months due	Comprehensive	DAPP/Lepto* Rabies Bordetella Lyme* Canine Influenza*	Heartworm test	Heartworm preventive Flea/Tick Control*	

* Varies with region of the country

Your clinic information here

<table>
<tr><td>C-section Discharge
Instructions</td><td>Date_____
Client _____
Patient _____</td></tr>
</table>

Restraint	❏ Please protect your pet when leaving the hospital by using either a leash and collar or a pet carrier. Excessive activity may result in injury, or a slower recovery than we would expect from a pet that is kept quiet during the healing process. ❏ Please remove the bandage covering the IV site on your pet's front leg upon arrival home.
Food and Water	With the excitement of returning home, your pet may be inclined to drink and eat excessively, which will most likely result in vomiting. **To avoid this, we ask that you remove your pet's food and water dishes for an hour until your pet has settled down. Then, only allow small amounts of food and water for the first day home.** ❏ Offer only half your pet's normal food and water tonight. Normal feeding may resume tomorrow. ❏ Do not offer food/water until_____. ❏ Feed _____ _____ times a day. ❏ Offer _____ to drink _____ times a day. ❏ Tube feed your puppies _____ cc/ml _____ times a day with _____. See handout. Keep them in a warm location. Their rectal temperature should be 96 to 98° F prior to feeding.
Eliminations	❏ Your pet may need to be reminded to go outside to urinate during the first evening home. Many patients may not have a bowel movement for 24 to 36 hours after surgery. This is normal. ❏ The puppies may need to be stimulated to urinate and defecate until mom is ready to care for them. ❏ The pup's urine should be very pale yellow in color and the stools should be soft, yellow and seedy looking.
Exercise and Activity	❏ Patients recovering from surgery or illness need limited activity to heal properly. Due to the effects of anesthesia, your pet may be groggy for the next 12 hours. Avoid access to stairs or situations that may lead to injury during this time. ❏ Your pet may resume normal activity in _____ days. ❏ NO swimming, bathing or grooming for 10 to 14 days. ❏ Your pet should be confined indoors, and taken outside on a short leash only for eliminations for _____ days. ❏ We recommend that you DO NOT leave your bitch unattended with the puppies until you are certain that she will not harm them. ❏ The pups should have their temperatures taken, urine color checked and weighed once daily at the same time every day. ❏ Early Neurologic Stimulation should be performed from day 3 to day 16 once daily on the pups.
Medications	❏ If dispensed, it is important to carefully follow the directions that are printed on the label. ❏ No medications dispensed. ❏ Medications dispensed for post op discomfort _____. Next dose due_____. ❏ Medications dispensed for increasing milk production Reglan® or Domperidone. ❏ Next dose _____ cc /tabs _____ times a day due at _____. ❏ Additional meds:_____. Next dose due_____ ❏ Worm the puppies & bitch once every other week with Strongid® for mom & Nemex® for pups starting at 2 weeks of age. ❏ **DO NOT ADMINISTER ASPIRIN WITHIN 2 WEEKS OF THE ABOVE PRESCRIBED MEDICATION**

Sutures and Bandages	In order for incisions to heal, your pet must not lick at the sutures, or the incision site. If your pet is licking, please notify us immediately. Please check the incision twice daily for any redness, swelling, or discharge. If it appears irritated or infected, please notify us immediately. Rechecks of post-op patients will be at no charge during regular office hours. ❏ Sutures/staples need to be removed 10 to 14 days after surgery. A short appointment is needed. ❏ Sutures are underneath the skin/gums, and will absorb over the next several weeks. They do not need to be removed. ❏ Apply warm compress to the surgical site 3 times daily for 10 minutes each time. ❏ Apply Tincture of Iodine to the umbilicus of each puppy 2 hours, 8 hours and 24 hours after birth. ❏ Clean the incision with hydrogen peroxide if necessary.
Appointments	Please make an appointment for the following: ❏ Suture removal in 10 to 14 days. ❏ Dewclaw removal and/or tail docks in _____ days. Appointment Time_____ ❏ Vaccinations and health exams in _____ weeks. Appointment Time_____
Monitor	A decrease in activity and/or appetite for the first 24 to 36 hours may be observed. However, if your pet exhibits any of the following symptoms, please notify the clinic immediately: ❏ Loss of appetite for over 36 hours ❏ Weakness or depression ❏ Refusal to drink for over 24 hours ❏ Vomiting and/or diarrhea ❏ The vaginal discharge should be small amounts of thick blood, changing to gray. If it is excessive or has a foul odor, call us.
Special Instructions	_____

AS ALWAYS, PLEASE CALL IF YOU HAVE ANY QUESTIONS OR CONCERNS.

Phone_____

I HAVE READ AND UNDERSTAND THE ABOVE DISCHARGE INSTRUCTIONS. THE DOCTORS AND STAFF HAVE ANSWERED MY QUESTIONS TO MY SATISFACTION.

_____(Signature of owner or authorized agent)

DISCHARGE BY:

❏ Doctor_____   ❏ Staff_____   ❏ Medication_____

Fresh Frozen Plasma Use for Neonatal Puppies

1. Keep all plasma frozen until use.
2. To thaw, carefully warm the plasma to body temperature. Only warm the tubes you will be using at each administration – keep the remaining tubes in the freezer. This is best done by warming to body temperature by placing tube against your body for heating, in a pocket, etc. Do NOT heat in warm water or microwave as this will denature/damage the proteins and render the product ineffective. Gently rock the tube during thawing; do not shake.
3. The dose is 5 cc per puppy 3 times over a 24 hour period. If this can be administered in the first 24 hours after birth, it can be given orally with a feeding tube. After the pups are 24 hours old, it must be given by subq or IO injection to be effective.
4. Draw 5 cc of warmed plasma into a syringe. Using a feeding tube (less than 24 hours old) or a 20 or 22 gauge needle (for pups over 24 hours old), inject the warmed plasma. If given subq, hold the skin pinched to prevent outflow from the injection site. If given by feeding tube, carefully follow instructions for feeding tube administration.
5. Repeat 2 more times in the next 24 hours. Change to subq injection if the pups have exceeded 24 hours of age before the doses are administered.
6. Please call if you have questions prior to administration of the plasma.

Pre-Natal Care for_____

Congratulations on completing your planned breeding. Her ovulation date was_____and she was bred on_____.

Please feed_____a high quality commercially prepared pregnancy or puppy food. Monitor her intake carefully for the first 5 weeks of her pregnancy to avoid excessive weight gain. It is common for many pregnant dogs to have a decrease in their appetite for a meal or two at the 3rd to 5th week of pregnancy. Please contact us if she refuses more than 3 meals. After the 5th week, she can have her meals increased to meet the demands of her pregnancy. We do not endorse feeding a raw meat diet or adding supplements to the diet during pregnancy as these can lead to a variety of health concerns. Please do not administer vaccines or any medications to your pet unless your veterinarian has prescribed them knowing she is bred - even ear drops can be dangerous during pregnancy if they contain a steroid.

So we can monitor her pregnancy, please make an appointment for the following:
- ❏ Suture removal in 10 to 14 days _____.
- ❏ Ultrasound in 26 to 30 days _____.
- ❏ Panacur should be used once daily from day 42 of pregnancy through day 14 of lactation to reduce the parasite load in the pups.
- ❏ X-rays in 55 to 60 days for puppy size, count and position _____.
- ❏ Surgery appointment for a scheduled C-section on _____.
- ❏ Her predicted date to whelp is _____. A rectal temperature of less than 99 degrees indicates she could whelp at any time.
- ❏ Please call for assistance if you see green, red, or black discharge prior to the delivery of the first pup, hard straining for over 1 hour with no pup delivered, more than 3 hours between pups, or any other concern that her labor is not progressing normally.
- ❏ The pups should be wormed every 2 weeks starting at 2 weeks of age. Examination and vaccinations should be done at 8 weeks of age, prior to placing in new homes.

As always, please call if you have any questions. Phone number _____.
Please feel free to contact_____on our staff for assistance.

Veterinary Clinic Name Here
Phone and website/email here

DISCHARGE CANINE SURGICAL INSEMINATION

DATE:	PATIENT'S NAME: OWNER'S NAME:
Restraint	❏ Please protect your pet when leaving the hospital by using either a leash and collar or a pet carrier. Excessive activity may result in injury, or a slower recovery than we would expect from a pet that is kept quiet during the healing process. ❏ **Do not lift your bitch with pressure under her abdomen as this is painful and may lead to semen escaping from her uterus.** ❏ Please remove the bandage covering the IV site on your pet's front leg upon arrival home.
Food and Water	With the excitement of returning home, your pet may be inclined to drink and eat excessively, which will most likely result in vomiting. **To avoid this, we ask that you remove your pet's food and water dishes for an hour until your pet has settled down. Then, only allow small amounts of food and water for the first day home.** ❏ Offer only half your pet's normal food and water tonight. Normal feeding may resume tomorrow. ❏ Often, there is a decrease in appetite 3 to 5 weeks after breeding.If your bitch refuses more than 3 meals, contact us. ❏ Feed your pet her normal diet. We recommend puppy or pregnancy. Upon confirmation of pregnancy, increase meal size by 20% but do not allow your dog to gain excessive weight during her pregnancy.
Eliminations	Your pet may need to be reminded to go outside to urinate during the first evening home. As she received IV fluids today, she may need to urinate more than usual tonight. Many patients may not have a bowel movement for 24 to 36 hours after surgery. This is normal.
Exercise and Activity	Patients recovering from surgery or illness need limited activity to heal properly. Due to the effects of anesthesia, your pet may be groggy for the next 12 hours. Avoid access to stairs or situations that may lead to injury during this time. ❏ Your pet may resume normal activity in 5 days. ❏ NO swimming, bathing or grooming for 10 to 14 days. ❏ Your pet should be confined indoors, and taken outside on a short leash only for eliminations for 3 days. ❏ Licking damages surgical sites and slows wound healing. Contact us if your pet is licking the surgical incision or IV site.
Medications	If dispensed, it is important to carefully follow the directions that are printed on the label. ❏ No medications dispensed. ❏ Please use the Betadine® on the enclosed gauze pads twice a day to cleanse the incision until healed. ❏ Medications dispensed for_____. Next dose due_____ ❏ Over-the-counter meds: _____. Next dose due_____ ❏ Over-the-counter meds: Aspirin Adult/Baby tabs times per day. Next dose due_____ ❏ DO NOT USE ASPIRIN WITHIN 2 WEEKS OF THIS USING THIS MEDICATION
Sutures and Bandages	In order for incisions to heal, your pet must not lick at the sutures, or the incision site. If your pet is licking, please notify us immediately. Please check the incision twice daily for any redness, swelling, or discharge. If it appears irritated or infected, please notify us immediately. Rechecks of post-op patients will be at no charge during regular office hours. ❏ Sutures/staples need to be removed 10 to 14 days after surgery. A short appointment is needed. ❏ Sutures are underneath the skin, and will absorb over the next several weeks. They do not need to be removed. ❏ Apply warm compress to the surgical site 3 times daily for 10 minutes each time. **Mild redness and swelling around the incision site is common post-op in surgical insemination patients,**

Appointments	Please make an appointment for the following: ❑ Suture removal in 10 to 14 days. ❑ Ultrasound exam in 26-30 days. ❑ X-rays in 55-60 days for puppy size & count ❑ Progesterone level on _____ to aid in scheduling your bitch's planned C-section **❑ Plan for a C-section if you expect 1-2 pups, over 10 pups, have a breed at risk or she has needed a previous C-section on _____** **❑ PREDICTED DATE TO WHELP (63 days from Ovulation) _____**
	A decrease in activity and/or appetite for the first 24 to 36 hours may be observed. However, if your pet exhibits any of the following symptoms, please notify the clinic immediately: ❑ Loss of appetite for over 36 hours ❑ Refusal to drink for over 24 hours ❑ Vomiting and/or diarrhea ❑ Weakness or depression
Special Instructions	_____

TUBE FEEDING DIRECTIONS:

MATERIALS:
1. Goat's milk, pasteurized, or commercial milk replacer
2. Feeding tube, silicon or red rubber feeding tube 8 to 14 French
3. Permanent magic marker
4. Syringe of appropriate size with catheter tip (10 or 60 cc)
5. Puppy scale – feed at a rate of 20 cc per 16 oz of body weight. Repeat every 3 to 6 hours, based on pups condition.
6. Retal thermometer.

STEPS:
1. Establish a well-lit warm location where you can hold the pup comfortably and all materials are within reach. Be attentive and do not rush.
2. Take the puppy's temperature rectally - do NOT feed unless the rectal temperature is between 96° F and 99° F. If the puppy's temperature is below 96° F, warm the pup before feeding.
3. On a safe surface, hold the pup with the neck extended. Hold the tapered end of the feeding tube even with the last rib of the largest pup to be fed. Lay the tube along the side of the pup, mark the tube even with the tip of the pup's nose.

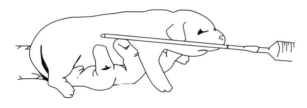

4. Fill the syringe with the calculated amount of formula or milk (20 cc/16 oz body weight or approximately 1 cc per ounce) plus 2 cc of air. Warm the formula to body temperature in a warm water bath – avoid microwaving.

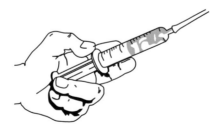

5. Attach the syringe to the feeding tube.
6. With the pup fully awake, warm (over 96° F rectal temp) lying horizontally on the chest, gently pass the tube over the pups tongue, left of center, applying gentle pressure to slide the tube up to the mark. Keep the pup's chin below his or her ears to prevent from passing the tube into the trachea. If resistance is met, remove tube and start over.
7. With your left hand if you are right handed, cup your left hand around the back of the pups head and hold the tube between your index and middle finger to prevent it from moving out of the correct position while feeding.

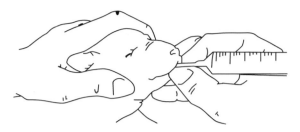

8. BEFORE FEEDING, firmly pinch the pup on the foot or tail. If the pup vocalizes, the tube placement is correct and you can proceed with feeding. If the tube is mistakenly in the trachea, the pup will struggle but will not be able to make any sound – STOP IMMEDIATELY, REMOVE THE TUBE AND START THE PROCESS OVER.

9. With your right hand, depress the plunger on the syringe, NOT too quickly, delivering the calculated amount, stopping sooner should milk reflux out of the pup's mouth or nose.

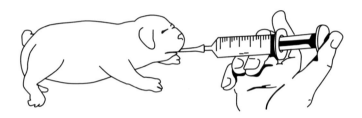

10. As you remove the tube, flex the tube on itself to prevent milk from being aspirated in to the pup's airway. Repeat for each pup. It is normal for the pup to swallow, knead, and make movements of the mouth as if nursing when the tube is in the esophagus positioned correctly.

11. Wash syringe and tube with hot soapy water and allow to air dry until next feeding.

12. Stimulate the external anal and urinary orifices to effect defecation and urination with a warm moistened cotton ball or washcloth.

Appendix D: For veterinarians

D-1. *Insemination procedure for fresh cooled semen*

Clinic Name

INSEMINATION PROCEDURE FOR FRESH COOLED SEMEN

THE ENCLOSED SEMEN IN VIALS SHOULD BE PLACED IN THE REFRIGERATOR UPON ARRIVAL ... DO NOT WARM OR FREEZE

PLEASE CONFIRM THE NAME OF THE OWNER AND STUD DOG CORRESPOND TO THAT YOU HAVE REQUESTED SEMEN FROM.

Enclosed please find fresh semen extended from _____(registered and/or call name of dog _____(breed) owned by _____.

His sperm count prior to the addition of extender is _____ x 10^6 with _____ % motility and _____ % normal.

The litter registration papers are:
❏ enclosed   ❏ will be sent under separate cover by the stud dog owner.

1. Examine one drop of the shipped semen on a warmed microscope slide. Leave the rest of the semen refrigerated. Evaluate the semen drop looking for sperm motility gradually changing from slow, sideward movement to rapid forward motility.

2. Attach the enclosed AI rod to the syringe and draw up the entire contents of the vial, without warming the semen. Let the bitch's body warm the semen.

3. When ready to proceed with the insemination, stand the bitch comfortably with an assistant or owner holding the head and supporting the hindquarters on their lap, with no pressure under the abdomen, or on a stairs or ramp. Gently, insert the rod dorsally, then cranially into the vagina and slowly push on the syringe plunger. Use only 1/2 cc of air to empty the AI rod. AVOID THE USE OF TOO MUCH AIR!

4. Withdraw the rod and internally or externally feather the bitch, simulating a tie. Avoid the use of latex in any contact with the semen. Keep her elevated, feather her for 5 to 6 minutes.

5. Crate the bitch for 30 minutes after insemination and do not allow her to urinate for 1 hour after insemination. Do not let her jump up for several hours.

6. If you have any questions, please call us.

Ovuplant Instructions

Setup for insertion:
1. Ovuplant
2. Ovuplant label for patient file
3. Sodium Bicarbonate injectable
4. TB syringe
5. Lidocaine
6. Nolvasan Surgical scrub, diluted
7. Cotton Balls
8. Sterile gloves
9. Hair clips
10. Towel for bitch to lay on
11. Non Sterile gauze squares

Instructions:
1. Open sterile supplies including Ovuplant on to open glove wrapper
2. Place the bitch in lateral recumbency with her right side down
3. Place hair clips on loose hair on tail and thighs if necessary
4. Prep vulva with Nolvasan
5. Inject lidocaine mixed 9:1 with sodium biocarbonate injectable along rim of tissue in right vulva lip adjacent to skin-mucosal margin midway between tip of vulva and dorsal commissure.
6. Partially depress plunger of Ovuplant to seat Ovuplant drug pellet into insertion needle, taking care not to push pellet out of tip of needle.
7. Part the lips of the vulva. Insert the Ovuplant with the needle directed ventrally. Start near dorsal commissure, directing the needle toward to the tip of the vulva (to reduce the chances of loss). Insert into mucosa adjacent to skin-mucosal margin, very superficially under the mucosa (do not insert deeply- do this so the drug pellet can be seen through the mucosal surface at insertion.) The ovuplant should end up halfway between the dorsal and ventral commissures of the vulva. This will aid in retrieval after the breeding.
8. Place a portion of a cotton ball in the vulva to minimize vaginal discharge after placement. The bitch will pass this when she urinates.
9. Record the location of the ovuplant for retrieval.
10. Remind the client the ovuplant must be removed after the breeding.

D-3. *Instructions for ovuplant removal*

Setup for removal:
1. Sterile gloves
2. 15 scalpel blade
3. Lidocaine and Sodium Bicarbonate injectable
4. TB syringe
5. Sterile saline flush in 3 ml syringe
6. Cotton balls
7. Nolvasan surgical scrub, diluted
8. Mini surgical pack
9. Gauze squares

Instructions to remove ovuplant:
1. Place the bitch in lateral recumbency with her right side down
2. Place hair clips on loose hair on tail and thighs if necessary
3. Prep vulva with Nolvasan
4. Identify location of Ovuplant by visualization and palpation along rim of tissue in right vulva lip adjacent to skin-mucosal margin midway between tip of vulva and dorsal commissure. In some cases, the Ovuplant has migrated.
5. Inject lidocaine near the area, taking care to avoid visually obliterating the ovuplant or physically disrupting it. Repeat Nolvasan prep.
6. Holding the right side of the vulva with support under it, make a superficial incision over the ovuplant, parallel to its plane.
7. Gently lift out the pellet or if it has broken down, curette out the white pasty material that represents the remaining drug pellet. Flush the area with saline.
8. Place a cotton ball in the vulva to minimize vaginal discharge. The bitch will pass this when she urinates.
9. Schedule ultrasound for 4 weeks.

D-4. *Puppy examination*

Veterinary Hospital Name here

Puppy Examination

Date _____ Clinician _____ Staff _____

Client Name _____ Client ID _____ Name of Dam _____

Puppy ID	Temp	Weight	Heart Rate	Resp Rate	MM Color	CRT	Urine Color/SG	Stool Character	Reflexes Present/Absent	Owner concerns	Feedings/Therapy Given	PE Findings
1												
2												
3												
4												
5												
6												
7												
8												
9												
10												
11												
12												
13												
14												
15												
16												

Neonate/Pediatric Sick Puppy SOAP:

Pet name_____ Pet ID _____ Age: _____ d/w/m/y

Client name_____ Client #_____Date_____

SUBJECTIVE:

Owner's concerns: _____

Last normal on_____ First symptom noted:_____

Other pets in litter/household affected/normal?_____

Human family members?: _____

How is your puppy's . . . ?

Attitude & Behavior: Normal/ Lethargic/ Depressed/ Overactive/Weak_____ _____days

Appetite: Normal/ Nursing/ Nursing a little/ Not nursing/ Eating a little/ Eating only table food/ Refusing all food_____ hours/days

Drinking: Normal/ Increased/ Decreased/ None_____ _____hours/days

Vomiting: Y/N Acute/ Chronic(<7d/>7d)____hours/days Regurgitation: Y/N ___ hours/days

    Appearance of Vomitus: Phlegm/ Blood/ Bile/ Parasites/ Food/Shape_____/ Hair/ Feces/ Odor

    Duration_____ Frequency_____ Time/hrs after eating: Varies/On empty stomach/Morning/

    Evening/_____hrs after meal

Stools: Normal/None/Diarrhea/Constipated_____ _____days

Diarrhea: Y/N Appearance of Stool: pasty/seedy/Blood Color: green-black-brown-yellow-white

    _____ Parasites_____/Hair/Mucus/Contents_____

    Normal/Hard/Soft/Pudding/Runny/Watery/None/Other_____

    Frequency_____/day   Size: Normal/small amounts/large   Straining

Weight: Normal/Increased/Decreased _____ _____ oz/kg/lbs

Cardiovascular: Normal/Panting/Coughing/Sneezing/Nasal discharge/Ocular Discharge ____

*Other:*_____ ____hours/days

OTHER SYMPTOMS: None/ Lethargic/ PU-PD/ No urine/ Weak/ Panting/ Cough/ Retch/ Gag/ Sneeze/

    Bloated/ Pain/ Haircoat changes

PREVIOUS RELATED ILLNESS: Y/N_____DETAILS_____

PREVIOUS BLOODWORK/FECAL: Y/N_____DETAILS_____

CURRENT or RECENT MEDICATIONS: Y/N Response?:_____DETAILS_____

WORMING HISTORY: Y/N_____DETAILS_____

VACCINATION HISTORY: Current/None/Overdue

*TRAVEL HISTORY:*_____DETAILS_____

*BEHAVIOR CHANGES:*_____

POSSIBLE CAUSES?: Diet change/Table scraps/Bones/Fat/Garbage/Plants/Item chewed

              Chemicals/foreign objects/Dead animal/Clothing/Missing toy etc

              Unsupervised indoors or outdoors/changes in household

OBJECTIVE: T_____(96°-102.5°) HR_____ (100-250) RR____ CRT_____ HYDRATION EST_____

MM: Normal Moist/ Dry/ tacky/ Pigmented/ Pink/ Pale/ Very pale/ Cyanotic/ Jaundice /Drooling

Status: Normal weight/ Thin/ Overweight/ Obese/ Painful/ Depressed/ Dehydrated/ Lateral recumbency/

    Nonresponsive

Mouth/Throat: Normal/ Cleft palate/ Brachygnatic? Y/N (normal)/ Glossitis/ Ulcers/Pharyngitis/Tonsillitis/

    Foreign body

    Under tongue: Normal/ Foreign body/ Can't examine

Skull: Open fontanelle Y/N _____ _____ cm x _____ cm

Nares: Normal/Discharge_____ Stenotic R/L Cleft nares R/L

Dental exam: Normal Retained Primary Teeth Malocclusion Gingivitis Y/N grade_____

Teething_____

Heart sounds: Normal/ Murmur Grade_____/ Gallop/ Muffled/ Arrhythmia_____

Lung sounds: Normal/Clear Crackles R/L Rales R/L Edema Congested R/L Other_____

    Tracheal cough/ Dyspnea/ Labored/ Open mouth breathing/ Distress

Lymph nodes: Normal Enlarged Submandibular/Generalized Peripheral _____

Abdominal Palpation: Normal/ Overweight Enlarged organ_____
Hernia: Umbilical/R inguinal/L inguinal   Tense/ Painful No/ cranial/ caudal/ throughout/ Fluid/Other_____
Umbilicus: Cord Present/ Absent Inflamed/ Discharge/ Herniated/ Intestines exposed
Bowel: Rectum patent Y/N GI sounds: Normal/None/Decreased/Increased
Urinary: Normal/ Anuric/ Dysuric/ Empty/ Full/ Hematuria/ Pollakiuria/ Pu-pd/ Stranguria/ Obstructed
External Genitals: Female Normal Y/N/ Inverted vulva/ Clitoris/ Vaginal Discharge _____
        Male: Testes present R/L Retained R/L Penis _____ Prepuce _____
Bladder: Full/ empty/ blocked/ stones
Kidneys: R Normal/abnormal/not palp L Normal/abnormal/not palp
Neuro: Open Fontanelle/Anisocoria/Head tilt/ Horner's/Nystagmus/Ataxia/Paresis/Paralysis/Seizures
        Proprioception: RF LF RR LR Normal/Decreased
        Other:_____
Eye exam: Normal Visual? Y/N Conjuctivitis OD OS Chemosis OD OS
        Corneal Ulcer OD OS Distichia OD OS   Discharge OD OS_____   Entropion/Ectropion OD
        OS FB OD OS PPMs OD____   OS____
        Schirmer OD___ OS___   IOP OD___ OS___ Nictitans Everted
        Follicular Conjunctivis OD____ OS Neonatal ophthalmia OD___ OS____
Ears: Normal Auditory? Y/N Discharge R/L_____ Mites Y/N
Musculoskeletal: Gait:_____ Lame/ Patellar Palpation RR/LR Ortolani R/L

ASSESSMENT/PRIMARY RULEOUTS: Other_____
PROGNOSIS: Excellent   Good   Guarded   Fair   Poor   Grave
PLAN: CBC/CS   UA   FECAL   Giardia   Culture   Parvo   Other_____
Rads: VD/LATERAL   THORAX/ABD   Ultrasound   OTHER_____

TREATMENT OPTIONS:
    Outpatient   Recommended by Dr./Owner declined hospitalization(AMA)
    Inpatient   Recommended by Dr./Medically appropriate/Owner request
    Referral_____
TEST RESULTS:_____
SURGERY:_____   See anesthesia/surgery report
HOSPITALIZE:
    Fluids: IV_____ cc/hr Total Dose _____
    SQ_____ CC/DOSE_____X/DAY Total dose_____
    Injections:_____ _____cc_____route_____x/day
        _____ _____cc_____route_____x/day
        _____ _____cc_____route_____x/day
        _____ _____cc_____route_____x/day

    Oral Meds:_____ cc/tab/capsule PO _____ x/day
        _____ cc/tab/capsule PO _____ x/day
        _____ cc/tab/capsule PO _____ x/day
        _____ cc/tab/capsule PO _____ x/day
    Feeding: NPO/BABY FOOD/ID/AD/LOW RESIDUE/MAX CAL/OTHER_____
        _____ Can/cups/cc _____ X/DAY
    Feeding tube/force feeding/hand feeding
    Drinking: Water/Ice/Electrolytes_____amount_____x/day

DISCHARGE/FOLLOW UP:_____

HANDOUTS:_____

DISPENSED: Meds_____
    Diet_____
    Other_____

DOCTOR_____ **Technician**_____

Breeding Soundness SOAP

Pet name_____ Client name_____ Client #_____ Pet ID #_____
Date_____
Pet's Registered name_____ Reg. Number_____Microchip#_____
DNA completed Y/N Date of last Brucella test_____ Test run – RSAT/Culture/AGID/PCR
Name of Owner/Stud dog/Bitch to be bred to_____
Day this heat cycle began_____ Is AI being done at our clinic? Y/N
Plan to use: Natural/ Fresh AI/ Fresh chilled AI/ Vaginal/ TCI/ Surgical

SUBJECTIVE:
Reason for Visit:_____
Describe your pet's overall health_____
Appetite: Normal/Eating a little/Eating only treats/Eating only table food/Refusing all food_____days
Drinking & Urination: Normal/Increased/Decreased/None_____ _____days
Vomiting: None/Describe_____ _____days
Attitude: Normal/Lethargic/Depressed/Overactive/Weak_____ _____days
Weight: Normal/Increased/Decreased _____
Stools: Normal/None/Diarrhea/Constipated_____ _____days
Cardiovascular: Normal/ Panting/ Coughing/ Sneezing/ Nasal discharge/ Ocular discharge_____days
Other:_____days

PREVIOUS ILLNESS: Y/N_____ DETAILS_____ MEDS_____
PREVIOUS BLOODWORK/FECAL: Y/N_____ DETAILS_____
    Brucella _____/ Progesterone_____/ Thyroid_____
    Culture_____/ Other_____
CURRENT MEDICATIONS: Y/N_____DETAILS_____
WORMING HISTORY: Y/N_____DETAILS_____
VACCINATION HISTORY: Current/None/due for DHLPP on_____/ RABIES due on _____
*TRAVEL HISTORY:*_____ DETAILS_____
*BEHAVIOR CHANGES:*_____
Other pets in household? Y/N/SEX_____ Health status of others in
household_____
PREVIOUS BREEDING HISTORY:
FEMALE: First breeding/Previously bred on _____/route_____
Outcome_____
Timing: None/Male/Vag cyt/Progesterone_____
Evaluated on palpation/ultrasound/x-ray
MALE: First/Last breeding dates/_____/ route_____
Outcome_____ Semen Analysis date/results _____

OBJECTIVE: T_____HR_____RR_____CRT_____HYDRATION EST_____
MM: Normal Moist Dry/tacky Pigmented Pink Pale Very pale Cyanotic Jaundice
Status: Normal weight/Thin/Overwt/Obese Painful/Depressed/Dehydrated/Lateral rec/Nonresponsive
Mouth/Throat: Can't examine Normal Other _____
Dental exam: Normal Tartar Y/N grade____ Gingivitis Y/N grade____ Teething Fractured teeth ___
Eye Exam: Normal Other: _____
Ear exam: Normal/NE/Otitis/_____
Heart sounds: Normal/Murmur Grade_____/ Gallop/ Muffled/ Arrhythmia_____
Lung sounds: Normal/Other _____
Lymph nodes: Normal Enlarged/Generalized Peripheral_____

Abdominal Palpation: Normal Overweight Tense Enlarged organ_____Painful Fluid Other_____
Urinary: Normal/Anuric/Dysuric/Empty/Full/Hematuria/Pollakiuria/Pu-pd/Stranguria/Obstructed
Neuro: WNL/ Proprioception: RF LF RR LR Normal/decreased Other _____
Othopedic:_____
Rectal: Prostate Normal/Enlarged/Symmetrical/Asymmetrical/NE/_____
Testes: R Normal/__x__x__cm diam/Enlarged/Small/Texture_____/Epididymis/Spermatic Cord____
       L Normal/__x__x__cm diam/Enlarged/Small/Texture_____/Epididymis/Spermatic Cord____
Prepuce: Normal/NE/_____/Penis: Normal/NE/_____
Vaginal Exam:_____
Mammary glands:_____
OFA/PENN HIP HISTORY_____
Eye Registry HISTORY_____
OTHER SCREENING_____
Breeding Counseling_____

PLAN: CBC/CSUA   FECAL T4/THYROID   CULTURE – source _____
ULTRASOUND   BIOPSY/Needle Aspirate   SEMEN ANALYSIS_____
VAG CYT_____ Vaginoscopy_____
Brucellosis serology/culture
PROGESTERONE QUANTITAVE/SEMIQUANTITATIVE   ESTROGEN   TESTOSTERONE
CHROMOSOME ANALYSIS OTHER_____
   Rads: VD/LATERAL   THORAX/ABD   OTHER_____
   Ultrasound_____ Referral_____

BREEDING PLAN:
Natural Fresh AI Fresh Chilled AI Frozen semen Surgical insemination/TCI Location: Here/Recipient__
Semen/stud dog located at_____/Semen to be received_____
SHIPPING ADDRESS_____
BILLING ADDRESS_____
Shipping arranged for BY OWNER OF DOG/ BITCH Package ID number_____ FedEx/
   UPS/Post office/other
SHIPPING BOX PROVIDED BY Shipping Veterinarian/RECIPIENT
PLAN:_____

Date:_____ Progesterone_____ Vag Cyt_____
Date:_____ Progesterone_____ Vag Cyt_____
Date:_____ Progesterone_____ Vag Cyt_____
Date:_____ Progesterone_____ Vag Cyt_____
BREEDING DATES:_____ _____ _____
ULTRASOUND DATE:_____ X-RAY DATE:_____
SURGERY:_____ See anesthesia/surgery report
WHELP DATE:_____ CESAREAN Y/N NUMBER OF PUPS____M____F
DISCHARGE/FOLLOW UP:_____
HANDOUTS:_____
Meds_____Diet_____Other_____
OWNER'S NAME_____ CREDIT CARD NUMBER_____
EXP DATE_____ SIGNATURE_____
DOCTOR_____ ESTIMATE:_____
BILLING COMPLETED_____ (DATE)_____ (STAFF INITIALS)
BOX CONTENTS CHECKLIST:
❏ SEMEN   ❏ AI PIPETTE   ❏ SYRINGE   ❏ INSEMINATION DIRECTIONS   ❏ ICE PACKS
❏ RETURN SHIPPING LABEL AND LETTER   ❏ AKC LITTER REGISTRATION

Semen Analysis: Date_____

PERCENT MOTILITY____% Speed Of Progression: 0 1 2 3 4 5 COLOR_____ VISCOSITY 1 2 3 4

VOLUME of Sperm Rich Fraction: (1)_____ ML x SPERM COUNT/ML (2)_____ x $10^{6/9}$ =
TOTAL SPERM COUNT (3) _____ x $10^{6/9}$

ABNORMAL MORPHOLOGY___% NORMAL _____% (4)

(MULTIPLY SPERM COUNT /ML (1) x VOLUME IN ML (2) = TOTAL SPERM COUNT = (3)

TOTAL NORMAL SPERM CELLS x $10^{6/9}$_____(5)

(MULTIPLY TOTAL SPERM COUNT (3) x % NORMAL + Immature MORPHOLOGY (4) = TOTAL NORMAL SPERM CELLS) (5) _____

Morphology
Head Defects: _____% Midpiece Defects: _____% Tail Defects: _____% Total
    Normal: _____%
Other: White Blood Cells _____ per 400x Red Blood Cells ____ per 400 x Cellular Debris light
    moderate heavy
Extender Used/Volume_____ Comments_____
Clinician_____ Technician_____

Table of normal puppy development from birth to 6 weeks of age				
What is normal?	Week 1	Week 2	Weeks 3-4	Weeks 5-6
Temperature, rectal	96 - 98° F	96-99° F	100° F	100 - 101° F
Ambient temperature	75 to 80°F	70 to 80° F	70 to 75° F	65 to 75°F
Heart rate & blood Pressure	200 to 240 beats per min; Blood pressure 61	200 to 240 beats per min, sinus rhythm	160 to 200 beats per min, sinus rhythm; blood pressure 139	Varies with breed
Respiratory rate	15 to 35 per min	15 to 35 per min	15 to 25 per min	15 to 25 per min
Mucus membranes Color/ CRT	Pink to hyperemic if recently nursed	Pink/1 second	Pink/1 second	Pink/1 second
Urine color	Very pale yellow, <1.020	Very pale yellow, <1.020	Pale yellow	Pale to moderate yellow
Weight	May lose up to 10% in the first 3 days. Birth weight: Toys 100-200 gms; Large 400-500 gms; Giant 700 gms	Gaining 5 to 10% daily, many double birth weight by day 10. Calculate weight gain of 2-4 gm/day/kg anticipated adult weight.	Calculate weight gain of 2 -4 gm/day/kg anticipated adult weight.	Calculate weight gain of 1 -4 gm/day/kg anticipated adult weight. Giant and large breeds gain at faster rate than small breeds.
Activity	Sleeps & eats 90% of time, twitch while sleeping	Sleeps & eats 90% of time, twitch while sleeping	Beginning to crawl, then stand and walk by day 21. Start to play when eyes open. Can sit.	Walking, climbing, playing, may bark, begin to explore environment, mouthing. Normal postural reflexes.
Attitude	Quiet, cry infrequently.	Quiet	Quiet, more active	Start to develop "personalities",
Body tone and reflexes	Flexor dominance for 1st 4 days, then extensor. Righting, rooting, weak withdrawal.	Extensor dominance, righting, rooting, crossed extensor. Withdrawal developing.	Approaching normal for adult. Suckling reflex & crossed extensor disappears.	Normal adult
Vision and hearing	No vision but blink with bright light. Limited hearing.	None to limited vision and hearing, menace present but slow initially. Limited hearing, waxy discharge.	Vision blurry, Pupillary light reflex present within 24 hours of eyelids opening, respond to sound. Startle reflex develops.	Approaching full vision and hearing
Teeth	None	None	Deciduous incisors & canine erupt	Deciduous premolars erupt
Breeder's interaction	Assure pups are nursing, supplement if necessary. Daily temp, weight, urine & stool character. Start Early Neurologic Stimulation day 3-16	Assure pups are nursing, supplement if necessary. Daily temp, weight, urine & stool character. Continue Early Neurologic Stimulation day 3-16	Continue to assure pups are thriving, begin to enrich environment by variation of toys, surfaces.	Continue to assure pups are thriving, continue to enrich environment. Lots of human interaction for socialization
Veterinary care	Assess & treat if not thriving, taildocks and dewclaws prior to 5th day	Assess & treat if not thriving. Dispense pyrantel pamoate to use on day 14 after birth.	Assess & treat if not thriving. Dispense pyrantel pamoate to use on day 28 after birth.	Veterinary wellness visit – assess pups for any abnormalities for breeder to sell pup with full disclosure. First vaccinations (DAPPv). Dispense pyrantel pamoate to use on day 42 after birth.
Food and water	Nursing only. If supplementing, 60 ml/ lb/24 hours divided by 12, fed every 2 hours.	Nursing only. If supplementing, 70 ml/ lb/24 hours divided by 8, fed every 3 hours.	Offer water, then gruel to start weaning. If supplementing, 90 ml/ lb/24 hours divided by 6, fed every 4 hours.	Teething. Many pups weaned, on full food and water, some still nurse for social interaction.

Small Animal Pediatric Medicine Tufts Animal Expo 2002 Johnny D. Hoskins, DVM, Ph.D. DocuTech Services, Inc. Baton Rouge, Louisiana, USA

Your hospital name here
Anesthesia Record

CLIENT NAME_____

CLIENT NUMBER_____

PET'S NAME_____

DATE_____

(PATIENT LABEL)

TEMP F	PULSE/ MIN	RESP/ MIN	BP_____ Hydration_____ AGE___	WEIGHT _____LB _____KG
PREMED	DOSE	ROUTE	TIME	RESPONSE
ET TUBE	SIZE	FR/MM	IV Cath size: G	Site:

❏ PRE-OP PAPERWORK ❏ PHOTO	❏ PRE-OP PHYSICAL WNL/ABN	❏ PRE-OP LAB _____date WNL/ABN	❏ PRE-OP EKG WNL/ABN	❏ READY TO DISCHARGE DR DISCHG Y/N TIME_____ DATE_____
❏ POST OP PAPERWORK	❏ CHARGES ENTERED	❏ POST OP MEDS RX/OTC/NONE	❏ TREATMENT SHEET	❏ OWNER CALLED TT_____/LM/NA/BZ

DATE	PROCEDURE_____	ADDITIONAL PROCEDURES ❏ Nail trim Y/N	❏ Microchip/Tattoo ❏ Dental/Extractions Y/N
DVM/TECH _____(Admit) _____(Procedure) _____(Surgeon)	❏ TESTES? Y/N ❏ HERNIA? Y/N ❏ RETAINED TEETH? Y/N ❏ IN HEAT Y/N	Vaccs to be administered/ None ❏ _____ ❏ _____	❏ Heartworm/Fecal ❏ Lump removal/Histopath Y/N ❏ Dewclaws ❏ _____

FLUIDS	FLUID START TIME	FLUIDS STOP TIME	Thermal Support:
ANESTHESIA	ANESTHESIA START TIME	ANESTHESIA STOP TIME	Shor-line/RICA board/BAER hugger Water circulating blanket/Rice/Other

TIME	SpO$_2$	CO$_2$	PULSE	RR	TEMP F	BP Systolic/ Diastolic	FLUID RATE/ VOLUME	ISO/ SEVO % RUN	NOTES (INCLUDES SURGERY START/ STOP TIME)

L   R

CANINE

L   R

FELINE

EXTUBATION TIME	POST OP MEDS/ROUTE	POST-OP RECTAL TEMP _____° F/C	RECOVERY

Anesthesia Record Page 2   PATIENT LABEL

TIME	SpO$_2$	CO$_2$	PULSE	RR	TEMP F	BP Systolic/ Diastolic	FLUID RATE/ VOLUME	ISO/ SEVO % RUN	NOTES (INCLUDES SURGERY START/ STOP TIME)

CANINE CESAREAN SECTION SURGERY REPORT

Your Hospital Name here:

Date_____

PATIENT LABEL

Clients name_____

Pet's name_____

Client number_____

Vital Signs:		TEMP F PULSE/ MIN_____ MM/Refill_____	RESP/ MIN_____	BP_____ Hydration_____ AGE_____	Weight today: _____Lb/kg Weight at breeding: _____Lb/kg
	ET TUBE	SIZE	FR/MM	IV Cath size: g	Site:
Drugs:	DOSE mg or ml administered:	Dosage calcula-tion:	ROUTE	TIME	RESPONSE
Solu-Medrol		1 cc/62 pounds BW of 125 mg/2 ml per vial	IV slow		
Atropine		1 cc/ 20 pounds BW of 1/120 gr/ml	SQ		
Metoclopramide		1 cc/37 pounds BW of 5 mg/ml	SQ		
Calcium (must be labeled for SQ use)		1 cc/10 pounds BW of 0.9 mEq/10 ml)	SQ in 2 sites		
Other					

Pre-surgical blood work was completed on_____ at _____Lab and was within normal limits/_____.

The EKG was WNL/_____.

The first day of estrus was _____ Bred on_____

Ovulation Date Estimated_____Predicted to whelp on:_____

Bred by Natural/Vaginal AI/TCI/Surgical using Fresh/Fresh chilled/ Frozen semen

Ultrasound revealed: _____ Radiographs revealed:_____

(See Table 6-2 and Appendix A-5 for sequence of events.)

Description of surgical procedure:

The dog was assessed for overall condition and labor and found to be_____.
An IV catheter was placed, the hair was clipped with a 40 Oster clipper. The dog was anesthetized with_____ and placed in dorsal recumbency. A sterile prep with Nolvasan® and sterile drape was applied. A ventral midline abdominal skin incision was made halfway between the pubis and umbilicus approximately_____ cm long with a #15 scalpel blade. The subcutaneous fat was sharply dissected off the underlying abdominal wall to clearly expose the fascia for the entire length of the skin incision to facilitate good apposition of the linea at closure. The linea was lifted up with thumb forceps, a stab incision was made thru the abdominal wall and the incision was completed with Metzenbaum scissors.

The R/L uterine horn was identified and exteriorized. An incision was made lengthwise on the antimesenteric border of the uterus. _____(#) pups were delivered including placentas. This was repeated for the R/L horn and_____(#) pups were delivered thru the same/new incision. The incision(s) were located at: _____.

The placentas were detached/easily removed/not removed/ _____.
Resorption sites were/were not noted in R/L horn_____.
Placentas/uterine samples were retained for pathology/culture/ _____.

The uterus was examined from vagina/cervix proximally to both ovaries to assure all pups
and placentas were removed and to assess integrity. The uterine incision(s) were sutured with
_____ in a continuous inverting baseball pattern. The uterine condition was
_____. The abdomen was irrigated with 1 L_____.

The abdominal wall was closed using_____ in a simple interrupted pattern in the linea.
The subcutaneous layer was closed using_____ in a simple continuous pattern. The
subcuticular layer was closed using _____in a simple continuous pattern. The skin was
closed using_____ in a _____ pattern.

#	ID	Suction	Spontaneous resps	Intubated	Caffeine	Dopram	APGAR 1 min	APGAR 5 min	Weight Oz/gm	Exam	Other
1											
2											
3											
4											
5											
6											
7											
8											
9											
10											
11											
12											
13											
14											
15											

Post-op recovery_____
Post-op pain meds by injection_____ Post-op pain meds dispensed for oral
use_____
Discharged on _____ Condition at discharge: _____
Comments_____
_____ (Surgeon's Signature)

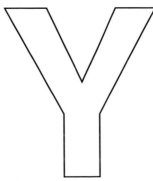

Date_____

PLACE PATIENT
LABEL HERE

Clients name_____
Pet's name_____
Client number_____

CANINE SURGICAL INSEMINATION SURGERY REPORT

Description of surgical procedure:
Presurgical blood work was completed on _____ at _____Lab and was within normal limits. The EKG was WNL.
The first day of estrus was _____ Ovulation Date Estimated_____ AM/PM
Progesterone Levels were:

Date	Time	Result ng/dl	Laboratory
	AM/PM	ng/dl	Lab_____
	AM/PM	ng/dl	Lab_____
	AM/PM	ng/dl	Lab_____
	AM/PM	ng/dl	Lab_____
	AM/PM	ng/dl	Lab_____
	AM/PM	ng/dl	Lab_____
	AM/PM	ng/dl	Lab_____
	AM/PM	ng/dl	Lab_____
			Ovulation Date Estimated
			Breeding Planned
			Whelping Date Estimated

At _____(time) on _____ (date), the dog was anesthetized with _____ and placed in dorsal recumbency with her caudal end elevated slightly above her cranial end. The hair was clipped with a 40 Oster clipper. A sterile prep with Nolvasan and sterile drape was applied. A ventral midline abdominal skin incision was made between the 3rd and 4th/ 4th and 5th nipples_____ cm long with a #15 scalpel blade/laser using a scalpel handle as a shield. The subcutaneous fat was sharply dissected off the underlying abdominal wall to clearly expose the fascia for the entire length of the skin incision to facilitate good apposition of the linea at closure. The linea was lifted up with thumb forceps, a stab incision was made thru the abdominal wall and the incision was completed with Metzenbaum scissors.

The uterine body was identified and exteriorized, and both uterine horns were partially exteriorized so as to visualize them. Ovaries were/were not visualized/palpated. The uterus was/was not normal _____.

Diagnostics _____.
Fresh/Fresh chilled shipped semen/Frozen was used from stud dog_____
owned_____ Sperm count_____ % motility **OR**

The frozen semen vial number used was_____
from ICSB/ICG-Synbiotics/Camelot/Canine Cryobank/_____
from _____ Veterinary Hospital in _____.
The semen was thawed according to the freezing centers enclosed guidelines
using_____ as thaw media.
The semen had an estimated _____% motility with _____ speed of progression and
_____ estimated % dead or immotile. (read by _____ Initals)
The uterine body was held off with digital pressure distal to the puncture site. A syringe with a 20
gauge catheter was used to introduce the semen into the uterine body/uterine horn just distal to the
ovary directing the semen into both horns. Pressure was maintained for 1 minute. The uterus was then
gently re-placed into the abdominal cavity while maintaining a digital barrier to the outflow of semen.

The abdominal wall was closed using_____ in a simple interrupted pattern in the linea.
The subcutaneous layer was closed using_____ in a simple continuous pattern. The
subcuticular layer was closed using _____in a simple continuous pattern. The skin was
closed using_____.

Post-op recovery_____
Pre-op pain meds _____ Post-op pain meds dispensed for home use_____
Discharged on _____ Ambulatory/Carried/In carrier/ Discharged to:_____
Date calculated to whelp on (63 days from ovulation)_____
Comments_____
❏ Staple Remover sent
_____ (Surgeon's Signature)

CANINE UTERINE BIOPSY/CULTURE/FLUSH REPORT

Date_____   PLACE PATIENT
Clients name_____   LABEL HERE
Pet's name_____
Client number_____
Dr._____ Tech_____
See anesthesia report

Presurgical blood work was completed on _____ and was/was not within normal limits.
EKG was completed on _____ and was/was not within normal limits.
Date first noticed estrus:_____
Progesterone levels were:

Date	Time	Result ng/dl	Laboratory
		ng/dl	
		ng/dl	
		ng/dl	
		ng/dl	

Significant Reproductive History:
Number of previous estrous cycles_____
Number of previous breedings_____   Timed?_____
Number of previous pregnancies?_____   Number of puppies?_____

The dog was anesthetized with _____ and placed in dorsal recumbency. The
hair was clipped with a 40 Oster clipper. A sterile prep with Nolvasan and sterile drape was applied.
A ventral midline abdominal skin incision was made halfway between the pubis and umbilicus
approximately _____ cm long with a #15 scalpel blade. The subcutaneous fat was sharply
dissected off the underlying abdominal wall to clearly expose the fascia for the entire length of the
skin incision to facilitate good apposition of the linea at closure. The linea was lifted up with thumb
forceps, a stab incision was made thru the abdominal wall and the incision was completed with
Metzenbaum scissors.
The uterine body was identified and exteriorized, and both uterine horns were partially exteriorized
so as to visualize them.
 Ovaries were/were not visualized/palpated/normal/abnormal_____.
The uterus was/was not normal_____
_____.
Cysts _____Adhesions_____.
# of biopsies done_____.
Location of biopsies_____.
Biopsy done as a wedge/with a 2/4/6 mm biopsy punch_____

Biopsies submitted to Cornell/_____ Lab for culture/ in formalin/in Bouins**_____.
Cultures taked for aerobic/anaerobic/mycoplasma culture sent to Cornell/_____ Lab
Fluid collected and submitted to Cornell/_____ Lab
The uterus was flushed through the biopsy site with a _____ Fr Red rubber feeding tube with
_____ cc of LRS/Normal saline/_____ to distend the uterine horns._____
The uterine biopsy sites were closed with 5-0 PDS suture/_____ in a Uttrech/_____
Pattern without penetration into the lumen of the uterus.
The abdomen was flushed with _____ cc LRS/Normal Saline/_____

The abdominal wall was closed using_____ in a simple interrupted pattern in the linea. The subcutaneous layer was closed using_____ in a simple continuous pattern. The subcuticular layer was closed using _____in a simple continuous pattern. The skin was closed using_____ in a _____ pattern.

Post-op recovery_____
Post-op pain meds by injection_____
Post-op pain meds dispensed for oral use_____
Other meds_____
Discharged on _____
Comments_____
❏ Staple Remover sent
_____(surgeon's signature)

Sequence of Events:
1. Presurgical blood work with/without progesterone level/Brucella/Pre-op exam
2. Premed with _____
3. Place IV catheter
4. Anesthetize with _____/ETT/ intubate/clip/prep/ move to surgery table
5. Place IV Catheter
6. Clip abdomen
7. Move to surgery table
8. Position on v-tray
9. Hook up to monitors and anesthetic machine
10. Prep for incision
11. Gown/gloves
12. Warm LRS in microwave
13. Make incision into abdominal wall
14. Evaluate uterus and ovaries
15. Make wedge or biopsy punch incisions – 3 or more if possible
16. Place 1 biopsy in sterile red top tube to grind up for culture
17. Place 1 biopsy in formalin for histopathology
18. Place 1 biopsy in sterile red top tube with Bouins** (2 cc) solution for histopathology
19. Culture inside of uterus with 3 culturettes – hand to Dr. without breaking sterile field
    • Aerobic – Aimes
    • Anaerobic – Porta-cul
    • Mycoplasma – Aimes without Charcoal
20. Flush uterine horns to distend.
21. Flush abdominal cavity.
22. Close uterus and abdomen

Equipment Checklist
1. Biopsy punches
2. 2 Aimes culturettes without charcoal
3. 1 Porta-cul with sterile swab
4. 3 sterile red top tubes for culture, fluid and bouins solution
5. Assorted red rubber feeding tubes
6. Surgery setup: Pack, trach tube, IV cath, Propofol, tape, gauze, eye ointment, flush, patient monitor, v-tray, towel, gloves (6.5), GOWN, 15 blade, 2-0 or 3-0 cutting suture, stapler and remover
7. 35 and 60 cc catheter tip syringe – keep in case to hand to Dr. without breaking sterile field
8. Sterile Stainless steel bowl
9. 1 L warmed LRS
10. 5-0 PDS suture

11. Sterile needles to handle biopsy tissue
12. Scissors to open sterile LRS
13. Plastic cassettes for tissues in solution
14. Small container of formalin
15. Bouin's solution, 3 cc syringe to transfer to red top tube
16. Mailing box with Styrofoam liner, frozen ice pack, newspaper, parafilm, BioHazard shipping bags, Small Styrofoam sleeve to keep anaerobic culture tube away from ice pack.
17. Cornell Laboratory requisition form
18. Fine tip Sharpie permanent marker to label sample vials

**Note – Bouin's must be carefully stored to prevent the solution from drying out into powder as in powder form, it has explosive properties.

D-12. *Algorithm for dystocia*

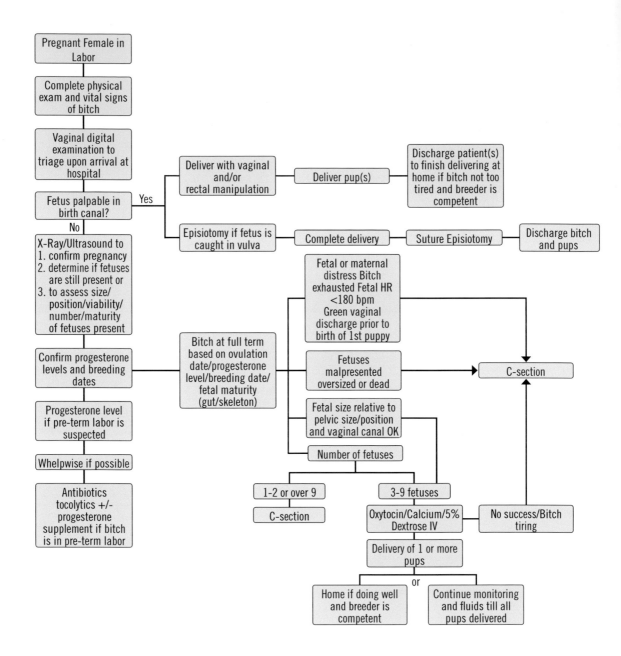

Pregnant Female in Labor
→ Complete physical exam and vital signs of bitch
→ Vaginal digital examination to triage upon arrival at hospital
→ Fetus palpable in birth canal?

Yes → Deliver with vaginal and/or rectal manipulation → Deliver pup(s) → Discharge patient(s) to finish delivering at home if bitch not too tired and breeder is competent

Episiotomy if fetus is caught in vulva → Complete delivery → Suture Episiotomy → Discharge bitch and pups

No →
X-Ray/Ultrasound to
1. confirm pregnancy
2. determine if fetuses are still present or
3. to assess size/ position/viability/ number/maturity of fetuses present

→ Confirm progesterone levels and breeding dates

→ Bitch at full term based on ovulation date/progesterone level/breeding date/ fetal maturity (gut/skeleton)

Fetal or maternal distress Bitch exhausted Fetal HR <180 bpm Green vaginal discharge prior to birth of 1st puppy → C-section

Fetuses malpresented oversized or dead → C-section

Fetal size relative to pelvic size/position and vaginal canal OK

→ Number of fetuses

1-2 or over 9 → C-section

3-9 fetuses → Oxytocin/Calcium/5% Dextrose IV → Delivery of 1 or more pups

No success/Bitch tiring → C-section

Delivery of 1 or more pups:
or
Home if doing well and breeder is competent
Continue monitoring and fluids till all pups delivered

Progesterone level if pre-term labor is suspected
→ Whelpwise if possible
→ Antibiotics tocolytics +/- progesterone supplement if bitch is in pre-term labor

D-13. *Drug formulary*

	Drug formulary					
Generic Drug Name	Trade Drug Name	Dose Range with Frequency and Route	Male Female Neonate or Pediatric	Drug Class and Indication	Comments	Reference or Source
Acyclovir	Zovirax®	10 mg per kg as suspension PO every 6 hours until 3 weeks of age.	Neonate	Antiviral. Canine Herpesvirus in the neonate.	Extralabel Drug Use*	Kampschmidt and others. Unpublished observation. Plumb 7th Edition.
Aglepristone	Alizine®	10 mg per kg (or 0.33 ml per kg per day at 30 mg/ml) administered on day 1, 2, 8, 15, and 29. This treatment can be combined with cloprostenol (at 1 mcg (micrograms) per kg SC once a day from day 3 to day 7) to increase uterine evacuation. Follow injection with massage of injection site. Maximum of 5 ml at any single injection site.	Female	Injectable progesterone blocker. To augment pyometra treatment by allowing the cervical os to open. 90% treatment success when used through day 29 of this protocol.	Not a US FDA Approved Drug+ Contraindicated during desired pregnancy.	Canine Pyometra: Pathogenesis, Therapy and Clinical Cases WSAVA 2002 Congress Prof. Stefano Romagnoli. Plumb 7th Edition.
Aglepristone	Alizine®	10 mg per kg SC (or 0.33 ml per kg per day at 30 mg/ml) repeated once 24 hours later. Administer 2 doses at 24 hour intervals SC, followed by massage of injection site. Maximum of 5 ml at any one injection site.	Female	Injectable progesterone blocker. Pregnancy termination.	Not a US FDA Approved Drug+ Contraindicated during desired pregnancy. Can be administered any day from confirmation of pregnancy up to day 45 of pregnancy. In mid pregnancy it can be used in bitches in which an unwanted pregnancy has been confirmed by ultrasound between days 22 and 30. 94% effective. May resorb fetuses or see vaginal discharge. The preparation is an oily alcohol solution.	Recent Advances in Small Animal Reproduction, P. W. Concannon, G. England and J. Verstegen. International Veterinary Information Service (www.ivis.org), Ithaca, New York, USA. Clinical Use of Anti-Progestins in the Bitch (23-Feb-2001) Fieni, Bruyas, Battut and Tainturier.

Altrenogest	Regu-Mate®	Female	Dosage	Extralabel Drug Use*	References

Drug	Product	Sex	Dosage	Extralabel Drug Use*	References
Altrenogest	Regu-Mate®	Female	0.088 mg per kg administered orally once daily, no later than 61 days post ovulation. Available as Altrenogest 0.22% (2.2 mg/ml) in oil. Give equine product (Regu-Mate®) at 2 ml per 100 lbs of body weight PO once daily for dogs.	Oral progestin. To manage luteal insufficiency that may lead to pre-term labor. Document luteal insufficiency and rule out infectious causes of pregnancy loss. Best to avoid during first trimester. Give equine product (Regu-Mate®) at 2 ml per 100 lbs of body weight PO once daily. Monitor pregnancy with ultrasound. Exogenous progesterone use is the experimental model for pyometra in the bitch, so monitor carefully. Considered safe during pregnancy. Client Information • The manufacturer lists the following people as those who should not handle the product: • Women who are or suspect that they are pregnant. • Anyone with thrombophlebitis or thromboembolic disorders or with a history of these events. • Anyone having cerebrovascular or coronary artery disease • Women with known or suspected carcinoma of the breast. • People with known or suspected estrogen-dependent neoplasias. • Women with undiagnosed vaginal bleeding. • People with benign or malignant tumor that developed during the use of oral contraceptives or other estrogen containing products. • Altrenogest can be absorbed after skin contact and absorption can be enhanced if the drug is covered by occlusive materials (e.g., under latex gloves, etc.). If exposed to the skin, wash	Root Kustritz MV. Small Animal Theriogenology. Package insert; Regu-Mate®, Matrix® - Intervet. Plumb 7th Edition. Purswell 1999.

Generic Drug Name	Trade Drug Name	Dose Range with Frequency and Route	Male Female Neonate or Pediatric	Drug Class and Indication	Comments	Reference or Source
					off immediately with soap and water. If the eyes are exposed, flush with water for 15 minutes and get medical attention. If the product is swallowed, do not induce vomiting and contact a physician or poison control center.	
Amoxicillin	Amoxi-Tabs®	10 to 22 mg per kg PO, IV every 12 hours.	All	Aminopenicillin. To treat susceptible infections in the neonate.	Considered safe during pregnancy.	Various. Plumb 7th Edition.
Amoxicillin	Amoxi-Tabs® Amoxi-Drops®	For susceptible UTI's: 10 to 20 mg per kg PO every 12 hours (up to every 6 hours) for 5 to 7 days. For susceptible systemic infections: 22 to 50 mg per kg PO every 8 hours for 7 days. For susceptible orthopedic infections: 22 to 30 mg per kg IV, IM, SC, or PO every 6 to 8 hours for 7 to 10 days. NOTE: Duration of treatment are general guidelines, generally treat for at least 2 days after all signs of infection are gone.	All	Aminopenicillin. To treat susceptible infections in the adult.	Considered safe during pregnancy.	Various. Greene and Watson 1998 Plumb 7th Edition.
Amoxicillin and Clavulanic acid	Clavamox®	12.5 to 25 mg per kg PO every 12 hours.	All	Potentiated aminopenicillin. To treat susceptible infections in neonates.	Considered safe during pregnancy.	Lee. Plumb 7th Edition.

Drug	Trade Name	Dosage	Species	Description	Pregnancy	References
Amoxicillin and Clavulanic acid	Clavamox®	For susceptible UTI's: 12.5 mg per kg PO every 8 to 12 hours for 5 to 7 days. For susceptible skin, soft tissue infections: 12.5 mg per kg PO every 12 hours for 5 to7 days (may need to extend to 21 days; do not exceed past 30 days); For susceptible deep pyodermas: 12.5 mg per kg PO every 12 hours for 14 to 120 days; For systemic bacteremia: 22 mg per kg PO every 8 to 12 hours for 7 days.	All	Potentiated aminopenicillin. To treat susceptible infections in adults.	Considered safe during pregnancy.	Plumb 7th Edition.
Amoxicillin + sulbactam	Unasyn®	Neonates: 50 mg per kg (Amoxicillin and sulbactam combined) IV every 4 to 6 hours as long as necessary. Adult dogs: For Gram (+) Positive Infections: 10 to 20 mg per kg PO every 12 hours; 5 mg per kg IM, SC every 12 hours; 5 mg per kg IV every 8 hours. For Gram (−) Negative infections: 20 to 30 mg per kg PO every 8 hours; 10 mg per kg IM or SC every 8 hours; 10 mg per kg IV every 6 hours. For susceptible UTI's: 12.5 mg per kg PO every 12 hours for 3 to 7 days;	All	Injectable potentiated aminopenicillin. To treat susceptible infections.	Can be administered IO, SC or IM in neonate. Considered safe during pregnancy. Reconstitute with 0.9% Sodium Chloride injection, 5% dextrose injection, sterile water for injection, Lactated Ringer's injection. If reconstituted with 10 ml of above solutions, makes 150 mg/ml. Once reconstituted at this concentration, is stable for 72 hours at refrigeration, 8 hours at room temperature. At 150 mg/ml, the typical neonate dose is 0.15 to 0.25 ml per dose based on weight of neonate.	Plumb 7th Edition. Aucoin 2000. Hawkins 2003.

Generic Drug Name	Trade Drug Name	Dose Range with Frequency and Route	Male Female Neonate or Pediatric	Drug Class and Indication	Comments	Reference or Source
		6.6 mg per kg IM or SC every 12 hours for 3 to 7 days. For susceptible soft tissue infections: 10 to 20 mg per kg PO, IM or SC every 8 hours for 7 days. For pneumonia, systemic infection: 22 mg per kg PO, IV or SC every 8 hours for 7 to 14 days. For susceptible sepsis, bacteremia: 20 to 40 mg per kg IV, IM or SC every 6 to 8 hours for as long as necessary.				
Atropine		0.04 mg per kg, SC as needed prior to induction of or during anesthesia. Using Atropine for small animal dose at 1/120 gr/ml or 0.54 mg/ml, this calculates to be 1 cc per 10 to 20 kg (20 to 40 lb).	Male, Female, Pediatric	Injectable anticholinergic. To prevent bradycardia during anesthesia.	Minimal or no response in neonates under 14 days of age. Bradycardia in the neonate should be treated with oxygen and warming. However, atropine is the drug of choice if the bitch becomes bradycardic during C-section.	Hellyer Veterinary Anesthesia & Analgesia Support Group 2012.
Azithromycin	Zithromax®	5 to 10 mg per kg PO once daily for 3 to 5 days.	All	Macrolide antibiotic. To treat susceptible infections.	Considered safe during pregnancy.	Plumb 7th Edition.
Bethanechol	Urecholine®	5 to 15 mg per dog PO every 8 hours or 0.5 to 1.0 mg per kg PO every 8 hours.	All	Cholinergic. To manage swallowing defects or to increase bladder contractility.	Use with caution. Principle contraindications are GI or urinary tract obstructions or wall integrity in question	Plumb 7th Edition.

Bromocriptine	Parlodel®	For estrous induction: 20 to 25 mcg (micrograms) per kg per day divided PO every 8 to 12 hours for 30 to 90 days until the start of proestrus.	Female	Dopamine agonist/pro-lactin inhibitor. Used to induce estrus.	Extralabel Drug Use* Contraindicated during desired pregnancy. Cabergoline has same effect with fewer side effects.	Plumb 7th Edition.
Bromocriptine	Parlodel®	To reduce size of mam-mary tumor pre-op: 10 mcg (micrograms) per kg PO every 8 hours for 5 to 8 days pre-op.	Female	Dopamine agonist/pro-lactin inhibitor. Used pre-op to reduce size of mammary tumor.	Extralabel Drug Use* Do not use in estrous bitch or during desired pregnancy.	Plumb 7th Edition.
Bromocriptine	Parlodel®	To augment pyometra treatment: 10 to 25 mcg (micro-grams) per kg every 8 to 12 hours PO for the first 8 days of pyometra therapy. The tablets are 2.5 mg (2500 mcg (micro-grams)), so for smaller bitches, 1 tablet should be dissolved in 10 cc of water (to make 250 mcg (micrograms)/ml), and stored in the refrigerator in a dark amber bottle. This should be shaken to resuspend before administered.	Female	Dopamine agonist/pro-lactin inhibitor. To augment medical treatment of pyometra.	Extralabel Drug Use* Contraindicated during desired pregnancy. Can use metoclopramide if necessary to manage nausea and vomiting.	Plumb 7th Edition.
Bromocriptine	Parlodel®	To manage false preg-nancy: 10 to 30 mcg (micro-grams) per kg PO every 8 to 12 hours for 16 days as needed.	Female	Dopamine agonist/pro-lactin inhibitor. To minimize symptoms of false pregnancy.	Extralabel Drug Use* Contraindicated during desired pregnancy. Evalu-ate to be certain bitch is not pregnant before initiating therapy. Can use metoclopramide if necessary to manage nausea and vomiting.	Plumb 7th Edition.

Generic Drug Name	Trade Drug Name	Dose Range with Frequency and Route	Male Female Neonate or Pediatric	Drug Class and Indication	Comments	Reference or Source
Bromocriptine	Parlodel®	To augment pregnancy termination: 10 to 25 mcg (micrograms) per kg PO every 8 hours to every 12 hours for 8 days or until progesterone level drops below 5 ng/dl. The tablets are 2.5 mg (2500 mcg (micrograms)), so for smaller bitches, 1 tablet should be dissolved in 10 cc of water (to make 250 mcg (micrograms) per ml), and stored in the refrigerator in a dark amber bottle. This should be shaken to resuspend before administered.	Female	Dopamine agonist/prolactin inhibitor. Used with cloprostenol to augment termination of pregnancy.	Extralabel Drug Use* Contraindicated during desired pregnancy. Bromocriptine may cause a plethora of adverse effects that are usually dose related and minimized with dosage reduction. Some more likely possibilities include: gastrointestinal effects (nausea, vomiting), nervous system effects (sedation, fatigue, etc.), and hypotension (particularly with the first dose, but it may persist).	Plumb 7th Edition.
Bupivacaine	Marcaine®	1 mg per kg up to a maximum dose of 2 mg per kg (1 mg/lb) as needed for pain management. Intra-lesion injection.	Male Female adults only NEVER in the neonate!	Local anesthetic. To manage pain as a local anesthetic. Slower onset of action (20 to 30 minutes) but longer duration of effect (3 to 5 hours) when compared to lidocaine.	Contraindicated in the neonate due to risk of cardiotoxicity. More potential for toxicity than lidocaine. Calculate doses very carefully. Never administer IV.	Neonatology A. P. Davidson 2009 SFT Proceedings.
Buprenorphine	Buprenex®	10 to 30 mcg (micrograms) per kg IV, IM or SC. (0.01 to 0.03 mg per kg) 10 mcg (micrograms) per kg post C-section.	All	Opiate partial agonist. To improve post-op analgesia. Safe to use AT induction to aid in analgesia for C-section – takes effect after pups are delivered IF surgeon is fast enough to deliver pups before the onset of action.	Controlled substance (CIII) Rarely causes respiratory depression: use with caution in patients with CNS or cardiovascular dysfunction.	Plumb 7th Edition. Mason DE. "Anesthesia for Cesarean Section." World Small Animal Veterinary Association World Congress Proceedings, 2006.

Buprenorphine	Buprenex®	0.02 mg per kg up to 4 times a day.	Puppy	Opiate partial agonist.	Controlled substance (CIII) Rarely causes respiratory depression: use with caution in patients with CNS or cardiovascular dysfunction.	Plumb 7th Edition. Veterinary Anesthesia & Analgesia Support Group.
Butorphanol Tartrate	Torbugesic® Torbutrol®	As an analgesic: SC, IM, IV, or PO up to 4 times a day. 1. 0.1 to 1 mg per kg IM, IV or SC every 1 to 3 hours 2. 0.2 to 0.4 mg per kg SC, IM or IV (use lower dose if given IV); Efficacy is 1 to 2 hours for moderate pain and 2 to 4 hours for mild pain. May give orally at 0.4 mg per kg to the nearest quarter tablet 3 times a day. 3. 0.5 to 1 mg per kg PO every 6 to 8 hours. As a pre-anesthetic: 1. 0.05 mg per kg IV or 0.4 mg per kg SC or IM. 2. 0.2 to 0.4 mg per kg IM (with acepromazine 0.02 to 0.04 mg per kg IM).	All	Opiate partial agonist. To manage pain, as a cough suppressant.	Controlled substance (C-IV) Causes more sedation than buprenorphine. Considered safe during pregnancy. Reduce dose in dogs with MDR-1 mutation.	Plumb 7th Edition. Hendrix and Hansen 2000 Mathews 1999 Morgan 1988 Reidesel Hardie 2000 Veterinary Anesthesia & Analgesia Support Group.

Generic Drug Name	Trade Drug Name	Dose Range with Frequency and Route	Male Female Neonate or Pediatric	Drug Class and Indication	Comments	Reference or Source
Cabergoline	Dostinex® (Pfizer) (human) Galastop® in liquid form in Europe	1. For estrus induction: 5 mcg (micrograms) per kg PO once daily for 10 days or until 2nd day of proestrus. Induces fertile proestrus in 4 to 25 days. 2. For treatment of pseudopregnancy: 5 mcg (micrograms) per kg once a day PO for 5 to 10 days. 3. To reduce lactation while treating mastitis: Administer for 2 to 3 days at 5 mcg (micrograms) per kg once daily) to reduce lactation can also speed recovery from mastitis. Pups must be weaned. 4. Pyometra ancillary treatment: 5 mcg (micrograms) per kg once a day PO for 5 to 10 days. Monitor response with ultrasound. 5. To assist with medical termination of pregnancy: 5 mcg (micrograms) per kg once a day PO for 5 to 10 days. Monitor response with progesterone testing. 6. To reduce the size of mammary tumors pre-op: 5 mcg (micrograms) per kg once daily for 5 to 8 days pre-op.	Female	Prolactin inhibitor/dopamine (D2) agonist. 1. For estrus induction (works ~70% of time). 2. To treat pseudopregnancy. 3. To reduce lactation during mastitis. 4. To aid in luteolysis in pyometra treatment. 5. To aid in pharmacologically induced abortion. 6. To reduce the size of mammary tumors pre-op.	Extralabel Drug Use* Contraindicated during desired pregnancy. Cabergoline is contraindicated in dogs and cats that are pregnant, unless abortion is desired (see indications). When using to induce estrus, it is recommended to wait at least 4 months after the prior cycle to allow the uterus to recover. Give this medication with food. Because of the dosage differences in animals versus human patients, and the strength of the commercially available tablet form of the product, a compounding pharmacist must usually reformulate this medication. Galastop liquid as an alternative.	Plumb 7th Edition.

					Extralabel Drug Use*	
Caffeine	NoDoz®	1 tablet dissolved in 1 cc water; 1 drop on the tongue of a neonate to stimulate respirations AFTER airways are clear. Repeat PRN once daily.	Neonate	Stimulant. As a Respiratory and cardiac stimulant of neonates.	Anecdotal. Used in human neonates once daily as a respiratory stimulant.	
Calcium	Cal-Pho-Sol®	Calcium glycerophosphate 50 mg and Calcium Lactate 50 mg Can be administered at a range of up to 1 cc per 10 pound of body weight SC up to 2 times a day.	Female	Essential cation nutrient. To improve uterine contractions during labor and at C-section. To improve maternal skills (anecdotal).	Considered safe during pregnancy. BE SURE THE PRODUCT YOU ARE USING IS LABELLED FOR SC ADMINISTRATION. THE WRONG FORM CAN CAUSE SERIOUS SKIN SLOUGHS. IF ADMINISTERING IV, GIVE VERY SLOWLY AND MONITOR EKG, STOP IF EKG CHANGES OR BITCH VOMITS.	Plumb 7th Edition.
Calcium gluconate	10% Calcium Gluconate or Calphosan SOLUTION ONLY (not Calphosan suspension)	0.5 to 1.0 cc per 10 pounds of body weight (0.1 mg per pound body weight) every 4 to 6 hours, SC divided into 2 locations, not to exceed 5 cc per location.	Female	Essential cation nutrient. To improve uterine contractions during labor and at C-section. To improve maternal skills (anecdotal).	Considered safe during pregnancy. BE SURE THE PRODUCT YOU ARE USING IS LABELLED FOR SC ADMINISTRATION. THE WRONG FORM (calcium chloride) CAN CAUSE SERIOUS SKIN SLOUGHS. IF ADMINISTERING IV, GIVE VERY SLOWLY AND MONITOR EKG, STOP IF EKG CHANGES OR BITCH VOMITS.	Plumb 7th Edition.

Generic Drug Name	Trade Drug Name	Dose Range with Frequency and Route	Male Female Neonate or Pediatric	Drug Class and Indication	Comments	Reference or Source
Calcium		Calcium gluconate 10%, warmed to body temperature, give IV at a rate of 50 to 150 mg per kg or 0.5 to 1.5 ml per kg over 20 to 30 minutes. An alternative IV treatment is 1% calcium glycerophosphate plus calcium lactate (Calphosan solution 1%) administered at 2.5 to 7.5 ml per kg, again over 20 to 30 minutes. With either protocol, STOP IF THE HEART RATE CHANGES. Best to use EKG to monitor administration.	Female	Essential cation nutrient. Used to treat postpartum eclampsia (hypocalcaemia).	Considered safe during pregnancy. If the 10% calcium gluconate solution is available, it can be diluted 50% with normal saline and administered SC every 8 hours until the oral calcium takes effect. Oral calcium treatment (500 mg EVERY 8 HOURS per 20 lbs) should be continued throughout lactation.	Plumb 7th Edition.
Calcium oral gel	Calsorb® gel	1 to 3 ml PO depending on severity of condition PO every 12 hours.	Female	Essential cation nutrient. To manage uterine inertia, aggression toward puppies.	170 mg/ml	Plumb 7th Edition.
Carnitine	Motility Plus™ Acetyl-L-Carnitine Quinicarn®	250 to 500 mg PO twice daily.	Male	Nutrient. To alter fat metabolism. May help with sperm motility.	Give with meals when possible to reduce likelihood of GI side effects.	Plumb 7th Edition.
Carprofen	Rimadyl®	4.4 mg per kg PO, IM or SC; may be given once daily or divided and given as 2.2. mg per kg twice daily; round dose to nearest half caplet increment. For postoperative pain, administer approximately 2 hours before the procedure, except for C-sections.	Female, Male	Non-steroidal anti-inflammatory. For pain and inflammation management.	Non-steroidal anti-inflammatory. To manage pain and inflammation. The manufacturer states that the safe use of carprofen in dogs less than 6 weeks of age, in pregnant dogs, dogs used for breeding purposes, or in lactating bitches has not been established. May cause GI liver	Plumb 7th Edition. Package Insert Rimadyl®–Pfizer.

		Injectable is dosed at the oral products dose, but administered SC.			and renal effects. In cases with long-term use, blood monitoring renal and hepatic function is recommended.	
Cefazolin	Ancef® Kefzol®	1. For systemic infections: 5 to 25 mg per kg IM or IV every 6 to 8 hours as long as necessary. 2. For sepsis, bacteremia: 15 to 25 mg per kg IV, IM or SC every 4 to 8 hours for 7 days or less.	All	First generation cephalosporin antibiotic. To treat bacterial infections susceptible to cephalosporins.	Cephalosporins have been shown to cross the placenta and safe use of them during pregnancy have not been firmly established, but neither have there been any documented teratogenic problems associated with these drugs. However, use only when the potential benefits outweigh the risks.	Plumb 7th Edition. Greene and Watson 1998.
Cefazolin	Kefzol® Keflex®	10 to 30 mg per kg SC or IO every 6 to 8 hours.	All	First generation cephalosporin antibiotic. To treat susceptible infections in neonates.	Considered safe during pregnancy.	Root Kustritz
Cephalexin	Ancef®	10 to 30 mg per kg every 8 to 12 hours PO.	All	First generation cephalosporin antibiotic. To treat bacterial infections susceptible to cephalosporins.	Considered safe during pregnancy. Administer to neonates via a stomach tube.	Plumb 7th Edition.
Ceftiofur	Naxcel®	2.5 mg per kg SC every 12 hours, 5 days maximum.	Neonate	Third generation cephalosporin. To treat susceptible infections in the neonate.	Drug of choice for neonates born with meconium in the fetal membranes. Causes minimal disruption of GI flora.	Davidson, Autumn. "Neonatology." Theriogenology. Albuquerque, 28 Aug. 2009.
Chloramphenicol	Cleocin®	22 mg per kg PO every 8 hours for up to 7 days total.	Puppies	Broad spectrum antibacterial. To treat susceptible infections – mycoplasma.	Contraindicated during pregnancy.	Poffenberger

Generic Drug Name	Trade Drug Name	Dose Range with Frequency and Route	Male Female Neonate or Pediatric	Drug Class and Indication	Comments	Reference or Source
Clindamycin	Antirobe®	1. For neosporosis, toxoplasmosis: 5 to 20 mg per kg IV, IM, SC, or PO every 12 hours for 15 days. 2. For neosporosis: 13.5 mg per kg PO every 8 hours for 21 days. Used concurrently with Trimethoprim/Sulfa at 15 mg per kg PO every 12 hours for 4 weeks.	All	Lincosamide antibiotic. To treat aerobes, anaerobes and Neosporum infection.	Considered safe during pregnancy.	Plumb 7th Edition. Greene and Watson 1998.
Clindamycin	Antirobe®	1. For infected wounds, abscesses and dental infections: 5.5 to 33 mg per kg PO every 12 hours. 2. For osteomyelitis: 11 to 33 mg per kg PO every 12 hours. Treatment may continue for up to 28 days. If no response after 3 to 4 days, discontinue.	All	Lincosamide antibiotic. To treat bacterial infections susceptible to clindamycin.	Considered safe during pregnancy. Because clindamycin is distributed into milk, nursing puppies or kittens of mothers taking clindamycin may develop diarrhea. However, in humans, the American Academy of Pediatrics considers clindamycin compatible with breast-feeding.	Plumb 7th Edition. Package insert – Antirobe®, Pfizer.
Clindamycin	Antirobe®	For chronic prostatitis: 5 to 10 mg per kg every 8 hours PO, IV or IM.	All	Lincosamide antibiotic. To treat bacterial infections susceptible to clindamycin.	Considered safe during pregnancy.	Plumb 7th Edition.
Cloprostenol	Estrumate®	For adjunctive treatment of open cervix pyometra: 1 to 5 mcg (micrograms) per kg (0.001 to 0.005 mg per kg) SC once per day. May require up to 2 to 3 weeks of treatment. When starting treatment, start with one-half the normal dosage and	Female	Prostaglandin F analog. To medically manage pyometra when Lutalyse® is not a viable option.	Extralabel Drug Use* Cloprostenol is contraindicated in pregnant animals when abortion or induced parturition is not desired. Combine with 4 weeks of antibiotics and supportive hydration to manage pyometra medically.	Plumb 7th Edition. Romagnoli 2002a.

Cloprostenol	Estrumate®	gradually increase to achieve the full dose within 2 to 3 days. To pharmacologically cause pregnancy termination at confirmation of pregnancy from days 24 to 28: 1.0 to 2.5 mcg (micrograms) per kg IM on day 1 and day 4 at confirmation of pregnancy with ultrasound. A third dose should be given on day 8 of treatment IF the progesterone level on day 4 is greater than 2 ng/dl and the ultrasound shows viable fetal structures. Larger breed dogs with larger litters should be dosed on the higher end of the dosage range. Can be combined with bromocriptine to improve efficacy. See chapter 9 and bromocriptine for dosage information.	Female	Prostaglandin F analog. To cause pregnancy termination	Extralabel Drug Use* Contraindicated during desired pregnancy. Most patients have nausea, vomiting and diarrhea after administration. Walking for 15 minutes after injection of cloprostenol and administering either metoclopramide or atropine diminishes symptoms. Do not administer IV. Other **oxytocic agents'** activity may be enhanced by cloprostenol. Cloprostenol should be used by individuals familiar with its use and precautions. Pregnant women, asthmatics or other persons with bronchial diseases should handle this product with extreme caution. Any accidental exposure to skin should be washed off immediately.	Verstegen – Society for Theriogenology Proceedings 2007.
Cosyntropin	Cortrosyn®	For testing (screening) for adrenal function: For ACTH stimulation: 1.5 mcg (micrograms) per kg IV; measure serum cortisol both prior to administered and 1 hour post-administration.	Male and female	Hormonal injectable diagnostic agent. For adrenal gland testing when the patient has infertility or other suspected metabolic disease.	Check with the diagnostic lab prior to use to assure you are following their protocol for testing. Laboratories vary in their protocols.	Plumb 7th Edition. Watson, Church et al. 1998. Behrend 2003.

Generic Drug Name	Trade Drug Name	Dose Range with Frequency and Route	Male Female Neonate or Pediatric	Drug Class and Indication	Comments	Reference or Source
		2. 5 mcg (micrograms) per kg with a maximum of 250 mcg (micrograms) IV. Once reconstituted, the solution may be frozen for up to six months for later use.				
DAP	Adaptil™	Collar is most useful application with most rapid onset. Topical by collar. Lasts 4 weeks.	Female	Pheromone behavior modifier. To improve maternal skills, calm pups.	Considered safe during pregnancy. Dog appeasing pheromone (DAP) is a synthetic derivative of bitch intermammary pheromone. Put collar on bitch 3 days prior to whelping.	Plumb 7th Edition.
Deslorelin	Ovuplant® 2.1 mg	Equine formulation – Pellet placed in submucosa of vulvar lip, removed after breeding to maintain pregnancy. See directions in chapter 9.	Female	Synthetic GnRH analog. To induce estrous in the intact female dog.	Not a US FDA Approved Drug + Contraindicated during pregnancy. Deslorelin increases the levels of endogenous luteinizing hormone (LH), thereby inducing ovulation. May block estrous if implanted during early proestrus – precede placement with progesterone test (should be < 1 ng/dl).	IVIS.
Deslorelin	Suprelorin® 4.7 mg and 9.4 mg	Inserted in the SC over the shoulders or SC near the umbilicus. Repeat in 6 to 12 months, based on formulation. If care is taken with technique and location of insertion, may be able to	Male and female post-puberty adults	Synthetic GnRH analog. To treat BPH in intact male dogs. Will cause sterility so should not be used in male dogs with future breeding potential.	Not a US FDA Approved Drug + Contraindicated during pregnancy. Pellet will remain in situ, encased in a protective synthetic sleeve. Experimental use in Europe for:	IVIS.

Drug		Dosage	Notes / Indications	Reference
		remove to reverse effects. Avoid implanting into fat. For male contraception, use a 4.7 mg implant SC every 6 months or 9.4 mg implant SC every 12 months.	1. To manage BPH. 2. To treat anal gland adenoma in the male dog. 3. To control of reproduction in male and female dogs. 4. To control roaming and to eliminate urine odor in male cats 5. To treat post-spaying urinary incontinence in the bitch. 6. To control mammary tumor metastatic disease in the bitch.	Urethral Sphincter Mechanism Incontinence Contributors: Linda Shell, DVM, DACVIM Plumb 7th Edition.
Diethylstilbestrol (DES)	Compounded	0.1 to 1.0 mg total dose (0.02 mg per kg; maximum of 1 mg) PO daily for 3 to 5 days and then tapered to 1 mg one to three times weekly for maintenance.	Female	Synthetic estrogen. To manage urinary incontinence in spayed females. Compounded Drug ∞ Should be replaced by estriol (Incurin™), an FDA approved product. Teratogenic - contraindicated during pregnancy. Aplastic anemia, thrombocytopenia, or neutropenia have NOT been observed in dogs treated with low-dose estrogen protocols. Estradiol cypionate (ECP) should never be given as treatment for urinary incontinence.	
Dihydrostreptomycin		Combine with minocycline (25 mg per kg PO once daily for 14 days) with dihydrostreptomycin (5 mg per kg IM every 12 hours for 7 days) and tetracycline (30 mg per kg PO every 12 hours for 21 days) with streptomycin (20 mg per kg IM once daily for 14 days).	Aminoglycoside antibiotic. Used to treat <u>Brucella canis</u>. Contraindicated during pregnancy. Dihydrostreptomycin and minocycline used n conjunction with surgical desexing to try to manage Brucellosis. Currently unavailable in the US.	Root Kustritz 2007.

Generic Drug Name	Trade Drug Name	Dose Range with Frequency and Route	Male Female Neonate or Pediatric	Drug Class and Indication	Comments	Reference or Source
Domeperidone	Equi-Tox®	0.05 to 0.1 mg per kg PO once or twice a day.	Female	Prokinetic/ Dopamine-2 agonist. Used to improve lactation by prolactin secretion stimulation effects.	Extralabel Drug Use* Equine (for fescue toxicity) and human (to improve lactation) use, scant canine data. Because domeperidone is potentially a neurotoxic substrate of P-glycoprotein, it should be used with caution in those herding breeds (e.g., Collies) that may have the gene mutation that causes a nonfunctional protein. Clients should understand the investigational nature of this drug. Formulation may cause salivation. Pregnant and lactating women should use caution handling the gel.	Plumb 7th Edition.
Doxapram	Dopram®-V	To stimulate respirations in newborns: 1. 0.05 cc IM in the caudal thigh or 2. 1 to 2 drops (1 to 2 mg) under tongue or 3. 1 to 5 mg IV in umbilical vein. Should be used with caution if product contains benzyl alcohol as a preservative.	Neonate	CNS/respiratory stimulant. For Neonatal Dogs and Cats: CNS stimulant – used stimulate respirations following dystocia or cesarean section.	The use of doxapram to initiate and stimulate respirations in newborns is controversial. Monitor for red "flush" of mucus membranes indicating anticipated respiratory effort, repeat if indicated. Most likely to be beneficial to increase respiratory efforts in newborns with ineffective respirations, combined with oxygen.	Plumb 7th Edition. Package Insert; Dopram®-V-Robins. Copley K: Parturition management: 15,000 whelpings later: An outcome based analysis. Theriogenology 2009; Vol. 1, Number 2: 297-307.

Ephedrine sulfate		4 to 5 mg per kg PO every 8 hours, repeated several hours prior to collection or breeding.	Male	Sympathomimetic bronchodilator/ vasopressor. Retrograde ejaculation	Extralabel Drug Use* Avoid in patients with arrhythmias, hypertension and glaucoma. Tachycardia and dry mouth are generally more pronounced with ephedrine than with PPA.	Plumb 7th Edition.
Epinephrine	Adrenalin®	For Cardiac resuscitation (asystole): 0.01 to 0.5 mg (0.5 to 5 ml) of 1:10,000 solution intratracheally or intravenously after ABC (Airway/breathing/ compressions) are initiated. May need to repeat every 3 to 5 minutes. If intratracheal or IV sites are inaccessible, the intracardiac (IC) route may be used. Neonates, when respiratory support and chest compression fails to elicit a heartbeat: 0.1 to 0.3 mg per kg IV or IO. IC dose is 0.5 to 5 micrograms per kg (0.0005 to 0.005 mg per kg).	All	Alpha and beta-adrenergic agonist. For cardiac resuscitation or anaphylaxis.	To convert a 1:1000 solution to a 1:10,000 solution for IV or intratracheal use, dilute 1 ml with 9 ml of normal saline for injection. Double the dose if intratracheal administration is necessary.	Plumb 7th Edition. Wingfield 1985. Traas 2009. Veterinary Anesthesia & Analgesia Support Group.
Erythromycin	Gallimycin®	For chronic prostatitis: 10 to 22 mg per kg every 8 hours PO long term as indicated by chronicity of disease.	Male, female	Macrolide antibiotic. To treat bacterial diseases susceptible to use of erythromycin.	Considered safe during pregnancy. May cause GI upset. May cause neurological signs in dogs with MDR1 mutation.	Plumb 7th Edition.
Estradiol cypionate	ECP®	NEVER use it in the dog as it may cause aplastic anemia. Previously used to interrupt pregnancy early.	Female	Natural estrogen salt.	Extralabel Drug Use* Contraindicated during desired pregnancy. Seek a safer alternate more effective treatment to prevent pregnancy.	Various.

Generic Drug Name	Trade Drug Name	Dose Range with Frequency and Route	Male Female Neonate or Pediatric	Drug Class and Indication	Comments	Reference or Source
Estrogens, conjugated	Premarin®	20 mcg (micrograms) per kg every 4 days PO.	Female	Conjugated synthetic estrogen. To manage spayed female incontinence.	Extralabel Drug Use* Contraindicated during pregnancy. Long-term therapy can cause anemia – avoid long term use.	Chew DC, Brown SA: Fixing the Dripping in Senior Female Dogs. Iams Senior Care 2004.
Estrogens, conjugated	Premarin®	20 mcg (micrograms) per kg every 12 hours a week for only 2 weeks PO.	Female	Conjugated synthetic estrogen. To manage puppy vaginitis.	Extralabel Drug Use* Contraindicated during pregnancy.	Threfall.
Fatty acids	Omega 3 Fatty Acid Supplement Multiple products	PO. See label of product.	Male	Nutrient. To improve semen quality.	Anecdotal evidence	Kampschmidt.
Fenbendazole	Panacur®	50 mg per kg PO once daily every 24 hours for 3 to 5 days in the neonate. 5 day course for Giardia.	Neonate	Broad spectrum anthelminthic. To remove ascarids, hookworms, whipworms, capillaria, some tapeworms, flukes, and giardia.	Considered safe during pregnancy. Treat or prevent intestinal parasites. Drug of choice to treat giardia during pregnancy. Better absorbed when administered with food.	Plumb 7th Edition.
Fenbendazole	Panacur®	To prevent transplacental and transmammary transmission of somatic *T. canis* and *A. caninum*: 50 mg per kg PO once daily from the 40th day of gestation to the 14th day of lactation.	Pregnant female	Broad spectrum anthelminthic. To remove ascarids, hookworms, whipworms, capillaria, some tapeworms, flukes, and giardia.	Extralabel Drug Use* Fenbendazole is considered safe to use in pregnant bitches and is generally considered safe to use in pregnancy for all species. Better absorbed when administered with food.	Treatment and Control of Gastrointestinal Helminths, Western Veterinary Conference 2002, Kevin R. Kazacos, D.V.M., Ph.D., Purdue University School of Veterinary Medicine, West Lafayette, Indiana, United States.
Finasteride	Proscar® Propecia®	0.1 to 0.5 mg per kg once daily PO.	Male	5 alpha reductase inhibitor. To manage benign prostatic hyperplasia. Clients should understand that therapy might be prolonged before efficacy can be determined and that regular dosing	Extralabel Drug Use* Contraindicated during pregnancy. Exposure Of Women - Risk To Male Fetus Women should not handle crushed or broken finasteride tablets when they are	Plumb 7th Edition. Root Kustritz and Klausner 2000; Kamolpatana, Johnston et al. 1998.

		Dosage	Species	Indication	Comments	Reference
				compliance is mandatory. Monitoring prostate size is required to assess efficacy.	pregnant or may potentially be pregnant because of the possibility of absorption of finasteride and the subsequent potential risk to a male fetus. Avoid use in sexually developing animals. Relatively expensive. Drug interactions: Anticholinergic drugs, adrenergic or xanthine-derivative bronchodilators may precipitate or aggravate urinary retention thereby negating the effects of the drug.	
Fluoroquinolones	Baytril®	5 to 20 mg per kg per day PO. ay be given once daily or divided and given twice daily. Treatment should continue for at least 2 to 3 days beyond cessation of clinical signs, to a maximum duration of therapy is 30 days. Avoid in young animals. For chronic prostatitis: 5 mg per kg PO every 12 hours.	Male and female, neonates under 4 weeks if needed, not appropriate for older pups.	Fluoroquinolone antibiotic. To treat bacterial diseases susceptible to fluoroquinolones	Avoid use in dehydrated patients. Enrofloxacin is labeled as contraindicated in small and medium breed dogs from 2 months to 8 months of age due to changes in the articular cartilage. Large and giant breed dogs may be in the rapid-growth phase for periods longer than 8 months of age, so longer than 8 months may be necessary to avoid cartilage damage. Some indication that it is safe up until the pup is 4 weeks old – no documentation.	Plumb 7th Edition. Baytril®; Package insert; Bayer.

Generic Drug Name	Trade Drug Name	Dose Range with Frequency and Route	Male Female Neonate or Pediatri	Drug Class and Indication	Comments	Reference or Source
					The safety of enrofloxacin in pregnant dogs has been investigated. Breeding, pregnant and lactating dogs receiving up to 15 mg per kg day demonstrated no treatment related effects. However, because of the risks of cartilage abnormalities in young animals, the fluoroquinolones are not generally recommended for use during pregnancy unless the benefits of therapy clearly outweigh the risks. Limited studies in male dogs at various dosages have indicated no effects on male breeding performance.	
Fluoroquinolone	Ciprofloxacin	Adjust dose based on reduced bioavailability.		Fluoroquinolone antibiotic. To treat susceptible infections.	In dogs, oral bioavailability of enrofloxacin is better than ciprofloxacin. See contraindication for young animals above.	Plumb 7th Edition.
Fluoroquinolone Marbofloxacin	Zeniquin®	1. For susceptible infections (urinary tract, skin and soft tissue): 2.75 to 5.5 mg per kg PO once daily. Give for 2 to 3 days beyond cessation of clinical signs (skin/soft tissue infections); and for at least 10 days (urinary tract). If no improvement noted after 5 days, reevaluate diagnosis. .	Male and female. Not young animals.	Fluoroquinolone antibiotic. For the treatment of susceptible bacterial infections in dogs and cats.	Same contraindications in young animals as fluoroquinolones related to cartilage erosions and arthropathy.	Plumb 7th Edition. Package insert; Zeniquin®-Pfizer.

Fresh frozen plasma	HemoPet	Maximum duration of treatment is 30 days 2. For chronic prostatitis: 4 mg per kg per day. Condition may require long term therapy but package insert states duration not to exceed 30 days.				Bouchard G, Plata-Madrid H, Youngquist RS, Buening GM, Ganjam VK, Krause GF, Allen GK, Paine AL. Absorption of an alternate source of immunoglobulin in pups. Am J Vet Res. February 1992; 53(2):230-233.
		16 cc per pup SC in divided doses over 24 hours in divided doses. SC or IO, 16 cc per pup divided, not to exceed stomach capacity (maximum capacity = 1 cc per 1 oz body weight) but can only use PO if given in first 12 hours after birth due to loss of absorption through the gut 12 hours or more post partum Must keep frozen until use. Warm gently to avoid damaging proteins.	Neonates	Blood product. To augment passive immunity in the neonate	Easiest to purchase in advance from commercial sources such as Hemopet. Can also be harvested from indigenous dogs in household or kennel. Donor dogs should be health screened prior to use. See client handout in appendix for handling instructions.	
Furosemide	Lasix®	0.2 ml furosemide IM up to every 8 hours, followed with potassium chloride PO.	Neonate	Loop diuretic. To manage neonates with anasarca.	Controversial treatment, often unsuccessful. Must first assure open airway. More information in Chapter 8.	Hoskins, Johnny D. "Small Animal Pediatric Medicine." Tufts Animal Expo. North Grafton MA. 2002.
Glycoaminoglycans	Glyco-flex® ICSB-CF Plus®	See product label.	Male	Nutritional supplement. To reduce inflammation.	Not documented but anecdotal evidence.	Hess, Milan. "Documented and anecdotal effects of certain pharmaceutical agents used to enhance semen quality in the dog." Theriogenology, Volume 66, Issue 3, 613-617.

Generic Drug Name	Trade Drug Name	Dose Range with Frequency and Route	Male Female Neonate or Pediatric	Drug Class and Indication	Comments	Reference or Source
GnRH	Cystorelin®	3.3 mcg (micrograms) per kg IM once daily for 3 days. An elevated progesterone level (>2 ng/ml) measured 1-2 weeks post treatment verifies successful completion of ovulation.	Female	Hypothalmic hormone. To treat persistent estrus due to cystic ovary. Suspect cystic ovary or ovarian tumor if estrus exceeds 30 days.	Extralabel Drug Use* Bitches may have recurrences of cystic ovaries on subsequent estrous cycles. Should confirm on ultrasound to rule out ovarian tumor. Advise client: Bitches are at increased risk of developing pyometra.	Purswell 1999 Plumb 7th Edition.
GnRH	Cystorelin®	1 to 3.3 mcg (micrograms) per kg IM 1 hour prior to collection. Can be used long-term. Repeated weekly for ongoing improved libido and spermatogenesis.	Male	Hypothalmic hormone. To improve libido prior to semen collection by creating a testosterone surge. Results variable.	Extralabel Drug Use* Avoid use in dogs with prostatic disease as it will increase testosterone levels.	Hess, Milan. "Documented and anecdotal effects of certain pharmaceutical agents used to enhance semen quality in the dog." Theriogenology, Volume 66, Issue 3, 613-617.
HCG	Chorulon®	100 to 1000 IU IM per pup twice a week for 4 to 6 doses to be administered over 2 to 3 weeks. Burns when given—brief vocalization post-op.	Male pups	Human hormone mimicking LH and FSH. To aid in testicular descent.	Extralabel Drug Use* Controversial use Monitor for anaphylaxis. Must complete series of injections prior to 16 weeks of age.	Feldman, Canine and Feline Endocrinology, 2nd edition.
HCG	Chorulon®	10 units per pound once daily for 3 consecutive days.	Female	Human hormone mimicking LH and FSH. To manage persistent estrus due to cystic ovary, by inducing ovulation. Suspect cystic ovary or ovarian tumor if estrus exceeds 30 days.	Extralabel Drug Use* Bitches may have recurrences of cystic ovaries on subsequent estrous cycles. Should confirm on ultrasound to rule out ovarian tumor. Risk of anaphylaxis. Bitch is at risk of developing pyometra due to cystic ovary.	Plumb 7th Edition.
Hydroxyethyl Starch 6% Hetastarch 6%	Vetstarch TM 6%	Shock bolus dose: 10 to 20 ml per kg IV per day by slow infusion.	Male and Female	Colloid volume expander. Used as a volume expander used to treat hy	Considered safe during pregnancy; no studies have been conducted	Plumb 7th Edition. Morgan 1997

	Dose	Species	Description	Notes	Reference
	Do not exceed 20 ml per kg over 24 hours. For IV use only.		povolemia where colloidal therapy required.	during labor and delivery but no untoward effects have been reported. Adverse Effects: hypersensitivity reactions, coagulopathies possible; too rapid administration to small animals may cause nausea/vomiting.	Davidson, Autumn. "Neonatology." Theriogenology. Albuquerque, 28 Aug. 2009.
Iodine, Tincture of	Alcohol with iodine solution. Apply to umbilicus of newborns every 8 hours by dipping cord until cord is dried, has fallen off and site healed.	Neonates	Iodine and alcohol. To prevent omphalitis, an infection of the umbilicus.	Used to dip the umbilical cord stump.	
Ivermectin	200 mcg (micrograms) per kg once a week from 3 weeks before to 3 weeks after parturition SC or PO. Administer 1 time per week from week 5 of pregnancy to week 3 of lactation.	Females	Avermectin antiparasiticide. This protocol will reduce roundworm and hookworm infections in the neonates by 98 to 100%	Extralabel Drug Use* Considered safe during pregnancy. Dogs who carry the MDR-1 gene should not be treated with this protocol. Not recommended for puppies under 6 weeks of age. Calculate dose very carefully.	Treatment and Control of Gastrointestinal Helminths, Western Veterinary Conference, 2002, Kevin R. Kazacos, D.V.M., Ph.D. Purdue University School of Veterinary Medicine, West Lafayette, Indiana, United States Plumb 7th Edition.
Ivomec®					
Kaolin and Pectin	1 to 2 ml per kg PO up to 6 times a day.	All	GI adsorbent and protectant combination. Adsorbent (only) anti-diarrheal products should be safe to use during pregnancy and lactation. At usual doses, kaolin/pectin generally have no adverse effects. Overzealous administration may lead to constipation. Purchase from a veterinary or farm store	Considered safe during pregnancy.	Plumb 7th Edition.

Generic Drug Name	Trade Drug Name	Dose Range with Frequency and Route	Male Female Neonate or Pediatric	Drug Class and Indication	Comments	Reference or Source
				source. Avoid human labeled product as most human over-the-counter products labeled as Kao-Pectate® now contain bismuth subsalicylate instead of kaolin and pectin. The FDA has not given bismuth subsalicylate a pregnancy risk category. There are no studies to show safety so these should NOT be used in neonates, pregnant bitches and lactating dams.		
Lidocaine	Xylocaine®	1. 1 to 4 mg per kg (0.5 to 2.0 mg per pound). To reduce burning at injection, mix 0.9 cc Lidocaine, 0.1 cc sodium bicarbonate, and 2 cc of sterile water. 2. Combine with bupivacaine and 0.003 mg per kg (0.0015 mg per lb) buprenorphine to extend the analgesic duration of local blocks to approximately 20 hours.	All	Local and topical anesthetic agent. Used to produce local anesthetic effect.	Considered safe during pregnancy. Useful for line blocks at C-section, episiotomy; also taildock and dewclaw removal on neonates. Do NOT combine with or interchange for bupivacaine for neonates due to potential toxicity.	Buprenorphine added to the local anesthetic for axillary brachial plexus block prolongs postoperative analgesia. Candido KD, Winnie AP, Ghaleb AH, Fattouh MW, Franco CD: Reg Anesth Pain Med. 2002 Mar-Apr; 27(2):162-7. Veterinary Anesthesia & Analgesia Support Group.
Levetiracetam	Keppra®	10 to 20 mg per kg every 8 to 12 hours. Titrate dose slowly up as needed.	Puppies	Anticonvulsant. Can be used pre-op to manage puppies with liver shunts and associated seizures.	For seizure control in patients with known or suspected portosystemic shunts and associated hepatic encephalopathy. Minimal side effects (drowsiness), but expensive.	Neurologic Manifestations Associated With Portosystemic Shunting, Michael Podell, MSc, DVM, Diplomate ACVIM (Neurology) ACVS 2007.

Megestrol acetate	Ovaban® Megace®	0.25 mg per pound PO once daily for 21 days, then 0.25 mg per pound once a week for long term management.	Male	Synthetic progestin. To manage dogs with benign prostatic hypertrophy.	Extralabel Drug Use* Contraindicated during pregnancy. Will decrease ejaculate volume, avoid use just prior to ejaculation.	Hutchison, Robert: "Canine Reproduction, Whelping and Neonatal Care." Lakeshore Pembroke Welsh Corgi Club. Crystal Lake, IL. 25 March 2005.
Megestrol acetate	Ovaban® Megace®	0.55 mg per kg PO once a day for 32 days if started 7 or more days prior to the onset of proestrus. Do not repeat more often than every 6 months.	Female	Synthetic progestin. To prevent estrous before the onset of proestrus.	Extralabel Drug Use* May increase risk of pyometra, mammary neoplasia and diabetes mellitus.	Plumb 7th Edition.
Megestrol acetate	Ovaban® Megace®	2.2 mg per kg PO once a day for 8 days if started on the first 3 days of estrus. (92% efficacy). Will not work if started later than day 3 of proestrus.	Female	Synthetic progestin. To prevent estrus after proestrus has started.	Extralabel Drug Use* May increase risk of pyometra, mammary neoplasia and diabetes mellitus.	Plumb 7th Edition.
Meloxicam	Metacam®	1. For surgical pain: 0.2 mg per kg (or less) IV or SC once; followed 24 hours later by 0.1 mg per kg (or less) IV, SC, PO repeat every 24 hours. 2. For chronic pain: 0.2 mg per kg (or less) PO once; 0.1 mg per kg (or less) PO repeat every 24 hours.	Male and Female	COX-2 Non-steroidal anti-inflammatory. To manage pain, fever, or inflammation.	No NSAIDs are labeled for use in pregnant or lactating bitches or pups under 6 weeks of age. Carefully measure dose (oral liquid); do not confuse the markings on the syringe (provided by the manufacturer) with mls or kgs. "A single NSAID dose postoperatively to normotensive bitches should improve patient comfort and is not thought to be of detriment to the neonates".	Plumb 7th Edition. 1 Mathews KA. Analgesia for the pregnant, lactating and neonatal to pediatric cat and dog. JVECC. 15(4) 2005, pp 273-284. Veterinary Anesthesia & Analgesia Support Group.

Generic Drug Name	Trade Drug Name	Dose Range with Frequency and Route	Male Female Neonate or Pediatric	Drug Class and Indication	Comments	Reference or Source
Methylprednisolone Sodium Succinate	Solu-Medrol	1 mg per pound of bitch's body weight IV SLOWLY. One dose only – at least 1 hour and preferably 18 to 24 hours prior to delivery of pups.	Female	Synthetic glucocorticoid. To increase surfactant in fetal lungs prior to delivery.	Extralabel Drug Use* Avoid use if bitch may have an infection.	Lopate.
Metoclopramide	Reglan®	0.1 to 0.4 mg per kg every 8 hours PO (liquid or tablet) or SC. For lactation – 0.5 to 1 mg per kg PO total daily dose, divided every 8 hours. Use the lowest effective dose to minimize side effects. The maximum dose should not exceed 5 mg per kg total daily dose – this is likely to induce extrapyramidal signs. May start treatment 1 to 2 days prior to whelping for bitches with a tendency to develop agalactia or on progesterone supplementation. May be used simultaneously with oxytocin to improve lactation as the 2 drugs act on different mechanisms.	Female	GI prokinetic agent/ Dopamine agonist. To aid in lactation induction and maintenance, GI stimulation and anti-emetic effect. Usually results are noted within 24 hours. Mechanism: prolactin secretion stimulation effects. To minimize the GI effects of prostaglandins such as Lutalyse® or Estrumate®.	Extralabel Drug Use* Considered safe during pregnancy. Contraindicated – GI obstruction. Metoclopramide is excreted into milk and may concentrate at about twice the plasma level, but there does not appear to be significant risk to nursing offspring. In dogs, the most common (although infrequent) adverse reactions seen are changes in mentation and behavior (motor restless and hyperactivity to drowsiness/ depression).	Plumb 7th Edition.

Metronidazole	Flagyl®	10 to 25 mg per kg PO once daily for 5 to 10 days in pups at least 12 weeks of age as the neonatal dose.	Male Female Pediatric	Antibiotic, antiparasiticide agent. To treat Giardia in the neonate.	Safety in the pregnant and lactating bitch not established. Should be strictly avoided during the first 3 weeks of pregnancy. Fenbendazole less likely to cause toxicity. Narrow safety margin – 65 mg per kg can cause neurotoxicity. Risk of neurotoxicity is increased in patients with liver dysfunction or on long term therapy. Diazepam may shorten recovery time when neurotoxicity has developed.	Hoskins, Johnny D. "Veterinary Pediatrics of the Puppy and Kitten." Atlantic Coast Veterinary Conference. Atlantic City, 2005.
Mibolerone	Cheque®	More information in chapter 9 Administered as noted below PO once daily. Maximum 24 months of continuous use.	Female	Androgenic, anabolic anti-gonadotropic hormone. To prevent estrous cycles. To treat bitches with short inter-estrous periods. To manage cystic endometrial hyperplasia by dosing 30 mcg (micrograms) per 25 pounds of body weight PO once daily for 6 months.	Compounded Drug ∞ Only available through compounding pharmacies. Teratogenic – Contraindicated during pregnancy. Need to monitor liver enzymes. Should not be used prior to first estrus. Must start 30 or more days prior to anticipated estrus. Do not confuse vaginal discharge with pyometra. Avoid use if patient has a history of liver disease or androgen dependent neoplasia.	Plumb 7th Edition. Hutchison. Fontbonne 2006.

Generic Drug Name	Trade Drug Name	Dose Range with Frequency and Route	Male Female Neonate or Pediatric	Drug Class and Indication	Comments	Reference or Source
Minocycline	Minocin®	Minocycline (25 mg per kg PO once daily for 14 days) with dihydrostreptomycin (5 mg per kg IM every 12 hours for 7 days) and tetracycline (30 mg per kg PO every 12 hours for 21 days) with streptomycin (20 mg per kg once daily for 14 days). May require long-term treatment.	Male and female	Tetracycline antibiotic. Combined with dihydro-streptomycin and surgical desexing to manage Brucella canis.	Combined with surgical desexing. Even long term treatment and desexing may not clear infection.

Contraindicated during pregnancy and in pups under 4 months. Avoid use in pups due to effects on bone and tooth development. | Root Kustritz, Margaret V. "Canine Brucellosis." Western Veterinary Conference, Las Vegas, 2007. |
| Misoprostol | Cytotec® | 1. For pyometra, 1 to 3 mcg (micrograms) per kg once daily instilled into the cranial vagina, near the cervical os.
2. For pregnancy termination: Pregnancy is confirmed with ultrasound, treatment is initiated no sooner than 30 days after breeding. 1 to 3 mcg (micrograms) per kg misoprostol given intravaginally twice daily concurrently with prostaglandin F₂alpha or aglepristone.

See Chapter 9 for more dosage information. Monitor efficacy with ultrasound. | Female | Prostaglandin E1 analog. To treat pyometra or medically terminate unwanted pregnancy. Combined with Prostaglandin F2 Alpha, to assist the cervix in opening to aid in medical therapy | Extralabel Drug Use* Contraindicated during desired pregnancy due to its abortifacient activity. Anecdotal reports on intravaginal use only at time of publishing.

Pregnant women to handle the drug with caution. | Plumb 7th Edition. Cain 1999. |

Morphine	Duramorph®	Female	Classic opiate analgesic. To improve post-C-section analgesia without loss of hindlimb function.	Epidurals MUST be done with only preservative free morphine. Costly as a result of form and delivery of drug. Performed after general anesthesia is induced, not as a substitute for general anesthesia. The epidural space is smaller in a pregnant than a non-pregnant dog	Plumb 7th Edition. Mason DE. "Anesthesia for Cesarean Section." World Small Animal Veterinary Association World Congress Proceedings, 2006. Veterinary Anesthesia & Analgesia Support Group.
	Epidural use- 0.1 mg per kg (0.045 mg per lb.) Total volume should not exceed 0.15 ml per kg.				
Oxytocin		Female	Hypothalamic hormone. To improve uterine contractions during labor. To treat post partum retained placentas and metritis if under 24 hours post partum.	Keep refrigerated. Assure the first pup has been born, there is not an obstructive dystocia, there are not ongoing strong contractions prior to administration. Overzealous use can cause uterine rupture and/or premature separation of placentae resulting in fetal death. More than 24 hours after parturition, the uterus responds poorly to oxytocin. Prostaglandins are indicated at this time if uterine contractility is required. Produces transient bradycardia if administered too rapidly IV>	Hutchison, Robert: "Canine Reproduction, Whelping and Neonatal Care." Lakeshore Pembroke Welsh Corgi Club. Crystal Lake, IL. 25 March 2005. Copley K: Parturition management: 15,000 whelpings later: An outcome based analysis. Theriogenology 2009; Vol. 1, Number 2: 297-307. Plumb 7th Edition.
	For labor and delivery: 0.1 ml per 10 pounds SC or IM The situations in which to avoid the use of oxytocin are: 1. Prior to the delivery of the first pup – if the cervix is closed or there is a malpresentation of a pup. 2. The bitch is already in hard labor 3. 2 doses have been administered in 20 minutes 4. If 2 to 3 doses do not succeed in delivering a pup, C-section should be recommended to the client. OR 0.25 USP U to 4 USP U SC or IM per dog per dose, at 45 to 60 min intervals, based on clinical response with uterine contraction monitoring.				

Generic Drug Name	Trade Drug Name	Dose Range with Frequency and Route	Male Female Neonate or Pediatric	Drug Class and Indication	Comments	Reference or Source
Oxytocin		For lactation: Inject oxytocin, then warm compress for 20 min, then put pups on to nurse: 0.5 unit SC every 2 hours X 4 doses, then 1 unit SC every 2 hours X 4 doses, then 2 units SC every 2 hours X 4 doses, then 3 units SC every 2 hours, then increase time between injections to 4, then 6 then 8 hours, then discontinue when lactating well.	Female	Hypothalamic hormone. To induce milk let-down in bitches with adequate milk production and who tolerate nursing. Can be combined with metoclopramide to promote milk production.	Does NOT aid in lactation, only in release of milk from the mammary gland.	Loar 1988. Copley.
Phenobarbital		Dogs < 3 months 0.5 mg per kg PO once daily, 1 mg per kg every 12 hours PO for dogs 3 to 6 months of age, 2 mg per kg every 12 hours PO for dogs over 6 months.	All	Barbiturate. To manage seizures in the neonate	Contraindicated during pregnancy. Consider hypoglycemia, porto-systemic shunt and hydrocephalus as underlying causes of seizures in the very young patient.	Hoskins, Johnny D. "Small Animal Pediatric Medicine." Tufts Animal Expo. North Grafton MA. 2002.
Phenylpropanolamine	Proin®	3 mg per kg PO every 12 hours, repeated several hours prior to collection or breeding.	Male	Sympathomimetic. To reduce retrograde ejaculation. Avoid long term use in patients with BPH or glaucoma.	Extralabel Drug Use* Side effects: restlessness, anorexia, tachycardia, hyper-excitability, tremors and GI upset. Hypertension possible.	Urethral Sphincter Mechanism Incontinence Linda Shell, DVM, DACVIM Fontbonne, Alain. "Infertility in the Bitch and in the Dog." World Small Animal Veterinary Association World Congress, Sydney, 21 Aug. 2007.

Drug	Trade	Dosage	Age/Sex	Indication	Notes	Reference
Piroxicam	Feldene®	0.3 mg per kg PO once a day. Narrow margin of safety. Give with food.	Male and female	Non-steroidal anti-inflammatory, anti-tumor. As an adjunct treatment of transitional Cell Carcinoma – bladder. May also be of benefit in squamous cell carcinomas, mammary adenocarcinoma, and transmissible venereal tumor (TVT).	∞ Compounded Drug Combined with long-term amoxicillin therapy to manage TCC. Do NOT combine with other NSAIDs. Narrow margin of safety – may require compounding to deliver a precise in dosage. Consider adding misoprostol at 3 mcg (micrograms) per kg, PO every 8 hours for dogs who tolerate NSAIDs poorly. Discontinue if severe irritation or ulceration occurs. Treat ulcers and if signs abate, may resume piroxicam with misoprostol.	Plumb 7th Edition. Frimberger 2000.
Potassium chloride		1 meq of potassium chloride PO every 3 hours for every 30 gms or 1 ounce of weight lost. 10% potassium chloride solution contains 1 meq in 1 ml (1 ml = 20 drops). See Chapter 8 more information.	Neonates	Electrolyte. To treat anasarca or Walrus puppy	Combine with furosemide therapy. Discontinue the potassium chloride when the furosemide is discontinued.	Hoskins, Johnny D. "Small Animal Pediatric Medicine." Tufts Animal Expo. North Grafton MA. 2002.
Prednisone		2.2mg per kg daily for 14 days, tapering slowly. Combined with appropriate antibiotic, anti-pruritics and astringent (Dome-boro®) soaks.	Puppies	Classic glucocorticoid. To treat strangles or juvenile cellulitis combined with antibiotics.	Contraindicated during pregnancy. Must combine with antibiotic therapy. May relapse if taper steroids too quickly.	MacDonald, John M. "Potpourri of Juvenile Dermatoses." Western Veterinary Conference, Las Vegas, 2002.

Generic Drug Name	Trade Drug Name	Dose Range with Frequency and Route	Male Female Neonate or Pediatric	Drug Class and Indication	Comments	Reference or Source
Progesterone in oil		2 to 3 mg per kg IM every 1 to 3 days, with dosage frequency based on response to therapy.	Female	Natural progesterone. Used ONLY when necessary to support pregnancy threatened by hypoluteoidism.	∞ Compounded Drug Considered safe during late pregnancy. Can alter fetal sexual development if given too early in pregnancy. Can monitor response to treatment with progesterone blood levels. Monitor for signs of pregnancy failure or pyometra, discontinue if all fetuses not viable.	Fontbonne, Alain. "Infertility in the Bitch." World Small Animal Veterinary Association World Congress, Prague, 11 Oct. 2006.
Propofol	Propoflo® Diprivan® Rapinovet®	Standard Induction: 1.0 to 6.0 mg per kg (0.5 to 3.0 mg per lb) IV over 30 to 90 seconds. C-section induction with no pre-op sedation: 3-8 mg per kg, to allow intubation, then maintain with SevofluraneR (preferred), isoflurane, or CRI propofol. CRI at 0.05 to 0.2 mg per kg per minute (0.025 to 0.1 mg per lb per minute), adjust as needed.	All	Short acting injectable hypnotic anesthetic agent. Used to induce general anesthesia.	After induction, change to Sevoflurane® or isoflurance after intubation and steady plane of anesthesia is attained Considered safe during pregnancy. Dose propofol to effect to minimize respiratory depression and hypotensive potential. Apnea possible if administered too rapidly.	Plumb 7th Edition. Mason DE. "Anesthesia for Cesarean Section." World Small Animal Veterinary Association World Congress Proceedings, 2006. Veterinary Anesthesia & Analgesia Support Group.
Prostaglandin F 2 alpha	Lutalyse®	To treat Pyometra – used with antibiotics, fluids, and bromocriptine or cabergoline. See more detail in chapter 9. LUTALYSE® 10 mcg	Female	THAM salt of natural occurring prostaglandin F2alpha. THAM salt of natural occurring prostaglandin F2alpha.	Extralabel Drug Use* Contraindicated during desired pregnancy. Follow size of uterus with ultrasound – look for a 50% decrease in uterine size within 3 to 4	Verstegen J, Dhaliwal G, Verstegen-Onclin K. Mucometra, cystic endometrial hyperplasia, and pyometra in the bitch: Advances in treatment and assessment

Drug	Brand	Dosage	Sex	Use	Notes	Reference
		(micrograms) per kg 3 to 5 times per day, SC. Slowly increase to 50 mcg (micrograms) per kg 3 to 5 times per day over 3 to 5 days, continue until resolved. May combine with metoclopramide and 15 minute walks after injections to minimize side effects of nausea, vomiting, salivation, and diarrhea.		Used to evacuate the uterus and lyse the corpus luteum which is supporting the pyometra hormonally.	days. Use for 7 to 10 days maximum. IF refractory, may improve response by stopping and restarting injections. Risk of DIC, uterine rupture (especially if cervix is closed at onset of treatment) or poor response to treatment. Not all patients will respond or breed back after treatment. Pregnant women should not handle; handle with caution in humans with asthma and women of childbearing age.	of future reproductive success. Theriogenology, Volume 70, Issue 3, Pages 364-374.
Prostaglandin F 2 alpha	Lutalyse®	To treat SIPS: 5C mcg (micrograms) per kg SC every 12 hours until RBCs are no longer seen on vaginal cytology.	Female	THAM salt of natural occurring prostaglandin F2alpha. To treat SIPS – Subinvolution of placental sites	Extralabel Drug Use* Contraindicated during desired pregnancy. Pregnant women should not handle; handle with caution in humans with asthma and women of childbearing age.	Plumb 7th Edition. Threfall, Walter. "Abnormal Conditions of the Bitch." AVMA, Honolulu. 16 July 2006.
Prostaglandin F 2 alpha	Lutalyse®	To improve semen collection: 50 to 100 mcg (micrograms) per kg (0.05 to 0.1 mg per kg) SC 15 min prior to semen collection. Once per collection, not more than 1 dose per day	Male	THAM salt of natural occurring prostaglandin F2alpha. Aids with sexual preparation - Improve ejaculate. May not have an erection and may have a small volume of ejaculate, but improves sperm count in many patients.	Extralabel Drug Use* Contraindicated during desired pregnancy. Pregnant women should not handle; handle with caution in humans with asthma and women of childbearing age. Side effects – panting, salivation, vomiting, urination, diarrhea, anxiety, restlessness, abdominal	Hess, Milan. "Documented and anecdotal effects of certain pharmaceutical agents used to enhance semen quality in the dog." Theriogenology, Volume 66, Issue 3, 613-617.

Generic Drug Name	Trade Drug Name	Dose Range with Frequency and Route	Male Female Neonate or Pediatric	Drug Class and Indication	Comments	Reference or Source
					pain, rarely collapse. Should be used with caution in brachycephalic dogs or older patients. Client should be advised of effects prior to administration.	
Prostaglandin F 2 alpha	Lutalyse®	To manage metritis – used with antibiotics and fluids. LUTALYSE 10 mcg (micrograms) per kg 3 times per day, SC. Slowly increase to 50 mcg (micrograms) per kg 3 to 5 doses per day over 3 to 5 days, continue until resolved. May combine with metoclopramide and 15 minute walks after injections to minimize side effects of nausea, vomiting, salivation, and diarrhea.	Female	THAM salt of natural occurring prostaglandin F2alpha. To manage metritis combined with antibiotics and supportive care.	Extralabel Drug Use* Contraindicated during desired pregnancy. Pregnant women should not handle; handle with caution in humans with asthma and women of childbearing age.	Verstegen J, Dhaliwal G, Verstegen-Onclin K. Mucometra, cystic endometrial hyperplasia, and pyometra in the bitch: Advances in treatment and assessment of future reproductive success. Theriogenology, Volume 70, Issue 3, Pages 364-374

Pseudoephedrine	Sudafed®	Male	4 to 5 mg per kg PO up to 3 times a day, 1 to 3 hours prior to ejaculation.	Oral sympathomimetic. To diminish retrograde ejaculation.	Extralabel Drug Use* Having the bladder full prior to ejaculation also aids in minimizing retrograde ejaculation.	Fontbonne, Alain. "Infertility in the Bitch and in the Dog." World Small Animal Veterinary Association World Congress, Sydney, 21 Aug. 2007.
Pyrantel pamoate	Nemex® Strongid T®	All	Dogs and puppies under 5 lbs: 10 mg per kg PO. For dogs and puppies weighing more than 5 lbs: 5 mg per kg PO. Starting when the pups are 2 weeks old, worm at 2, 4, 6, 8, 10 and 12 weeks of age.	Pyrimidine anthelmintic. To treat or prevent ascarids, hookworms and stomach worms.	Considered safe during pregnancy. Important to educate and protect clients against zoonotic diseases. All pups and dams should be treated. See www.capcvet.org for more information on preventing zoonoses.	Plumb 7th Edition. www.capcvet.org
Selamectin	Revolution®	Female	Apply topically to the bitch at 6 mg per kg at 6 and 2 weeks before whelping and at 2 and 6 weeks after whelping. (Week 3 and 7 of pregnancy and week 2 and 6 of lactation.)	Topical avermectin antiparasiticide. This protocol reduced roundworm burdens in puppies by 98%, and reduced egg shedding by 99.7% in the dams.	Extralabel Drug Use* Considered safe during pregnancy. Avoid in dogs who carry the MDR-1 mutation.	Kazacos, KR: "Treatment and Control of Gastrointestinal Helminths." Western Veterinary Conference. Las Vegas. 2002.
Simethicone	GasX® Phazyme®	Neonates	Several drops PO as needed to relieve gas and bloating. Available OTC in several forms.	Oral anti-foaming agent. To relieve intestinal and gastric gas.	Symptomatic only – should determine and treat underlying cause. Surfactant.	Various
Sucralfate	Carafate®	Any	0.5 gm (small dogs) to 1 gm PO every 8 hours.	Gastroprotectant. To manage oral, esophageal, gastric, and duodenal ulcers. Also useful for non-specific gastritis and esophagitis.	Probably safe during pregnancy as only 3 to 5% absorbed. Best given on an empty stomach. Suspension works better – can dissolve tablets prior to use. Check formulary to assess timing when used with other drugs, as may decrease absorption of certain pharmaceuticals.	Plumb 7th Edition.

Generic Drug Name	Trade Drug Name	Dose Range with Frequency and Route	Male Female Neonate or Pediatric	Drug Class and Indication	Comments	Reference or Source
Sulfadimethoxine	Albon®	50 mg per kg PO first dose, then 25 mg per kg in pups 2 to 6 weeks of age once every 24 hours for 5 to 10 days.	Pediatric	Sulfonamide antimicrobial. To control coccidia in the neonate.	Use caution in patients with dehydration, diminished renal or hepatic function, or urinary obstruction. Can cause KCS. Contraindicated in Doberman Pinschers.	Plumb 7th Edition.
Tetracycline	Panmycin®	Minocycline (25 mg per kg PO once daily for 14 days) with dihydrostreptomycin (5 mg per kg IM every 12 hours for 7 days) and tetracycline (30 mg per kg PO every 12 hours for 21 days) with streptomycin (20 mg per kg IM once daily for 14 days).	Male and female	Tetracycline antibiotic. To help manage canine brucellosis when combined with other antibiotics and desexing.	Avoid use in the last half of pregnancy and in pups without full adult dentition as it affects tooth and bone development. To manage canine brucellosis in conjunction with surgical desexing. Even long term treatment and desexing may not clear infection.	Root Kustritz, Margaret V. "Canine Brucellosis." Western Veterinary Conference, Las Vegas, 2007.
Terbutaline	Brethine®	0.03 mg per kg PO or SC every 4 to 8 hours as needed to control preterm labor contractions. OR 0.03 mg per kg IV by continuous infusion to effect OR 2.5 to 5 mg total dose PO every 8 to 12 hours. Dose may be titrated to effected based on tocodynometry.	Pregnant female	Tocolytic/beta-adrenergic agonist. To quiet inappropriate or premature uterine activity. Discontinue the drug 48 hours before predicted delivery date to allow the bitch to initiate normal labor and delivery.	Extralabel Drug Use* Considered safe during pregnancy. To quiet excessive uterine activity associated with premature labor. Can be combined with progesterone and antibiotics if indicated. Maternal pulse should be evaluated for tachycardia prior to and 1 hour after each terbutaline dose.	Adams, Ana. "Increasing Conception Rates and Litter Sizes." Western Veterinary Conference, Las Vegas, 2004. Copley K: Parturition management: 15,000 whelpings later: An outcome based analysis. Theriogenology 2009: Vol. 1, Number 2: 297-307.
Tramadol	Ultram®	1 to 5 mg per kg PO every 8 to 12 hours.	Female post-op	Synthetic mu-receptor opiate agonist. To manage post-op pain.	No documentation but experience shows safe use in bitches post-surgical AI and post-C-section.	Hardie, Lascelles et al. 2003 Plumb 7th Edition.

Trimethoprim-sulfa	Tribrissen® Bactrim®	15 mg per kg in the neonate PO every 12 hours. Dose is calculated by adding the combined amount of the 2 drugs.	Neonate	Potentiated sulfonamide antimicrobial. To treat bacterial infection susceptible to this drug class.	May have CNS and GI effects. Avoid in pregnant bitches or those intended for breeding – teratogen.	Plumb 7th Edition.
Trimethoprim-sulfadiazine or Trimethoprim-Sulfa-methoxazole	Tribrissen® Bactrim®	30 mg per kg every 12 hours PO, IV or SC for chronic prostatitis. Dose is calculated by adding the combined amount of the 2 drugs.	Male	Potentiated sulfonamide antimicrobial. To treat bacterial infections susceptible to this drug class.	Avoid in pregnant bitches or those intended for breeding. Monitor closely for side effects of keratoconjunctivitis sicca, hypersensitivity (type 1 or type 3) acute neutrophilic hepatitis with icterus, vomiting, anorexia, diarrhea, fever, hemolytic anemia, urticaria, polyarthritis, facial swelling, polydipsia, crystalluria, hematuria, polyuria, cholestasis, hypothyroidism, anemias, agranulocytosis, thrombycytopenia, idiosyncratic hepatic necrosis in dogs. Stop if any develop.	Plumb 7th Edition.
Vitamin A analogs		No therapeutic dose recommended. Avoid excesses and liver during pregnancy.	Female	Fat soluble vitamin.	Contraindicated during pregnancy as a teratogen – may cause cleft palates.	
Vitamin K	Mephyton®	0.01 to 0.1 mg SC or IM one time only. Useful when there is spontaneous hemorrhage or if there is excessive bleeding at taildock or dewclaw removal.	Neonate	Fat-soluble vitamin. To minimize neonatal hemorrhage.	Considered safe during pregnancy. Neonates under 48 hours old are deficient in thrombin and may show signs of hemorrhage associated with sepsis, trauma, or other illness.	Plumb 7th Edition. Macintire, Douglass K. "Pediatric Emergencies." Western Veterinary Conference, Las Vegas, 2004.

Many drugs used in veterinary medicine are not labeled for the indication, species, route, or dosage used. There are 3 general categories: Extra-label drug use, Non US FDA Approved Drugs, and Compounded drugs. These drugs may have anecdotal, not evidence-based criteria for use. All 3 are associated with liability to the prescriber. Consider the risk-benefit ratio of the product, what is "best" for the patient, the alternative treatment options, the relationship of the prescriber to the client, your professional liability insurance status, and the informed consent laws in your state before prescribing. Keep good records including the rationale for use of the product. Economic decisions are not the basis for selection and use of one of these products. These products are to be used for prevention, treatment, and control purposes only when a non-food producing animal's health is threatened.

* Drug Use (ELDU) or Off Label Drug use: Extra-label drug use is the practice of prescribing pharmaceuticals for an unapproved indication, in an unapproved species, or in an unapproved dose or route of administration. See AMDUCA at: http://www.fda.gov/AnimalVeterinary/GuidanceComplianceEnforcement/ActsRulesRegulations/ucm085377.htm ELDU applies if a product is used for an indication not in the approved labeling. In this case, the prescriber has the responsibility to be well-informed about the product, to base its use on firm scientific rationale and on sound medical evidence, to maintain records of the products use and effects, and to have the client's informed consent regarding ELDU and treatment alternatives. In addition, a valid veterinary-client-patient relationship (VCPR) must exist. Prior to ELDU, the prescriber must verify there is no approved animal drug that is labeled for such use in the species, or that contains the same active ingredient in the required dosage form and/or concentration that would otherwise be appropriate for the patient. ELDU of an FDA approved drug may be used if either there is no approved animal drug that is labeled for such use, or that contains the same active ingredient in the required dosage form and concentration or alternatively, an approved animal drug for that species and condition exists, but a veterinarian finds, within the context of a VCPR, that the approved drug is clinically ineffective for its labeled use. The decision cannot be made on an economic basis.

+ Not a US FDA Approved Drug: A drug or pharmaceutical that has not been approved or submitted for approval by the US FDA. The FDA's evidence-based system of drug approval and the OTC monograph system play essential roles in ensuring drugs are both safe and effective. See: http://www.fda.gov/Drugs/GuidanceComplianceRegulatoryInformation/EnforcementActivitiesbyFDA/SelectedEnforcementActionsonUnapprovedDrugs/default.htm

∞ Compounded Drug: A compounded drug is a pharmaceutical or chemical product altered or manipulated that results in a product used as medication. This category may create the greatest liability for the prescribing practitioner. Perform due diligence on the compounding pharmacy prior to use of their services and products. Be certain the compounding pharmacy is not manufacturing the product is prescribed.
See: http://www.fda.gov/ICECI/ComplianceManuals/CompliancePolicyGuidanceManual/ucm074656.htm.

D-14. *Algorithm for prostate disease*

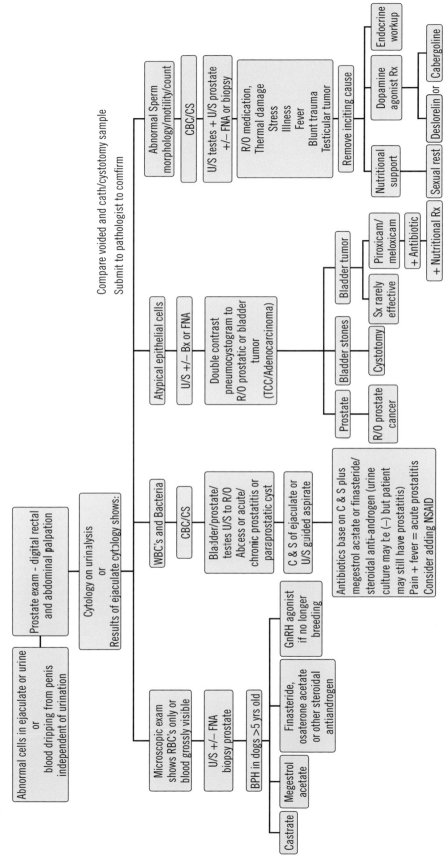

Abnormal cells in ejaculate or urine
or
blood dripping from penis independent of urination

Prostate exam - digital rectal and abdominal palpation

Cytology on urinalysis
or
Results of ejaculate cytology shows:

Compare voided and cath/cystotomy sample
Submit to pathologist to comfirm

Microscopic exam shows RBC's only or blood grossly visible

U/S +/- FNA biopsy prostate

BPH in dogs >5 yrs old

Castrate

Megestrol acetate

Finasteride, osaterone acetate or other steroidal antiandrogen

GnRH agonist if no longer breeding

WBC's and Bacteria

CBC/CS

Bladder/prostate/testes U/S to R/O Abcess or acute/chronic prostatitis or paraprostatic cyst

C & S of ejaculate or U/S guided aspirate

Antibiotics base on C & S plus megestrol acetate or finasteride/steroidal anti-androgen (urine culture may be (−) but patient may still have prostatitis)
Pain + fever = acute prostatitis
Consider adding NSAID

Atypical epithelial cells

U/S +/- Bx or FNA

Double contrast pneumocystogram to R/O prostatic or bladder tumor (TCC/Adenocarcinoma)

Prostate

R/O prostate cancer

Bladder stones

Cystotomy

Bladder tumor

Sx rarely effective

Piroxicam/meloxicam
+ Antibiotic
+ Nutritional Rx

Abnormal Sperm morphology/motility/count

CBC/CS

U/S testes + U/S prostate +/- FNA or biopsy

R/O medication, Thermal damage
Stress
Illness
Fever
Blunt trauma
Testicular tumor

Remove inciting cause

Nutritional support

Dopamine agonist Rx

Endocrine workup

Sexual rest

Deslorelin or Cabergoline

D-15. Page 1. *Algorithm for female infertility*

Infertile ♀

♀ Not cycling or cycling @ >12 month intervals

- Under 2 yrs.
  - Carefully examine external genitals and complete physical exam for masculine traits including prominent os clitoris (Looks "doggy")
  - Wait until > 2 yrs of age Then →
- Over 2 yrs
  1. CBC/CS/UA
  2. Progesterone test
  3. Weekly vaginal cytologies + monthly progesterone assays to monitor for silent heat
  4. Ultrasound with radiologist to look for ovaries and uterus
  5. Drugs – including accidental ingestion/ exposure
  6. Karyotype if not cycling
  7. Thyroid and TSH + T$_4$
  8. 2 LH levels @ >24hr interval or single AMH test to check for presence of ovaries
  9. Inadequate nutrition
  10. Excess stress or work 2° to housing or performance
  11. Last resort–R/O Hermaphroditism or Pseudohermaphroditism Exploratory laparotomy with biopsy of gonads

♀ Cycling @ 6-12 mo intervals

PE

1. Thyroid (low)
2. Adrenal Hyperadreno corticism
3. Hyperprolactinemia
4. Exposure to hormone therapy including accidental ingestion/ exposure
   a. Androgens
   b. Progestagens
   c. Anabolic steroids
5. Ovarian cysts
6. Environmental causes
   a. Low lighting
   b. Poor nutrition
   c. Overcrowding

Timing
Sperm count and morphology

♀ Cycling < every 120 to 160 days esp German Shepherd Rottweiler or Basset Hound

- Progesterone > 5 ng/ml short - interestrous periods
  - Rx Mibolerone or magestrol acetate to increase interestrous period
- Premature decline in progesterone during diestrus
- Progesterone <5 ng/ml for 30 days
  - R/O Split cycle
  - Wait till it comes in and breed that cycle

→ Granulosal cell tumor
- Dx by seeing cornified epithelium for 6 wks
- Induce ovulation

→ Cystic ovary
- Ultrasound guided aspiration of fluid from ovarian cyst(s) Test progesterone level in aspirated fluid
- GnRH or HCG +/– Deslorelin implant when < 70% anucleated cells on cytology & U/S shows preovulatory follicles

or

Breed next cycle-eggs too old in most cases to be fertile in this cycle

D-15. Page 2. *Algorithm for female infertility*

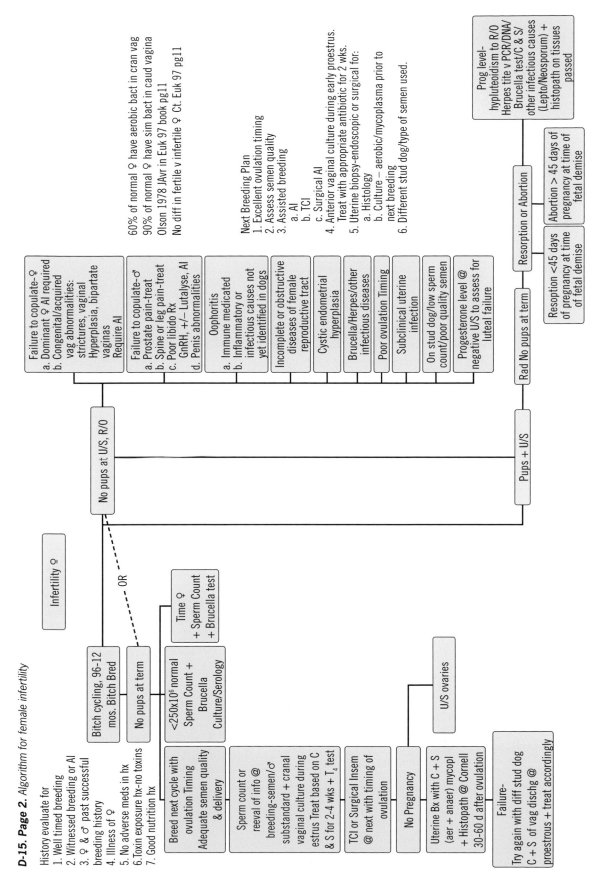

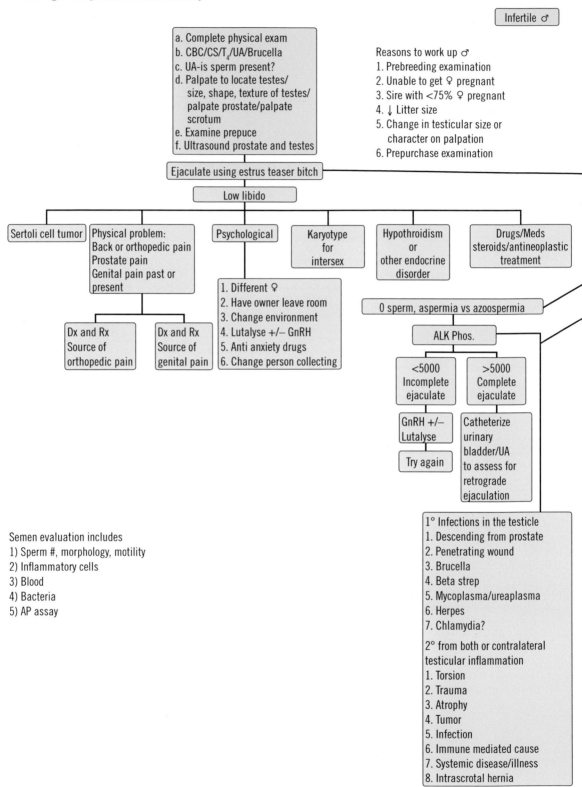

Infertile ♂

a. Complete physical exam
b. CBC/CS/T$_4$/UA/Brucella
c. UA–is sperm present?
d. Palpate to locate testes/
   size, shape, texture of testes/
   palpate prostate/palpate
   scrotum
e. Examine prepuce
f. Ultrasound prostate and testes

Reasons to work up ♂
1. Prebreeding examination
2. Unable to get ♀ pregnant
3. Sire with <75% ♀ pregnant
4. ↓ Litter size
5. Change in testicular size or
   character on palpation
6. Prepurchase examination

Ejaculate using estrus teaser bitch

Low libido

Sertoli cell tumor

Physical problem:
Back or orthopedic pain
Prostate pain
Genital pain past or
present

Psychological

Karyotype
for
intersex

Hypothroidism
or
other endocrine
disorder

Drugs/Meds
steroids/antineoplastic
treatment

Dx and Rx
Source of
orthopedic pain

Dx and Rx
Source of
genital pain

1. Different ♀
2. Have owner leave room
3. Change environment
4. Lutalyse +/− GnRH
5. Anti anxiety drugs
6. Change person collecting

0 sperm, aspermia vs azoospermia

ALK Phos.

<5000
Incomplete
ejaculate

>5000
Complete
ejaculate

GnRH +/−
Lutalyse

Catheterize
urinary
bladder/UA
to assess for
retrograde
ejaculation

Try again

Semen evaluation includes
1) Sperm #, morphology, motility
2) Inflammatory cells
3) Blood
4) Bacteria
5) AP assay

1° Infections in the testicle
1. Descending from prostate
2. Penetrating wound
3. Brucella
4. Beta strep
5. Mycoplasma/ureaplasma
6. Herpes
7. Chlamydia?

2° from both or contralateral
testicular inflammation
1. Torsion
2. Trauma
3. Atrophy
4. Tumor
5. Infection
6. Immune mediated cause
7. Systemic disease/illness
8. Intrascrotal hernia

Differential Diagnosis for:

Testicle ↑ in size - Active disorder
1. Active orchitis
2. Recent torsion
3. Sertoli cell tumor

Testicle ↓ in size - Degenerative disorder
1. Chronic orchitis
2. Previous trauma or torsion
3. Leydig cell tumor
4. Epididymis - sperm granuloma - can be bilateral

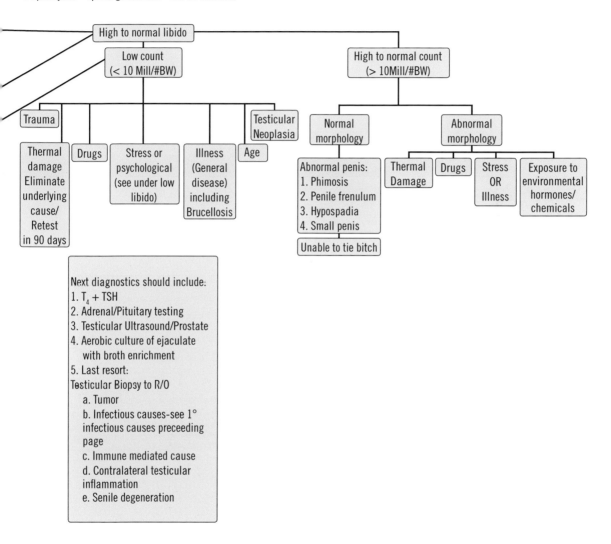

D-16. Page 2. *Algorithm for male infertility*

Hx ♂
1) ♀ - a) Estrus detection
      b) # of times ♀ bred
      c) Methods of Preg Dx
2) Controlled trial to proven ♀?
3) Libido, Use and Frequency
4) # of Pups/litter
5) Hx of illness, urination, defecation, toxins and trauma
6) Medications, hormones/gluco corticoids
7) Family Hx of reproductive performance of father + littermates

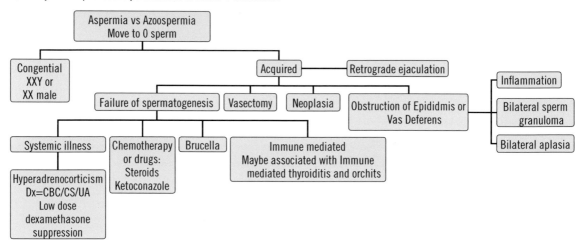

Definitions:
Teratospermia - Morphologicaly abnormal sperm < 80% normal
Asthenospermia - < 25% sperm of sperm have normal motility, congenitial = Ciliary dyskinesis usually caused by contamination by water, lubes, powder, and disinfectants
Oligospermia - low sperm count
Aspermia or azospermia = no sperm
Hematospermia - blood in ejaculate

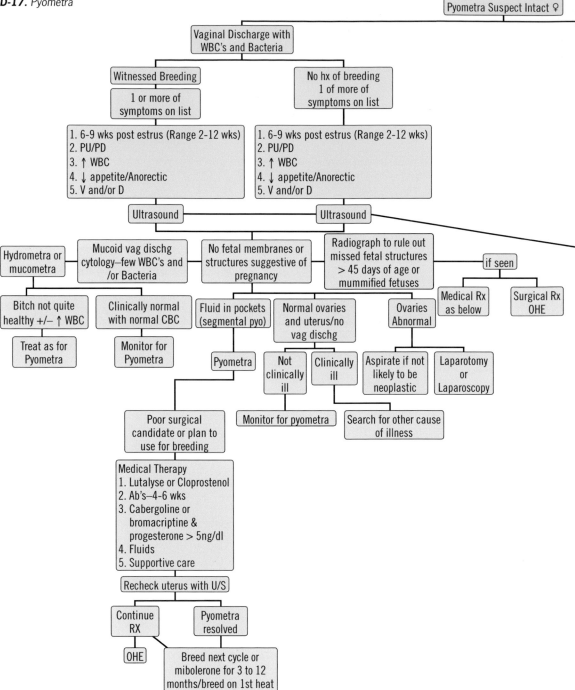

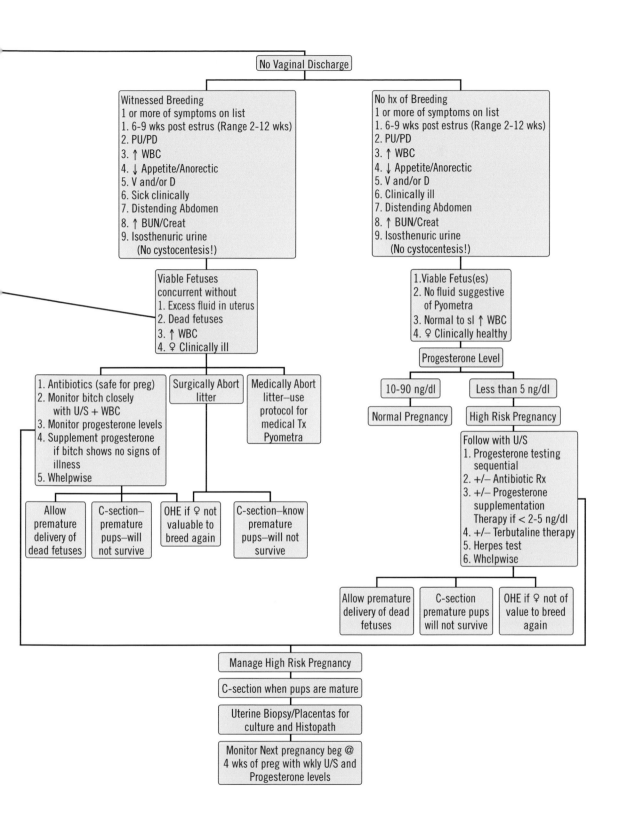

No Vaginal Discharge

Witnessed Breeding
1 or more of symptoms on list
1. 6-9 wks post estrus (Range 2-12 wks)
2. PU/PD
3. ↑ WBC
4. ↓ Appetite/Anorectic
5. V and/or D
6. Sick clinically
7. Distending Abdomen
8. ↑ BUN/Creat
9. Isosthenuric urine
   (No cystocentesis!)

No hx of Breeding
1 or more of symptoms on list
1. 6-9 wks post estrus (Range 2-12 wks)
2. PU/PD
3. ↑ WBC
4. ↓ Appetite/Anorectic
5. V and/or D
6. Clinically ill
7. Distending Abdomen
8. ↑ BUN/Creat
9. Isosthenuric urine
   (No cystocentesis!)

Viable Fetuses
concurrent without
1. Excess fluid in uterus
2. Dead fetuses
3. ↑ WBC
4. ♀ Clinically ill

1. Viable Fetus(es)
2. No fluid suggestive
   of Pyometra
3. Normal to sl ↑ WBC
4. ♀ Clinically healthy

Progesterone Level

10-90 ng/dl

Normal Pregnancy

Less than 5 ng/dl

High Risk Pregnancy

1. Antibiotics (safe for preg)
2. Monitor bitch closely
   with U/S + WBC
3. Monitor progesterone levels
4. Supplement progesterone
   if bitch shows no signs of
   illness
5. Whelpwise

Surgically Abort
litter

Medically Abort
litter—use
protocol for
medical Tx
Pyometra

Follow with U/S
1. Progesterone testing
   sequential
2. +/− Antibiotic Rx
3. +/− Progesterone
   supplementation
   Therapy if < 2-5 ng/dl
4. +/− Terbutaline therapy
5. Herpes test
6. Whclpwise

Allow
premature
delivery of
dead fetuses

C-section—
premature
pups—will
not survive

OHE if ♀ not
valuable to
breed again

C-section—know
premature
pups—will not
survive

Allow premature
delivery of dead
fetuses

C-section
premature pups
will not survive

OHE if ♀ not of
value to breed
again

Manage High Risk Pregnancy

C-section when pups are mature

Uterine Biopsy/Placentas for
culture and Histopath

Monitor Next pregnancy beg @
4 wks of preg with wkly U/S and
Progesterone levels

Index

C

Cabergoline (Dosinex®; Galastop®)
  client information sheet for, 364
  for estrous induction, 246
  for false pregnancy/whelping, 252
  formulary for, 410
  for mastitis, 131
  for pyometra, 258, 259, 260
  for unwanted pregnancy, 271
Caffeine (NoDoz®), formulary for, 411
Cal-Pho-Sol® (calcium), formulary for, 411
Calcium
  for aggression toward puppies, 135
  for C-section surgery, 109
  contraindications to in delivery, 92
  for eclampsia, 136-137
  formulary for, 411-412
  post-partum, 129
  for post-partum dystocia, 152
Calcium gluconate
  to assist vaginal delivery, 91
  formulary for, 411
Calsorb® gel (calcium), formulary for, 412
Canine Eye Registration Foundation (CERF) exams, 16-17
Canine genome, 13
Canine health, OFA certificates for, 27
Canine Health Foundation, 13
Canine health information, sharing, 12
Canine herpesvirus (CHV), 158-160
  in failed pregnancies, 236-239
  in fetal loss, 80
  managing outbreak of, 238
  in neonates, 193
  prevention of, 238-239
  symptoms of, 237
  testing for, 237-238
  transmission of, 238
  vaccination for during pregnancy, 68-69
Canine parvovirus. See Parvovirus
Cannibalism, 162
Capstar® (nitenpyram), during pregnancy, 161
Carafate® (sucralfate), formulary for, 437
Carbapenems, 173
Carcinoma, inflammatory mammary, 272-273
Cardiac auscultation, 17
Cardiac compressions, in neonatal resuscitation, 124
Cardiac disease, neonatal testing for, 185
Carnitine (Motility Plus™; Acetyl-L-Carnitine Quinicarn®), formulary for, 412
Carprofen (Rimadyl®), formulary for, 412-413
Caseload, working with breeders, 5-6
Castration
  for benign prostatic hypertrophy, 295
  bilateral, 308
  for testicular tumors, 304-305
  unilateral, 310
Cefazolin (Acef®; Kefzol®)
  in C-section, 109
  dosages of for neonates, 178
  formulary for, 413
  for pyometra, 258
Cefotaxime, neonate dosages of, 178
Ceftiofur (Naxcel®)
  in C-section, 109
  formulary for, 413
  for septicemia, 192

for sick neonates, 173
Cellulitis, juvenile, 193-194
Central nervous system inflammation, 203
Cephalexin (Ancef®)
  dosages of for neonates, 178
  formulary for, 413
  for hypoluteoidism, 241
  for pyometra, 258
Cephalosporins
  for juvenile cellulitis or strangles, 193-194
  for orchitis, 305
Cervical plug passing, 87
Cesarean section, 5
  anesthesia in, 110-112, 113
  benefits and risks of, 104
  delivery of puppies in, 116-118
  discharge after, 125-126
  discharge instructions for client, 373-374
  in dystocia, 102-103
  evaluating need for, 354
  final decision for, 112
  fluids and nutritional support after, 125
  incision closure in, 118-120
  indications for, 101-102
  items to take for, 363
  last steps before, 112
  for maternal or fetal dystocia, 95
  monitoring during, 113
  neonatal resuscitation in, 121-124
  number of, 219
  planning protocols for, 105-106
  postoperative drugs in, 120-121
  preparation for, 106-107, 108-110
  procedure in, 97, 100
  puppy survival rates in, 101-102
  reason to proceed to, 89-90
  reducing risks of, 112
  sequence of events in, 99-100
  set up for, 97-99, 340-342
  staff's role in, 106
  surgery report for, 393-394
  surgical approach in, 113-116
  surgical prep for, 113
  techniques for, 106-108
  umbilical care after, 124-125
Chemotherapy, for mammary tumors, 278
Cheque® drops, 249
Cheque® (mibolerone), formulary for, 429
Chest wall defects, 201-202
CHIC website, 12, 13
Chloramphenicol (Cleocin®)
  dosages of for neonates, 178
  formulary for, 413
Chorukin®, formulary for, 424
Chorulon®, formulary for, 424
Cimetidine, interfering with spermatogenesis, 308
Ciprofloxacin, formulary for, 422
Clavamox®
  formulary for, 404-405
  for hypoluteoidism, 241
  for pyometra, 258
Clavulanate potassium, 192
Clavulanic acid
  in C-section, 109
  dosages of for neonates, 178
  formulary for, 404-405

Galastop® (cabergoline), formulary for, 410
Gallimycin® (erythromycin), formulary for, 419
Gastrointestinal function testing, neonatal, 186
Gastroschisis, 197-198, 199
GasX® (simethicone), formulary for, 437
Gene-based DNA tests, 28
Genetic bottlenecking, 10
Genetic defects, 10
  counseling on, 29-30
  "outcrossing," 33
  screening for, 11-12
Genetic disorders, 155-157
  classifying, 10-11
  counseling for, 32-33, 35
  screening for, 16
Genetic diversity, loss of, 34
Genetic incompatibilities, 242
Genetic information, sharing, 12
Genetic screening, 8, 11-12, 16
Genetic selection, 8
Genetics, individual breed, 13
Genotype, selection based on, 8
Genotypic screening
  counseling breeders about, 29-33
  tests available for, 27-29
Giardia infection, 190
Gloves, latex or vinyl, 85
Glyco-flex®, formulary for, 423
Glycogen storage disease, 169
Glycosaminoglycans
  formulary for, 423
  for male infertility, 322
Gonadotropin-releasing hormone (GnRH)
  formulary for, 424
  in semen collection procedure, 289
Gonadotropin-releasing hormone (GnRH) agonists
  for benign prostatic hypertrophy, 296
  interfering with spermatogenesis, 308
Goodwinol ointment, 195

H
Hand-rearing, 206-207
The Harriet Lane Handbook, 176
HCG, formulary for, 424
Health care, post-partum, 128
Heart defects, 197
Heartworm microfilaria, 161
Heartworm prevention
  post-partum, 128
  during pregnancy, 70
Heat lamps, 85
  for sick neonates, 166
Heating pads, 85
  for sick neonates, 166
Hematospermia, 320
HemoPet, formulary for, 423
Hemorrhage, post-partum, 133
Hemostats, 85
Hepatic function tests, neonatal, 186
Hermaphrodites, 225
Herpes virus. See Canine herpesvirus (CHV)
Hetastarch, formulary for, 424-425
Hip dysplasia
  in breeding stock, 21-22
  follow-up for, 23
  screening for, 20-21

Hip joint laxity measurement, 24
Holter monitoring, 25
Hookworms, 160-161
Hormonal abnormalities, in infertility, 226
Hormone level tests, 25
Hot water bottles, 167
Housetraining, 146
Housing, at weaning, 211-212
Husbandry
  neonatal problems of, 193
  skills for, 147
Hybrid dogs, 13
Hydrocephalus, 203-204
Hydrometra, 264
Hydroxyethyl starch, formulary for, 424-425
Hygiene, for sick neonates, 176
Hyperadrenocorticism
  in male infertility, 294
  in oligospermia, 318
Hyperglycemia, during pregnancy, 78
Hypoadrenocorticism, in male infertility, 294
Hypocalcemia
  in maternal aggression, 135, 162
  post-parturient, 136-137
Hypodermic needles, 85
Hypoglycemia
  during pregnancy, 78
  in seizures, 202
Hypoluteoidism, 81-82, 240
  treatment of, 241-242
  when to treat, 240-241
Hypospadia, 199, 311
Hypothyroidism, in low sperm counts, 318
Hypoxia, in seizures, 204

I
Ice cream, vanilla, in vaginal delivery, 90
ICSB-CF Plus®, formulary for, 423
Immunity, passive
  failure of, 156-157
  in neonates, 173-175
Immunosuppression, in neonates, 163
Impetigo, 193
Inborn errors of metabolism, 155-156
  testing for, 184
Inbreeding, 33
Inbreeding coefficient, 221
Incubators, 166, 167
Infectious diseases, 157-161
Infertility
  evaluation for, 316
  female, 223-224
    algorithm for, 442-443
    causes of, 219, 222-226, 240-280
    diagnostic workup for, 221-222
    drugs causing, 242
    environmental causes of, 226
    reproductive tract disorders in, 261-269
  immunologic, 232
  male
    algorithm for, 444-446
    causes of, 282
    diagnostic workup for, 293-301
    evaluation for, 282-289
    penile disorders in, 311-316
    scrotal disorders in, 310

signs of, 282
 sperm count and morphology in, 290-293
 sperm disorders in, 316-322
 sperm production disorders in, 317-322
 spermatocele in, 307
 testicular disorders in, 301-310
 treatment protocols for, 322-323
 in missed breedings, 229-230
 treatment protocols for, 316-317
 vaginitis in, 231
Insemination. *See* Artificial insemination
Inter-estrous, prolonged, 246
Intersex, 222-225, 314
Intraosseous (IO) fluids
 set up for, 338
 for sick neonates, 170-171
Intravenous (IV) fluids, 170
 for C-section surgery, 108
Iodine, 85
 tincture of, 425
Iohexol clearance test, 187
Isoflurane, in C-section, 111
Itraconazole, 298
Ivermectin (Ivomec®)
 formulary for, 425
 for heartworm, 161
 for parasitic disease, 160-161
 during pregnancy, 70
Ivomec® (ivermectin)
 formulary for, 425

K
K-Y Jelly®, 85
Kaolin and pectin, formulary for, 425-426
Kefzol® (cefazolin), formulary for, 413
Keppra® (levetiracetam), formulary for, 426
Ketamine, 113
Ketoconazole, interfering with spermatogenesis, 308
Kitten formula, homemade, 362

L
L-carnitine, 322-323
Labor
 normal, stages of, 88
 premature, 81-82
 prolonged, 152
Laboratory services/vendors, 339
Laboratory tests, for C-section surgery, 108
Lactated Ringer's solution, 172
Lactation
 disorders that reduce, 189
 improving, 153
 nutrition and, 163
Lasix® (furosemide), formulary for, 423
Legg-Calve-Perthes, 22
Legg-Calve-Perthes disease screening, 22
Levetiracetam (Keppra®), formulary for, 426
Leydig cell tumors, 303
Libido, sperm production and
 low, 317
 low to no, 317-318
 normal to low, 318-323
Lice, 161
Lidocaine (Xylocaine®)
 in C-section, 111
 formulary for, 426

Line breeding, 33-34
Linked marker tests, 27, 28-29
Litters
 evaluating, 7
 registering, 215
 size of
 genetics in, 220-221
 health and, 219
 maximizing, 219-221
 small, 219
 veterinary care of, 45
Liver shunts, screening for, 20
Longevity, 16
Low birth weight, 144, 163
Lutalyse® (prostaglandin F2 alpha)
 formulary for, 434-436
 for hydrometra, 264
 for metritis, 132, 264
 for pyometra, 256-257, 258, 259, 260
 in semen collection procedure, 289
 for SIPS, 137
 for unwanted pregnancy, 270, 271
Luteolytic compounds, 242
Lymphoid follicular hyperplasia, penile, 314

M
Mammary gland
 tumors of, 271-273
 diagnosing and staging, 274
 medical treatment for, 278
 postoperative complications of, 277-278
 primary, 273
 prognosis for, 278-279
 risk factors for, 273
 surgical treatment for, 274-277, 279-280
Mammary glands
 inflammatory carcinoma of, 272-273
 male, evaluation of, 284
Marbofloxacin, formulary for, 422-423
Marcaine® (bupivacaine), formulary for, 408
Mastitis
 gangrenous, 131
 post-partum, 130-131
 sick neonates in, 158
Matador, 34
Maternal aggression, 135-136
Maternal skills, inadequate, 193
Mating schemes, 33-34
Megace® (megestrol acetate), formulary for, 427
Megaesophagus, 191
Megestrol acetate (Ovaban®; Megace®)
 for benign prostatic hypertrophy, 296
 for estrous prevention, 251
 formulary for, 427
Meloxicam (Metacam®), formulary for, 427
Mephyton® (vitamin K), formulary for, 439
Metabolic diseases, congenital, 155-156
Metabolic Screening Laboratory, 184
Metacam® (meloxicam)
 in C-section, 100, 121
 formulary for, 427
Metestrus, 51
Metestrus I, 47
Metestrus II, 47
Methoxyflurane, contraindicated, 113
Methylprednisolone, formulary for, 428

for estrous prevention, 251
formulary for, 427
Ovarian cysts, 228-229
functional, 226, 227
Ovarian remnant syndrome, 263-264
Ovariectomy, 268-269
Ovaries
aplasia or agenesis of, 225
neoplasia of, 229, 261-262
Ovariohysterectomy, 133, 225
for mammary tumors, 273, 275-278, 279-280
for SIPS, 265
for uterine prolapse, 265
for uterine segmental aplasia, 265
for uterine stump pyometra, 268-269
Oviduct pathology, 219-220, 232
Ovulation
failure of, 231
progesterone levels during, 50-51
Ovuplant® (deslorelin)
client information sheet for, 364
for estrous induction, 246-249
formulary for, 416
instructions for, 382
removal instructions for, 383
Oxacillin, 305
Oxygen therapy
in neonatal resuscitation, 124
for sick neonates, 164-165
Oxytocin
after C-section, 120-121
for agalactia, 134-135
to assist vaginal delivery, 91-92
contraindications to, 91, 92
dosages and rules for use of, 92
formulary for, 431-432
for milk letdown, 153
post-partum, 128
for uterine prolapse, 137
in uterine torsion, 265

P

Padgett, George, 12
Pain, with sperm production, 317-318
Palpation, in pregnancy diagnosis, 72-73
Panacur® (fenbendazole)
formulary for, 420
during pregnancy, 70
Pancreatic function tests, neonatal, 186
Panmycin® (Tetracycline), formulary for, 438
Paraneoplastic syndrome, 306
Paraphimosis, 313
Paraprostatic cysts, 299, 300
Parasitic infections
in failed pregnancies, 240
in fetal loss, 80
in neonates, 160-161
Parentage tests, 27, 28
Parenteral feeding, 154
Parlodel® (bromocriptine)
formulary for, 407-408
for pyometra, 258
Parvovirus, canine, 160
in diarrhea, 190
in failed pregnancies, 239
Patellar luxation

diagnosis of, 17-18
grading, 18-19
Pediatric care. *See* Neonates; Puppies
Pedigree analysis, 12
Penile frenulum, persistent, 311-312
Penis
disorders of, 311-314, 311-316
of ejaculation, 315-316
erectile, 314-315
evaluation of, 284
foreign bodies in, 312
hypoplasia of, 311
neoplasms of, 314
trauma to, 312
PennHIP®, 24
"Perfect dog," 35
Performance traits, evaluation of, 16
Pet breeders, 3
working with, 4-5
Pet puppies, health and temperament of, 11
Phazyme® (simethicone), formulary for, 437
Phenobarbital
for epilepsy, 204
formulary for, 432
Phenotype
abnormalities of, 14-16
selection based on, 8, 13-14
Phenotypic screening, 16-19
for arrhythmias, 19
based on physical evaluation, 14-16
for deafness, 19
disease-based, 16-27
laboratory tests in, 25-27
for liver shunts, 20
radiographic and ultrasound findings in, 20-25
Phenylpropanolamine (Proin®), formulary for, 432
Pheromone collar. *See* Adaptil™); Dog Appeasing Pheromone (DAP)
Phimosis, 313
Physical examination
before C-section, 107
general findings on, 14-16
before placement, 212
post-partum, 128
for sick neonates, 180-182
PIO fluids, for sick neonates, 172
Piroxicam (Feldene®)
formulary for, 433
for mammary tumors, 278
Placement (of puppies), 214-215
Placenta
expulsion of, 88
failure to form and maintain, 232
retained, 131-132
separation of, 88
Plasma
administration of, 175
fresh frozen, 174
formulary for, 423
instructions for thawing and using, 375
in sick neonates, 175
harvesting, 174
Pneumonia
in neonate, 190
treatment of, 190
Polygenetic disease, counseling for, 32-33

of uterine stump, 268-269
Pyrantel pamoate (Nemex®; Strongid T®), 85, 145, 146
  dosages of for neonates, 179
  formulary for, 437
  post-partum, 128, 129
Pyrethroids/permethrins, during pregnancy, 161

R

Radiation therapy, interfering with spermatogenesis, 308
Radiographic tests
  for elbow dysplasia, 22-23
  for hip dysplasia, 20-22
  for Legg-Calve-Perthes disease, 22
PennHIP®, 24
Radiography
  for bitch with dystocia, 89
  before C-section, 107-108
  in neonates, 185-186
  for pregnancy diagnosis, 75-76
Rapid card/slide agglutination test (RSAT), 79
Rapinovet® (propofol), formulary for, 434
Rear leg abnormalities, 202
Record keeping
  retrievable system of, 7
  skills for, 147-149
Referrals, veterinarian's role in, 6
Reglan® (metoclopramide)
  for agalactia, 134
  formulary for, 428
Regu-Mate® (altrenogest), formulary for, 403
Regurgitation, in neonates, 191
Renal function tests, neonatal, 187
Reproduction, normal, 2
Reproductive care, skills to provide, 5
Respiratory support, neonatal, 121-124
Retained pups, 132-133
Retrograde ejaculation, 315
Revolution® (selamectin)
  formulary for, 437
  during pregnancy, 161
Rimadyl® (carprofen)
  in C-section, 100
  formulary for, 412-413
Rotenone, 195
Roundworms, 160-161

S

Schistosomus reflexus, 200-201
Scrotal hernia, 307
Scrotum
  dermatitis of, 310
  disorders of, 310
  palpation of, 283
  thermal damage to, 306
  trauma to, 310
  tumors of, 310
Sebaceous adenitis, 26-27
Seizures, neonatal, 202
  causes of, 202-203
  treatment of, 203-204
Selamectin (Revolution®)
  formulary for, 437
  for heartworm, 161
  during pregnancy, 161
Semen
  with abnormal components, 321-322

analysis of, 283
  sperm count and morphology in, 290-293
  supplies for, 284-286
collection of, 59-62, 284
  with erectile dysfunction, 315
  for freezing, 360-361
  ideal location for, 286
  owner and handler in, 286
  procedures in, 287-289
  staff and doctors' role in, 286
  supplies for, 284-286
  teaser bitch in, 286-287
  timing of, 327
freezing, 326
  location for, 327
  technique for, 327-329
fresh, 326
fresh chilled
  checklist for shipping, 337
  collection of, 60-62
  handling, 58-60
  insemination using, 358-360, 381
fresh chilled extended, 326
frozen, 39, 327
  breeding with, 50, 329-330
  handling and use of, 62-63
  insemination using, 361
  liability for, 329
impaired delivery of, 232
packaging, 59-62
poor quality of, 231
type and deposition of, 220
when to collect, 327
Semen report, 343
Seminoma, testicular, 303
Sepsis, in neonates, 157-158, 192-193
Septicemia, in neonates, 158, 192-193
Sertoli cell tumors, 303, 304
  interfering with libido and spermatogenesis, 317
Serum
  administration of, 175
  collection of, 174
Sevoflurane, 111
Sexual immaturity, in ejaculation disorders, 316
Sexual maturity, failure to achieve, in males, 314
Sexual overuse, in ejaculation disorders, 316
Shoulder osteochondrosis screening, 23-24
Shoulders, evaluation of, 23-24
Sick newborn appointment scheduling, 351
Simethicone (GasX®; Phazyme®), formulary for, 437
Singleton puppy, raising, 207
SIPS (subinvolution of placental sites), 138, 264-265
Skin biopsies, 26-27
Skin disease, bacterial, 193
Snuggle Safe®, 85, 167
SOAP (subjective/objective/analysis/plan), 177
  breeding soundness form, 387-389
  neonatal visit form, 385-386
Sodium succinate, formulary for, 428
Solu-Medrol®
  formulary for, 428
  in neonatal resuscitation, 123
Sperm, 290
  agglutination of, 293
  disorders of, 316-322
  gross appearance of, 290

knowing when to intervene in, 93
normal, 86-88
supplies for, 85-86
at veterinary hospital, 89-96
Whelping area, 149-151, 154-155
preparing, 84-86
Whelping calendar, 344
WhelpWise™, 96, 240
White coat syndrome, 286
Worming
in neonates, 145, 146
before placement, 212-213
post-partum, 128, 129-130

X

X-linked recessive disease, counseling for, 31-32
XX sex reversal, 225
Xylazine, 113
Xylocaine® (lidocaine), formulary for, 426

Z

Zeniquin®, formulary for, 422-423
Zithromax® (azithromycin), formulary for, 406
Zoonotic disease, in puppies, 215
Zovirax® (acyclovir), formulary for, 402